Strategic Management of Health Care Organizations

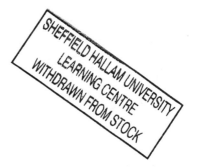

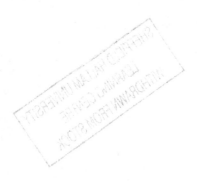

Blackwell
Publishing

Strategic Management of Health Care Organizations

Fifth Edition

Linda E. Swayne
University of North Carolina at Charlotte

W. Jack Duncan
University of Alabama at Birmingham

Peter M. Ginter
University of Alabama at Birmingham

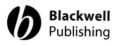

Blackwell
Publishing

© 2006 by Linda E. Swayne, W. Jack Duncan, Peter M. Ginter

BLACKWELL PUBLISHING
350 Main Street, Malden, MA 02148-5020, USA
9600 Garsington Road, Oxford OX4 2DQ, UK
550 Swanston Street, Carlton, Victoria 3053, Australia

First published 2006 by Blackwell Publishing Ltd

1   2006

Library of Congress Cataloging-in-Publication Data

Swayne, Linda E.
   Strategic management of health care organizations / Linda E. Swayne,
W. Jack Duncan, Peter M. Ginter.—5th ed.
      p. cm.
   Includes bibliographical references and index.
   ISBN-13: 978-1-4051-2432-4 (hard cover : alk. paper)
   ISBN-10: 1-4051-2432-6 (hard cover : alk. paper)
   1. Health facilities—Administration.   2. Strategic planning.   I. Duncan, W. Jack
(Walter Jack)   II. Ginter, Peter M.   III. Title.

RA971.S924 2006
362.1′068—dc22

                                              2005004897

A catalogue record for this title is available from the British Library.

Set in 10/12pt Book Antique
by Graphicraft Limited, Hong Kong
Printed and bound in the United Kingdom
by TJ International, Padstow, Cornwall

The publisher's policy is to use permanent paper from mills that operate a sustainable forestry policy, and which has been manufactured from pulp processed using acid-free and elementary chlorine-free practices. Furthermore, the publisher ensures that the text paper and cover board used have met acceptable environmental accreditation standards.

For further information on
Blackwell Publishing, visit our website:
www.blackwellpublishing.com

Contents

Preface

More than fifteen years ago, the three of us agreed that health care was entering "whitewater change" and that health care strategic management might benefit from a strategic perspective drawing upon the experience and strategic thinking and planning processes first developed in the business sector. At that time, we wrote in the Preface of the first edition, "Clearly health care has had difficulty in dealing with a dynamic environment, holding down costs, diversifying wisely, and balancing capacity and demand." It was clear to us that only a structured strategic thinking and planning approach that recognized the value of emergent thinking could make sense of that rapidly changing environment. Such an approach still seems applicable.

Health care has continued to experience significant environmental change including technological breakthroughs in gene research and therapy and bioengineering, economic and competitive pressures that have altered the industry, phenomenal growth in the use of the system that will only continue as the "boomers" age into retirement, and health care professionals that are in short supply.

In addition in that first edition we stated, "Today health care organizations that do not have a clear strategy are doomed to mediocrity at best – and failure at worst – resulting in poor quality of life for the community." Health care organizations that did not develop that clear strategy are gone – more than 1,400 hospitals have closed their doors. The financing of health care has significantly evolved and the industry has undergone two decades of restructuring with a multitude of new types of organizations and services. The health care environment has indeed changed.

Changes in this Edition

Along with the health care industry, this text has evolved as well. Its evolution in many ways mirrors the changes that have taken place in the health care industry and its management. As a result, this edition brings strategic thinking to the forefront and clearly differentiates strategic thinking, strategic planning, and managing the strategy (managing the strategic momentum). These concepts represent the central elements of our new conceptual model of strategic management and we believe that it better reflects the realities of developing and managing strategies.

Broadly, the new model depicts strategic management as the processes of strategic thinking, consensus building and documentation of that thinking into a strategic plan, and managing the strategic momentum. Through the management of the strategic plan, new insights and perspectives emerge and the strategic thinking, planning, managing process is reinitiated. Therefore, strategic managers must become strategic thinkers with the ability to evaluate the changing environment, analyze data, question assumptions, and develop new ideas. Additionally, they must be able to develop and document a plan of action through strategic planning. Once a strategic plan is developed, managers must maintain the strategic momentum of the organization. As strategic managers attempt to carry out the strategic plan they evaluate its success, learn more about what works, and incorporate new strategic thinking.

It is our view that strategic control is integral to managing the strategic momentum and can not be thought of as a separate process. Therefore, in this edition, control concepts have been integrated into the strategy development chapters under the heading of "Managing the Strategic Momentum" and the separate chapter on control found in previous editions has been eliminated. We believe that this approach better reflects how strategic control works in organizations – as a part of managing the strategy, not as an afterthought or add on.

This edition contains updated text with new examples throughout as well as new and updated perspectives. In addition, of the twenty cases, twelve of them are a change from the fourth edition: three of them are updated – the Health Care Industry Note, Midwest Medical Group or MMG, and Riverview the HMA facility – and nine of them are new to this edition. Eight cases have been recommended as "classics" to be maintained. Several international health care cases have been included that will require students to expand their thinking. We believe that merely reading the cases, even without analyzing them, can be a useful exercise because students are introduced to a wide variety of organizations and their approaches to strategic management. This provides additional insight.

Features Retained

Strategic management is highly subjective, often requiring significant intuitive powers. However, the intuitive powers are not easily learned (or taught). A major task of the future strategic thinker is to develop objective or analytical means –

a logical sequence – to strategic planning and then through experience develop the intuition to consider strategic issues. We have used the analogy of the map and the compass to express this approach. A map enables you to start your own personal journey toward strategic thinking. This text has a number of logical sequences or "maps," although we have never claimed that they are the only way to approach strategic management. Students of strategic management need to study a wide variety of organizations and situations to gain a greater insight – their own compass – into strategic management.

Some of the more important features that have been retained in this edition include:

- Each chapter begins with an *Introductory Incident* to provide a practical example of the concepts discussed in the chapter.
- *Learning Objectives* direct attention to the important points or skills introduced in the chapter.
- Models, examples, and exhibits are included to assist in learning chapter material.
- Six or more *Perspectives* drawn from actual health care organizations' current experiences provide insight. These sidebars enable the student to relate to particular concepts presented in the chapter.
- A *Chapter Summary* highlights the most important topics covered in each chapter.
- *Key Terms and Concepts* present the essential vocabulary and terminology relative to the chapter's material.
- *Questions for Class Discussion* aid the reader in reviewing the important material and thinking about the implications of the ideas presented.
- *Notes* contain the references used in development of the chapter materials.
- *Additional Readings* offer the student further up-to-date or classic sources on topics related to the material discussed in each chapter.
- *Appendices* assist readers by presenting a methodology for case analysis and a review for making oral professional presentations.

Feedback from users of previous editions has reinforced our belief that these features aid in providing an informative, interesting, and pedagogically sound foundation for understanding and embracing strategic management of health care organizations.

Through our own teaching, research, and consulting in the health care field, we have applied the process outlined in this text to physician practices, hospitals, local and state public health departments, long-term care facilities, and physical therapy practices. We have students who report back to us saying that they lead strategic planning in their organizations using the process with great success. The process works.

Author Order

In developing and writing this book, as with all our joint projects, we have created a team in its truest sense. Recognizing that each of us makes a unique contribution and provides leadership, we are once again rotating the order in which the authors are listed. For the first and second editions, the authors were listed as Duncan, Ginter, and Swayne; for the third and fourth editions the authors were listed as Ginter, Swayne, and Duncan.

Acknowledgements

A number of people have provided inspiration, ideas, and considerable effort to produce the fifth edition. We are indebted to many individuals for their assistance and encouragement. First, we would like to thank Gary Kohut and Carol Baxter for writing Appendix B – Oral Presentations for Health Care Professionals. Strategic management does not work if it is not communicated.

A special note of thanks to Dean Claude C. Lilly of the Belk College of Business at The University of North Carolina at Charlotte, to Dean Max Michael, MD of the School of Public Health at the University of Alabama at Birmingham, and to Dean Robert Holmes of the School of Business at the University of Alabama at Birmingham, who have all continued to be supportive of our efforts.

We especially thank the organizations whose experiences are the cases for this book. We are grateful for their willingness to enhance the education of health care students. In addition, we thank the authors who crafted the organizations' experiences into cases for students to read and analyze to practice strategic thinking and strategic management skills. The Industry Note (Case 1) sets the stage for the analysis of the nineteen cases that follow. Each case was selected to provide lively discussion and a variety of alternative solutions. The *Instructor's Manual* (available on CD from Blackwell Publishing) contains teaching notes for each of the cases. Case writing is a difficult art, requiring many hours of library research, personal interviews, and detailed analysis. The case contributors in this text are masters at their craft. We believe that the students will benefit from their work.

Finally, but most importantly, we thank our families who have supported and encouraged us as we worked on still another writing project. Thank you all for your understanding.

Paul Stringer, the copy editor, has done his best to perfect this text. If there are any errors, they are ours.

Linda E. Swayne   W. Jack Duncan   Peter M. Ginter

Strategic Management

Part 1 contains ten chapters addressing the philosophy and activities of strategic management. Chapter 1 introduces definitions for strategic management and its activities – strategic thinking, strategic planning, and strategic momentum. The chapter discusses the need and rationale for strategic management in today's turbulent health care environment and traces its historical foundations. In addition, Chapter 1 presents a conceptual model or map that guides strategic thinking, focuses on important areas for strategic planning, and initiates and sustains strategic momentum.

Chapter 2 contains strategic thinking and planning maps for investigating the external environment – both the general environment and the health care industry environment. Chapter 3 narrows the focus by providing strategic thinking maps for conducting service area competitor analysis – the more immediate environment for a specific health care organization. Assessment of the internal environment is accomplished through strategic thinking maps for a health care value chain and analysis of the organization's resources, capabilities, and competencies, as examined in Chapter 4.

The directional strategies – mission, vision, values, and goals – are examined in Chapter 5. Developing a mission forces members of an organization to strategically think about its distinctiveness today; developing a vision forces them to think about their hopes for its future; and building awareness of organizational values makes members cognizant of the things that should be cherished and not compromised as the mission and vision are pursued. Organizational goals establish clear targets and help focus activities.

Strategy formulation is concerned with making strategic decisions using the information gathered during situational analysis. Chapter 6 provides the decision logic for strategy formulation and demonstrates that strategic decisions are connected in an "ends–means" chain. Each decision along the decision chain more explicitly defines the strategy and must be consistent with upstream and

downstream decisions. Chapter 7 discusses how to evaluate the strategic alternatives within each strategy type in the decision chain. These evaluation methods
do not make the strategy decision but, rather, are constructs or maps for helping
strategists think about the organization and its relative situation, thus enabling
them to understand the potential risks and rewards of their strategic choices.

Strategic momentum entails putting strategies to work (managerial actions that
accomplish the strategy), strategy evaluation and control, and strategic awareness.
Implementation requires that strategic managers shape and coordinate the value
chain components and ensure that the organization's action plans are directly tied
to selected strategies. Chapter 8 addresses the development of implementation
plans through either maintaining or changing the pre-service, point-of-service, and
after-service strategies. Strategic managers should determine the essential characteristics of service delivery to ensure it best contributes to accomplishment of
the strategy. Chapter 9 examines the role of organizational culture, organizational
structure, and strategic resources in implementing strategy. These value chain components determine the organizational context and are vital in effective strategy
implementation. Chapter 10 demonstrates how strategy may be translated into
organizational objectives and action plans. It is the divisions, organizations, and
functional units that must carry out strategy and strategic managers must review
objectives and action plans to ensure that they are coordinated and make best
use of human, physical, and financial resources. Each of these chapters points out
the need to maintain strategic momentum by thinking, planning, and doing, and
then rethinking, new planning, and doing.

CHAPTER **1**

The Nature of Strategic Management

"Somehow there are organizations that effectively manage change, continuously adapting their bureaucracies, strategies, systems, products, services and cultures to survive the shocks and prosper from the forces that decimate others . . . they are the masters of what I call renewal."

Robert H. Waterman, Jr.
The Renewal Factor

Introductory Incident

The Tale of Two Cities Continues

"It was the best of times, it was the worst of times, it was the age of wisdom, it was the age of foolishness. . . ."[1] Likewise, it was the best of times for insured US citizens needing health care; the best health care in the world was available and continued to improve. Yet it was the worst of times for some, as 2004 was the fourth consecutive year of double-digit increases in health insurance premiums plus the number of uninsured and underinsured continued to increase.

In this age of wisdom, medical advances are astounding. Scientists may soon have a new diagnostic technique that uses scans by beams of fast-moving neutrons, making it possible to "see" aberrant cells even before the smallest tumor forms.[2] Nevertheless, in this age of foolishness,

over 22 percent of the total US population continues to smoke cigarettes, a behavior that greatly increases a person's risk of developing cancerous tumors and heart conditions.[3] The US health care system continues to flounder between the best and the worst, between wisdom and foolishness, as do the two cities in this tale, Boston and Nashville.

Boston

Not-for-profit Harvard Pilgrim, the state's largest insuror, was placed into receivership by the Attorney General in 2000 after losses of over $225 million, but by 2002 it was in the black again, albeit without the full state reserve requirements. Meanwhile, CareGroup, the health system – including the prestigious Beth Israel Deaconess hospital – was troubled.

▶

One of its six hospitals, the 199-bed Deaconess Waltham hospital, was expected to lose $9 million and was to be closed after the state required 90-day notice period. No other hospital group was interested in buying the hospital. Developer Roy MacDowell acquired the property in a controversial deal and turned the site into a "medical mall" that includes urgent care, inpatient behavioral care, acute care, a cancer treatment center, a wound recovery unit, and various other small practices.

CareGroup, which lost $163 million in two years, was expected to be in technical default; however, under the new CEO, the projected $102 million loss for Beth Israel Deaconess was only a $59 million loss. Helped by pressure from the Massachusetts Attorney General, who was overseeing Harvard Pilgrim's turn-around, the new CEO cut supply costs, laid off workers, reformed the board, and started to rebuild the relationship with doctors.[4]

At the beginning of 2003, things looked rosy for Boston: CareGroup and Partners (the other large hospital group that includes Massachusetts General and Brigham and Women's) were headed in the right direction. Because of their size and clout, the hospitals pushed through large payment increases from Harvard Pilgrim, Tufts Health Plan, and Blue Cross. The increases helped the hospitals' bottom lines; the health plans remained viable as they passed most of the increases along to employers – some of whom could not pay the higher costs and dropped health care coverage for employees.

At the end of 2003, reports started to point out that not everything was rosy. Health care costs in Boston – already 30 percent higher than other metropolitan areas – had not been decreased by the hospital mergers. Although Beth Israel and Deaconess, formerly two hospitals in the CareGroup, may have saved on costs by merging their two clinical units into one, Partners' Massachusetts General and Brigham and Women's were still operating as two hospitals. In 1999, hospitals were responsible for 36 percent of the increase in Boston's health care costs; by year end 2002, hospitals accounted for 51 percent of the increase.[5] Critics claimed that the real reasons for the mergers were to give the groups more bargaining power with the health plans and to weaken local health care institutions. When health plans were forced to make higher payments to hospitals, the result was more expensive care and increased employer costs.[6] The New England Healthcare Institute pointed out that the state was losing its dominant position as a health care employer. Although New England still had the highest concentration of health care workers in the country – a concentration 25 percent above the national average – the percentage of health care jobs in the region continued to slip.[7]

By 2003, Partners HealthCare, the most financially secure of Boston's big hospital groups, posted an $8.7 million operating loss for the last quarter of fiscal 2003, and the yearly profit was only about half as much as the previous year. CareGroup hospitals generally improved their financial performance for the year, but they still showed losses. By the end of the year the health plans had started to push back on hospital payments; after months of negotiations, Tufts Health Plan's renewed contract with Partners included incentives for excellent care provided by physicians. Harvard Pilgrim brought in Nashville's American Healthways to provide disease management for its subscribers and Blue Cross's new contract with Partners included incentives for using new technology to reduce errors and for cost containment.[8] Urged by employers, the three big health plans launched websites that allowed consumers to search for the top-ranked hospitals for their condition. Beginning July 2004 for some employees, and by January 1, 2005 for all employees, Tufts and Harvard Pilgrim grouped the area's hospitals and physicians into tiers. Employees pay steep surcharges for choosing to receive care from hospitals or physicians in the second or third tiers. None of Boston's big teaching hospitals was included in first tier providers.[9] The trend started by the health plans may continue to gain momentum.

Nashville

Encouraged by groups such as the Nashville Health Care Council (NHCC), health care companies in Nashville are capitalizing on the woes of the rest of the industry. Nashville's thriving health care sector, instead of focusing on hospitals, has focused on businesses that provide services to hospitals and health plans to help them perform better. Several years ago, the Nashville Chamber of Commerce predicted that the US health care system would have to make massive changes if it were

▶

to serve the population without bankrupting the country. To that end, the Chamber started NHCC to act as the center of a network for people interested in developing entrepreneurial health services companies. NHCC is an association of health care industry leaders working together to further establish Nashville's position as the health care industry capital of the US by creating a supportive operating environment for existing, start-up, and relocating health care businesses.

Among those companies thriving in Nashville is American Healthways, a disease management service company that enlisted Boston's Harvard Pilgrim and other health plans across the country to search for ways to hold down health costs. Another is Caremark Rx, a drug benefits services company that helps health plans control drug costs. HealthStream, a provider of learning systems for the health care industry, and HealthTrio, a provider of e-health and business-application technology for managed care, help hospitals ensure high quality among professionals and help insurors provide consumer information, respectively. Vanderbilt University's Center for Better Health, started in 2002 to help physicians and hospitals improve quality and lower costs, recently teamed up with Accenture, a consulting company, to start a research-based initiative to aid the health care industry in collaborating on information technology.[10]

Nashville's hospitals are not sharing equally in the vital health care sector's rewards, however. HCA, Inc., the nation's largest for-profit hospital chain based in Nashville, announced increased reserves for doubtful accounts that contributed to a 31 percent decrease in net income for the first quarter of 2004.[11] Additionally, Nashville-based Iasis Healthcare, Vangard Health Systems, and LifePoint Hospitals increased reserves as the percent of bad debt rose across the country.[12] HCA has been hit with a class action lawsuit brought by disgruntled uninsured patients claiming that, to try to make up for bad debt, HCA hospitals charge them more for care than the industry norm and several times more than the rates paid by insured patients. Across town, Saint Thomas Hospital has similar lawsuits.

Nashville maintains that it will remain the "Silicon Valley of Health Care" because of its rich history of entrepreneurship, strong managerial talent, and access to venture capital funding.

Nashville's leadership claims that the changing health care environment will only contribute to its health care sector strength and that it is the best of times. In the age of rising costs and increasing quality demands, is it, then, the worst of times only for the hospital sector? Are hospitals the dinosaurs of today's health care world? If so, forming a herd, like Partners or HCA, may not slow the march toward extinction – after all, two dinosaurs in a herd eat just as much as two solo dinosaurs. Perhaps extinction can be averted if these behemoths grow smaller and more flexible and learn how to survive in different environments. In the landscape of the future, there may no longer be two cities about which a health care tale can be told. Rather, there may be a tale of the megalopolis.

Notes

1. Charles Dickens, *A Tale of Two Cities* (November 1859).
2. P. Weiss, "Neutrons May Spotlight Cancers," *Science News* 166, no. 8 (August 21, 2004), p. 125.
3. J. A. Grunbaum, L. Kann, S. Kinchen, J. Ross, J. Hawkins, R. Lowry, W. A. Harris, T. McManus, D. Chyen, and J. Collins, "Youth Risk Behavior Surveillance – United States 2003," *Morbidity and Mortality Weekly Report* 53, no. SS02 (May 21, 2004), p. 1.
4. S. Bailey, "A Hospital Heals Itself," *Boston Globe* (September 6, 2002), p. E-1.
5. C. Stein, "Tomorrow's HMO Is Here, But Will Consumers Buy It?" *Boston Globe* (June 9, 2003), p. E-1.
6. R. Abelson, "Merged Hospitals Gain Both Power and Critics," *New York Times* (September 26, 2002), p. C-1.
7. L. Kowalczyk, "Study Sees Challenges to N.E. Healthcare Growth," *Boston Globe* (February 18, 2003), p. E-1.
8. L. Kowalczyk, "Partners, Blue Cross Reach Agreement," *Boston Globe* (August 11, 2004), p. C-2.
9. L. Kowalczyk, "Health Plans Set Care Surcharges. Tiered System Tied to Provider Costs," *Boston Globe* (March 25, 2004), p. A-1.
10. "Vanderbilt, Accenture Launch Health Care Information Research Project," *Nashville Business Journal* (January 12, 2004), pp. 1, 63.
11. R. Moore, "Bad Debt Bites HCA," *Nashville Business Journal* (September 10, 2004), p. 3.
12. D. Raiford, "Hospitals 'Wheel of Misfortune' Begins to Spin More Quickly," *Nashville Business Journal* (July 25, 2003), pp. 1, 58.

Source: Terrie Reeves, PhD, University of Wisconsin at Milwaukee.

Learning Objectives

After completing this chapter the student should be able to:

1. Explain why strategic management has become crucial in today's dynamic health care environment.

2. Trace the evolution of strategic management and discuss its conceptual foundations.

3. Describe and explain the concept of strategic thinking maps.

4. Define and differentiate between strategic management, strategic thinking, strategic planning, and managing the strategic momentum.

5. Understand the necessity for both the analytic and emergent models of strategic management.

6. Understand how an organization may realize a strategy that it never intended.

7. Understand the benefits of strategic management for health care organizations.

8. Understand the importance of systems approaches.

9. Explain the links between the different levels of strategy within an organization.

10. Describe the various leadership roles of strategic management.

Managing in a Dynamic Environment

The dramatic changes in the health care industry that began in the 1980s, marked by the implementation of Medicare's prospective payment system in 1983, continue well into the first decade of the twenty-first century. As a result, both public and private health care institutions continue to face a turbulent, confusing, and often threatening environment. Significant change comes from many sources including: federal, state, and local health care legislative and policy initiatives; international as well as domestic economic and market forces; demographic shifts and lifestyle changes; technological advances; and health care delivery changes within the industry. Certainly, the health care systems in Boston and Nashville, described in the Introductory Incident, as well as other domestic and international health care institutions, have had to adapt to these changes and in the future may have to reinvent themselves once again. As suggested in the introductory quote, organizations will have to effectively manage change and become "masters of renewal" in this dynamic environment.

Coping with Change

How can health care leaders deal with important, complex, and sometimes conflicting issues and trends? Which ones are most important or most pressing?

Furthermore, what new issues will emerge? It is likely that there will be new opportunities and threats to health care organizations that have yet to be identified or fully assessed. Even more sobering, it seems certain that there will be more change in the health care industry in the next ten years than there has been in the past ten.

Dealing with rapid, complex, and often discontinuous change requires leadership. Successful health care organizations have leaders who understand the nature and implications of external change, the ability to develop effective strategies that account for change, and the will as well as the ability to actively manage the momentum of the organization. These activities are collectively referred to as "strategic management." The clearest manifestation of leadership in organizations is the presence of strategic management and its activities. Strategic management is fundamental in leading organizations in dynamic environments. Strategic management provides the momentum for change.

Organizational change is a fundamental part of survival. Because strategic managers understand the relationship between change and survival, there have been many management approaches to changing organizations. As health care leaders change and manage their organizations, they chart new courses into the future. In effect, they create new beginnings, new chances for success, new challenges for employees, and new hopes for patients. Therefore, it is imperative that health care managers understand the changes taking place in their environment; they should not simply be responsive to them, but strive to create the future. Health care leaders must see into the future, create new visions for success, and be prepared to make "quantum improvements" (see Perspective 1–1).

The Foundations of Strategic Management

In the political and military context, the concept of strategy has a long history. For instance, the underlying principles of strategy were discussed by Sun Tzu, Homer, Euripides, and many other early strategists and writers. The English word strategy comes from the Greek *stratēgōs*, meaning "a general," which in turn comes from roots meaning "army" and "lead."[1] The Greek verb *stratēgeō* means "to plan the destruction of one's enemies through effective use of resources."[2] As a result, many of the terms commonly used in relation to strategy – objectives, mission, strengths, weaknesses – were developed by the military.

Long-Range Planning to Strategic Planning

The development of strategic management begins with much of the business sector adopting long-range planning. Long-range planning developed in the 1950s in many organizations because operating budgets were difficult to prepare without some idea of future sales and the flow of funds. Post-WWII economies were growing and the demand for many products and services was accelerating. Long-range forecasts of demand enabled managers to develop detailed marketing and distribution, production, human resources, and financial plans for their growing organizations. The objective of long-range planning is to predict for some

Perspective 1–1

Good to Great in Health Care

Several years ago Jim Collins's book, *Good to Great: Why Some Companies Make the Leap . . . and Others Don't,* came on the business scene. Collins studied 1,435 good companies and then analyzed why 11 of the companies became great. Chip Caldwell & Associates began a "good to great" project in health care and studied 44 health care organizations ranging in size from 15 to 854 beds. An additional project conducted by the group assessed 226 healthrelated organizations in Los Angeles County, California. For each organization they measured changes in cost per case mix adjusted discharge. Those organizations that finished in the 75th percentile or higher were labeled quantum improvers and those in the bottom quartile were labeled nonstarters.

About 20 percent of the quantum improvers were already in a favorable cost position and about 20 percent of the nonstarters were already in an un-favorable cost position. The researchers observed that this meant that the quantum-improvers were becoming better faster and the nonstarters were becoming worse faster. In other words, the performance gap was increasing and health care firms not applying quantum-improver strategies risked being left behind by organizations that were raising the bar and redefining the playing field. Some important principles of the quantum improvers are that they:

1. Set nonnegotiable goals. Quantum improvers perform a gap analysis and determine areas where improvement is possible and necessary. They determine where the biggest differences are from established benchmarks and focus on the vital few areas that will make the biggest positive difference to the organization. Nonstarters receive gap information, debate it for six months, seek more data, and agree to talk some more. Quantum improvers interpret the results as an immediate call for action. Strategic leaders step up at defining moments, keep the organization on path, and demonstrate that failure to act is not an option.
2. Focus on key businesses. Health care organizations cannot be all things to all people. Organizations have to develop a "stop doing" list to include those services that are least profitable and must be eliminated. Doing away with any service is very hard in health care because no one wants to eliminate a service that is helping people even if it is very expensive. Focusing on those services that support the core mission and separating financial issues from emotional issues may make the decision to eliminate a service easier and more objective.
3. Use a tight-loose-tight approach. Begin with a tight understanding of the preferred direction for the organization, then delegate the understanding to a group of leaders who have flexibility in determining how they will achieve the direction, and finally, monitor with tight accountability to make sure that the selected approach is working.

Quantum improvers have a culture of accountability but not a punitive culture. They are not threat driven. Rather than punish those who do not achieve, assistance is provided by upper leadership until the desired results are accomplished. As Collins notes, great organizations do not have miracle moments of change; instead they emphasize committed, controlled, and practical leadership.

Source: Shannon K. Pieper, "Good to Great in Healthcare: How Some Organizations Are Elevating Their Performance," *Healthcare Executive* 19, no. 3 (2004), pp. 20–6.

specified time in the future the size of demand for an organization's products and services and to determine where demand will occur. Many organizations have used long-range planning to determine facilities expansion, hiring forecasts, capital needs, and so on.

As industries became more volatile, long-range planning was replaced by strategic planning because the assumption underlying long-range planning is that the organization will continue to produce its present products and services – thus, matching production capacity to demand is the critical issue. However, the assumption underlying strategic planning is that there is so much economic, social, political, technological, and competitive change taking place that the leadership of the organization must periodically evaluate whether it should even be offering its present products and services, whether it should start offering different products and services, or whether it should be operating and marketing in a fundamentally different way.

Although strategies typically take considerable time to implement, and thus are generally long range in nature, the time span is not the principal focus of strategic planning. In fact, strategic planning, supported by the management of the strategy, compresses time. Competitive shifts that might take generations to evolve instead occur in a few short years.[3] Therefore, it is preferable to use "long range" and "short range" to describe the time it will take to accomplish a strategy rather than to indicate a type of planning.

Strategic Planning to Strategic Management

The 1960s and 1970s were decades of major growth for strategic planning in business organizations. Leading companies such as General Electric were not only engaged in strategic planning but also actively promoted its merits in the business press. The process provided these firms with a more systematic approach to managing business units and extended the planning and budgeting horizon beyond the traditional 12-month operating period. In addition, business managers learned that financial planning alone was not an adequate framework.[4] In the 1980s the concept of strategic planning was broadened to strategic management. This evolution acknowledged not only the importance of the dynamics of the environment and that organizations may have to totally reinvent themselves but also that continuously managing and evaluating the strategy are keys to success. Thus, strategic management was established as an approach or philosophy for managing complex enterprises.

Strategic Management in the Health Care Industry

Strategic management concepts have been employed within health care organizations only in the past 25 to 30 years. Indeed, many of the management methods adopted by health care organizations, both public and private, were developed in the business sector. In many respects health care has become a complex business using many of the same processes and much of the same language as the most sophisticated business corporations.

Although the values and practices of for-profit business enterprises in the private sector have been advocated as the appropriate model of managing health care organizations, a legitimate question arises concerning the appropriateness of the assumption that business practices may always be appropriate to the health care industry. Certainly, not all the "big ideas" (Perspective 1–2) have delivered what was promised, even in business.[5] However, strategic management, especially when customized to health care, does seem to provide the necessary processes for health care organizations to cope with the vast changes that have been occurring.

Strategic Management Versus Health Policy Planning

In the past, individual health care organizations had few incentives to employ strategic management because typically they were independent, freestanding, not-for-profit institutions, and health services reimbursement was on a cost-plus basis. Yet, there has been substantial health planning in the United States. Efforts at health planning were initiated by either state or local governments and implemented through legislation or private or nongovernmental agencies. For the most part, these planning efforts were disease oriented; that is, they were categorical approaches directed toward specific health problems (e.g., the work of the National Tuberculosis Association that stimulated the development of state and local government tuberculosis prevention and treatment programs).[6]

As a result, a variety of state and federal health planning or policy initiatives have been designed to (1) enhance quality of care – through studies of outcomes measures; (2) provide or control access to care – through the Hospital Survey and Construction Act (better known as the Hill-Burton Act), Medicaid, Medicare, state certificate of need (CON) laws; and (3) contain costs – through the National Health Planning and Resource Development Act, implementation of DRGs and RBRVSs, and the Balanced Budget Act of 1997 that slashed Medicare by $115 billion over five years. Exhibit 1–1 presents the year for major cost and control events since 1900.

These health planning efforts are not strategic management. Health planning is the implementation of federal and state health policy and affects a variety of health care organizations. As explained in Perspective 1–3 the intent of *health policy* is to provide the context for the development of the health care infrastructure as a whole. In contrast, strategic management is organization specific. Strategic management helps an individual organization respond to state and federal policy and planning efforts, as well as to a variety of other external forces.

The Dimensions of Strategic Management

There are many ways to think about strategic management in organizations. In fact, Henry Mintzberg identified ten distinct schools of thought concerning organizational strategy.[7] As described in Exhibit 1–2, three of these approaches were prescriptive or analytical (rational): the design (conceptual) school, the planning

1950s	1960s	1970s
• Theory "Y" • Management by Objectives • Quantitative Management • Diversification	• Managerial Grid • T-Groups • Matrix Management • Conglomeration • Centralization/Decentralization	• Zero-Based Budgets • Participative Management • Portfolio Management • Quantitative MBAs
1980s	**1990s**	**2000s?**
• Theory Z • One-Minute Managing • Organization Culture • Intrapreneuring • Downsizing • MBWA (Management by Wandering Around) • TQM/CQI	• Customer Focus • Quality Improvement • Reengineering • Benchmarking • Resource-Based View	• Six Sigma • Balanced Score Card • Transformational Leadership • Self-Managed Teams • Dynamic Capabilities • Virtual Organizations

Management fads? Management techniques? Management fads is usually the flippant answer. However, each of these management approaches was a genuine attempt to change and improve the organization – to focus efforts, to improve the quality of the products and services, to improve employee morale, to do more with less, to put meaning into work, and so on. Some of the approaches worked better than others; some stood the test of time and others did not. Yet, it would be too harsh to simply dismiss them as fads or techniques. The goals for all of these management approaches were to manage and shape the organization – to make it better, to make it an excellent organization. One of the things that has distinguished all of these "fads" is the enthusiasm and commitment they have engendered among managers and workers. For many, these approaches have significantly increased the meaning of work – no small accomplishment in an era in which people are increasingly hungry for meaning. And certainly organizations need to create meaning.[1]

When management approaches such as these fail, it is usually because they become an end in themselves. Managers lose sight of the real purpose of the approach and the process becomes more important than the product. Managers start working for the approach rather than letting the approach work for them.

Important Thoughts for the Future
What will be the "management fads" of the next decade? Will you be a part of these attempts to make the organization better or will you simply dismiss them as fads? Perhaps benchmarking, quality improvement, or strategic thinking will turn your organization around. One of these approaches may help make your organization truly excellent or save it from decline.

Is strategic management just another fad? Will it stand the test of time? If strategic management becomes an end in itself, if its activities do not foster and facilitate thinking, it will not be useful. However, if strategic management helps managers think about the future and guide their organizations through this turbulent decade, strategic management will have succeeded.

1. J. Daniel Beckham, "The Longest Wave," *Healthcare Forum Journal* 36, no. 6 (November/December 1993), pp. 78, 80–2.

Exhibit 1–1: Major Health Care Cost and Control Events

Year	Health Care Cost and Control Events
1906	Pure Food and Drug Act passed
1910	Managed care born in Tacoma, Washington when two physicians contract to provide medical care to a lumber company
1910	First group health insurance policy is issued covering Montgomery Ward retail employees
1910	Abraham Flexner publishes *Medical Education in the United States and Canada* setting standards for medical schools
1913	The American College of Surgeons is founded and creates minimum standards for hospitals
1918	The American College of Surgeons begins hospital inspections – only 89 of 692 inspected met minimum standards
1921	Federal Veterans' Bureau (now the Department of Veterans Affairs) is created
1929	First Blue Cross plan is formed by 1,250 teachers in Dallas for hospital care from Baylor Hospital
1932	Not-for-profit Blue Cross and Blue Shield organizations begin offering group health insurance
1933	The organization to become Kaiser Permanente is created based on prepayment of medical insurance per covered life
1935	Social Security Act passed
1943	IRS rules that employer contributions to group health insurance premium are not taxable to employees
1945	Kaiser Permanente HMO is opened to public enrollment
1946	Centers for Disease Control (CDC) is created
1946	The Hill-Burton Act passes, creating public-backed financing for hospital construction
1951	The Joint Commission on Accreditation of Hospitals is formed
1954	Disability benefits are included in Social Security Coverage
1963–1969	During the Johnson administration Congress enacts 51 pieces of health care legislation
1964	Surgeon General releases landmark report on dangers of smoking
1965	Medicare and Medicaid programs enacted to provide health care for elderly and low-income Americans
1970s	State legislatures enact certificate of need (CON) legislation
1972	Senate creates peer standards review organizations
1974	HMO Act designed to promote growth of health maintenance organizations takes effect

Exhibit 1–1: (cont'd)

Year	Health Care Cost and Control Events
1977	VHA established by 30 hospital CEOs – first national cooperative of not-for-profit health care organizations
1979	"Healthy People" released, the Surgeon General's first report on health promotion and disease prevention
1980	National health care spending as a portion of GDP is 8.9 percent
1980	HMO enrollment at 9.1 million
1982	Medicare risk-contract legislation enacted for HMOs
1983	Prospective Payment System (PPS) based on diagnosis-related groups (DRGs) mandated for hospitals under Medicare
1989	"Stark I" legislation prohibits physician self-referrals for lab services
1989	Medicare represents 68 percent of physicians' income
1989	Omnibus Budget Reconciliation Act reforms Medicare physician payment
1990	National health care spending as a portion of GDP is 12.2 percent
1990	Ryan White Act passes providing federal assistance for low-income AIDS patients and for AIDS testing and counseling
1991	National Committee for Quality Assurance begins accrediting managed care organizations
1992	HCFA adopts resource-based relative value scale (RBRVS), which increases payments to primary care physicians and reduces payments to specialists
1992	Buyers Health Care Action Group, an employer purchasing group, forms in Minneapolis
1993	Managed care enrollment exceeds 50 percent of those with job-based coverage
1993	Oregon's Medicaid health care rationing "experiment" approved
1993	Family and Medical Leave Act passed
1993	President Bill Clinton introduces American Health Security Act, a health-reform plan based on managed competition
1994	Oregon passes Death with Dignity Act giving residents the right to obtain prescriptions for self-administered lethal medications from physicians
1995	Blue Cross of Washington and Alaska becomes the first major insuror to reimburse for alternative medical treatments such as acupuncture and homeopathy
1995	Major federal crackdown on health care fraud begins

Exhibit 1–1: (*cont'd*)

Year	Health Care Cost and Control Events
1996	Health Insurance Portability and Accountability Act (HIPAA) passes
1997	An estimated 44 million Americans are uninsured
1997	Balanced Budget Act slashes Medicare budget by $115 billion over five years and authorizes Medicare + Choice to provide broader coverage options, includes CHIP (Children's Health Insurance Program)
1998	First HMO malpractice lawsuit filed by a consumer under landmark Texas law
1998	HMO enrollment at 78.8 million
1998	PPO enrollment hits 90 million surpassing that of HMOs
1999	Aetna Inc. purchases Prudential HealthCare giving it coverage of one in ten Americans
2002	Almost 50 percent of major teaching hospitals lose money because of Medicare cuts
2006	Projected national health care spending as a portion of GDP to be 15.8 percent

Source: VHA, Inc. and Deloitte & Touche, *Health Care 2000: A Strategic Assessment of the Health Care Environment in the United States* (Irving, TX and Detroit, MI: VHA and Deloitte & Touche, 2000), pp. 2–11.

(formal) school, and the positioning (analytical) school. Six schools of thought were descriptive (emergent, intuitive) and dealt with philosophical approaches to strategic management: the entrepreneurial school (a visionary process), the cognitive school (a mental process), the learning school (an emergent process), the political school (a power process), the cultural school (an ideological process), and the environmental school (a passive process). The final school of thought, the configurational school, specifies the stages and sequence of the process and attempts to place the findings of the other schools in context.[8]

Analytical Versus Emergent Approaches

Given the careful reasoning of the proponents of these various approaches to strategic management, it is safe to assume that there is no one best way to think or learn about strategy making in complex organizations. Analytical or rational approaches to strategic management rely on the development of a logical sequence of steps or processes (linear thinking). Emergent models, on the other hand, rely on intuitive thinking, leadership, and learning and are viewed as being a part of managing. Both approaches are valid and useful in explaining an

Perspective 1–3
What is Health Policy?

Health policy determines the rules of the game that apply to all consumers and providers in the field. It is the development and maintenance of an infrastructure to efficiently enhance the health of the public.

An infrastructure need not imply a governmentally financed health care system nor the delivery of services by a governmental entity. What it does imply is a set of institutions that meet the preferences of most of the society. These institutions can take many forms ranging from unfettered markets to the provision of services by governments.

The role of health policy is to determine the preferences of the society and to develop and fine tune institutions that can efficiently meet those preferences. This may mean defining the ground rules under which insurors and providers compete. It may mean defining those services that will be provided by only a single provider, and then deciding whether that provider will be a public or private organization. It will certainly mean revisiting these decisions as new ways of doing things and new problems emerge.

The Congress and the state legislatures set health policy. In addition, the administrative authority given to executive branches and their agencies sets policy. Therefore, the Center for Medicare and Medicaid Services determines much of the health policy for federal Medicare and Medicaid. The Centers for Disease Control and Prevention, the Food and Drug Administration, and the Occupational Health and Safety Administration set and enforce health and safety standards. State Departments of Health, Insurance, and Environmental Quality set health policy within their own spheres of influence.

There are many analytic tools that come into play in helping to determine the rules that are adopted. These include economics, law, political science, epidemiology, medicine, and health services research. Health policy questions are sometimes very broad and at other times very specific. Some important questions include:

- Is health care a right or an individual responsibility?
- Can the human costs of poor health be quantified?
- Can higher tobacco taxes reduce deaths from lung cancer?
- Does managed care reduce health care costs? Does it reduce quality?
- Would higher incomes or more health services do more to improve health status?
- Who pays if employers are required to provide health insurance?

Source: Michael A. Morrisey, PhD, Director, Lister Hill Center for Health Policy and Department of Health Care Organization and Policy, University of Alabama at Birmingham.

organization's strategy. However, neither the analytical approach nor the emergent assumption, by itself, is enough. David K. Hurst explained:

> "The key question is not which of these approaches of action is right, or even which is better, but when and under what circumstances they are useful to understand what managers should do. Modern organizational life is characterized by oscillations between periods of calm, when prospective rationality seems to work, and periods of turmoil, when nothing seems to work. At some times, analysis is possible; at other times, only on-the-ground experiences will do."[9]

As a result, both approaches are required. It is difficult to initiate and sustain organizational action without some predetermined logical plan. Yet in a dynamic

Exhibit 1–2: Strategy Formation Schools of Thought

School of Thought	Basic Process	Brief Description
Design School	A conceptual process, simple, judgmental, deliberate (prescriptive)	Strategy formation as a process of informal design, essentially one of conception, process of fitting the organization to its environment
Planning School	A formal process, staged, deliberate (prescriptive)	Formalized the design approach, describing strategy as a more detached, sequential, and systematic process of formal planning
Positioning School	An analytical, systematic process, deliberate (prescriptive)	Focuses on the selection of strategic positions considered generically, emphasizes the content of strategy, selection of the optimal strategy
Entrepreneurial School	A visionary process, intuitive, largely deliberate (descriptive)	Strategy is associated with the vision of single leader, focuses on personal intuition, judgment, wisdom, experience, insight
Cognitive School	A mental process, overwhelming (descriptive)	Strategy is viewed as a cognitive process of concept attainment, an understanding of the strategist's mind, how individuals handle information to develop strategies
Learning School	An emergent process, informal, messy (descriptive)	The world is too complex to develop clear plans or visions, hence strategies must emerge in small steps or stages, strategy is a process of doing and learning
Political School	A power process, conflictive, aggressive, messy, emergent (descriptive)	Strategy is a process of exploiting power within organizations and by organizations with regard to their external environment
Cultural School	An ideological process, constrained, collective, deliberate (descriptive)	Strategy is rooted in the culture of the organization and thereby depicts it as collective, cooperative, and based on the beliefs shared by the members of the organization
Environmental School	A passive process, emergent (descriptive)	Strategy formation is a passive process and power over it rests not in the organization but the force in the environment
Configurational School	An episodic process, integrative, sequenced (contextual)	Strategy is composed of behavioral typologies, stages, episodes, or cycles

Source: From Henry Mintzberg, "Strategy Formation Schools of Thought," in *Perspectives on Strategic Management*, James W. Frederickson ed., pp. 105–197. Copyright © 1990 by HarperBusiness. Reprinted by permission of HarperCollins Publishers, Inc.

environment, such as health care, managers must expect to learn and establish new directions as they progress. In reality the methods are both complementary and contradictory – the analytical approach is similar to a map, whereas the emergent model is similar to a compass. Both may be used to guide one to a destination but in some cases they may indicate different routes. Maps are better in known worlds – worlds that have been charted before. Compasses are helpful when leaders are not sure where they are and have only a general sense of direction.[10]

Managers may use the analytical approach to develop a map as best they can from their understanding of the external environment and by interpreting the capabilities of the organization. Once the journey begins, through managing the strategic momentum, new understandings and strategies may emerge and old maps (plans) must be modified. Harvard Professor Rosabeth Moss Kanter concluded from her research that pacesetter organizations "did not wait to act until they had a perfectly conceived plan; instead, they create the plan by acting."[11] Therefore, managers must remain flexible and responsive to new realities – they must learn. However, the direction must not be random or haphazard. It must be guided by some form of strategic sense – an intuitive, entrepreneurial sensing of the "shape of the future" that transcends ordinary logic. The concept of the compass provides a unique blend of thinking, performance, analysis, and intuition.[12]

Therefore, what is needed is some type of model that provides guidance or direction to strategic managers, yet incorporates learning and change. If strategy making can be approached in a disciplined way, then there will be an increased likelihood of its successful implementation. A model or map of how strategy may be developed will help organizations view their strategies in a cohesive, integrated, and systematic way.[13] Models are abstractions that attempt to identify, simplify, and explain processes, patterns, and relationships inherent within a phenomenon. As a result, models are quite useful because they circumvent the need to store masses of data and allow us to recognize the logic underlying a series of interdependent activities. Without a model or map, managers run the risk of becoming totally incoherent, confused in perception, and muddled in practice.[14]

Combining the Analytical and Emergent Views into a Single Model

In this text, a series of "strategic thinking maps" are presented. These maps are designed to ignite strategic thinking as well as strategic planning and foster new thinking and planning when required. The strategic thinking maps will start the journey to develop a comprehensive strategy for the organization, yet the maps cannot anticipate every contingency. Managers learn a great deal about the strategy as they are managing it because today's plans and decision templates will not be adequate for solving all of tomorrow's problems. Therefore, strategic managers will have to think, analyze, use intuition, and reinvent as they go. As the physicist David Bohm observed, the purpose of science is not the "accumulation of knowledge" but rather the creation of "mental maps" that guide and shape our perception and action.[15]

Exhibit 1–3: Strategic Thinking Map of Strategic Management

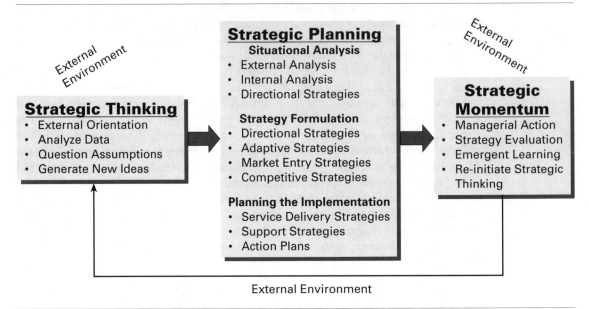

A model or map that accounts for both the analytical and the emergent views of strategic management, and that illustrates the interrelationships and organizes the major components is presented in Exhibit 1–3. This strategic thinking map serves as a general model for health care strategic managers and provides the framework for much of the discussion in this book. As illustrated in Exhibit 1–3, strategic management has three elements – strategic thinking, strategic planning, and strategic momentum. These activities are interdependent; activities in each element affects, and are affected by, the others.

As suggested in Exhibit 1–3, strategic managers must become strategic thinkers with the ability to evaluate the changing environment, analyze data, question assumptions, and develop new ideas. Additionally, they must be able to develop and document a plan of action through strategic planning. Strategic planning has three parts – situational analysis, strategy formulation, and strategy implementation. Strategic planning is a decision-making and documentation process that creates the strategic plan. Once a strategic plan is developed, strategic managers must manage the strategic momentum of the organization. As strategic managers attempt to carry out the strategic plan they evaluate its success, learn more about what works, and incorporate new strategic thinking. As indicated by the double-headed arrows, any one element of the model may initiate a rethinking of another element. For example, planning the implementation may provide new information that necessitates taking another look at strategy formulation. Similarly, managing the strategic momentum may provide new insights for implementation planning, strategy formulation, or the situational analysis.

The distinction among the terms strategic thinking, strategic planning, and strategic momentum is important and all three activities must occur in truly strategically managed organizations. Therefore, each term within the model presented in Exhibit 1–3 is explored more closely by examining what it is, why it is important, and who within the organization should be responsible for it.

Strategic Thinking

The first element depicted in Exhibit 1–3 is strategic thinking and is the fundamental intellectual activity underlying strategic management. It has been observed that leaders, similar to great athletes, must simultaneously play the game and observe it as a whole.[16] This skill is similar to leaving the playing field and going to the pressbox to observe the game and see its broader context. Thus, strategic managers must be able to keep perspective and see the big picture – not get lost in the action. But to truly understand the big picture, one must not only go to the pressbox to observe the "game," but also must have a "quiet room" to periodically think about it, to understand it, and perhaps to change the strategy or players.

Strategic thinking is an individual intellectual process, a mindset, or method of intellectual analysis that asks people to position themselves as leaders and see the "big picture." Vision and a sense of the future are an inherent part of strategic thinking. Strategic thinkers are constantly reinventing the future – creating windows on the world of tomorrow. James Kouzes and Barry Posner in *The Leadership Challenge* have indicated: "All enterprises or projects, big or small, begin in the mind's eye; they begin with imagination and with the belief that what is merely an image can one day be made real."[17] Strategic thinkers draw upon the past, understand the present, and envision an even better future. Strategic thinking requires a mindset – a way of thinking or intellectual process that accepts change, analyzes the causes and outcomes of change, and attempts to direct an organization's future to capitalize on the changes. More specifically, strategic thinking:

- acknowledges the reality of change,
- questions current assumptions and activities,
- builds on an understanding of systems,
- envisions possible futures,
- generates new ideas, and
- considers the organizational fit with the external environment.

Strategic thinking generates ideas about the future of an organization and ways to make it more relevant – more in tune with the world. Strategic thinking assesses the changing needs of the organization's stakeholders and the changing technological, social and demographic, economic, political/regulatory, and competitive demands of its world.

Strategic thinkers are always questioning: "What are we doing now that we should stop doing?" "What are we not doing now, but should start doing?" and "What are we doing now that we should continue to do but perhaps in a fundamentally different way?" For the strategic thinker, these questions are applicable to everything the organization does – its products and services, internal processes, policies and procedures, strategies, and so on. Kouzes and Posner suggest making a list of all practices in the organization that fit the description "That's the way we've always done it around here." For each one, ask "How useful is this for stimulating creativity and innovation? If your answer is 'absolutely essential,' then keep it. If not, find a way to change it."[18] Strategic thinkers examine assumptions, understand systems and their interrelationships, and develop alternative scenarios of the future. Strategic thinkers forecast external technological, social and demographic changes, as well as critical changes in the political and regulatory arenas.

WHY ENGAGE IN STRATEGIC THINKING?

The fundamental reason to engage in strategic thinking is that the world is undergoing dramatic change. In health care especially, change has become so rapid, so complex, so turbulent, and so unpredictable that it is sometimes called chaos or *whitewater change*.[19] As a result, many heath care markets have entered an era of *hypercompetition* – rapidly escalating competitive activity. Richard D'Aveni explains that in hypercompetition the frequency, boldness, and aggressiveness of dynamic movement by players accelerates to create a condition of constant disequilibrium and change.[20] We are moving irrevocably beyond an awareness of "turbulent environments" to a recognition of our participation in a truly chaotic world.[21] Health care leaders will have to cope with whitewater change and position their organizations to take advantage of emerging opportunities while avoiding external threats. Strategic managers need some type of intellectual process to consider this change if their organizations are to remain relevant – some way to consider how to renew or reinvent themselves. This intellectual process is strategic thinking.

If an organization operates in an environment where there is little change then leaders probably have less need to be concerned with strategic thinking. However, today, just as in health care, there are few industries that are not experiencing massive change – technological, economic, social, political, regulatory, and competitive – that can devastate a successful organization or propel a struggling one to greatness. Moreover, to assume that what an organization is currently doing will always be valuable and relevant is the type of arrogance that has destroyed many organizations. As the premise of James Mapes's book *Quantum Leap Thinking* indicates, "If you think the way you have always thought and do what you have always done, you will get the results you have always gotten."[22] Even the old ways of thinking and performing that were effective in the past may not achieve the results you have always accomplished in the hypercompetition of health care today.

As the world changes, so do the "rules for success." New technologies, changing social values, shifting demographics, hostile political environments, complex regulations, turbulent economic conditions, and hypercompetition call for new approaches, new products and services, and new ways to deliver them.

Everyone a Strategic Thinker

Strategic thinking provides the foundation for strategic management. However, strategic thinking is not just the task of the CEO, health officer, or top administrator of the organization. For strategic management to be successful, everyone must be encouraged to think strategically – think as a leader. *Leadership* is a performing art – a collection of practices and behaviors – not a position.[23] Everyone, even the lowest paid employees, should be encouraged to think strategically and consider how to reinvent what he or she does. For example, understanding that a nursing home's image is based in the customer's perception of cleanliness can motivate custodians to think strategically and reinvent the way the nursing home is cleaned. Strategic thinking is supported by the continuous management of the strategy and documented through the periodic process of strategic planning.

Strategic Planning

Strategic planning is the next activity in the general model of strategic management illustrated in Exhibit 1–3. *Strategic planning* is the periodic process of developing a set of steps for an organization to accomplish its mission and vision using strategic thinking. Therefore, periodically, strategic thinkers come together to reach consensus on the desired future of the organization and develop decision rules for achieving that future. The result of the strategic planning process is a plan or *strategy*. More specifically, strategic planning:

- provides a sequential, step-by-step process for creating a strategy,
- involves periodic group strategic thinking (brainstorming) sessions,
- requires data/information, but incorporates consensus and judgment,
- establishes organizational focus,
- facilitates consistent decision making,
- reaches consensus on what is required to fit the organization with the external environment, and
- results in a documented strategic plan.

The process of strategic planning defines where the organization is going and sometimes where it is not going. It defines the organization and provides focus. At the same time, the plan sets direction for the organization and – through a common understanding of the vision and broad goals – provides a template for everyone in the organization to make consistent decisions that move the organization toward its envisioned future.

Strategic planning, in large part, is a decision-making activity. Although these decisions are often supported by a great deal of quantifiable data, strategic decisions are fundamentally judgmental. Because strategic decisions cannot always be quantified, managers must rely on "informed judgment" in making this type of decision. As in our own lives, generally the more important the decision, the less quantifiable it is and the more we will have to rely on the opinions of others

Exhibit 1–4: Strategy and Vision

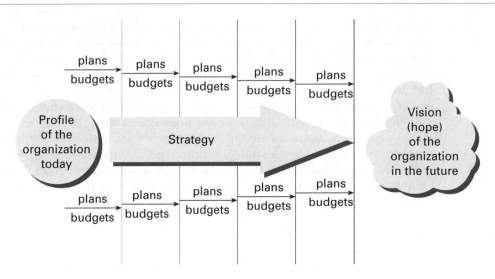

and our own best judgment. For example, our most important personal decisions – where to attend college, whether or not to get married, where to live, and so on – are largely judgments. Similarly, the most important organizational decisions, such as entering a market, introducing a new service, or acquiring a competitor, although based on information and analysis, are essentially judgments.

Decision consistency is central to strategy; when an organization exhibits a consistent behavior it has a strategy. The requirements of decision consistency suggest that a strategy is the means an organization chooses to move from where it is today to a desired state some time in the future. Thus, strategy also may be viewed as a set of guidelines or a plan that will help assure consistency in decision making and serve as a map to the future. Strategic plans indicate what types of decisions are appropriate or inappropriate for an organization. As illustrated in Exhibit 1–4, strategy is the link between understanding today and hope for the future – it is the road map to that future. Developing the road map (strategic plan) requires situational analysis, strategy formulation, and planning the implementation of the strategy.

Analyzing and understanding the situation is accomplished by three separate strategic thinking activities: (1) external environmental analysis; (2) internal environmental analysis; and (3) the development or refinement of the organization's directional strategies. The interaction and results of these activities form the basis for the development of strategy. These three interrelated activities drive the strategy.

A closer look at these three interrelated strategic thinking and planning activities is presented in Exhibit 1–5. These influences must be understood before a strategy can be formulated, as they represent the organization's situation. Forces in the external environment suggest "what the organization *should* do." That is,

Exhibit 1–5: Analyzing and Understanding the Situation

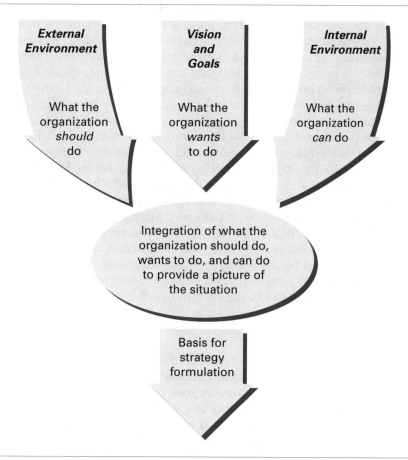

Source: Adapted from Fred Luthans, Richard M. Hodgetts, and Kenneth R. Thompson, *Social Issues in Business: Strategic and Public Policy Perspectives*, 6th edn. © 1990, p. 13. Adapted by permission of Prentice-Hall, Inc., Upper Saddle River, NJ.

success is a matter of being effective in the environment – doing the "right" thing. Strategy is additionally influenced by the internal resources, competencies, and capabilities of the organization and represents "what the organization *can* do." Finally, strategy is driven by a common mission, common vision, and common set of organizational values and goals – the directional strategies. The directional strategies are the result of considerable thought and analysis by top management and indicate "what the organization *wants* to do." Together, these forces are the essential input to strategy formulation. They are not completely distinct and separate; they overlap, interact with, and influence one another.

Chapter 2 provides strategic thinking maps for examining the general and health care external environment and Chapter 3 addresses service area competitor analysis. Chapter 4 discusses the internal environment and provides strategic thinking maps for evaluating the organization's strengths and weaknesses and the creation of competitive advantage. The development of the directional strategies through strategic thinking maps is explored in more detail in Chapter 5.

Whereas situational analysis involves a great deal of strategic thinking – gathering, classifying, and understanding information – strategy formulation involves decision making that uses the information to create a plan. Hence, strategy formulation involves *directional, adaptive, market entry,* and *competitive* strategy decisions and, typically, these decisions are made in strategic planning sessions. Strategic maps for strategy formulation are presented in Chapters 6 and 7.

Once the strategy for the organization has been formulated (including directional, adaptive, market entry, and competitive), implementation plans that accomplish the organizational strategy are developed. These implementation plans are made up of strategies developed in the key areas that create value for an organization – service delivery and support activities – and are typically discussed as part of strategic planning. Strategies must be developed that best deliver the products or services to the customers through pre-service, point-of-service, and after-service activities. In addition to service delivery strategies, strategies must be developed for value adding support areas such as the organization's culture, structure, and strategic resources. Strategy implementation is discussed further in Chapters 8 through 10.

WHY ENGAGE IN STRATEGIC PLANNING?

An assumption underlying strategic thinking is that, because of external change, organizations must periodically consider changing what they do or how they do it. Hence, there must be some process or mechanism for organizations to renew themselves, reinvent who they are, revamp their products and services, change their rules, procedures, policies and strategies, and reconsider their mission, vision, and values. Strategic planning is that process. Strategic planning provides the structure to consider issues and reach consensus on how the organization should proceed. Having a periodic structured process initiates a reconsideration, discussion, and documentation of all the assumptions. Without a planned process managers never quite get to it. Without a process, ideas are not discussed, conclusions are not reached, decisions are not made, strategies are not adopted, and strategic thinking is not documented.

A GROUP PROCESS

Strategic planning for organizations is typically a group process. It involves a number of key participants working together to develop a strategy. Although strategic planning provides the structure for thinking about strategic issues, effective strategic planning also requires the exchange of ideas, sharing perspectives, developing new insights, critical analysis, and give-and-take discussion.

The CEO can develop a strategy. An isolated planning department can develop a strategy. However, such approaches run into trouble during implementation, as there is no common "ownership" of the plan or the tasks associated with it. On the other hand, for most organizations, it is not possible for everyone to be a full participant in the strategic planning process. Decision making is protracted if everyone must have a say – and a consensus may never be reached. A few key players – senior staff, top management, or a leadership team – are needed to provide balanced and informed points of view. Often representatives of important functional areas are included as well. An effective leader will incorporate a variety of individuals with different backgrounds and perspectives to provide input to the process. Some participants may be mavericks and nudge the group in new ways. If everyone is pre-programmed to agree with the leader, participation is not required – but neither will an actionable plan be realized.

Strategic Momentum

The third element of strategic management shown in Exhibit 1–3, *strategic momentum*, concerns the day-to-day activities of managing the strategy to achieve the strategic goals of the organization. Thus, once plans are developed, they must be actively managed and implemented to maintain the momentum of the strategy. Strategic thinking and periodic planning should never stop; they become ingrained in the culture and philosophy of a strategically managed organization. As part of managing the strategy, strategic momentum:

- is the actual work to accomplish specific objectives,
- concerns decision-making processes and their consequences,
- provides the style and culture,
- fosters anticipation, innovation, and excellence,
- evaluates strategy performance through control,
- is a learning process, and
- relies on and reinforces strategic thinking and periodic strategic planning.

Strategic planning activities are common in all types of organizations. Top managers come together to develop a strategic plan, often using strategic thinking, and many important issues are discussed and documented. However, sometimes a strategic plan is created and everyone enthusiastically returns to the organization only to find "business as usual" – nothing really changes, the strategic momentum is lost, and plans are never implemented. As next year rolls around, it is once again time for the annual strategic planning retreat and the cycle repeats itself. This is an example of strategic planning without strategic momentum. Alan Weiss, in his irreverent book, *Our Emperors Have No Clothes*, explains that in these situations the problem is that, "Strategy is usually viewed as an annual exercise at best, an event that creates a 'product,' and not a process to be used to actually run the business."[24]

Strategic momentum ensures an ongoing philosophy for developing and managing the plans, actions, and control of the organization. It attempts to continually orchestrate a fit between the organization's external environment (political, regulatory, economic, technological, social, and competitive forces) and its internal

| **Perspective 1–4**

To Manage Is to
Control – To Control
Is to Manage | To control means to regulate, guide, or direct. To manage means to control, handle, or direct. Therefore, management is control and control is management. The very act of managing suggests controlling the behavior or outcome of some process, program, or plan. Vision, mission, values, and strategies are types of controls. Similarly, policies, proced-ures, rules, and performance evaluations are clearly organizational con-trols. All of these are attempts to focus organizational efforts toward a |

defined end. Yet, if these tools are improperly used, employees may perceive control to be dominating, overpowering, dictatorial, or manipulative.

When processes are poorly managed, control runs afoul as well. It is interpreted as domination when management enforces too much control and manages too closely by controlling subprocesses or too many details. Management requires the right touch. If control is too great, we create hopeless bureaucracy. If control is too weak, we have a lack of direction causing difficulty in accomplishing organizational goals. When there is too much management (control), then innovation, creativity, and individual initiative will be stifled; when there is too little, chaos ensues. Management should focus efforts but not be dictatorial or manipulative.

Given how easy it is to overdo management (control), a general rule of thumb is that "less is best." Setting direction and empowering people to make their own decisions on how best to achieve the vision seems to work. Effective management (control) is essential if organizations are to renew themselves; how-ever, overmanaging (overcontrolling) can destroy initiative and be viewed as meddling, often reducing motivation as well.

situation (culture, organization structure, resources, products and services, and so on). In some cases orchestrating the fit may mean responding to external forces; in other cases the organization may attempt to actually shape its environment (change the rules for success). External change is inevitable; often the shifts may be subtle, other times they can be discontinuous and extremely disruptive. When such dramatic changes occur, new opportunities emerge and new competencies are born, while others die or are rendered inconsequential. Inevitably, the basic rules of competing and survival will change.[25] Therefore, strategic thinking and periodic planning do not cease. Strategic momentum is how an organization constructively manages change, evaluates strategy, and reinvents or renews the organization. As Henry Mintzberg has indicated, ". . . a key to managing strat-egy is the ability to detect emerging patterns and help them take shape."[26] Perspective 1–4 provides an additional perspective concerning managing and attempting to "control" the behavior of the organization.

Managing the strategic momentum must be both externally and internally ori-ented. Thus, it represents a back and forth process of analysis and evaluation to continuously monitor the environment and adapt the organization.[27] Strategic man-agers focus on anticipating external change, fostering innovation in the services and processes of the organization, shaping the organization's culture, develop-ing organizational systems, managing the strategic resources, and promoting excel-lence. At the same time, strategic managers pursue the vision and broad goals providing everyone in the organization a template for making consistent decisions.

Evaluation occurs as a part of managing strategically. The performance of the strategy is monitored as it is implemented. Evaluation is directed toward the implementation strategies, the organization's general strategy, situational analysis, and strategic thinking. As strategic managers monitor various organizational processes, they learn what is effective and take corrective action as necessary. Evaluation is an inherent part of not only strategic thinking and strategic planning, but also strategic momentum; therefore, it will be addressed within the discussion of each element of the strategic management map.

WHY MANAGE STRATEGIC MOMENTUM?

For many organizations strategic planning is the easiest part of strategic management and the planning process receives the greatest attention. However, plans must be implemented to create momentum and to realize strategic intent. Poor implementation or lack of implementation has rendered many strategic plans as worthless. Whereas the strategic plan and its underlying strategic thinking must be viewed as important, they fall apart without implementation and the decision-making guidelines provided for managers at all levels in the organization. If the strategy is not actively managed, it will not happen.

Sometimes it is difficult for managers to plan or envision the long-term future of an organization in a dynamic environment. Managers often need to react to unanticipated developments and new competitive pressures. Different environmental characteristics and different organizational forms require new and different ways of defining strategy.[28] Strategy becomes an intuitive, entrepreneurial, political, culture-based, or learning process. In these cases, maps are of limited value. Managers must create and discover an unfolding future, using their ability to learn together in groups and interact politically in a spontaneous, self-organizing manner. However, learning is difficult in organizations. Learning requires engagement, mastering unfamiliar ideas, and adopting new behaviors. Engaged learning demands that executives share leadership, face harsh truths, and take learning personally. It requires them to fundamentally change the way they manage.[29] It requires strategic thinking.

When there are provocative atmospheres conducive to complex learning, organizations may change and develop new strategic direction. In such an environment, the destination as well as the route may turn out to be unexpected and unintended. As a result, strategy emerges spontaneously from the chaos of challenge and contradiction, through a process of real-time learning and politics.[30] For these uncharted, complex situations, a compass indicating a general direction, steadied by leadership, may be more appropriate than a map of known events, territories, and ideas.

Clearly, rational strategies do not always work out as planned (an *unrealized strategy*). In other cases, an organization may end up with a strategy that was quite unexpected as a result of having been "swept away by events" (an *emergent strategy*). Leadership, vision, and "feeling our way along" (learning through strategic awareness) often provide a general direction without a real sense of specific objectives or long-term outcomes.

Exhibit 1–6: Intended Versus Realized Strategy

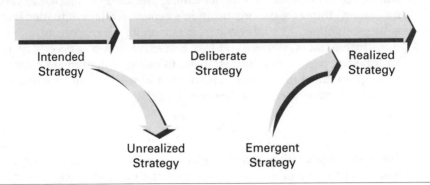

Source: Henry Mintzberg, "Patterns in Strategy Formation," *Management Science* 24, no. 9 (1978), p. 934.

Exhibit 1–6 presents three outcomes for an organization. These outcomes may be summarized as follows:

1. *Intended strategies* that are realized (*deliberate strategies*).
2. *Intended strategies* that are not realized, perhaps because of unrealistic expectations, misjudgments about the environment, or changes during implementation (*unrealized strategies*).
3. *Realized strategies* that were never intended, perhaps because no strategy was developed at the outset or perhaps because the strategies somehow were displaced along the way (*emergent strategies*).[31]

Obviously, health care organizations formulate strategies and realize them to varying degrees. For instance, as a part of a deliberate strategy to broaden their market, improve service to the community, and retain referral patients, many community hospitals began offering cardiac services such as catheterization and open heart surgery.[32] As a result, some of these hospitals have built market share and increased profitability. Other community hospitals have not fared as well. Their managers had unrealistic expectations concerning the profitability of cardiac services and the number of procedures required. A large volume is crucial to cardiac services because it allows the hospital to order supplies in bulk and provides physician experience that produces better outcomes and shorter lengths of stay. In addition, some community hospital managers misjudged the level of reimbursement from Medicare, thereby further squeezing profitability. The strategies of those community hospitals that left the cardiac services market were not realized.

Still other community hospitals seemed to move into a full range of cardiac services without an explicit strategy to do so. In an effort to retain patients and enhance their images, these hospitals began by offering limited cardiac services but shortly found that they were not performing enough procedures to be "world class." They added services, equipment, and facilities to help create the required volume and, without really intending to at the outset, ended up with emergent strategies that resulted in significant market share in cardiac services.

Mintzberg added several possible outcomes to those presented in Exhibit 1–6. For example, he discussed strategies that, as they were realized, changed form and became, in part at least, emergent; emergent strategies that were formalized as deliberate ones; and intended strategies that were over-realized.[33] It is quite possible that a strategy may be developed and subsequently realized. However, we must be realistic enough to understand that when we engage in strategic management the theoretical ideal (strategy developed, then realized) may not, and in all probability will not, be the case. A great deal may go wrong. The possibilities include the following:

1. There is a reformulation of the strategy during implementation as the organization gains new information and feeds that information back to the formulation process, thus modifying intentions en route (a function of strategic control).
2. The external environment is in a period of flux and strategists are unable to accurately predict conditions; the organization may therefore find itself unable to respond appropriately to a powerful external momentum.[34]
3. Organizations in the external environment implementing their own strategies may block a strategic initiative, forcing the activation of a contingency strategy or a period of "groping."

STRATEGIC MOMENTUM – AN ORGANIZATION-WIDE ACTIVITY

As with strategic thinking, everyone plays a role in maintaining strategic momentum. Everyone in the organization should be working for the strategy and understand how their work contributes to the accomplishment of the strategic goals. As Max DePree has suggested, "Leaders are obligated to provide and maintain momentum."[35] The only legitimate work in an organization is work that contributes to the accomplishment of the strategic plan. Although organizations may accomplish superior results for a brief period of time, it takes the orchestration of management as well as leadership to perpetuate these capabilities far into the future.[36]

The Benefits of Strategic Management

The three activities of strategic management – strategic thinking, strategic planning, and strategic momentum – will provide many benefits to health care organizations. However, because strategic management is a philosophy or way of managing an organization, its benefits are not always quantifiable. Overall, strategic management:

- ties the organization together with a common sense of purpose and shared values;
- improves financial performance in many cases;[37]

- provides the organization with a clear self-concept, specific goals, and guidance as well as consistency in decision making;
- helps managers understand the present, think about the future, and recognize the signals that suggest change;
- requires managers to communicate both vertically and horizontally;
- improves overall coordination within the organization; and
- encourages innovation and change within the organization to meet the needs of dynamic situations.

Strategic management is a unique perspective that requires everyone in the organization to cease thinking solely in terms of internal operations and their own operational responsibilities. It insists that everyone adopt what may be a fundamentally new attitude, an external orientation and a concern for the big picture. It is basically optimistic in that it integrates "what is" with "what can be."

In our view, health care leaders require a comprehensive strategic management approach for guiding their organizations through societal and health care industry changes that will occur in the future. We believe that the strategic management concepts, activities, and methods presented in this text will prove to be valuable in coping with these changes. In addition, the internal, non-quantifiable benefits of strategic management will aid health care organizations in better integrating functional areas to strategically utilize limited resources and to satisfy the various publics served. Strategic management is the exciting future of effective health care leadership.

What Strategic Management Is Not

Strategic management should not be regarded as a technique that will provide a "quick fix" for an organization that has fundamental problems. Quick fixes for organizations are rare; successful strategic management often takes years to become a part of the values and culture of an organization. If strategic management is regarded as a technique or gimmick, it is doomed to failure. Similarly, strategic management is not just strategic planning or a yearly retreat where the leadership of an organization meets to talk about key issues only to return to "business as usual." Although retreats can be effective in refocusing management and for generating new thinking, strategic management must be adopted as a philosophy of leading and managing the organization.

Strategic management is not a process of completing paperwork. If strategic management has reached a point where it has become simply a process of filling in endless forms, meeting deadlines, drawing milestone charts, or changing the dates of last year's goals and plans, it is not strategic management. Effective strategic management requires little paperwork. It is an attitude, not a series of documents. Similarly, strategic management is not initiated merely to satisfy a regulatory body's or an accrediting agency's requirement for a "plan." In these situations, no commitment is made on the part of key leadership, no participation is expected from those in the organization, and the plan may or may not be implemented.[38]

Strategic management is not a process of simply extending the organization's current activities into the future. It is not based solely on a forecast of present trends. Strategic management attempts to identify the issues that will be important in the future. Health care strategic managers should not simply ask the question, "How will we provide this service in the future?" Rather, they should be asking questions such as, "Should we provide this service in the future?" "What new services will be needed?" "What services are we providing now that are no longer needed?"

A Systems Perspective

The problems facing organizations are so complex that they defy simple solutions. Understanding the nature of the health care environment, the relationship of the organization to that environment, and the often-conflicting interests of internal functional departments requires a broad conceptual paradigm. Yet, it is difficult to comprehend so many complex and important relationships. Strategic managers have found general systems theory or a *systems approach* to be a useful perspective for organizing strategic thinking.

A system may be defined literally as "an organized or complex whole: an assemblage or combination of things or parts forming a complex or unitary whole."[39] More simply, a system is a set of interrelated elements. Each element connects to every other element, directly or indirectly, and no subset of elements is unrelated to any other subset. Further, a system must have a unity of purpose in the accomplishment of its goals, functions, or desired outputs.[40] Understanding the complex whole through a systems approach:

- aids in identifying and understanding the "big picture;"
- facilitates the identification of major components;
- helps identify important relationships and provides proper perspective;
- avoids excessive attention to a single part;
- allows for a broad scope solution;
- fosters integration; and
- provides a basis for redesign.

The use of the systems approach requires strategic managers to define the organization in broad terms and to identify the important variables and interrelationships that will affect decisions. By defining systems, strategic managers are able to see the "big picture" in proper perspective and avoid devoting excessive attention to relatively minor aspects of the total system.[41] A systems approach permits strategic managers to concentrate on those aspects of the problem that most deserve attention and allows a more focused attempt at a resolution. As Peter Senge has indicated, systems approaches help us see the total system and how to change the pieces within the system more effectively and intelligently.[42] Perspective 1–5 provides additional insight into the use of systems approaches to see the big picture.

Perspective 1–5

Mu-Shin
Management

Drawing upon the sport of karate, *Harvard Business Review* Senior Executive Editor Suzy Wetlaufer explains the art of systems thinking. She suggests that the karate paradoxical mind-set mu-shin is the same mind-set that is needed by organizational leaders. Mu-shin directs adherents to "look at everything, see nothing." Or to put it another way, absorb the world in all its messy details, but keep your mind free, uncluttered. Masters of karate consider the acute mental clarity created by mu-shin a prerequisite for flawless execution. Similarly, organizational leaders must be able to see the big picture uncluttered by many details of managing large complex organizations. As Ms. Wetlaufer suggests, executives must look at everything, yet, to act intelligently, must see nothing – to be blind to the distractions of hundreds of little questions so that one or two big answers become blindingly clear. This mu-shin mind-set can be difficult to achieve as managers often tend to get "pulled" into – and ultimately mired in – the detail and minutiae of management. Therefore, it is necessary for managers to "take a step back" and see the bigger picture.

Source: Suzy Wetlaufer, "Mastering Mu-Shin Management," *Harvard Business Review* 78, no. 5 (September–October 2000), p. 10.

Recognizing the importance of a systems framework, health care managers commonly refer to "the health care system" or "the health care delivery system" and strive to develop logical internal organizational systems to deal with the environment. In a similar manner, health care strategic managers must use systems to aid in strategic thinking about the external environment. The community and region may be thought of as an integrated system with each part of the system (subsystem) providing a unique contribution. Many contemporary health care strategies are driven by a systems approach as evidenced by the growth of health care systems, networks, cooperatives, and alliances.

The Level and Orientation of the Strategy

A systems perspective will be required to specify the level of the strategy and the relationship of the strategy to the other strategic management activities. Therefore, the organizational level and orientation should be carefully considered and specified before the strategic planning begins. For example, strategies may be developed for large, complex organizations or small, well-focused units. The range of the strategic decisions that are considered in these two organizations is quite different, but both can benefit from strategic management.

A clear specification of the "level" of thinking will determine the type and range of decision to be made in strategic planning. For example, a large integrated health care system may develop strategy for a number of levels – a corporate level, divisional level, organizational level, and a unit level. As illustrated in Exhibit 1–7, when considered together these strategic perspectives create a hierarchy of strategies and must be consistent and support one another. Each strategy provides the "means" for accomplishing the "ends" of the next higher level. Thus, the functional unit level provides the means for accomplishing the ends of the

Exhibit 1–7: The Link Between Levels of Strategic Management

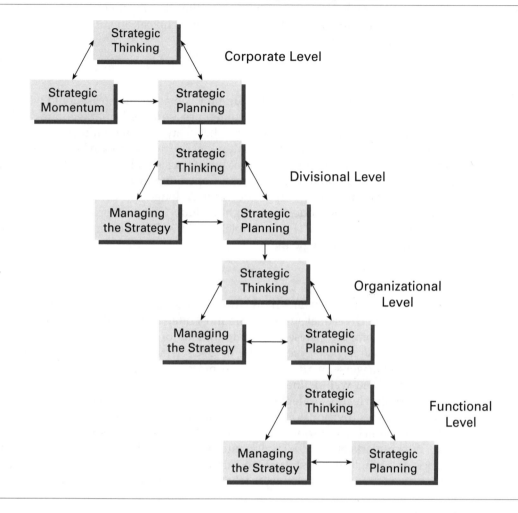

organizational level. The organizational level, in turn, provides the means for accomplishing the ends of the divisional level. Finally, the divisional level is the means to the ends established at the corporate level. As illustrated in Exhibit 1–7, part of the context for lower order strategy is provided by the strategic planning of higher order strategies.

Trinity Health, formed by the consolidation of Mercy Health Services and Holy Cross Health System, is the third largest Catholic health system in the United States and is an example of a health care organization that should develop strategy for all four perspectives. As of 2005, Trinity had over $5.1 billion in assets, $4.1 billion in revenues, and comprised 45 hospitals, 402 outpatient facilities, 31 long-term care facilities, 28 home health offices, and 20 hospice programs located in 7 US states. Clearly, strategies should be developed for the entire system (corporate level – Trinity Health), for each major division (business level – Eastern Division), for each distinct organization within the division (Saint Joseph Mercy Health System), and within the various units (clinical operations – Saint Joseph Mercy Saline Hospital).

CORPORATE-LEVEL STRATEGY

Corporate-level strategies address the question "What business(es) should we be in?" Such strategies consider multiple, sometimes unrelated, markets and typically are based on return on investment, market share or potential market share, and system integration. For Trinity Health, clearly the corporate perspective is an important one. The question of "What businesses should we be in?" has resulted in several semi-autonomous "businesses" operating in a number of different markets, including hospitals, outpatient facilities, long-term care, home health, and hospices. Key strategic questions might include "What other types of businesses should Trinity consider?" For example, would wellness or mental health centers be an appropriate strategic move?

DIVISION-LEVEL STRATEGY

Divisional-level strategies are more focused and provide direction for a single business type. Divisional strategies are most often concerned with positioning the division to compete. These semi-autonomous organizations are often referred to as SBUs (*strategic business units*) or SSUs (*strategic service units*). Therefore, strategic managers for these units are most concerned with a specified set of competitors and well-defined markets (service areas).

For Trinity Health, strategies must be developed for the hospital division, outpatient facilities division, long-term care division, and so on. For the hospital division key strategic questions may include "How many hospitals are optimal?" or "Which markets should Trinity enter with a new hospital?" This perspective concerns a single business type and its markets. Therefore, it is quite different from the corporate perspective of what businesses Trinity should be in.

ORGANIZATION-LEVEL STRATEGY

Within a division, individual organizational units may develop strategies as well. These *organizational-level strategies* typically concern one organization competing within a specific well-defined service area. For example, each hospital in Trinity's hospital division may develop a strategic plan to address its own particular market conditions. Key strategic questions for this level of strategy may include "What combination of hospital services is most appropriate for this market?" and "What strategies are the competitors using to increase market share?"

UNIT-LEVEL STRATEGY

Unit-level strategies support organizational strategies through accomplishing specific objectives. Unit operational strategies may be developed within departments of an organization such as clinical operations, marketing, finance, information systems, human resources, and so on. Unit strategies address two issues. First, they are intended to integrate the various subfunctional activities. Second, they are designed to relate the various functional area policies with any changes in the functional area environment.[43] In addition, linkage strategies are directed toward integrating the functions themselves and creating internal capabilities across functions (for example, quality programs or changing the organization's culture).

STRATEGY HIERARCHY

Strategic management may be employed independently at any organizational level of the organization. However, it is much more effective if there is a top-down support and strategies are integrated from one level to the next. For some organizations, of course, there is no corporate or divisional level, such as with a free-standing community hospital or independent long-term care organization. For these organizations the question of scope and perspective and integration of the strategy is much more straightforward.

The Importance of Leadership

Ultimately, strategic decision making for health care organizations is the responsibility of top management. The CEO is a strategic manager with the preeminent responsibility for positioning the organization for the future. The leader must be able to inspire, organize, and implement an effective pursuit of a vision and maintain it even when sacrifices are required.[44] If the CEO does not fully understand or faithfully support strategic management, it will not happen.

Leadership Roles Throughout the Organization

In the past, strategy development was primarily a staff activity. The planning staff would create the strategy and submit it for approval to top management. This process resulted in plans that were often unrealistic, did not fully consider the realities and resources of the divisions or departments, and separated planning from leadership.

Over the past decade, many large formal planning staffs have been dissolved as organizations learned that strategy development cannot take place in relative isolation. Therefore, the development of the strategy has become a line job with each manager responsible for the strategic implications of his or her decisions. The coordination and facilitation of strategic planning typically may be designated as the responsibility of a key manager (often the CEO) but the entire leadership team is responsible for strategy development and its management. The rationale underlying this approach is that no one is more in touch with the external environment (regulations, technology, competition, social change, and so on) than the line manager who must deal with it every day and lead change. The leadership

1970s

An expert at strategic planning, knowledgeable in all strategic planning functions. Will be required to develop a strategic planning process for corporate and divisional units. An ability to build and manage a staff of planning specialists as they perform strategic analysis and complete the strategy formulation and selection process.

1980s

A strategic planning specialist who can guide the CEO as well as direct reports to explore and identify the strategic alternatives available, evaluate them, and select the most beneficial for the organization. Will be responsible for conducting strategic analysis and providing input to the CEO and direct reports.

1990s

Knowledge of strategic planning models and responsible for establishing and monitoring the strategic planning schedule, handling the logistics of planning group meetings, providing strategic analysis and assessments to the strategic planning group, and documenting and distributing strategic planning group meeting results. Assist the CEO to establish, articulate, communicate, and educate those responsible for putting into practice strategies that pay off. Major efforts will be in establishing the criteria for effective strategy and ensuring that they are applied.

2000s

Line managers with functional responsibility wanted to be a part of leadership team. Must be a strategic thinker and able to foster strategic thinking in others. Must be able to facilitate a strategic thinking workgroup as well as be a participating member. Must be creative and a consensus builder. Must be able to lead strategy development as well as its implementation. Applicant should be able to function as an extension of the CEO to make strategic management effective in fulfilling the vision for the organization.

team must coordinate the organization's overall strategy and facilitate strategic thinking throughout the organization. As a result, the organization's key top managers act as an extension of the CEO to ensure that an organized and used planning process ensues.[45] Perspective 1–6 illustrates the changing role of the strategic planner over the past decades.

Leadership plays an important role in strategy development. Strategies cannot be created entirely by analysis, but their development can be enhanced by a logical approach. Therefore, planners have critical roles to play.[46] Planners can:

- pose the right questions rather than find the right answers;
- provide alternative conceptual interpretations of situations;
- act as catalysts, encouraging managers to think about the future in creative ways;
- help identify and provide information concerning important issues and emerging strategies;
- clarify and express the strategies in terms sufficiently clear to render them operational;

- break down strategies into substrategies, ad hoc programs, and action plans specifying what must be done to realize each strategy;
- consider the effects of the strategic changes on the organization's operations; and
- communicate and control the strategy.[47]

In organizations that have seriously adopted strategic management, managers understand the organization's strategy and take leadership roles. Increasingly, organizations are finding it unworkable for a single leader at the top to understand the full complexity of the industry and organization, build consensus throughout the organization, and make all the important decisions. Instead, many health care organizations are fostering leadership development throughout the organization. The many changes that have taken place in the work environment in the past decade have brought the challenges and opportunities of leadership down to the individual employee – contributors with no positional authority, who are not designated as "leader" but who have leadership challenges presented to them on a daily basis.[48] As part of the job, every manager must be concerned with change, innovation, and excellence. Each must ask the critical questions "Should we be doing this in the future?" "How should we be doing this?" "What new things should we be doing?" Strategic thinking, strategic planning, and maintaining strategic momentum are the clearest manifestations of leadership in organizations. As outlined in Perspective 1–7, strategic managers must develop the "habits" of leadership.

Perspective 1–7

Habits of a Successful Strategic Leader

Strategic leaders:

- Develop and communicate an exciting vision for the future.
- Involve people from all levels and backgrounds in meaningful strategic management processes.
- Manage "tomorrow" rather than "today." The leader's job is assuring a future for the organization rather than current operations.
- Manage by wandering around (MBWA). Leaders understand the employees and their problems because he or she talks to them on a regular basis.
- Allow people to make mistakes. Innovation in products, services, and management processes requires that people take chances. Sometimes people will fail, but there is little chance for success without attempts to achieve it.
- Build leaders throughout the organization. CEOs should encourage others in the organization to take responsibility for setting direction and aligning people, as well as inspiring and motivating others.
- Trust others in the organization to make the best decisions they can and do not "micromanage."
- Make heroes out of people who innovate and contribute to the development and accomplishment of the strategic plan.
- Allow time for the process to work.
- Lead by example.
- Empower employees to solve problems.

Lessons for Health Care Managers

Strategic management is a complex and difficult task. Yet, the model of strategic management presented in this chapter provides a useful framework or map for conceptualizing and developing strategies for an organization. The model may be applied to a variety of types of health care organizations operating in dramatically different environments. The model is useful for both large and small organizations and facilitates strategic thinking at all levels of the organization.

The twenty-first century will place a higher premium on effective strategic management and leadership than ever before. Yet, no single approach may be adequate to understand social and organizational processes. Indeed, different organizational situations may call for dramatically different leadership styles.[49] The strategic thinking map presented in this text is designed to provide the essential logic of the activities involved in strategic management and therefore is based on both the analytical (rational) as well as the emergent (learning) approaches for understanding strategy making in organizations. The analytical model provides an excellent starting point for understanding the concept of strategy and a foundation for comparing and contrasting strategies. However, the strategic thinking map does not perfectly represent reality and must not be applied blindly or with the belief that "life always works that way."

Strategic management is not always a structured, well-thought-out exercise. In reality, thought does not always precede action, perfect information concerning the environment and organization never exists, and rationality and logic are not always superior to intuition and luck. Sometimes organizations "do" before they "know." For instance, intended strategies are often not the realized strategies. Sometimes managers are able to just "muddle through." Or, managers may have a broad master plan or logic underlying strategic decisions, but, because of the complexity of the external and internal environments, incremental adjustments or guided evolution is the best they can do.[50] Managers must realize that, once introduced, strategies are subject to a variety of forces, both within and outside the organization. Sometimes we learn by doing. Yet, without a plan (a map) it is difficult to start the journey, difficult to create any type of momentum for the organization, and difficult to have consistent decision making. Thus, strategic managers begin with the most rational plan that can be developed and continue to engage in strategic thinking. Effective strategic managers become adept at "freezing" and "unfreezing" their thinking and strategic plans as the situation changes.

Summary and Conclusions

This chapter discussed the nature and activities of strategic management. Strategic thinking, strategic planning, and strategic momentum are all a part of strategic management. Many changes are taking place in the environment that will profoundly affect the success of health care organizations; therefore, strategic thinking and strategic planning are essential. Strategic momentum is required to provide an ongoing philosophy of strategic management that aligns service delivery and support activities to the strategic plan, evaluates against the plan, and yet acknowledges the importance of external change and learning (strategic thinking).

In exploring the nature of strategic management, it is important to note that strategic management decisions are largely judgmental, yet are crucial to the success of the organization. Strategic thinking, strategic planning, and strategic momentum attempt to achieve a fit between the demands of the external environment and the organization's internal capabilities. When an organization makes consistent decisions and exhibits a consistent behavior, it has a strategy. A strategy may also be viewed as a guideline or plan to help assure decision consistency in the future. The concept of strategic management has been successfully used by business organizations, the military, and in government agencies. Health care managers are finding it essential for their organizations, as well. Strategic management is organization specific and very different from health policy.

Strategic planning may be either formal or informal. However, models or theories of complex phenomena are useful in understanding the various activities involved and their interrelationships. Models provide an abstract overview and conceptual anchors for managers to consider as they struggle to deal with complexity. Without some conceptual framework it would be difficult to begin strategic thinking and planning. However, strategic plans may be both analytical and emergent. Health care managers must understand that, although the analytical approach provides a framework for thinking about the organization and its future, they must deal with powerful internal and external forces that in many cases are beyond their control. As Mintzberg has said, "Practice is always more complicated – and more interesting – than theory . . ."

A model of strategic management was presented that included strategic thinking, strategic planning, and strategic momentum. The model of strategic management is not itself reality but rather a framework or map for dealing with reality. Accurate modeling of the behavior of an organization is unlikely. In reality, the elements of strategic management may be blended together as the strategy is formed and reformed through leadership, intuition, and organizational learning. Indeed, implementing the strategy may actually create an entirely new, unintended strategy.

The strategic planning portion of the model incorporates situational analysis, strategy formulation, and strategy implementation. The strategic thinking activities within situational analysis combine to influence strategy formulation. Strategy formulation in turn affects planning the implementation. Finally, the strategy must be managed, evaluated, and modified as needed. Strategic momentum is an iterative process that may incorporate new understandings of the situation, change the fundamental strategy, or modify strategy implementation. Strategic momentum essentially continues strategic thinking and strategic planning.

Strategic management may be applied at various levels within the organization. Thus, strategic management often involves developing strategies at the functional unit level to achieve strategies at the organization level. Organization strategies help achieve divisional strategies. Divisional strategies, in turn, are the means to achieving corporate ends. At any level, however, strategic management must not be separated from leadership.

Key Terms and Concepts in Strategic Management

Analytical Approach
Corporate-Level Strategy
Deliberate Strategies
Divisional-Level Strategy
Emergent Strategy
Health Policy
Hypercompetition
Intended Strategies
Managing the Strategy

Map/Compass
Organizational-Level Strategy
Rational Approach
Realized Strategies
Situational Analysis
Strategic Business Unit (SBU)
Strategic Management
Strategic Momentum
Strategic Planning

Strategic Service Unit (SSU)
Strategic Thinking
Strategy
Strategy Formulation
Strategy Implementation
Systems Approach
Unit-level Strategies
Unrealized Strategies
Whitewater Change

QUESTIONS FOR CLASS DISCUSSION

1. Explain why strategic management has become crucial in today's dynamic health care environment.
2. What is the rationale for health care organizations' adoption of strategic management?
3. Trace the evolution of strategic management. Have the objectives of strategic management changed dramatically over its development?
4. How is strategic management different from traditional health policy?
5. Compare and contrast the analytical model of strategic management with the emergent, learning model. Which is most appropriate for health care managers?
6. Why are conceptual models of management processes useful for practicing managers?
7. What is a strategic thinking map? How are strategic thinking maps useful? What are their limitations?
8. What are the major activities of strategic management? How are they linked together?
9. Differentiate among the terms strategic management, strategic thinking, strategic planning, and strategic momentum.
10. Who should be doing strategic thinking? Strategic planning? Managing the strategic momentum?
11. Explain whitewater change and hypercompetition. Why are these occurring? What effect will they have on the management of health care organizations?
12. Is strategic thinking enough? Why do we engage in strategic planning? What are the elements of strategic planning?
13. What is meant by realized strategies? How can strategies be realized if they were never intended?
14. What can go wrong with well-thought-out strategies that were developed using all the steps in strategic planning?
15. Explain and illustrate the possible benefits of strategic management. What types of health care institutions may benefit most from strategic management?
16. Why is a "systems approach" helpful to strategic managers?

17. At what organizational level(s) may a strategy be developed? If at more than one level, how are these levels linked by the planning process?
18. How has the role of the strategic planner changed over the past several decades? What new skills will be essential for the strategic planner?
19. What is meant by the statement "Strategic leaders should try to create the future"?
20. Select a health care organization you are familiar with and discuss the demands of strategic management for the organization.

NOTES

1. Jeffrey Bracker, "The Historical Development of the Strategic Management Concept," *Academy of Management Review* 5, no. 2 (1980), pp. 219–224.
2. Ibid.
3. Bruce D. Henderson, "The Origin of Strategy," *Harvard Business Review* 67, no. 6 (November–December 1989), p. 142.
4. Bracker, "The Historical Development of the Strategic Management Concept," pp. 219–224.
5. Margarete Arndt and Barbara Bigelow, "The Transfer of Business Practices into Hospitals: History and Implications," in John D. Blair, Myron D. Fottler, and Grant T. Savage (eds) *Advances in Health Care Management* (New York: Elsevier Science, 2000), pp. 339–368.
6. Ernest L. Stebbins and Kathleen N. Williams, "History and Background of Health Planning in the United States," in William A. Reinke, *Health Planning: Qualitative Aspects and Quantitative Techniques* (Baltimore: Johns Hopkins University, School of Hygiene and Public Health, Department of International Health, 1972), p. 3.
7. Henry Mintzberg, "The Design School: Reconsidering the Basic Premises of Strategic Management," *Strategic Management Journal* 11, no. 3 (1990), pp. 171–195.
8. Ibid.
9. David K. Hurst, *Crisis and Renewal: Meeting the Challenge of Organizational Change* (Boston: Harvard Business School Press, 1995), pp. 167–168.
10. Ibid.
11. Rosabeth Moss Kanter, "Strategy as Improvisational Theater," *MIT Sloan Management Review* (Winter 2002), p. 76.
12. Ian H. Wilson, "The 5 Compasses of Strategic Leadership," *Strategy & Leadership* 24, no. 4 (1996), pp. 26–31 and Dusya Vera and Mary Crossan, "Strategic Leadership and Organizational Learning," *Academy of Management Review* 29, no. 2 (2004), pp. 222–240.
13. Robert S. Kaplan and David P. Norton, "Having Trouble with Your Strategy? Then Map It," *Harvard Business Review* 78, no. 5 (September–October 2000), pp. 167–176.
14. Hurst, *Crisis and Renewal*, p. 7.
15. Peter M. Senge, *The Fifth Discipline: The Art & Practice of The Learning Organization* (New York: Currency Doubleday, 1990), pp. 239–240.
16. Ronald A. Heifetz and Marty Linsky, "A Survival Guide for Leaders," *Harvard Business Review* (June 2002), pp. 65–74.
17. James M. Kouzes and Barry Z. Posner, *The Leadership Challenge: How to Keep Getting Extraordinary Things Done in Organizations* (San Francisco: Jossey-Bass Publishers, 1995), p. 93.
18. Ibid., p. 55.
19. H. B. Gelatt, "Future Sense: Creating the Future," *Futurist* 27, no. 5 (September–October 1993), pp. 9–13 and Stuart L. Hart and Sanjay Sharma, "Engaging Fringe Stakeholders for Competitive Imagination," *Academy of Management Executive* 18, no. 1 (2004), pp. 7–18.
20. Richard A. D'Aveni, "Coping with Hypercompetition: Utilizing the New 7S's Framework," *Academy of Management Executive* 9, no. 3 (1995), pp. 45–60.
21. Ruben F. W. Nelson, "Four-Quadrant Leadership," *Planning Review* 24, no. 1 (1996), pp. 20–25, 37.
22. James J. Mapes, *Quantum Leap Thinking* (Beverly Hills, CA: Dove Books, 1996).
23. Kouzes and Posner, *The Leadership Challenge*, p. 30.
24. Alan Weiss, *Our Emperors Have No Clothes* (Franklin Lakes, NJ: Career Press, 1995), p. 20.
25. Michael A. Mische, *Strategic Renewal: Becoming a High-Performance Organization* (Upper Saddle River, NJ: Prentice Hall, 2001), p. 21.
26. Henry Mintzberg, *Mintzberg on Management* (New York: The Free Press, 1989), p. 41.
27. Jim Begun and Kathleen B. Heatwole, "Strategic Cycling: Shaking Complacency in Healthcare

Strategic Planning," *Journal of Healthcare Management* 44, no. 5 (September–October 1999), pp. 339–351.

28. John C. Camillus, "Reinventing Strategic Planning," *Strategy & Leadership* 24, no. 3 (1996), pp. 6–12.

29. Jane Linder, "Paying the Personal Price for Performance," *Strategy & Leadership* 28, no. 2 (March–April 2000), pp. 22–25.

30. Ralph Stacey, "Strategy as Order Emerging from Chaos," *Long Range Planning* 26, no. 1 (1993), pp. 10–17.

31. Henry Mintzberg, "Patterns in Strategy Formation," *Management Science* 24, no. 9 (1978), p. 945.

32. Mary Wagner, "Cardiac Services Find a New Home in Community Hospitals," *Modern Healthcare* (October 29, 1990), pp. 23–31.

33. Mintzberg, "Patterns in Strategy Formation," p. 946.

34. Ibid.

35. Max DePree, *Leadership Is An Art* (New York: Doubleday, 1989), p. 14.

36. Craig R. Hickman, *Mind of a Manager, Soul of a Leader* (New York: John Wiley & Sons, 1992), p. 261.

37. After almost four decades of research, the effects of strategic planning on an organization's performance are still unclear. Some studies have found significant benefits from planning, although others have found no relationship, or even small negative effects. For an extensive survey of the strategic planning/financial performance literature, see Lawrence C. Rhyne, "The Relationship of Strategic Planning to Financial Performance," *Strategic Management Journal* 7, no. 5 (September–October 1986), pp. 423–436, and Brian K. Boyd, "Strategic Planning and Financial Performance: A Meta-analytic Review," *Journal of Management Studies* 28, no. 4 (July 1991), pp. 353–374.

38. Begun and Heatwole, "Strategic Cycling," pp. 339–351.

39. David I. Cleland and William R. King, *Systems Analysis and Project Management* (New York: McGraw-Hill Book Company, 1983), pp. 19–20.

40. Joseph K. H. Tan, *Health Management Information Systems: Methods and Practical Applications*, 2nd edn (Gaithersburg, MD: Aspen Publishers, 2001), p. 25.

41. Cleland and King, *Systems Analysis and Project Management*, pp. 19–20.

42. Senge, *The Fifth Discipline*, p. 7.

43. Dan E. Schendel and Charles W. Hofer, "Introduction," in D. E. Schendel and C. W. Hofer (eds) *Strategic Management: A New View of Business Policy and Planning* (Boston: Little, Brown, 1979), p. 12.

44. Russell L. Ackoff, "Transformational Leadership," *Strategy & Leadership* 27, no. 1 (1999), pp. 20–25.

45. Donald L. Bates and John E. Dillard, Jr., "Wanted: A Strategic Planner for the 1990s," *Journal of General Management* 18, no. 1 (1992), pp. 51–62.

46. Henry Mintzberg, "The Fall and Rise of Strategic Planning," *Harvard Business Review* 72, no. 1 (January–February 1994), pp. 107–114.

47. Ibid.

48. Horst Bergmann, Kathleen Hurson, and Darlene Russ-Eft, "Introducing a Grass-roots Model of Leadership," *Strategy & Leadership* 27, no. 6 (1999), pp. 15–20.

49. Daniel Goleman, "Leadership that Gets Results," *Harvard Business Review* 78, no. 2 (March–April 2000), pp. 78–90.

50. Bjorn Lovas and Sumantra Ghoshal, "Strategy as Guided Evolution," *Strategic Management Journal* 21, no. 9 (2000), pp. 875–896.

ADDITIONAL READINGS

Bettis, Richard (ed.) *Strategy in Transition* (Malden, MA: Blackwell Publishing, 2004). Outstanding scholars from around the globe examine how business models have developed and evolved. Patterns of success and failure in emerging markets, the changing nature of capital, and corporate governance are a few of the topics examined. Emphasis is placed on the lessons learned in the past that can provide insights into future success.

Cashman, Kevin, *Awakening the Leader Within: A Story of Transformation* (Hoboken, NJ: John Wiley & Sons, 2003). This is the story of Bensen Quinn, a fictitious CEO, who faces a number of challenges in his personal and professional life. As the story progresses, six essential leadership principles are presented. The author carefully places reflection boxes throughout the book to help readers examine their own lives. Readers are encouraged to consider the connection between their vision and their current behavior. This book challenges everyone to think about what can be gained if one commits to new habits and behaviors and what will be lost if they do not commit to change. You do not have to be a CEO to find meaning in this book. As the author notes "Regardless of your particular career role, you are the CEO of your life."

Chakravarthy, Bala, Guenter Mueller-Stewens, Peter Lorange, and Christoph Lechner (eds) *Strategy Process: Shaping the Contours of the Field* (Malden, MA: Blackwell Publishing, 2003). Although most believe there is a relationship between accomplishing a strategy and organizational success, there remains much unknown about the process whereby executives shape, execute, evaluate, and change strategies. The book is comprehensive and thought provoking. Contributors represent a diverse group of scholars in the field of strategic management.

Duncan, W. Jack, Peter M. Ginter, and Linda E. Swayne (eds) *Handbook of Health Care Management* (Cambridge, MA: Blackwell Publishers, 1997). The Handbook contains 15 chapters on highly relevant topics written by as many different experts in health care management and leadership. The book is organized into three major sections: the management of relationships (stakeholders, customers, alliances, and strategic management), key organizational processes (teams, leadership, change and innovation, organizational design, and motivation), and tools for managers to develop and maintain efficient and effective organizations (finance, economics, information systems, marketing, and quality). The invited authors make important contributions to our understanding of effective health care management.

Johnston, Robert and J. Douglas Bate, *The Power of Strategy Innovation: A New Way of Linking Creativity and Strategic Planning to Discover Great Business Opportunities* (New York: AMACOM, 2003). This book describes how creativity and the identification of visionary opportunities should be an integral part of all strategic thinking. Although more traditional strategic planning processes emphasize analytical analysis, Johnston and Bate advocate an innovative approach that relies on divergent–convergent iterations to generate ideas. The iterative process is called the discovery process and involves a series of stages – staging, aligning, exploring, creating, and mapping. The discovery process is shown to be particularly applicable to organizations in rapidly changing environments.

Lloyd, Donald J., *Healthcare 2010: A Journey to the Past* (Murfreesboro, TN: StarLight Press, 1999). Donald Lloyd begins in the year 2010 and looks back at the changes in health care delivery in the first decade of the twenty-first century. This innovative approach provides a fascinating "history" about the development of his vision for a better way to deliver health care. Lloyd suggests that over-regulation of providers, too much administrative bureaucracy, and widespread dissatisfaction of physicians, consumers, and legislators will lead to managed care's demise. Because managed care failed to live up to its promises to reduce cost, improve access, and enhance the quality of care, it will be replaced by a whole new system of delivery. The centerpiece of this system is a partnership between government and private enterprise and the result is a total reinvention of health care delivery.

Martin, Vivien, *Leading Change in Health and Social Care* (New York: Routledge Publishing, 2003). A practical guide for anyone in, or taking on, a leadership role at any level of health care or social service organizations. The emphasis of the book is on how to make change happen and the importance of the leader as an agent of change. A number of tools are presented that are designed to make change easier for those who must introduce it and those who must live with it. Perhaps most important, the book makes a number of suggestions on how change can be preserved as well as introduced.

Mintzberg, Henry, *The Rise and Fall of Strategic Planning* (New York: Free Press, 1994). In this classic work, Mintzberg makes a convincing argument that strategic planning has failed. Strategy cannot be planned because planning is about analysis and strategy is about synthesis. He argues that managers must preconceive the process by which strategies are created. Mintzberg suggests that informal learning and personal vision are the important elements of strategy formation. He exposes three fallacies of traditional strategic planning: discontinuities can be predicted; strategists can be detached from the operation; and the process can be formalized.

Wilson, Ian, *The Subtle Art of Strategy* (Westport, CT: Praeger Publishing, 2004). The author looks at examples of where strategic planning has failed and attempts to understand the reasons for the failures. Using examples and illustrations, Wilson reformulates strategic planning as a long-term, holistic art form. The book provides a different and interesting way of thinking about strategy and strategic management that is both practical and theoretically sound.

CHAPTER 2

Understanding and Analyzing the General Environment and the Health Care Environment

"When written in Chinese, the word 'crisis' is composed of two characters – one represents danger and one represents opportunity."

Anonymous

Introductory Incident

Tax Exempt Status for Hospitals Under Scrutiny

About 85 percent of the 5,000 hospitals in the United States are not-for-profit, but some of them are facing legal challenges to maintain their tax exempt status. State regulators in Illinois ruled that Provena Covenant Medical Center was no longer considered a charitable organization and thus lost its property tax exemption valued at $1.1 million annually.[1] Aggressive collection practices were cited. According to Provena, "the State of Illinois revoked the tax exemption for one of our hospitals. The State's decision was restricted to property taxes and that issue is under appeal."[2] The hospital has so far paid almost $2 million in property taxes for 2002 and 2003.

Against a tight economy and a deteriorating bottom line, hospitals across the country have been advised to increase their collections of bad debts. Many hospitals have hired collection agencies that are paid fees based on a percentage of the amount collected. The agencies are aggressive in their efforts, sometimes with intimidating phone calls and letters, but also with other tactics, such as threatening to report patients with Hispanic-sounding last names to the immigration authorities or the practice of "body attachment" that makes a patient with an unpaid balance subject to arrest for not appearing in court.[3]

Richard Scruggs, the attorney known for his class-action suits and billion dollar settlements against the tobacco industry, filed federal class-action lawsuits in June 2004 against 18 hospitals in 11 states on behalf of uninsured patients. He alleged that the hospitals did not deserve tax exempt status because of their aggressive collection practices and their lack of charity care as they overcharged uninsured patients. Scruggs considers the actions by the hospitals to be a "breach of contract" based on the agreement that the not-for-profits have with the government to receive tax exempt status in return for treating uninsured patients.[4]

At issue is the practice by many hospitals to charge uninsured patients full price whereas insured patients, especially those working for large employers, have a negotiated price that is significantly lower. In addition, government payors (Medicare and Medicaid) require the greatest discounts. Hence, the "full price" may be three or four times that charged to insured patients. As the economy declines, there are more uninsured. More and more small businesses are dropping health care insurance for employees; employees who still receive coverage for themselves are opting not to cover their families.

One of the hospitals being sued, Advocate Health Care in Chicago, defended its charity care noting that it has provided more than $1 billion in uncompensated and charity care in the past nine years. Under IRS regulations, to be declared not-for-profit, hospitals have to demonstrate that they "provide a community benefit."

The lawsuits claim that hospitals in Illinois, Minnesota, Ohio, Texas, Georgia, Alabama, Florida, and Tennessee used creative accounting practices to grossly distort the small amount of charity care they provide to uninsured patients. "Instead, the hospitals charge the uninsured 'sticker' prices for health care, an amount higher than any other patient group, and then, when the uninsured can't pay, harass the uninsured through, among other tactics, aggressive collection efforts such as garnishment of wages and bank accounts, seizures of homes, and personal bankruptcies," Scruggs said.[5]

Since June 2004, there have been 39 suits filed against 340 hospitals in 20 states. Trinity Health, operator of 12 hospitals in Michigan, is included. For the fiscal year ended June 30, 2003, Trinity Health reported net income of $110.9 million and an operating margin of 2.3 percent above average compared with other large Catholic health systems, according to Trinity. The system said it provided $438.4 million in community health care services in fiscal '03, including $224.5 million in unpaid cost of Medicare and $79.0 million in unpaid cost of Medicaid.[6]

Rep. Bill Thomas (R, California), chair of the House Ways and Means Committee, is planning hearings on federal tax exemptions for not-for-profit hospitals.

Notes

1. Philip Betbeze, "Aggressive Collections," *HealthLeaders*, July 1, 2004.
2. Thomas H. Hansen, Provena Health, Letter to Editor of *Time* Magazine, dated October 15, 2004. www.provenahealth.com/news.
3. Philip Betbeze, "Aggressive Collections."
4. *Wall Street Journal*, June 17, 2004.
5. Holbrook Mohr, "Nonprofit Hospitals Face Lawsuits," *Detroit Free Press*, June 18, 2004.
6. Kim Norris, "Charity Suits Name 2 Hospitals: Trinity, Beaumont Accused," *Detroit Free Press*, July 22, 2004.

Learning Objectives

After completing this chapter the student should be able to:

1. Appreciate the significance of the external environment's impact on health care organizations.

2. Understand and discuss the specific goals of environmental analysis.

3. Point out some limitations of environmental analysis.

4. Describe the various types of organizations in the general and health care environments and how they create issues that are of importance to other organizations.

5. Identify major general and industry environmental trends affecting health care organizations.

6. Identify key sources of environmental information.

7. Discuss important techniques used in analyzing the general and health care environments.

8. Conduct an analysis of the general and industry external environments for a health care organization.

9. Suggest several questions to initiate strategic thinking concerning the general and industry environments as a part of managing the strategic momentum.

The Importance of Environmental Influences

Fifty years ago the delivery of health care was a relatively uncomplicated relationship of facilities, physicians, and patients working together. Government and business stood weakly on the fringes, having little significant influence. Today, a multitude of interests are directly or indirectly involved in the delivery of health care. For instance, the for-profit provider segment has grown dramatically; private-sector businesses are largely responsible for the development and delivery of drugs and medical supplies; and government agencies regulate much of the actual delivery of health care services. As a result, in their quest for competitive advantage, organizations are pouring increasingly more money into collecting and organizing information about the world in which they operate.[1]

Ultimately, strategic thinking is directed toward positioning the organization most effectively within its changing external environment. Peter Drucker writes, "The most important task of an organization's leader is to anticipate crisis. Perhaps not to avert it, but to anticipate it. To wait until the crisis hits is already abdication. One has to make the organization capable of anticipating the storm, weathering it, and in fact, being ahead of it."[2] Therefore, to be successful, health care organization leaders must have an understanding of the external environment in which they operate; they must anticipate and respond to the significant shifts taking place within that environment. Strategic thinking, and the incorporation of that thinking into the strategic plans for the organization, is now more important than ever. Futurist Joel Barker has suggested that "in times of turbulence the ability to anticipate dramatically enhances your chances of success. Good anticipation is the result of good strategic exploration."[3] Organizations that fail to anticipate change, ignore the external forces, or resist change will find themselves out of touch with the needs of the market, especially because of antiquated technologies, ineffective delivery systems, and outmoded management. Institutions that anticipate and recognize the significant external forces and modify their strategies and operations accordingly will prosper.

The introduction of an early recognition system to identify external opportunities and threats is a major task for health care managers. This task has evolved because of the growing impact of economic factors, new technologies, increasing government influence, new centers of power, demographic shifts, changes in motivation for work, and changes in values and lifestyles, as well as changes in the kind and extent of competition. Therefore, strategic thinking must be directed toward "reading" the many shifts occurring in the external environment and determining which are important to the success of the organization. As discussed in the Introductory Incident, should hospitals be concerned about the shift taking place in tax exempt status?

One of the greatest challenges for health care organizations is identifying the changes that are most likely to occur and then planning for that future. Interviews with health care professionals and a review of the health care literature suggest that health care organizations will have to cope with change in some or all of the following areas: legislative/political, economic, social/demographic, technological, and competitive.[4]

Legislative/Political Changes

- More regulation of health plan activity is expected, including legislation to curb health plan abuse, disclosure rules, mandates for clinical protocols, and privacy of medical records.
- Incremental legislative reform can be assumed, rather than large-scale health or social programs; legislative efforts to reduce escalating health care costs.
- Health care will become the political "hot potato" that it was during the early 1990s because of medical inflation, pressure to control the cost of Medicare, and so on.

Economic Changes

- Moderate but consistent increases in the cost of health care are anticipated, accounting for 15 percent of the gross domestic product (GDP).
- Employers will become more unwilling to shoulder the entire burden of increasing costs for health care insurance and health care for their employees.

- Over 15 percent of Americans are without health insurance – a number that is predicted to be 48 million by 2009.
- Forced mobility of patients from one health care provider to another will increase because of changes in the health plan selected by employers.

Social/Demographic Changes

- An aging population and increased average life span will place capacity burdens on some health care organizations while a lessening of demand threatens the survival of others. By 2020, the US population over the age of 65 is expected to reach 53.7 million.
- The Hispanic population, many of whom do not speak English or speak it poorly, will continue to grow. Hispanics could become the largest minority child population as early as 2010. By 2050, one out of four Americans will be Hispanic.
- A more ethnically diverse and better-educated population will develop.
- An increase in income disparity is expected – a critical factor in determining health care delivery.
- "Tiered" access to health care is anticipated, with the division between the tiers becoming more extreme.
- There are predictions of critical shortages of nonphysician health care professionals and primary care physicians, yet a surplus of physicians within some specialties and in some geographic regions.

Technological Changes

- The high costs of purchasing new, sophisticated, largely computer-based technologies to meet the demand for high-quality health care will continue to rise.
- Significant advances in medical information technology are anticipated, such as automation of basic business processes, clinical information interfaces, data analysis, and telehealth.
- New technologies will emerge in the areas of drug design, imaging, minimally invasive surgery, genetic mapping and testing, gene therapy, vaccines, artificial blood, and xenotransplantation (transplantation of tissues and organs from animals into humans).

Competitive Changes

- Further consolidation will be seen within the health care industry because of cost pressures and intensified competition.
- The disintegration of some health care networks can be expected.
- Health care corporations will continue to expand into segments that have less regulation, and into businesses outside of the traditional health care industry.
- The importance of market niche strategies and services marketing will increase.
- Outpatient care and the development of innovative alternative health care delivery systems will continue to grow.
- The decreasing viability of many of the nation's small, rural, and public hospitals means there will be a reconfiguration of the rural health care delivery system.

- Increasing numbers of physician executives will have leadership roles in health care organizations.
- More emphasis will be on preventive care through wellness programs and healthy behavior.
- An increased emphasis will be placed on cost containment and measurement of outcomes of care (cost/benefit).
- A changing role for public health is expected, moving back to "core" activities (prevention, surveillance, disease control, assurance) and away from the delivery of primary care.
- A shortage of 800,000 nurses will occur by 2020.
- Pressure to reduce the costs of administration of health care will increase.

Major Industry Shifts

Such legislative/political, economic, social/demographic, technological, and competitive changes over the past three decades have shaped the health care industry and have contributed to the creation of a new language to describe it. Perspective 2–1 examines the growing list of health care acronyms and abbreviations that characterize the nature of industry change. Major industry shifts are perhaps most obvious in two related areas – the evolution of the financing of care and the restructuring of the industry's organizations.

Perspective 2–1
The Changing Language of Health Care

- AHC (academic health center) or AMC (academic medical center): a group of related institutions including a teaching hospital, a medical school and its affiliated faculty practice plan, as well as other health professional schools.
- CMS (Center for Medicare and Medicaid Services): part of the US Department of Health and Human Services, the contracting agency for health maintenance organizations (HMOs) that seek direct contractor/provider status for provision of Medicare and Medicaid benefits. (Formerly HCFA.)
- CON (certificate of need): laws in some states require a CON to determine whether the state will permit a hospital or a physician's practice to add beds, operating rooms, or expensive pieces of technology (see Perspective 2–4).
- DRG (diagnosis related group): a classification system using 383 major diagnostic categories that assign patients into case types. It is used to facilitate utilization review, analyze patient case mix, and determine hospital reimbursement. For example, the classification DRG 320 indicates a kidney and urinary tract infection.
- DSH (disproportionate share hospital): programs that provide for additional payments to hospitals that serve a large number of low-income inpatients.
- EMR (electronic medical record): A medical document stored in a machine-readable format. Data are entered into the record via many different sources, including computerized entry and various document imaging systems. Also called an electronic patient record.

▶

- EPO (exclusive provider organization): although structurally similar to a preferred provider organization (PPO) in that an EPO can simply be a network of health care providers, the plan beneficiaries cannot go out of the network or they must pay the entire cost of services. EPO physicians are reimbursed only for services actually provided to plan beneficiaries (rather than a capitated rate).
- FFS (fee for service): refers to a provider that charges the patient according to a fee schedule set for each service or procedure performed; the patient's total bill will vary by the number of services or procedures actually performed.
- HEDIS (healthplan employer data and information set): a set of standardized measures of health plan performance that allows comparisons of quality, access, satisfaction, membership, utilization, financial information, and management.
- HIPAA (Health Insurance Portability and Accountability Act): enacted in 1996, it includes five primary sections or "titles." Title 1: Health Care Access, Portability, and Renewability. Title 2: Preventing Health Care Fraud and Abuse; Administrative Simplification. Title 3: Tax-Related Health Provisions. Title 4: Application and Enforcement of Group Health Plan Requirement. Title 5: Revenue Offsets.
- HMO (health maintenance organization): an organization interposed between providers and payors that attempts to "manage the care" on behalf of the health service consumer and payor. HMOs are responsible for both the financing and delivery of comprehensive health services to an enrolled group of patients.
- IDS (integrated delivery system): IDSs combine and own, or closely coordinate, multiple stages of health care delivery. The integration usually includes many steps in the full spectrum of health services delivery, including physicians, hospitals, and long-term care facilities.
- IPA, IPO (independent practice association, independent practice organization): a legal entity composed of physicians who have organized for the purpose of negotiating contracts to provide medical services. Typically, physicians maintain their independent businesses but come together as a group to negotiate with payors. A super IPA has many IPAs rolled into one to contract with payors.
- JCAHO (Joint Commission on Accreditation of Healthcare Organizations): the major accrediting body for many health care organizations. Hospitals must be JCAHO accredited to receive Medicare and Medicaid funds; thus, the organization has great importance in the health care delivery system.
- LOS (length of stay): length of stay is also known as the average length of stay (ALOS) or the arithmetic mean of length of stay (AMLOS). It is the average number of days patients stay in the hospital for a specific DRG (diagnosis related group).
- MCO (managed care organization): any organization whose goal is to eliminate excessive and unnecessary service, thereby keeping health care costs manageable.
- MSO (management service organization): a legal corporation formed to provide practice management services to physicians. At one extreme, an MSO could own one practice or several hundred practices. At the other extreme, an MSO may not own any physician practices or provide management services. In that case, the MSO would be strictly an entity that signs managed care contracts for an affiliated provider group. Typically, an MSO will require a commitment of 10 to 40 years from the physician or group practice contracting for its services.
- NCQA (National Committee for Quality Assurance): a private, not-for-profit organization, NCQA is governed by a board of directors that includes employers, labor representatives, consumers, health plans, quality experts, policy makers, and representatives from organized medicine.
- NIH (National Institutes of Health): one of the agencies of the Public Health Service, which is a part of the Department of Health and Human Services of the US federal government. The NIH is responsible for medical and behavioral research for the United States.
- NP (nurse practitioner): a nurse who serves as the initial contact into the health care system and coordinates community-based services necessary for health promotion, health maintenance, rehabilitation,

or prevention of disease and disability. Nurse practitioners work interdependently with other health professionals to provide primary health care in many communities.

- OON (out of network): describes health care services received from providers who do not participate in a managed care program's contracted network of providers. Typically, patients pay all costs out of pocket (no reimbursement).
- OSHA (Occupational Safety and Health Act): a comprehensive plan for regulating workplace safety.
- PA (physician assistant): an allied health professional who, by virtue of having completed an educational program in the medical sciences and a structured clinical experience in surgical services, is qualified to assist the physician in patient care activities. Physician assistants may be involved with patients in any medical setting for which the physician is responsible, including the operating room, recovery room, intensive care unit, emergency department, hospital outpatient clinic, and the physician's office.
- PBM (pharmacy benefit management).
- PCP (primary care physician): a physician responsible for coordinating and managing the health care needs of members. PCPs may be trained in primary care, pediatrics, obstetrics/gynecology, internal medicine, or family medicine. They determine hospitalization and referral to specialists for their patients.
- PHO (physician–hospital organization): an organization designed to integrate a hospital and its medical staff to contract with payors as a single entity. Physicians retain their independence. A super PHO has many PHOs rolled into one to contract with payors.
- PMPM (per member per month): under capitation, the amount paid to care for each member per month, regardless of the number and extent of services used by the member.
- POS (point-of-service): combines a health maintenance organization insurance plan with traditional insurance. "Point-of-service" refers to members deciding whether to go in or out of the network. The employee belongs to a managed care plan but can opt for the traditional plan anytime. POS members usually pay less when they stay within the HMO network but can avoid restrictions. When they choose the traditional insurance plan, typical coverage requires them to meet a deductible and 70 to 80 percent of health care costs are paid. Sometimes POS is called an "HMO with an escape hatch."
- PPO (preferred provider organization): an entity through which various health plans or carriers contract to purchase health care services for patients from a selected group of providers, typically at a better per-patient cost.
- PPS (prospective payment system): a system designed to control costs for Medicare and Medicaid patients. Rather than reimbursing on a retrospective cost-plus system, PPS legislation in 1983 reimbursed hospitals on a prospective (predetermined) basis. For example, a hospital would know that it would receive a set amount to treat a broken hip. If the patient could be treated at a cost lower than the reimbursed amount, the hospital could keep the "profit." On the other hand, if the hospital spent more than the reimbursable amount, for whatever reason, it had to absorb the loss.
- PSO (provider-sponsored organization): integrated groups of doctors and hospitals that assume managed care (often Medicare) risk contracts.
- RBRVS (resource-based relative value scale): a national fee system for Medicare payments to physicians. The fee schedule is designed to shift payment patterns from a number of more costly specialties (such as those in surgery) to primary care.
- SNF (skilled nursing facility): an institution that provides inpatient skilled nursing care and rehabilitative services and has transfer agreements with one or more hospitals.
- TPA (third-party administrator): a firm that performs administrative functions such as claims processing and membership for a self-funded health care insurance plan or a start-up managed care plan.
- UR (utilization review): the review of services delivered by a health care provider to evaluate the appropriateness, necessity, and quality of the prescribed services.

Financing of Health Care and Managed Care

Because of health care cost escalation during the 1970s and 1980s, Medicare's prospective payment system (PPS) was implemented in 1983. As a result of PPS, the financing of health care delivery today is quite different than it was in the mid-1980s. PPS shifted national priorities from insisting on high-quality care regardless of cost to reducing or holding health care delivery costs in check. The health care system was characterized by cost shifting among patients, providers, physicians, payors, employers, and the government.[5] As a result, national health care expenditures have continued to increase, rising from $190 billion in 1978 to an estimated $2.2 trillion in 2008 and $3.1 trillion in 2012. Total health care spending as a percent of GDP leveled off at about 13.7 percent at the end of the 1990s but is expected to be 16.2 percent of GDP by 2008 and 17.7 percent in 2012. Another significant result of PPS has been a shift from inpatient to outpatient services, with outpatient visits increasing from 285 million in 1989 to over 500 million at the beginning of the 2000s.

The evolution of managed care systems, including PPOs and HMOs, is the most visible sign of the change in competition and the financing of health care. Although often referred to as health care providers, these organizations are actually interposed between providers and payors and attempt to "manage the care" on behalf of the health service consumer and payor. By the first decade of the twenty-first century, system emphasis was on consumer choice, reducing errors, and competition among health plans for patients.[6] As a result HMO market penetration varied dramatically throughout the United States, largely related to the level of competition. In 2004, HMO penetration varied from a low of under 3 percent in states such as Mississippi, North Dakota, Wyoming, and Alaska to over 40 percent in California, Connecticut, and Massachusetts. In addition, over 95 percent of all urban hospitals were affiliated with HMOs. Now more than 70 percent of major employers offer managed care plans and over 80 percent of inpatient care is covered by some fixed-price, managed care payment system.

As well as changing the financing of health care, managed care has fostered industry restructuring and the growth of integrated health systems. Yet, despite the profound effect that managed care had on how providers were organized and how health care was financed, by year 2000, it had only a modest effect on how health care organizations actually deliver medical care. The "revolution" in health care was related more to the "business" of health care than to its delivery.[7] As a result, in the first decade of the twenty-first century there has been a renewed interest in quality, reducing medical errors, and improving hospital practices.

Restructuring of the Industry's Organizations

Significant restructuring of the industry began in the early 1990s and continues today, though at a somewhat slower pace. The large number of failures of health care organizations, on the one hand, and the large numbers of mergers, acquisitions, alliances, and cooperatives, on the other, indicate the magnitude of the restructuring that has taken place. This volatility has given rise to many types of new organizational forms and strategies. As health services researchers have noted:

> Nowhere has this [change] been felt more than in the multitude of different organizations that make up the health care industry. Historical, regulatory, and geographic boundaries that traditionally divided the various sectors of the industry have toppled, creating new opportunities for organizations to expand outside their traditional domains.... Changing technology and population demographics have given rise to a multitude of organizational types providing niche services or products at various points along the continuum of care. Health care insurors and government payors have shifted more of the risk of health costs to providers and patients. This sharing and shirking of risk has spawned a plethora of new organizational forms as providers seek to gain greater coordination and control over cost and utilization.[8]

The peak of the merger and acquisition activity by hospital companies appears to have occurred in 1996 when 768 hospitals were involved in 235 separate merger or acquisition deals. Since 1996 there has been a steady decline in the level of hospital mergers or acquisitions but there are still significant numbers of hospitals involved in this type of activity. In 2003, 100 hospitals were involved in 68 mergers or acquisitions.

Consolidation is taking place in every segment of the health care industry, not just hospitals. Physician medical groups, long-term care, home health, HMOs, rehabilitation, psychiatric, and so on are involved. Even academic medical centers have not escaped restructuring. The academic medical center as an independent, not-for-profit institution of higher learning, research, and patient care may be a thing of the past. Accustomed to having the most difficult cases referred to them, academic medical centers that are not part of a managed care system find they are being left out as they deal with high-cost patients. Institutions that were either state supported or private-university affiliated are seeking alternatives to management and even ownership. They are reengineering themselves into lean, cost-efficient, less bureaucratic, more market-responsive organizations and are renegotiating relationships with the universities, state governments, medical schools, and others to attain greater flexibility and the ability to innovate.

Examples of organizations reading shifts in the external environment and being open to change include the development and growth of outpatient clinics specializing in various alternative medicine approaches such as chiropractic therapy, alternative wound care, nonsurgical cardiac care, and mind/body medicine. Changes in the health care delivery system, institutional support, and the public's attitudes are environmental shifts that have provided these opportunities in nontraditional medicine.[9] As discussed in Perspective 2–2, another, more recent, shift in the external environment to which health care organizations must successfully respond is terrorism and disaster preparedness.

Perspective 2-2

Health Care
Facility Disaster
Preparedness:
Planning for
Emerging Threats

At a time when many health care organizations are struggling to remain solvent, the specter of terrorism continues to shape the health care delivery system. Since the September 11, 2001 terror attacks, the anthrax mailings, and the increasing threat of infectious disease outbreaks from agents such as SARS and pandemic flu, the national agenda has focused on the ability of health care organizations to respond to emergencies, both terrorist related and naturally occurring. Increasingly, federal agencies such as the Health Resources and Services Administration and the Joint Commission on Accreditation of Healthcare Organizations identify emergency preparedness as a major initiative for hospital accreditation. However, planning and holding disaster preparedness exercises by hospitals and communities across the nation reveal that large gaps exist in the health care system, such that many institutions lack the capacity or the capability to respond to an incident that produces multiple victims. Additionally, emergency planning intensifies the financial burden already plaguing health care organizations. Recent evidence from nationally based disaster preparedness exercises indicates that disaster response mandates are insufficiently funded and hospitals must make up the difference in cost from operating revenues – while still maintaining the full array of patient services.

The challenges faced by health care institutions adapting to the current environment are manifold; however, all problem areas must be examined and solutions must be identified prior to an emergency situation. The failure to do so will severely hinder community response and may result in unnecessary casualties. Some of the fundamental issues that affect the preparedness level of any health care system are as follows:

- The health care delivery system is burdened with increased patient utilization and severe staff shortages as well as decreased medical and financial resources. Care must be taken by hospital planners to maximize response capability without taxing the already fragile situation.
- Hospitals will be the "first receivers" as patients exposed to bioterror or infectious disease agents seek care in hospital emergency departments as serious symptoms begin to emerge. Because emergency departments are already overcrowded and hospitals operate at capacity on a daily basis, a successful planning initiative must consider surge capacity, or a means to free up patient care areas and resources to care for large numbers of affected individuals.
- Even a small event with minimal casualties can overload the hospital response system. Therefore, plans should be regional in nature. Integration and coordination of the spectrum of response agencies in the community will enable the combination of existing resources to provide for the optimum outcome.
- Existing information technologies, such as those that facilitate data transfer, real-time situational analysis, diagnostics, and surveillance must be utilized to manage the flow of information before, during, and after an event to improve coordination, incident management, and response.
- Training must be ongoing. Hospital staff members must be familiar with the incident command structure of the facility and all the policies and procedures associated with emergency event response. An emergency plan must be constantly evaluated through exercises to identify strengths and weaknesses and to keep it current and realistic.

Source: Rachel D. Vásconez, MPH, University of Alabama at Birmingham, from Dan Hanfling, Klaus O. Schafer, and Carl W. Armstrong, "Making Healthcare Preparedness a Part of the Homeland Security Equation," *Topics in Emergency Medicine* 26, no. 2 (April–June 2004), pp. 128–143 and John L. Hick, Dan Hanfling, Jonathan L. Burstein, Craig DeAtley, Donna Barbisch, Gregory M. Bogdan, and Stephen Cantrill, "Health Care Facility and Community Strategies for Patient Care Surge Capacity," *Annals of Emergency Medicine* 44, no. 3 (2004), pp. 253–261.

Efficiency Versus Effectiveness

The key to strategic management and, indeed, to the organization's success is to "do the right thing" (*effectiveness*) and not just "do things right" (*efficiency*). Organizational effectiveness has an external orientation and suggests that the organization is well positioned to accomplish its mission and realize its vision and goals. Efficiency, on the other hand, has an internal orientation and suggests that economies will be realized in the use of capital, personnel, or physical plant. However, if an organization is doing the wrong thing, no amount of efficiency or good management will save it from decline. Health care organizations, of course, should strive to be both effective and efficient. With the continued pressure on health care organizations to reduce costs, a great deal of emphasis has been placed on efficiency; in fact, it may be critical to survival. However, effectiveness is primary; first we must understand what we *should* be doing.

Overall, efficiency and effectiveness must be balanced. Efficiency is established through the institution of routines directed toward achieving a high level of performance; however, routines are aimed at maintaining the status quo and preventing change. Sometimes highly structured "routines get us into ruts, dull our senses, stifle our creativity, constrict our thinking, remove us from stimulation, and destroy our ability to compete. Yet some routines are essential to a definable, consistent, measurable, and efficient operation."[10] Effectiveness, especially in a dynamic environment, requires learning and change. One of the costs of a learning organization may be lowered performance in the short run. The dynamics of the learning process hamper performance by discouraging the establishment of routine, whereas the demands of performance inhibit learning by institutionalizing routine.[11] Therefore, strategic managers must carefully balance efficiency, routines, and the requirements for performance with effectiveness, disorder, learning, and lowered short-term performance. Health care strategic managers must be careful not to allow routines and efforts directed toward efficiency to smother creativity, the organization's external orientation, or its ability to respond to change – its opportunity to be effective.

The External Nature of Strategic Management

Strategic thinking, strategic planning, and strategic momentum should be directed toward positioning the organization most effectively within its changing environment. Environmental analysis is a part of the situational analysis section of the strategic thinking map presented in Exhibit 1–3. The conclusions reached in environmental analysis will affect the directional strategies and internal analysis. *Environmental analysis* is largely strategic thinking and strategic planning and consists of understanding the issues in the external environment to determine the implications of those issues for the organization.

Environmental analysis requires externally oriented strategic managers. Strategic managers search for opportunities – ways to radically alter the status quo, create something totally new, or revolutionize processes. They search for opportunities to do what has never been done previously or to do known things in a new way. The fundamental nature of strategic management requires the awareness and understanding of outside forces. Strategic managers encourage adoption of new ideas in the system, maintain receptivity to new ways, and expose themselves to broad views. Strategic managers, through environmental analysis, can remove the protective covering in which organizations often seal themselves.[12] Effective environmental analysis occurs through strategic thinking. This chapter concerns methods to assess the general environment and the health care environment and Chapter 3 focuses on analysis methods to evaluate the service area and competitors within it.

Determining the Need for Environmental Analysis

Based on extensive experience in business, A. H. Mesch developed a series of questions to determine if an organization needs environmental analysis. The questions include:

1. Does the external environment influence capital allocation and decision-making processes?
2. Have previous strategic plans been scrapped because of unexpected changes in the environment?
3. Has there been an unpleasant surprise in the external environment?
4. Is competition growing in the industry?
5. Is the organization or industry becoming more marketing oriented?
6. Do more and different kinds of external forces seem to be influencing decisions, and does there seem to be more interplay between them?
7. Is management unhappy with past forecasting and planning efforts?[13]

These questions concern the general and health care industry environments as well as the service area. Answering "yes" to any of the questions suggests that management should consider some form of environmental analysis. Answering "yes" to five or more of the questions indicates that environmental analysis is imperative. In today's dynamic environment, most health care managers would probably answer "yes" to more than one of these questions and should therefore be performing environmental analysis – assessing trends, events, and issues in the general environment, the health care industry environment, and the service area.

External environmental analysis attempts to identify, aggregate, and interpret environmental issues as well as provide information for the analysis of the internal environment and the development of the directional strategies. Therefore, environmental analysis seeks to eliminate many of the surprises in the external environment. Organizations cannot afford to be surprised. As one writer has pointed out, "to the blind all things are sudden." However, while certain repetitive patterns, such as seasons, may be predictable, the forecasting of discontinuities, such as technological innovation or price increases, is virtually impossible.[14] Yet, strategic managers who practice environmental analysis are so "close" to the environment that by the time change becomes apparent to others, they have already detected the signals of change and have explored the significance of the changes. These managers are often called visionaries; however, vision is often the result of their *strategic awareness* – thoughtful detection and interpretation of subtle signals of change. Such strategic managers are able to eliminate "predictable surprises" for the organization – surprises that shouldn't have been. These mangers are able to avoid disasters by recognizing the threat, making it a priority in the organization, and mobilizing the resources required to address it.[15]

The lack of forecasting and planning success sometimes is the result of directing processes internally toward efficiency rather than externally toward effectiveness. Such planning systems have not considered the growing number and diversity of environmental influences. Early identification of external changes through environmental analysis will greatly enhance the planning efforts in health care organizations. For example, as it became clear that health care reform was moving toward some form of managed care or managed competition (in the health care industry environment and service area), many physician group practices and solo practitioners joined together to create large physician-driven health care organizations that could compete for prepaid health care contracts. These physicians viewed such organizations as a way to evolve competitively to ensure their survival.

The Goals of Environmental Analysis

Although the overall intent of environmental analysis is to position the organization within its environment, more specific goals may be identified. The specific goals of environmental analysis are:

1. to classify and order issues and changes generated by outside organizations;
2. to identify and analyze current important issues and changes that will affect the organization;
3. to detect and analyze the weak signals of emerging issues and changes that will affect the organization;
4. to speculate on the likely future issues and changes that will have significant impact on the organization;
5. to provide organized information for the development of the organization's internal analysis, mission, vision, values, goals, and strategy; and
6. to foster strategic thinking throughout the organization.

There is an abundance of data in the external environment. For it to be meaningful, managers must identify the sources as well as aggregate and classify the data into information. Once classified, important issues that will affect the organization may be identified and evaluated. This process encourages managers to view environmental changes as external issues that may affect the organization.

In addition to the identification of current issues, environmental analysis attempts to detect weak signals within the external environment that may portend a future issue. Sometimes based on little hard data, managers attempt to identify patterns that suggest emerging issues that will be significant for the organization. Such issues, if they continue or actually do occur, may represent significant challenges. Early identification aids in developing strategy.

Strategic managers must go beyond what is known and speculate on the nature of the industry, as well as the organization, in the future. This process often stimulates creative thinking concerning the organization's present and future products and services. Such speculation is valuable in the formulation of a guiding vision and the development of mission and strategy. The bulleted list of external trends and issues at the beginning of this chapter provides some of the emerging and speculative trends and issues that strategic managers will begin to incorporate into their thinking today.

When strategic managers – top managers, middle managers, and front-line supervisors – throughout the organization are considering the relationship of the organization to its environment, innovation and a high level of service are likely. Strategic thinking within an organization fosters adaptability, and those organizations that adapt best will ultimately displace the rest.

The Limitations of Environmental Analysis

Environmental analysis is important for understanding the external environment, but it provides no guarantees for success. The process has some practical limitations that the organization must recognize. These limitations include the following:

- Environmental analysis cannot foretell the future.
- Managers cannot see everything.
- Sometimes pertinent and timely information is difficult or impossible to obtain.
- There may be delays between the occurrence of external events and management's ability to interpret them.
- Sometimes there is a general inability on the part of the organization to respond quickly enough to take advantage of the issue detected.
- Managers' strongly held beliefs sometimes inhibit them from detecting issues or interpreting them rationally.[16]

Even the most comprehensive and well-organized environmental analysis processes will not detect all of the changes taking place. Sometimes events occur that are significant to the organization but were preceded by few, if any, signals. Or the signals may be too weak to be discerned.

Perhaps the greatest limiting factor in external environmental analysis is the preconceived beliefs of management. In many cases, what leaders already believe about the industry, important competitive factors, or social issues inhibits their ability to perceive or accept signals for change. Because of managers' beliefs, signals that do not conform to what he or she believes may be ignored. What an individual actually perceives is dramatically determined by paradigms (ways of thinking and beliefs). And any data that exist in the real world that do not fit the paradigm will have a difficult time permeating the individual's filters. He or she will simply not see it.[17] As creativity expert Edward De Bono explains, "We are unable to make full use of the information and experience that is already available to us and is locked up in old structures, old patterns, old concepts, and old perceptions."[18] Despite long and loud signals for change, in some cases organizations do not change until "the gun is at their heads," and then it is often too late.

The External Environment

Organizations and individuals create change. Therefore, if health care managers are to become aware of the changes taking place outside of their own organization, they must have an understanding of the types of organizations that are creating change and the nature of the change. Exhibit 2–1 illustrates the concept of

Exhibit 2–1: The External Environment of a Health Care Organization

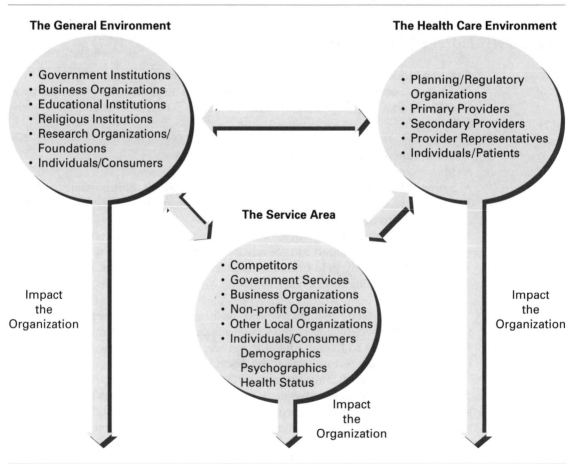

The General Environment

- Government Institutions
- Business Organizations
- Educational Institutions
- Religious Institutions
- Research Organizations/ Foundations
- Individuals/Consumers

The Health Care Environment

- Planning/Regulatory Organizations
- Primary Providers
- Secondary Providers
- Provider Representatives
- Individuals/Patients

The Service Area

- Competitors
- Government Services
- Business Organizations
- Non-profit Organizations
- Other Local Organizations
- Individuals/Consumers
  Demographics
  Psychographics
  Health Status

Impact the Organization

Impact the Organization

Impact the Organization

the external environment for health care organizations. In this chapter we will explore the types of changes initiated in the general environment and the health care industry environment.

Components of the General Environment

All types of organizations and independent individuals generate important issues – and subsequently change – within the general environment. For example, a research firm that is developing imaging may introduce a new technology that could be used by a variety of other organizations in very diverse industries such as hospitals (magnetic resonance imaging) and manufacturing (robotics). The members of the *general environment* may be broadly classified in a variety of ways depending on the strategic management needs of the organization analyzing the environment. These groups of organizations and individuals make up the broad context of the general environment:

1. Government institutions,
2. Business organizations,
3. Educational institutions,
4. Religious institutions,
5. Research organizations and foundations, and
6. Individuals and consumers.

Organizations and individuals in the general environment, acting alone or in concert with others, initiate and foster the "macroenvironmental" changes within society. These organizations and individuals generate technological, social, regulatory, political, economic, and competitive change that will, in the long run, affect many different industries (including health care) and may even directly affect individual organizations. Therefore, external organizations engaged in their own processes and pursuing their own missions and goals will affect other industries, organizations, and individuals.

In the general environment, changes usually affect a number of different sectors of the economy (industry environments). For example, passage of the prescription drug bill during the George W. Bush presidency affected a variety of organizations as well as individuals. Similarly, the early health care reform initiatives of the Clinton administration would have affected virtually all institutions in the general environment, not just health care organizations. Market forces, not politicians, speeded much of health care change during the 1990s, although two pieces of legislation were passed from the Clinton health care reform efforts – HIPAA and CHIP.

The Health Insurance Portability and Accountability Act (HIPAA) of 1996 was passed to protect those who already had health insurance from losing it if they changed jobs, create a pilot program for medical savings accounts, increase the deductibility of health insurance for the self-employed, and provide tax breaks to increase the use of long-term care insurance.[19] Compliance was legislated for

February 2000; however, by 2004 there were still issues to be resolved regarding security and privacy of patient medical information as it became standardized and electronically available. The final rule adopting HIPAA standards for the security of electronic protected health information was not published in the Federal Register until February 20, 2003.[20]

The Balanced Budget Act of 1997 incorporated the Children's Health Insurance Program (CHIP) to provide insurance coverage for low-income children who did not qualify for Medicaid. Many of the 10 million children who have no health insurance are from working families with incomes too high to qualify for Medicaid but too low for them to afford private health insurance. CHIP is a jointly funded federal/state program that gives the states three options: states can expand their Medicaid program to cover these children, create a separate program, or employ a combination of the two. Fifteen states and the District of Columbia have expanded their Medicaid programs, 16 states created separate state programs, and the remaining 19 states developed combination programs.[21]

Government organizations that foster changes in the general regulatory climate or businesses that develop breakthroughs in computer technology contribute to environmental changes that, although perhaps not specifically related to health care, may have a significant and long-lasting impact on the delivery of health care. For instance, although initially developed in the business sector, innovations in computer systems and information processing technologies have significantly affected the delivery of health care – e-health.

The organization itself may be affected directly by the technological, social, regulatory, political, economic, and competitive change initiated and fostered by organizations in the general environment. In the aggregate, these alterations represent the general direction of societal change that may affect the success or failure of any organization. Therefore, an organization engaging in strategic management must try to sort out the fundamental changes being generated in the external environment and detect the major shifts taking place. A shift in consumer attitudes and expectations about health care is an example of a societal change that may affect the success or failure of health care organizations. Demographic changes are somewhat more predictable and the growing number of seniors in the US population will impact every aspect of the macroenvironment as well as the health care environment.

Typically, as information is accumulated and evaluated by the organization, it will be summarized as environmental issues affecting the industry or organization. The identification and evaluation of the issues in the general environment are important because the issues will accelerate or retard changes taking place within the industry yet may affect the organization directly as well.

Components of the Health Care Environment

Organizations and individuals within the *health care environment* develop and employ new technologies, deal with changing social issues, address political change, develop and comply with regulations, compete with other health care organizations, and participate in the health care economy. Therefore, strategic managers should view the health care environment with the intent of understanding the nature of all these issues and changes. Focusing attention on all the major change areas facilitates the early identification and analysis of industry-specific environmental issues and trends that will affect the organization. The environmental analysis techniques and methods presented in this chapter help pinpoint important general and industry issues. However, in today's environment a more focused service area competitor analysis is typically required as well (see Chapter 3).

The wide variety of health care organizations makes categorization difficult. However, the health care system may be generally grouped into five segments:

1. Organizations that regulate primary and secondary providers;
2. Organizations that provide health services (primary providers);
3. Organizations that provide resources for the health care system (secondary providers);
4. Organizations that represent the primary and secondary providers; and
5. Individuals involved in health care and patients (consumers of health care services).[22]

Exhibit 2–2 lists the types of organizations and individuals within each segment and provides examples. The categories of health care organizations listed under each of the health care segments are not meant to be all-inclusive, but rather to provide a starting point for understanding the wide diversity and complexity of the industry.

Exhibit 2–2: Organizations in the Health Care Environment

Organizations that Regulate Primary and Secondary Providers
- Federal regulating agencies
  Department of Health and Human Services (DHHS)
  Center for Medicare and Medicaid Services (CMS)
- State regulating agencies
  Public Health Department
  State Health Planning Agency (e.g., certificate of need [CON])
- Voluntary regulating groups
  Joint Commission on Accreditation of Healthcare Organizations (JCAHO)
- Other accrediting agencies (CAHME, CEPH)

Primary Providers (Organizations that Provide Health Services)
- Hospitals
  Voluntary (e.g., Barnes/Jewish/Christian Health System)
  Governmental (e.g., Veteran's Administration Hospitals)
  Investor-owned (e.g., HCA–The Healthcare Company, Tenet)
- State public health departments
- Long-term-care facilities
- Skilled nursing facilities (e.g., Beverly Enterprises, Mariner Post-Acute Network, ManorCare)

Exhibit 2–2: (cont'd)

- Intermediate care facilities
- HMOs and IPAs (e.g., Care America, Aetna Health Care, United Healthcare)
- Ambulatory care institutions (e.g., Ambulatory Care Centers, Ranchos Los Amigos Rehabilitation Center)
- Hospices (e.g., Hospice Care, Inc., Porter Hospice, Grace House of Minneapolis)
- Physicians' offices
- Home health care institutions (e.g., CareGivers Home Health, Arcadia Home Health Care, Visiting Nurses Association [VNA], Interim Home Care)

Secondary Providers (Organizations that Provide Resources)
- Educational institutions
  Medical schools (e.g., Johns Hopkins, University of Alabama at Birmingham [UAB])
  Schools of public health (e.g., The University of North Carolina at Chapel Hill, Harvard)
  Schools of nursing (Presbyterian School of Nursing)
  Health administration programs (University of Washington, The Ohio State University)
- Organizations that pay for care (third-party payors)
  Government (e.g., Medicaid, Medicare)
  Insurance companies (e.g., Prudential, Metropolitan)
  Businesses (e.g., Microsoft, Ford Motor Company)
  Social organizations (e.g., Shriners, Rotary Clubs)
- Pharmaceutical and medical supply companies
  Drug distributors (e.g., Bergen Brunswig, Walgreen, McKesson)
  Drug and research companies (e.g., Bristol Myers Squibb, Merck, Pfizer, Hoffman-LaRoche, Eli Lilly, Upjohn, Warner Lambert)
  Medical products companies (e.g., Johnson & Johnson, Baxter International, Abbott Labs, Bausch & Lomb)

Organizations that Represent Primary and Secondary Providers
- American Medical Association (AMA)
- American Hospital Association (AHA)
- State associations (e.g., Illinois Hospital Association, New York Medical Society)
- Professional associations (e.g., Pharmaceutical Manufacturers Association [PMA], American College of Healthcare Executives [ACHE], American College of Physician Executives [ACPE], Medical Group Management Association [MGMA])

Individuals and Patients (Consumers)
- Independent physicians
- Nurses
- Nonphysician professionals
- Nonprofessionals
- Patients and consumer groups

Source: Adapted from Beaufort B. Longest, Jr., *Management Practices for the Health Professional*, 4th edn (Norwalk, CT: Appleton & Lange 1990).

ORGANIZATIONS THAT REGULATE

A number of organizations regulate primary and secondary health care providers. These organizations may be generally categorized into four groups: federal regulating agencies, state regulating agencies, voluntary regulating groups, and accrediting groups.

Federal involvement in the regulation of the health care industry has increased in the past 30 years. The passage of legislation to begin and supervise the Medicare and Medicaid programs in the mid-1960s and the 1974 enactment of the National Health Planning and Resource Development Act dramatically increased the federal government's participation in the regulation of health care.[23] Important federal health care regulating organizations include the Department of Health and Human Services (DHHS) and the Center for Medicaid and Medicare Services (CMS), formerly known as the Health Care Financing Administration (HCFA). Federal legislation can have a profound long-term impact on the health care industry, such as did the Medicare Prescription Drug Improvement and Modernization Act discussed in Perspective 2–3.

In a similar manner, state governments have become concerned about the provision of health care and have created a variety of organizations and agencies to regulate health care within the states. For example, many states enacted certificate of need (CON) legislation in order to regulate provider growth and viability (see Perspective 2–4). Similarly, state Medicaid agencies have attempted to ensure health care access to the poor.

In addition to federal and state government regulating agencies, there are a number of voluntary regulatory groups such as the American Association of Blood Banks (AABB) and accrediting agencies such as the Joint Commission on Accreditation of Healthcare Organizations (JCAHO). In addition, a number of separate discipline accrediting agencies such as the American Dietetic Association, the National League of Nursing, and the Commission on Accreditation of the American Dental Association provide regulation. With a growing emphasis on quality, the role of these types of organizations likely will expand in the future.

PRIMARY PROVIDERS

There are a number of ways to classify the wide and diverse range of *primary providers* – those that "touch" the patient and the most visible component of the health care system. (Note: primary and secondary providers should not be confused with primary, secondary, and tertiary levels of hospital care.) Exhibit 2–2 suggests one approach that has nine, sometimes overlapping, groups: hospitals; state public health departments; long-term care facilities; intermediate care facilities; HMOs, PPOs, and IPAs; ambulatory care institutions; hospices; physicians' offices; and home health care institutions. These types of organizations make up the delivery portion of the health care industry.

In the past, hospitals have been the dominant segment, but as the industry becomes more specialized and fragments further, other primary providers have grown in importance. In 2002, hospitals accounted for 31 percent of personal health

Perspective 2–3

Really, What Is the Effect of Specialty Hospitals?

When President Bush signed the Medicare Prescription Drug Improvement and Modernization Act, he signed off on changes to the Stark II law as well. A temporary (18 month) ban on physician investment in new specialty hospitals when the investing doctors referred patients to the facility was put into effect and then extended to January 1, 2007. The law grandfathered specialty hospitals already in existence and under development. At the same time the ban provided some breathing room for acute care hospitals facing competition from specialty hospitals.

Some find this political action puzzling. Although the number of specialty hospitals in the United States has tripled since 1990, the total number of cardiac, orthopedic, surgical, and women's hospitals represents only 2 percent of the total number of acute care hospitals nationwide. Apparently, the concern is really over physician investment. Of the 100 specialty hospitals in existence or under development, 70 percent have physician owners.

Many health care observers agree that there is no overwhelming evidence to suggest that physician ownership has a negative impact on Medicare and Medicaid programs. Before the Stark law was enacted, studies were carried out to analyze the effects of physicians having financial relationships with clinical laboratories and other designated health services. These studies found that when physicians had financial relationships with laboratories they ordered significantly more laboratory services than did physicians without a financial interest. Congress admits that it has not sufficiently studied or collected data on the issue.

Advocates for specialty hospitals argue that physician investment actually improves quality by giving doctors control over treatment and provides tangible incentives to improve the quality of care. Opponents argue that physician-owned specialty hospitals will adversely affect the viability of acute care hospitals because they siphon off more lucrative specialty care patients. To date, however, data do not exist to resolve the controversy. Specialty hospitals are viewed by opponents as patient prospectors who skim off the best-insured patients in areas with the most generously reimbursed procedures. Moreover, these "boutique" hospitals tend to be for-profit entities and are jointly owned by doctors. Advocates say that specialty hospitals are being unfairly targeted, claiming that physicians are merely responding to market forces and delivering services more efficiently than general acute care hospitals.

Although the ban on specialty hospitals does not apply to existing hospitals and those under development, the changes to the Stark law do affect them. For example, existing specialty hospitals are prohibited from increasing the number of physician investors. Questions such as "What happens when a physician investor retires or dies?" remain unanswered.

Source: Christopher J. Gearon, "A Different Nice?" *Hospital & Health Networks* 78, no. 2 (2004), pp. 16–18 and Sarah Swartzmeyer and Carrie Norbin Killoran, "Specialty Hospital Ban Was Premature, Studies Would Have Shown Whether Those Facilities Help or Harm Healthcare," *Modern Healthcare* 34, no. 21 (January 21, 2004), pp. 21–23.

care expenditures compared with 36.8 percent in 2000, 39.5 percent in 1995, and 41.7 percent in 1990.[24] Managed-care organizations have already had a significant influence in the 1990s but may have reached maturity. Total enrollment in HMOs dropped after 27 years of growth (since InterStudy began collecting data in 1973). On January 1, 1999 there were 81.3 million Americans enrolled in HMOs; on January 1, 2000 the number had dropped to 80.9 million.[25]

A certificate of need (CON) is a process that begins with a state body surveying the health care needs of its population and using that information to determine whether a hospital or physician's practice will be given permission to add beds, operating rooms, or expensive pieces of technology. In 2005, 36 states and the District of Columbia had some form of CON review; three of the states limited the review to long-term care.

CON statutes came into existence during the 1960s. A federal law enacted in 1974 provided grant funding for states to operate CON programs, effectively expanding the number of states that used CON. CON laws were aggressively adopted by states in an effort to encourage consolidation of small (and presumably inefficient) hospitals and reduce expensive duplication of medical services. At its peak, all states except for Louisiana had a CON program. Under President Ronald Reagan, federal officials began to cut funding for state CON programs in 1981 and by the end of the 1980s federal funding ended. Fourteen states have repealed CON laws and others have lessened the impact by restricting CON to long-term care.

Hospitals generally are in favor of CON laws because they believe that without them, medical specialists and for-profit organizations supported by Wall Street investors would build outpatient centers and specialty hospitals to effectively skim the paying patients. Community hospitals would struggle to keep open some services such as emergency rooms and labor and delivery rooms because of the loss of paying patients.

Proponents of the CON process argue that it is a way to control health care costs. In addition, they believe that because health care is "different," increased competition will not lead to reduced costs. Opponents of CON believe that it favors hospitals (which they believe is unfair and illegal), stifles new business and innovation, and, because the health care market is changing, CONs are no longer needed. The arguments against CON persuaded the state of Ohio to deregulate its CON program for same-day surgery centers. Within one year there were 103 new centers built. Opponents are concerned that so much proliferation will dilute the quality of medical care. They worry that by spreading procedures across many providers, none will have the critical mass necessary to develop and maintain expertise, thereby diminishing the quality of health care.

Critics argue that the state-appointed council that determines the "need" is subject to industry politics, especially because many of the large hospitals have a representative on the council. This enables the large hospital to limit competition.

Michael Morrisey, Lister Hill Center for Health Policy at University of Alabama Birmingham, stated that "in a standard economic model, CON would be viewed as a barrier to entry and by artificially restricting the supply of a health care service, current providers would be able to charge higher prices, and be less motivated to innovate." In addition, they would likely devote resources to maintaining their "franchise" through a restrictive CON. He noted that proponents of CON argue that health care is not price competitive and that regulation of supply is necessary to control costs. His review of the research that has been done finds that CON has not resulted in lower hospital costs. In fact, he found that hospitals in states with CON had costs that were 20.6 percent higher.

Because each state determines its own CON statutes, the variations are significant, making it very difficult to assess whether CON has contributed to higher costs. There is some agreement that CON has limited the number of beds; some researchers have found that the restricted supply led to higher costs per day and per admission and higher hospital profits.

There has been no definitive research to settle the argument. Thus, each side continues to provide "evidence" for the benefits and limitations of CON.

Source: Michael A. Morrisey, "State Health Care Reform: Protecting the Provider," in R. Feldman (ed.) *American Health Care: Government, Markets and the Public Interest* (Oakland, CA: Independent Institute, 2000), pp. 229–266 and Christopher J. Conover and Frank A. Sloan, "Does Removing Certificate-of-Need Regulations Lead to a Surge in Health Care Spending?" *Journal of Health Politics, Policy and Law* 23, no. 3 (June 1998), pp. 455–481.

SECONDARY PROVIDERS

Essentially composed of support organizations for primary providers, the *secondary provider* component includes educational institutions, organizations that pay for health care, and pharmaceutical and medical equipment and supply companies. Educational institutions, through their medical schools, nursing schools, schools of public health, and allied health care programs, educate a variety of health care personnel. Organizations that pay for care (third-party payors) include the government (principally through Medicare and Medicaid), commercial insurance companies, and employers. The pharmaceutical and medical equipment and supply organizations make up a particularly important segment supporting the research and material needs of primary providers. These organizations include drug distributors, drug production and research companies, and medical products companies.

REPRESENTATION OF THE PRIMARY AND SECONDARY PROVIDERS

The various providers of health care are typically represented by associations created for the purpose of fostering the disciplines and representing the interests of their constituencies. Examples include national associations such as the American Medical Association, the American Hospital Association, the Pharmaceutical Manufacturers Association, and so on. In addition, there are a variety of state and local health care associations.

INDIVIDUALS AND PATIENTS

The final segment of the health care industry includes individuals working within the industry (either independently or in health care organizations), patients, and consumer groups. Individuals working within the industry create the culture of the industry and are the source of many issues. Patients are the reason that health care organizations exist. In the past this group was treated as a mere component of the health care system; in today's competitive environment the needs and wants of the users of health services are driving the system. Patients create important issues for health care managers. In addition, groups of consumers such as the American Association of Retired Persons (AARP) and the American Cancer Society make their voices heard about health care issues. As indicated in the discussion of the general environment, the US population is aging and these mature consumers are profoundly affecting the delivery of health care (see Perspective 2–5).

The Process of Environmental Analysis

There are a variety of approaches to conducting an environmental analysis. Regardless of the approach, four fundamental processes are common to environmental analysis efforts (see Exhibit 2–3): (1) *scanning* to identify signals of

Perspective 2–5

What Influences
the Mature
Consumer?

The 2000 census counted more than 60 million people 55 years of age and older; the number is expected to double in size and constitute 33 percent of the US population by 2030. Not only are older consumers increasing in absolute and relative terms, they account for a disproportionately larger share of health care spending.

The older population is a prime customer for health care because:

- Nearly every hospital and physician provides services for the elderly under Medicare;
- The elderly are predictable in their utilization and reimbursement for most hospital and physician services;
- Discretionary income is available for additional services;
- The elderly customer is loyal to both physician and hospital;
- Price insensitivity exists for health care;
- The older consumers have the time and opportunity to use health services;
- An average of four chronic health conditions per elderly person require ongoing care;
- Older consumers have high personal interest in their own health.

Not all seniors are alike however. The Center for Mature Consumer Studies at Georgia State University found that seniors are clustered into four distinct groups: (1) Healthy Hermits – seniors who are in relatively good health yet are somewhat withdrawn socially (20 million); (2) Ailing Outgoers – seniors who are in relatively poor health yet determined to remain socially active (18 million); (3) Frail Recluses – inactive individuals with health problems (18 million); and (4) Healthy Indulgers – relatively wealthy and healthy and focused on making the most of life (7 million). Depending on the cluster, elderly consumers will make health care choices differently. For example, Ailing Outgoers are more influenced by low fees/prices charged by hospitals, more likely to consider senior discounts and engage in special deals through group or membership programs, and prefer ads that have people of similar age. On the other hand, Healthy Indulgers prefer to be able to receive a variety of health services in one place and want staff to willingly explain various health services. In addition, they are more likely to seek personal referrals in choosing a hospital – from people their own age. Frail Recluses value convenience.

The growing elderly market offers significant opportunities to those who understand its different segments and offer services that fit the different clusters.

Source: George F. Moschis, Danny N. Bellenger, and Carolyn Folkman Curasi, "Before Targeting the Elderly Market, Find Out How They Make Choices," *Marketing Health Services* 23, no. 4 (Winter 2003), pp. 16–21.

environmental change, (2) *monitoring* identified issues, (3) *forecasting* the future direction of the issues, and (4) *assessing* the organizational implications of the issues.[26]

Scanning the External Environment

As suggested earlier in this chapter, the external environment is composed of a number of organizations and individuals in the general and health care environments. Some of the organizations and individuals in the external environment have little direct involvement with the health care industry while others are directly

Exhibit 2–3: Strategic Thinking Map of the Environmental Analysis Process

Scanning

- View external environmental information
- Organize information into desired categories
- Identify issues within each category

Monitoring

- Specify the sources of data (organizations, individuals, or publications)
- Add to the environmental database
- Confirm or disprove issues (trends, developments, dilemmas, and possibility of events)
- Determine the rate of change within issues

Forecasting

- Extend the trends, developments, dilemmas, or occurrence of an event
- Identify the interrelationships between issues and between environmental categories
- Develop alternative projections

Assessing

- Evaluate the significance of the extended (forecasted) issues to the organization
- Identify the forces that must be considered in the formulation of the vision, mission, internal analysis, and strategic plan

involved. The distinction is not always clear. These organizations and individuals, through their normal operations and activities, are generating changes that may be important to the future of other organizations. Changes in the general environment are always "breaking through" to the health care environment, as when laser technology was developed outside of the health care industry and was quickly adopted within the industry. This phenomenon sometimes is referred to as "environmental slip".

The environmental scanning process acts as a "window" to these organizations. Thus, these general environment strategic issues may shape the entire health care industry or have a direct impact on any one health care organization. Through this window, managers engaged in environmental scanning carry out three functions. They:

1. view external environmental data;
2. organize external information into several desired categories; and
3. identify issues within each category.

Thus, *strategic issues* are trends, developments, dilemmas, and possible events that affect an organization as a whole and its position within its environment. Strategic issues are often ill-structured and ambiguous and require an interpretation effort (forecasting and assessment).[27]

The scanning function, conceptualized in Exhibit 2–4, serves as the organization's "window" or "lens" on the external world. The scanning function is a process of moving the lens across the array of external organizations in search of current and emerging patterns or issues. Using the lens, the viewer can focus on diverse and unorganized data generated by external organizations and individuals, and compile and organize it into meaningful categories. Thus, issues generated in the external environment are organized through the scanning process. Prior to this interpretation process, change is diverse, unorganized, sporadic, mixed, and undefined. The scanning process categorizes, organizes, accumulates, and, to some extent, evaluates issues. This organized information is then used in the monitoring function.

INFORMATION CATEGORIES

To monitor and further analyze issues, they must be organized into logical categories. Categories not only aid in tracking but also facilitate the subsequent assessment of the issues' impact on the organization. The categories most used to classify issues are technological, social, political, regulatory, economic, and competitive. Issues, of course, are not inherently technological, social, and so on. However, using this approach helps managers to understand the nature of the issues and to evaluate their impact. In addition, such classification helps aggregate information and organize it for the identification of important issues that may affect the organization. Through the aggregation and organization process, patterns may be identified and evidence accumulated to support an issue.

INFORMATION SOURCES

There are a variety of sources for environmental information. Although organizations create change, they themselves are often difficult to monitor directly. However, various secondary sources (published information) are readily available to most investigators, allowing them to monitor other organizations. Essentially, people and publications both outside and inside the organization serve as the lens to the external world. These sources are outlined in Exhibit 2–5.

Typically, within the organization, there are a variety of experts who are familiar with issues created outside the organization and who may be the best sources

Exhibit 2–4: The Concept of Scanning the External Environment

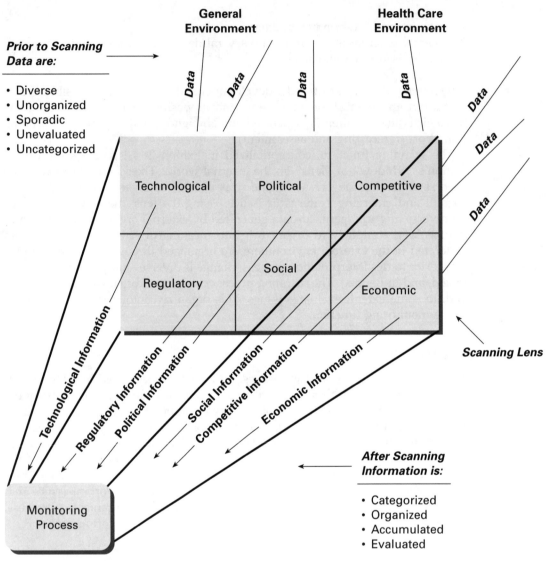

Scanning As the Organization's Lens

The scanning process allows the organization to focus on technological, political, competitive, regulatory, social and economic issues, trends, dilemmas, and events important to the organization. The "viewing process" must sort diverse, unorganized data. This process also filters out data not relevant to the mission of the organization.

Exhibit 2–5: Information Sources

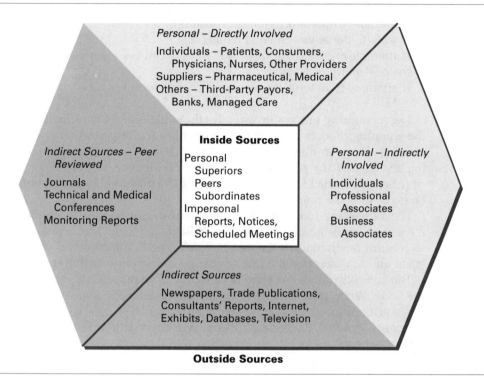

Personal – Directly Involved

Individuals – Patients, Consumers,
   Physicians, Nurses, Other Providers
Suppliers – Pharmaceutical, Medical
Others – Third-Party Payors,
   Banks, Managed Care

Inside Sources

Personal
  Superiors
  Peers
  Subordinates
Impersonal
  Reports, Notices,
  Scheduled Meetings

Indirect Sources – Peer Reviewed

Journals
Technical and Medical
  Conferences
Monitoring Reports

Personal – Indirectly Involved

Individuals
Professional
  Associates
Business
  Associates

Indirect Sources

Newspapers, Trade Publications,
Consultants' Reports, Internet,
Exhibits, Databases, Television

Outside Sources

of such information. Outside the health care organization, nonmembers and patients may be considered important direct sources. Indirect sources are mostly newspapers and journals, the Internet, television, libraries, and public and private databases.

Environmental scanning is perhaps the most important part of environmental analysis because it forms the basis for the other processes. In the scanning activity, issues and changes are specified and sources identified. It is from this beginning that a database for decision making will be built. It is crucial that managers understand the thinking that led to the development and selection of strategic and tactical issues from among those identified in the scanning process. It is therefore advantageous if as many managers as possible take part in scanning. An important aspect of environmental scanning is that it focuses leaders' attention on what lies outside the organization and enables them to create an organization that can adapt to and learn from that environment.[28]

Monitoring the External Environment

The *monitoring* function is the tracking of trends, issues, and possible events identified in the scanning process. Monitoring accomplishes four important functions:

1. It researches and identifies additional sources of information for specific issues delineated in the scanning process that were determined to be important or potentially important to the organization.
2. It adds to the environmental database.
3. It attempts to confirm or disprove issues (trends, developments, dilemmas, and the possibility of events).
4. It attempts to determine the rate of change within issues.

The monitoring process investigates the sources of the information obtained in the scanning process and attempts to identify the organization or organizations creating change and the sources reporting change. Once the organizations creating change and the publications or other information sources reporting change have been identified for a given health care organization, special attention should be given to these sources.

The monitoring function has a much narrower focus than scanning; the objective is to accumulate a database around an identified issue. The database will be used to confirm or disconfirm the trend, development, dilemma, or possibility of an event and to determine the rate of change taking place within the environment.

The intensity of monitoring is reflected in management's understanding of the issue. When managers believe they understand the issue well, less monitoring will be done. However, when environmental issues appear ill-structured, vague, or complex, the issues will require a larger amount of data to arrive at an interpretation.[29]

Forecasting Environmental Change

Forecasting environmental change is a process of extending the trends, developments, dilemmas, and events that the organization is monitoring. The forecasting function attempts to answer the question, "If these trends continue, or if issues accelerate beyond their present rate, or if this event occurs, what will the issues and trends 'look like' in the future?"

Three processes are involved in the forecasting function:

1. Extending the trends, developments, dilemmas, or occurrences of an event;
2. Identifying the interrelationships between the issues and environmental categories; and
3. Developing alternative projections.

Assessing Environmental Change

Information concerning the environment, though abundant, is seldom obvious in its implications. Strategic managers must interpret and intuit the data they receive. After all, facts do not speak for themselves; one has to make sense of the facts, not just get them straight.[30] Therefore, *assessing* environmental change is a process that is largely nonquantifiable and therefore judgmental. The assessment process includes evaluation of the significance of the extended (forecasted) issue on the organization; identification of the issues that must be considered in the internal analysis; development of the vision and mission; and formulation of the strategic plan.

The complexity of what is found and the grossness of most of the data that is collected are not consistent with traditional decision-making methods.[31] There are few procedures for incorporating "fuzzy" issues into the planning process.[32] In addition, even when exposed to identical issues, different managers may interpret their meaning quite differently. Different interpretations are a result of a variety of factors including perceptions, values, and past experiences.

An excellent example of organizations attempting to assess the significance of an issue on the organization occurred in late 1996 when HIPAA was signed into law. Some health care organizations did not wait for all the regulations to be written before they began to process electronically and reaped rewards. The assessment or interpretation of a strategic issue is often represented by general labels such as opportunity or threat. These labels capture the strategic leadership's belief about the potential effects of environmental events and trends. Other dimensions may be used, such as positive/negative, gain/loss, and controllable/uncontrollable.

Unfortunately no comprehensive conceptual scheme or computer model can be developed to provide a complete assessment of environmental issues. The assessment process is not an exact science, and sound human judgment and creativity may be bottom-line techniques for a process without much structure. The fundamental challenge is to make sense out of vague, ambiguous, and unconnected data. Analysts have to infuse meaning into data; they have to make the connections among discordant data such that signals of future events are created. This involves acts of perception and intuition on the analyst's part. It requires the capacity to suspend beliefs, preconceptions, and judgments that may inhibit connections being made among ambiguous and disconnected data.[33]

Environmental Analysis Tools and Techniques

Several different strategic thinking frameworks and techniques may be used to examine the general and health care environments. These frameworks, which are informal and generally not overly sophisticated, have been variously described as "judgmental," "speculative," or "conjectural."[34] Indeed, environmental analysis is largely an individual effort and is directed to person-specific interests. Environmental analysis usually is not limited to just one of the environmental analysis processes, but rather encompasses scanning, monitoring, forecasting, and assessing. The remainder of this chapter will discuss environmental analysis frameworks that identify trends and issues in the general and health care environments. An approach and techniques for more specific market segmentation and competitive analysis will be discussed in Chapter 3.

Simple Trend Identification and Extrapolation

Trend identification and extrapolation is a matter of plotting environmental data and then, from the existing data, anticipating the next occurrence. Perhaps because of its relative simplicity, trend extrapolation is a widely practiced analysis method. Obviously, such a method works best with financial or statistical data. Environmental issues are rarely presented as a neat set of quantifiable data; rather, environmental issues are ill-structured and conjectural. Thus, in many cases, trend identification and extrapolation in environmental analysis is a matter of reaching consensus on the existence of an issue and speculating on the likelihood of its continuance.

Trend identification and extrapolation was applied by Vern Cherewatenko, MD, when he was operating Washington State's largest independent practice association (55 doctors, 130 employees, 75,000 patients, $10 million in revenues). He realized that in 1997 the IPA was losing $7 for every patient seen or about $80,000 per month and the trend was continuing! He determined that the insurance companies, including Medicare and the state's workers comp, were reimbursing at about half of the practice's costs and the trend was not changing. For example, a vasectomy was billed at $550 with all its proper coding and he was reimbursed $180 after any number of hassles back and forth with the insuror. Dr. Cherewatenko and his partner bailed out of the IPA and began "SimpleCare," a cash-based practice where they spend more time with patients and charge them about half of the former billing amount.[35] SimpleCare has expanded into a national network of cash-based practices.

In the case of Lake Villa Nursing Home, demographic trends as well as others are of interest. As illustrated in Exhibit 2–6, the trend identification and extrapolation process includes the identification of issues by environmental category, the designation of an issue as an opportunity or threat, and the determination of its probable impact on the organization. Additionally, managers may assess the likelihood that the trend, development, or dilemma will continue or that the event will occur, and then identify the sources for additional information.

These issues may then be plotted on the chart shown in Exhibit 2–7. The assumption is that the issues to the right of the curved line in the exhibit have a significant impact (high impact) on the organization and are likely to continue or occur (high probability) and should be addressed in the strategic plan.

The formats illustrated in Exhibits 2–6 and 2–7 are useful for organizing environmental data and providing a starting point for speculating on the direction and rate of change for identified trends. However, as with Dr. Cherewatenko's move to a cash-based practice, trend extrapolation of environmental issues requires extensive familiarity with the external environment (the issues) and a great deal of sound judgment.

Exhibit 2–6: Trend/Issue Identification and Evaluation by Lake Villa Nursing Home

Trend/Issue	Opportunity/ Threat	Evidence	Impact on Our Organization (1–10)	Probability of Trend Continuing (1–10)
Aging Population	Opportunity	1 in 5 Americans will be at least 65 by 2030	9	9
Wealthier Elderly	Opportunity	Income of those 60+ has increased 10% faster than any other group	7	6
Local Competition	Threat	Over past 5 years, number of nursing homes in the service area has increased from 5 to 7	7	9

10 = High probability of occurring
 1 = Low probability of occurring

Exhibit 2–7: Environmental Trends/Issues Plot

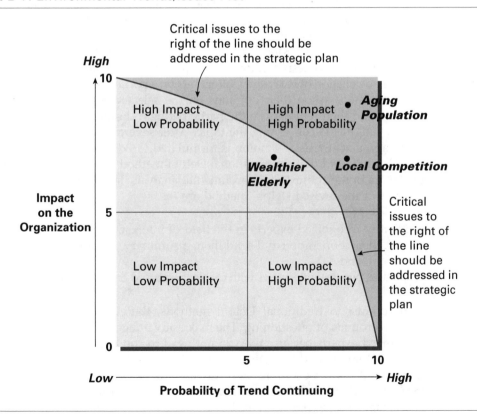

Solicitation of Expert Opinion

Expert opinion is often used to identify, monitor, forecast, and assess environmental trends. Experts play a key role in shaping and extending the thinking of leaders. For example, health care experts have concluded that these managerial skills will be essential throughout the remainder of the decade: the ability to deliver quality care at reasonable cost, the ability to enhance the health status of the community, the ability to gain the respect of the business and medical communities, and the ability to improve outcomes and satisfaction. Health care leaders can use these opinions to stimulate their strategic thinking and begin developing human resources strategies.

To further focus leaders' thinking and generate additional perspectives concerning the issues in the external environment, there are a number of more formal expert-based environmental analysis techniques. These strategic thinking frameworks help solicit and synthesize the opinions and best judgments of experts within various fields.

THE DELPHI METHOD

The Delphi method is a popular, practical, and useful approach for analyzing environmental data. The Delphi method may be used to identify and study current and emerging trends within each environmental category (technological, social, economic, and so on). More specifically, the *Delphi method* is the development, evaluation, and synthesis of individual points of view through the systematic solicitation and collation of individual judgments on a particular topic. In the first round, individuals are asked their opinions on the selected topic. Opinions are summarized and then sent back to the participating individuals for the development of new judgments concerning the topic. After several rounds of solicitation and summary, a synthesis of opinion is formulated.[36]

S. C. Jain found that the traditional Delphi method has undergone a great deal of change in the context of environmental analysis. Jain suggests that the salient features of the revised Delphi method are to:

1. identify recognized experts in the field of interest;
2. seek their cooperation and send them a summary paper (based on a literature search); and
3. conduct personal interviews with each expert based on a structured questionnaire.[37]

In contrast to traditional Delphi methods, there is no further feedback or repeated rounds of questioning. The major advantage is that it is easier to recruit recognized experts because they do not need to commit as much of their time.

The Delphi method is particularly helpful when health care managers want to understand the opportunities and threats of a specific environmental issue. For example, a Delphi study was designed to define the role and responsibilities of sports medicine specialists in the United Kingdom. A mail questionnaire was sent to a random sample of 300 members of the British Association of Sport and Exercise Medicine. The original questionnaire contained 300 attributes and allowed participants to modify their responses based on feedback from other participants. The study concluded that sports medicine was an evolving specialty in the United Kingdom. The study, however, was recognized as the first systematic attempt to define the role and responsibilities of the sports medicine specialist and should be a valuable resource in the future development of career pathways for physicians.[38]

NOMINAL GROUP TECHNIQUE, BRAINSTORMING, AND FOCUS GROUPS

The nominal group technique (NGT), brainstorming, and focus groups are interactive group problem identification and solving techniques. In *nominal group technique*, a group is convened to address an issue, such as the impact of consolidation within the health care industry or the impact of an aging population on hospital facilities. Each individual independently generates a written list of ideas surrounding the issue. Following the idea-generation period, group members take turns reporting one idea at a time to the group. Typically, each new idea is recorded on a large flip chart for everyone to consider. Members are encouraged to build on the ideas of others in the group. After all the ideas have been listed, the group discusses the ideas. After the discussion, members privately vote or rank the ideas. After voting, further discussion and group generation of ideas continue. Typically, additional voting continues until a reasonable consensus is reached.[39]

A *brainstorming* group is convened for the purpose of understanding an issue, assessing the impact of an issue on the organization, or generating strategic alternatives. In this process, members present ideas and are allowed to clarify them with brief explanations. Each idea is recorded, but evaluation is generally not allowed. The intent of brainstorming is to generate fresh ideas or new ways of thinking. Members are encouraged to present any ideas that occur to them, even apparently risky or impossible ideas. Such a process often stimulates creativity and sparks new approaches that are not as risky, crazy, or impossible as first thought.[40]

NGT and brainstorming could be used to understand and respond to the moratorium on specialty-hospital physician investment and referral mandated by the Medicare Prescription Drug Improvement and Modernization (MMA) Act on December 8, 2003 (effective through June 8, 2005). Under the moratorium a doctor was not allowed to refer a patient to certain specialty hospitals in which the physician had an ownership or investment interest and the hospital was not allowed to bill Medicare or any other entity for services provided as a result of a prohibited referral. Hospitals under development as of November 18, 2003 were excluded from the moratorium, which applied specifically to hospitals engaged exclusively in the care and treatment of patients with cardiac or orthopedic conditions, surgical patients, and patients receiving other specialized types of services that CMS designated.[41]

Obviously, managers of specialty hospitals and their competitors faced a great deal of uncertainty as to how the moratorium might "play out." Specialty hospitals would have to decide whether or not to continue with plans for the development and expansion of new facilities after June 2005. Brainstorming groups would be useful in carefully thinking about the various options facing specialty hospitals during the moratorium.

Similar to the process of brainstorming, *focus groups* bring together 10 to 15 key individuals to develop, evaluate, and reach conclusions regarding environmental issues. Focus groups provide an opportunity for management to discuss particularly important organizational issues with qualified individuals. Hospitals and large group practices have used focus groups of patients to better understand the perceived strengths and weaknesses of the organization from the patient's view. For example, Johns Hopkins was considering the establishment of an integrated delivery system under one umbrella name. Focus groups of physicians, present and past patients, nonpatients, and others convinced them to change plans (see Perspective 2–6). Focus groups can provide new insights for understanding the issues and suggest fresh alternatives for their resolution.

Dialectic Inquiry

Dialectic inquiry is a "point and counterpoint" process of argumentation. The nineteenth-century German philosopher Hegel suggested that the surest path to truth was the use of a dialectic process – an intellectual exchange in which a thesis is pitted against an antithesis. According to this principle, truth emerges from the search for synthesis of apparently contradictory views.[42]

More specifically, in environmental analysis, dialectic inquiry is the development, evaluation, and synthesis of conflicting points of view (environmental issues) through separate formulation and refinement of each point of view.[43] For instance, one group may argue that health care costs will be declining between 2005 and 2010 (thesis) because of the prospective payment system, pressure by businesses and labor, market-based health care reform, physician reimbursement reform, and so on. Another group may present a case that the trend toward rising health care costs will continue (antithesis) because of hospital failures, the high cost of new technology, failure of health care reform initiatives, and so on. Debating this issue will unearth the major factors influencing health care costs and the implications for the future.

Any health care provider can utilize this technique by assigning groups to debate specific external issues. The groups make presentations and debate conflicting points of view concerning the environment. After the debate, the groups attempt to form a synthesis of ideas concerning the likely future.[44]

Stakeholder Analysis

Stakeholder analysis is based on the belief that there is a reciprocal relationship between an organization and certain other organizations, groups, and individuals. They are referred to as stakeholders: that is, organizations, groups, and individuals

Perspective 2–6

Johns Hopkins Uses Focus Groups to Understand Consumer Perceptions

Although *US News and World Report* ranks Johns Hopkins among the best in the country, "locals" (who are 75 percent of its patients) often perceive it as a place of last resort. Hopkins wanted to better understand the rational and emotional value of the Johns Hopkins name among consumers and physicians. In addition, strategists wanted to know whether the Hopkins name could be extended to primary sites or other hospitals.

The research was carried out in a number of phases. First, 14 focus groups of consumers from seven regions of Maryland and southern Pennsylvania were conducted to understand what people "knew" about Hopkins. Results verified Hopkins's excellent image for medical quality and top-notch physicians, but it was perceived as inaccessible, expensive, impersonal, and in a bad location. Further, consumers did not understand the benefits of a "health care delivery system" (perceiving it as an HMO). Consumers were mixed on extending the Hopkins name as they thought it was somewhat akin to a "Good Housekeeping seal of approval" on the one hand, but would imply higher costs and dilute the Hopkins name on the other.

An additional 14 focus groups were conducted to understand the emotional value of the Hopkins name. A variety of groups were included: current patients, individuals who had attended a Hopkins seminar but never been a patient, individuals who had had no contact with Hopkins, physicians who referred to Hopkins, and Hopkins Medicine leadership. In these focus groups individuals were asked to do a variety of exercises that led to positive, mixed, and negative conclusions about the emotional value of the name. The positive conclusions were: the community had pride and respect for Hopkins as an institution in the city, there was security in knowing that Hopkins had the highest quality doctors and nurses as well as latest technology, the research and teaching tradition led to hope and pride in innovation, and the former patients group perceived compassion and excellence in patient care. The mixed response was for "patients coming from all over the world." Some saw this as indicative of providing quality care, whereas others saw it as Hopkins serving only important people or people from outside Baltimore. The negatives were that Hopkins was a big, powerful institution and thus overpriced, and Hopkins was elitist and discriminating (interpreted by the focus groups as intimidating, unwelcoming, and overwhelming).

The focus groups led to the following conclusions:

- Protect the hospital's strong brand image for medical excellence in complex cases and discovery.
- Use care in extending the hospital's name to other parts of the system as the positive associations are with the main campus.
- Position Hopkins as a "family of hospitals and doctors" under the leadership of Johns Hopkins rather than an "integrated delivery system."
- Use Johns Hopkins Medicine as an endorser of other faculties.
- Emphasize the accessibility of members of Johns Hopkins Medicine.
- Expand the Hopkins brand from a "place of last resort" to cover the broad range of services.
- Soften the intimidating and unwelcoming image perceived by current and potential customers.

Source: Michael P. Harnett and Carol A. Bloomberg, "Johns Hopkins Brand Research: Case Study," *Healthcare Growth Strategies 2001* (Santa Barbara, CA: COR Health LLC, 2000), pp. 15–18.

Exhibit 2–8: A Stakeholder Map for a Large Multispecialty Group Practice

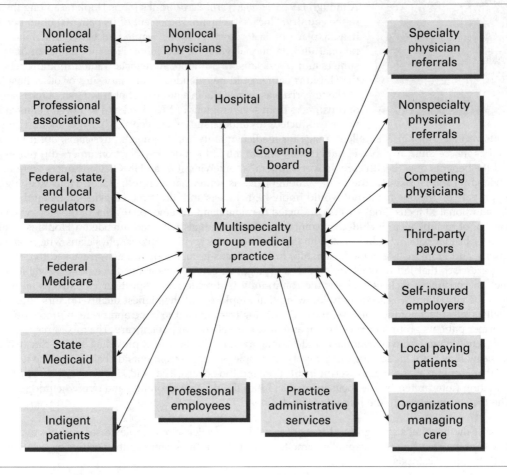

that have an interest or "stake" in the success of the organization. Examples of possible health care stakeholders, shown as a "stakeholder map," are presented in Exhibit 2–8.

Stakeholders may be categorized as internal, interface, and external. Internal stakeholders are those who operate primarily within the bounds of the organization, such as managers and other employees. Interface stakeholders are those who function both internally and externally, such as the medical staff and the corporate officers of the parent company. External stakeholders operate outside the organization and include such entities as suppliers, third-party payors, competitors, regulatory agencies, the media, the local community, and so on.[45] Such stakeholders have been referred to as the "organization ecosystem" – organizations that affect and are affected by the creation and delivery of the organization's product or service. Part of stakeholder analysis is to systematically identify the organizations with which their future is most closely intertwined and determine the dependencies that are most critical.[46]

Some of these stakeholders are almost always powerful or influential; others are influential regarding only certain issues; still others have little influence or power. If the stakeholders can be identified and evaluated, then the "forces" affecting the organization may be specified. The needs and wants of these constituencies may dramatically affect the strategy of an organization.[47]

Stakeholders can impact the strategic management process by demanding to participate or certain groups might be invited to participate (physicians, directors from a community-based board of directors, and so on). Some stakeholders (patients, employees, insurance companies) may not be a direct part of strategic management but their interests are clearly considered as part of the scanning process.

Management usually relies on its collective judgment to provide an accurate assessment of the relative power of the important stakeholders. It can be a critical error not to understand how the stakeholders perceive their own power and how they would contribute to the strategy formulation process. Blair and Buesseler point out that an organization does not choose its stakeholders; rather, the stakeholders choose themselves.[48]

To know how these self-selected stakeholders view their power offers an opportunity to know how to negotiate with them. In one study, all other groups rated physicians as having greater power than the physicians rated their own power.[49] The board of directors, however, rated its influence as very high; all other groups did as well. Despite the recent emphasis in health care on developing a customer orientation, patients did not believe they had much influence; nor did any other group rate them as possessing very high influence. A patient may complain to a physician about some aspect of a hospital experience and expect some action; however, the physician will probably feel relatively unable to cause any change. Because those who feel they have power in an organization are more likely to support its mission and strategic plan, it is no wonder that leaders have to be diligent in involving the medical community.

Typically, managers tend to focus attention on known, salient, or powerful stakeholders to help protect existing competitive advantages. However, there is growing evidence that "fringe" stakeholders are important as well – particularly for developing new ways of thinking. Stuart Hart and Sanjay Sharma suggest that "the knowledge needed to generate competitive imagination and to manage disruptive change increasingly lies outside the organization, at the periphery" of the organization's established stakeholder network.[50] Therefore, strategic thinkers must be open to fringe ideas and nontraditional thinking developed by fringe players. At first, these stakeholders may apear to be poor, weak, isolated, nonlegitimate or radical.[51] In reality, they may be strong purveyors of change.

Stakeholders should be viewed as partners who create value through problem solving that results in a corporate community. From a profit-centered model to a social responsibility-centered model, corporate governing boards are now moving toward collaborative working relationships or a corporate community model. This shift has occurred as capital assets (factories, land, money) have declined relative to the value of information or knowledge. Knowledge cannot be used up and the "more that is dispensed, the more you generate."[52] Stakeholder collaboration does more than gain political clout – it encourages joint problem solving to increase valuable knowledge. A health care organization can benefit from knowing its stakeholders and being the beneficiary of input from such valuable stakeholders.

Scenario Writing and Future Studies

Many businesses regularly use scenarios. The popularity of scenario analysis is due in large part to the inability of other, more quantitative forecasting methods to predict and incorporate major shifts in the environment and provide a context for strategic thinking. Scenarios avoid the need for single-point forecasts by allowing users to explore several alternative futures.[53] Scenario analysis is an alternative to conventional forecasting that is better suited to an environment with numerous uncertainties or imponderables – where there is no map.

A *scenario* is a coherent story about the future, using the world of today as a starting point. Based on data accumulated in the scanning and monitoring processes, a scenario or narrative that describes an assumed future is developed. The objective of scenarios and future studies is to describe a point of time in the future as a sequence of time-frames or periods of time. Scenario writing often requires generous assumptions. Few guidelines indicate what to include in the scenario. In most cases several plausible scenarios should be written. It is an all-too-common mistake to envision only one scenario as the "true picture of the future."[54] Most authorities advocate the development of multiple scenarios. However, to avoid decision makers focusing only on the "most likely" or "most probable" scenario, each scenario should be given a distinctive theme name, such that they appear equally likely.

Multiple scenarios allow the future to be represented by different cause–effect relationships, different key events and their consequences, different variables, and different assumptions. The key question is: "If this environmental event happens (or does not happen), what will be the effect on the organization?" The use of multiple scenarios was particularly helpful as organizations considered the probable impact of health care reform legislation on their organizations. Exhibit 2–9 presents a brief summary of three scenarios or alternative futures for health care between now and 2010. The scenarios were developed by the Institute for the Future to provide a description of critical factors that will influence health and health care in the first decade of the twenty-first century.

Selecting the Strategic Thinking Framework

The purpose of analyzing the general and health care environments is to identify and understand the significant shifts taking place in the external environment. Exhibit 2–10 summarizes the primary focus, advantages, and disadvantages of each strategic thinking framework.

Exhibit 2–9: Three Future Health Care Scenarios

Scenario One: **Stormy Weather**
None of the fundamental problems of cost, quality, or access are resolved by 2005. Between 2005 and 2010, managed care fails to deliver reduced costs or push quality resulting in a backlash by consumers and providers. Legislation is enacted to negate the authority of managed care. Medicare cherry-picking by risk insurance plans leaves the sickest patients to be covered by conventional indemnity plans. A few major provider groups emerge; physicians and hospitals fear leaving their group. In a tight labor market, large employers continue to offer health benefits to employees; smaller employers are less able to pay for the increased costs. Health care spending reaches 19 percent of GDP and 22 percent of the population is uninsured. New technology continues to offer improved, less invasive alternatives and is demanded by baby boomers – a knowledgeable group that expects to participate in their own health care decisions. No social consensus develops to limit end-of-life care. Information technologies require huge investment but lead to disappointing results in terms of cost savings. The public health sector minimally meets its mandated functions. People worry about losing health benefits and most are unhappy with the increased out-of-pocket costs. Medicaid strains state budgets; Medicare strains the federal budget – especially as early boomers begin to access the system in 2010. Health care reform is in the forefront of public policy once again.

Scenario Two: **Long and Winding Road**
Large employers maintain price pressure on health plans and require greater contribution by employees. The increased out-of-pocket costs cause employees to reduce their use of health care services. Health plans tighten control through closed networks that pressure providers for clinical price controls. Providers attempt to resist the insurance "hassles" with very limited success. The 1998 federal budget bill includes Medicare and Medicaid cost containment as it does each year following. The public health system continues to compete with the private sector on health service delivery. Health care costs reach 16 percent of GDP and 16 percent of the population is uninsured. The system remains tiered with 20 percent in public coverage or uninsured, 60 percent in restrictive managed care, and 20 percent in high-end, indemnity insurance programs. Cost-based reimbursement is curtailed; large integrated providers have not materialized. Physicians tend to practice in small groups (although there are no solo practices). Comprehensive health care reform does not rise to the top of the public policy agenda because the system is managing to "muddle on through . . ."

Scenario Three: **Sunny Side of the Street**
Competition drives excess capacity from the system and providers and patients work together to improve health. Newly trained physicians have lowered income expectations. Providers with best practices survive; consolidation occurs and excess capacity (especially hospital beds) is eliminated. Prospective payment covers all outpatient services. Clinical information systems improve care processes and outcomes. The electronic patient record becomes a reality. Technology focuses on improved outcomes and reduced costs. Therapy trade-off can be made based on cost-effectiveness. Public health will engage in public–private partnerships and will focus on assessment, development of policy, and assurance. Health care costs are 15 percent of GDP, and 10 percent of the population is uninsured. The systems are in place to minimize unnecessary variations in health care practices, operate efficiently, track outcomes to lead to further improvements, and handle the aging of baby boomers. Insurors are rewarded for improving the health of a population and focusing on long-term health care decisions.

Source: Institute for the Future, *Health and Health Care 2010: The Forecast, The Challenge* (San Francisco: Jossey-Bass Publishers, 2000), pp. 10–14.

Exhibit 2–10: Primary Focus, Advantages, and Disadvantages of Environmental Techniques

Technique	Primary Focus	Advantage	Disadvantage
Simple Trend Identification and Extrapolation	Scanning Monitoring Forecasting Assessing	• Simple • Logical • Easy to communicate	• Need a good deal of data in order to extend trend • Limited to existing trends • May not foster creative thinking
Delphi Method	Scanning Monitoring Forecasting Assessing	• Use of field experts • Avoids intimidation problems • Eliminates management's biases	• Members are physically dispersed • No direct interaction of participants • May take a long time to complete
Nominal Group Technique	Scanning Monitoring Forecasting Assessing	• Everyone has equal status and power • Wide participation • Ensures representation • Eliminates management's biases	• Structure may limit creativity • Time consuming
Brainstorming	Forecasting Assessing	• Fosters creativity • Develops many ideas, alternatives • Encourages communication	• No process for making decisions • Sometimes gets off track
Focus Groups	Forecasting Assessing	• Uses experts • Management/expert interaction • New viewpoints	• Finding experts • No specific structure for reaching conclusions
Dialectic Inquiry	Forecasting Assessing	• Surfaces many subissues and factors • Conclusions are reached on issues • Based on analysis	• Does not provide a set of procedures for deciding what is important • Considers only a single issue at a time • Time consuming
Stakeholder Analysis	Scanning Monitoring	• Considers major independent groups and individuals • Ensures major needs and wants of outside organizations are taken into account	• Emerging issues generated by other organizations may not be considered • Does not consider the broader issues of the general environment
Scenario Writing	Forecasting Assessing	• Portrays alternative futures • Considers interrelated external variables • Gives a complete picture of the future	• Requires generous assumptions • Always a question as to what to include • Difficult to write

The approach selected for evaluating the general and health care environments will depend on such factors as the size of the organization, the diversity of the products and services, and the complexity and size of the markets (service areas). Organizations that are relatively small, do not have a great deal of diversity, and have well-defined service areas may opt for a simple strategic thinking framework that may be carried out in house, such as trend identification and extrapolation, in-house nominal group technique or brainstorming, or stakeholder analysis. Such organizations may include independent hospitals, HMOs, rural and community hospitals, large group practices, long-term care facilities, hospices, and county public health departments.

Health care organizations that are large, have diverse products and services, and have ill-defined or extensive service areas may want to use a strategic thinking framework that draws on the knowledge of a wide range of experts. As a result, these organizations are more likely to set up Delphi panels and outside nominal groups or brainstorming sessions. In addition, these organizations may have the resources to conduct dialectics concerning environmental issues and engage in scenario writing. Such approaches are usually more time consuming, fairly expensive, and require extensive coordination. Organizations using these approaches may include national and regional for-profit health care chains, regional health care systems, large federations and alliances, and state public health departments. Ultimately, the strategic thinking framework selected for environmental analysis may depend primarily on the style and preferences of management. If used properly, any of the frameworks can be a powerful tool for identifying, monitoring, forecasting, and assessing issues in the general and health care environments.

Issues in the Health Care Environment

The health care industry is faced with many dynamic issues and will have to deal with a host of new developments in the rapidly changing external environment. Strategic managers of health care organizations should assess these issues and others unique to their organizations to provide a foundation for understanding the complexity of health care delivery and to furnish a backdrop for developing strategy. An excellent example of identifying environmental issues, recognizing opportunity, and building a strategy around that opportunity is provided by Accordant Health Services, Inc., an independent disease management company involved with 15 chronic diseases (see Perspective 2–7).

For the foreseeable future, the health care environment will continue to generate numerous complex issues. Using a format similar to that shown in Exhibit 2–6, a list of current issues can be generated. This format can provide a useful summary of environmental issues and encourage managers to cite specific evidence supporting their beliefs concerning those issues. For instance, the high cost of technology is commonly cited as a health care issue, but what is the specific evidence indicating that it is still an issue or is continuing as an issue? Individual health care managers will have to assess the likelihood that these issues will continue and what their impact will be for individual organizations.

Perspective 2–7

Accordant Health Services, Inc.

Accordant Health Services, Inc., was started by Steve Schelhammer in 1995 because he believed that the complications and catastrophic crises associated with chronic diseases were manageable or preventable and that patients with these diseases wanted to participate in their own health care. Many insurors have in-house programs for some of the more common chronic diseases such as diabetes and asthma. However, there are additional complex chronic diseases that do not occur as frequently in the population. These diseases could be managed with greater cost and clinical effectiveness by outsourcing this function to a disease management company.

Accordant, an AdvancePCS company based in Greensboro, NC, has grown to become the nation's largest independent provider of health improvement services, touching the lives of more than 75 million health plan members and managing approximately $28 billion in annual prescription drug spending. AdvancePCS offers health plans a wide range of health improvement products and services designed to improve the quality of care delivered to health plan members and manage costs.

By 2005, Accordant was providing disease management programs for 15 complex, chronic diseases: multiple sclerosis, Parkinson's disease, lupus, myasthenia gravis, sickle cell anemia, polymyositis, cystic fibrosis, chronic inflammatory demyelinating polyradiculoneuropathy (CIDP), amyotrophic lateral sclerosis (ALS), scleroderma, dermatomyositis, hemophilia, gaucher disease, rheumatoid arthritis, and seizure disorder. In 2003, Accordant earned Full NCQA Patient- and Practitioner-Oriented Disease Management Accreditation for all 15 of its disease management programs – more than any other organization nationwide.

According to Accordant, "Effective chronic disease management is the application of continuous quality improvement to the whole spectrum of care. We recognize that a disease management program stressing prevention, education, and support can positively impact both the customer's cost of care and the patient's quality of life."

Accordant's quarterly disease specific assessments stratify a health plan's population of patients for severity of illness and risk of adverse events. The company relies on its expert "tele-web" system that integrates Internet and call-center technologies to enable flexible, intelligent, and customized information sharing among patients, providers, and health plans. Chronic, progressive diseases such as multiple sclerosis, hemophilia, cystic fibrosis, lupus, myasthenia gravis, and rheumatoid arthritis cause physical and lifestyle impairment. For some MS patients, the web is an important way to communicate with someone who can answer questions and who understands their disease, because they no longer can speak. Other patients prefer to call the 1–800 number to talk to one of the nurses that are on duty 24 hours a day.

Using Accordant's disease management program, the following services are available to insurors:

- Risk stratification of diagnosed members;
- Disease-specific education resulting in better self-management;
- 24-hours per day 1–800 number for enrolled members;
- Development of individual care plans;
- Disease management reports;
- Demographic oriented reports;
- Outcomes reports – reports relating to clinical/functional status;
- Distribution of reports – health plan and physician.

Patients are offered education and resources:

- Self-motivating methods to help them recognize early signs of problems.
- Self-motivating techniques to help them maintain their health.

▶

- Educational resources to help them learn more about their disease.
- Information on the latest medical breakthroughs.

Through Accordant's services, one-on-one relationships with patients are built by regular contact with them as nurses monitor and assess patients' health status and provide targeted education, support, and guidance for both patients and their caregivers. In addition, Accordant nurses communicate frequently with treating physicians to keep them up to date on the clinical status and specific health care needs of patients. Accordant's Medical Advisory Board is comprised of national medical experts who participate in the development and continuous quality improvement of the company's programs.

Accordant focuses on managing complex chronic diseases with the goal of improving clinical, patient satisfaction, and cost-of-care outcomes. According to Steve Schelhammer, "We work with the patients' existing medical community to facilitate access to coordinated, preventive care and provide better management of crises. For the purpose of outcomes reporting, key disease-specific data points are collected for each patient. Accordant tracks and reports financial, functional, clinical, and patient satisfaction outcomes for all diseases. We stand behind our methodology and provide performance-based contracts, sharing risk for cost and quality outcomes."

Source: Accordant company documents.

Strategic Momentum – Validating the Strategic Assumptions

The strategic plan is based in part on an analysis of the external environment. Initially this analysis provides the basic beliefs or assumptions that management holds concerning various issues in the external environment. Once strategic management is adopted as the operating philosophy of managing, strategic thinking, strategic planning, and strategic momentum require frequent validation of the strategic assumptions to determine whether issues in the external environment have changed and to what extent. Continued strategic thinking is vital to maintaining strategic momentum.

The strategic thinking map presented in Exhibit 2–11 provides a series of questions designed to detect signals of new perspectives regarding these assumptions. The questions examine management's understanding of the external environment and the effectiveness of the strategy. The board of directors, strategic managers, or others may use these questions as a beginning point to confirm the assumptions underlying the strategy. Such strategic thinking questions may indicate the emergence of new external opportunities or threats that will affect the organization and may suggest areas where additional information will be required in future planning efforts. Current, accurate information may mean survival for many health care organizations. Questions concerning the external environment may reveal that a group practice knows far too little about the views of its major constituents (stakeholders) or the existence of new technologies or social trends. A validation (or invalidation) of the strategic assumptions reinvigorates strategic thinking and provides a basis for investigating whether to change the strategy.

Exhibit 2–11: Strategic Thinking Questions for Validation of the Strategic Assumptions

1. Has the organization's performance been adversely affected by unexpected or new trends or issues in the general environment?
2. Has the organization's performance been adversely affected by unexpected or new trends or issues in the health care environment?
3. Have new opportunities emerged as a result of new trends, issues or events in the external environment?
4. Is the strategy acceptable to the major stakeholders?
5. Are there new technological developments that will affect the organization?
6. Have there been social or demographic changes that affect the market or strategy? Changes in ethnic mix? Language barriers? Family structure?
7. Are there new regulations or has the political environment changed?
8. Are there new local, state, or federal regulations or laws being introduced, debated or passed that will affect operations or performance?
9. Are there new economic issues?
10. Have new competitors outside the industry considered entering or actually entered into health related areas?
11. Is the strategy subject to government response?
12. Is the strategy in conformance with the society's moral and ethical codes of conduct?

Summary and Conclusions

This chapter is concerned with understanding and analyzing the general environment and health care industry environment. To be successful, organizations must be effectively positioned within their environment. Organizations involved in making capital allocations, experiencing unexpected environmental changes or surprises from different kinds of external forces, facing increasing competition, becoming more marketing oriented, or experiencing dissatisfaction with their present planning results should engage in environmental analysis.

The goal of environmental analysis is to classify and organize the general and health care industry issues and changes generated outside the organization. In the process, the organization attempts to detect and analyze current, emerging, and likely future issues. The gathered information is used for internal analysis; development of the vision and mission; and formulation of the strategy for the organization. In addition, the process should foster strategic thinking throughout the organization.

Although the benefits of environmental analysis are clear, there are several limitations. Environmental analysis cannot foretell the future; nor can managers hope to detect every change. Moreover, the information needed may be impossible to obtain or difficult to interpret, or the organization may not be able to respond quickly enough. The most significant limitation may be managers' preconceived beliefs about the environment.

This chapter provides a comprehensive description of the broad external environment for health care organizations. The environment includes organizations and individuals in the general environment (government institutions and agencies, business firms, educational institutions, research organizations and foundations, and individuals and consumers) and organizations and individuals in the health care environment (organizations that regulate, primary providers, secondary providers, organizations that represent providers, and individuals and patients).

Organizations and individuals in both the general and health care environments generate changes that may be important to health care organizations. Typically, such change is classified as technological, social, political, regulatory, economic, or competitive. Such a classification system aids in aggregating information concerning the issues and in determining their impact. Sources for environmental issues are found both inside and outside the organization and are direct as well as indirect.

The steps in environmental analysis include scanning to identify signals of environmental change, monitoring identified issues, forecasting the future direction of issues, and assessing organizational implications. Scanning is the process of viewing and organizing external information in an attempt to detect relevant issues that will affect the organization. Monitoring is the process of searching for additional information to confirm or disprove the trend, development, dilemma, or likelihood of the occurrence of an event. Forecasting is the process of extending issues, identifying their interrelationships, and developing alternative projections. Finally, assessing is the process of evaluating the significance of the issues. The information garnered from external environmental analysis influences internal analysis, the development of the vision and mission, and formulation of the strategy for the organization.

Several strategic thinking frameworks were discussed to conduct the scanning, monitoring, forecasting, and assessing processes. These methods include simple trend identification and extension, solicitation of expert opinion, dialectic inquiry, stakeholder analysis, and scenario writing. In addition, several relevant issues in the health care environment were explored. Finally, as part of strategic momentum, strategic thinking questions were presented to evaluate the strategic assumptions generated from the external environmental analysis. The next chapter will focus on service area competitive analysis.

Key Terms and Concepts in Strategic Management

Assessing	Focus Groups	Scanning
Brainstorming	Forecasting	Scenarios
Delphi Method	General Environment	Secondary Provider
Dialectic Inquiry	Health Care Environment	Stakeholder Analysis
Efficiency/Effectiveness	Monitoring	Strategic Awareness
Expert Opinion	Nominal Group Technique (NGT)	Strategic Issues
External Environmental Analysis	Primary Provider	Trend Identification

QUESTIONS FOR CLASS DISCUSSION

1. What types of changes are likely to occur in the health care environment in the next several years? Explain how any major shift in an industry creates a wide range of changes throughout the industry.
2. Why is environmental analysis important for an organization?
3. Describe the "setting" for health care management. Is the setting too complex or changing too rapidly to accurately predict future conditions?
4. Most health care managers would answer "Yes" to many of A. H. Mesch's questions to determine whether an organization needs environmental analysis. Are there other questions that seem to indicate that health care organizations should be performing environmental analysis?
5. What are the specific goals of environmental analysis?
6. What are the limitations of environmental analysis? Given these limitations, is environmental analysis worth the effort required? Why?
7. Why is it important to be able to identify influential organizations in the external environment? How may these organizations be categorized?
8. What four processes are involved in environmental analysis? What are their subprocesses?
9. How does the scanning process create a "window" to the external environment? How does the window concept help in understanding organizations and the types of information they produce?
10. Why is the process of environmental analysis as important as the product?
11. What are some important technological, social, political, regulatory, economic, and competitive issues that are affecting health care today?
12. Which of the environmental analysis strategic thinking frameworks are most useful? Why?
13. Using Exhibit 2–8 as an example, develop a "stakeholder map" for a health care organization in your metropolitan area or state. On this map show the important health care organizations and indicate what impact they may have on the industry.
14. Which of the scenarios in Exhibit 2–9 do you think is most likely? Why? Based on today's trends, issues, dilemmas, and so on, develop your own scenario of health care in 2010.
15. A strategic plan is based on a set of beliefs and assumptions that management holds in terms of the environment. What are some of those assumptions for a health care organization in your community?
16. What are an organization's strategic assumptions? How may the strategic assumptions be evaluated as part of managing the strategic momentum?
17. Go beyond your immediate data and speculate on the major forces that will affect the delivery of health care after the year 2010.

NOTES

1. Kathleen M. Sutcliffe and Klaus Weber, "The High Cost of Accurate Knowledge," *Harvard Business Review* 81, no. 5 (2003), p. 75.
2. Peter F. Drucker, *Managing the Nonprofit Organization: Principles and Practices* (New York: HarperCollins Publishers, 1990), p. 9.
3. Joel A. Barker, *Future Edge: Discovering the New Paradigms of Success* (New York: William Morrow, 1992), p. 28.
4. This partial list of issues in the health care industry results from tracking the strategic issues in health care in the professional and trade literature as well as numerous interviews with both public and private health care professionals by the authors. Also, issues were included from Institute for the Future, *Health and Health Care 2010: The Forecast, The Challenge* (San Francisco: Jossey-Bass Publishers, January 2000).
5. Michael E. Porter and Elizabeth Olmsted Teisberg, "Redefining Competition in Health Care," *Harvard Business Review* 82, no. 6 (June 2004), pp. 65–76.
6. Ibid.
7. Linda T. Kohn, "Organizing and Managing Care in a Changing Health System," *Health Services Research* 35, no. 1 (April 2000), pp. 37–52.
8. James B. Goes, Leonard Friedman, Nancy Seifert, and Jan Buffa, "A Turbulent Field: Theory, Research, and Practice on Organizational Change in Health Care," in John D. Blair, Myron D. Fottler, Grant T. Savage (eds) *Advances in Health Care Management* (New York: Elsevier Science, 2000), pp. 143–144.
9. John Burns, "Market Opening Up to the Non-Traditional," *Modern Healthcare* 23, no. 32 (August 9, 1993), pp. 96–98.
10. James M. Kouzes and Barry Z. Posner, *The Leadership Challenge: How to Keep Getting Extraordinary Things Done in Organizations* (San Francisco: Jossey-Bass Publishers, 1995), p. 44.
11. David K. Hurst, *Crisis and Renewal: Meeting the Challenge of Organizational Change* (Boston: Harvard Business School Press, 1995), p. 49.
12. Kouzes and Posner, *The Leadership Challenge*, pp. 47–48.
13. A. H. Mesch, "Developing an Effective Environmental Assessment Function," *Managerial Planning* 32 (1984), pp. 17–22.
14. Henry Mintzberg, "The Fall and Rise of Strategic Planning," *Harvard Business Review* 72, no. 1 (1994), pp. 107–114 and Mie Augier and Saras D. Sarasvathy, "Integrating Evolution, Cognition, and Design: Extending Simonian Perspectives to Strategic Organization," *Strategic Organization* 2, no. 2 (2004), pp. 169–204.
15. Michael D. Watkins and Max H. Bazerman, "Predictable Surprises: The Disasters You Should Have Seen Coming," *Harvard Business Review* 81, no. 3 (2003), pp. 72–80.
16. J. O'Connell and J. W. Zimmerman, "Scanning the International Environment," *California Management Review* 22 (1979), pp. 15–22.
17. Barker, *Future Edge*, p. 86.
18. Edward De Bono, *Serious Creativity: Using the Power of Lateral Thinking to Create New Ideas* (New York: HarperBusiness, 1992), p. 17. See also Bradley L. Kirkman, Benson Rosen, Paul E. Tesluk, and Christina B. Gibson, "The Impact of Team Empowerment on Virtual Team Performance: The Moderating Role of Face-to-Face Interaction," *Academy of Management Journal* 47, no. 2 (2004), pp. 175–192.
19. "Bill Makes Health Insurance Portable," *Congressional Quarterly Almanac*, 104th Congress, 2nd Session (1996), pp. 6-28–6-39.
20. Nilay B. Patel, "A Guide to the Final Installment of the HIPAA Trilogy: The Security Regulation," *Journal of Health Care Compliance* 6, no. 4 (2003), pp. 13–19.
21. Karl Kronebush and Brian Elbel, "Simplifying Medicaid and SCHIP," *Health Affairs* 23, no. 3 (2004), pp. 233–247.
22. Beaufort B. Longest, Jr., *Management Practices for the Health Professional*, 4th edn (Norwalk, CT: Appleton & Lange, 1990), pp. 12–28.
23. Ibid., p. 23.
24. http://www.hcfa.gov/stats/NHE-Proj/proj1998/tables/table2.htm. Centers for Medicare and Medicaid Services, Office of the Actuary, 2004.
25. Vince Gallaro, "Drop in Uninsured and Drop in HMO Ranks," *Modern Healthcare* 30, no. 41 (October 2, 2000), pp. 2–3.
26. Liam Fahey and V. K. Narayanan, *Macroenvironmental Analysis for Strategic Management* (St. Paul: West Publishing, 1986).
27. James B. Thomas and Reuben R. McDaniel, Jr., "Interpreting Strategic Issues: Effects of Strategy and the Information-Processing Structure of Top Management Teams," *Academy of Management Journal* 33, no. 2 (1990), p. 288.
28. P. T. Terry, "Mechanisms for Environmental Scanning," *Long Range Planning* 10 (1977), p. 9.

29. Thomas and McDaniel, "Interpreting Strategic Issues," pp. 289–290.
30. Sutcliffe and Weber, "The High Cost of Accurate Knowledge," p. 75.
31. W. R. Dill, "The Impact of Environment on Organizational Development," in S. Mailick and E. H. VanNess (eds) *Concepts and Issues in Administrative Behavior* (Englewood Cliffs, NJ: Prentice-Hall, 1962).
32. Harold Klein and W. Newman, "How to Use SPIRE: A Systematic Procedure for Identifying Relevant Environments for Strategic Planning," *Journal of Business Strategy* 5 (1980), pp. 32–45.
33. Fahey and Narayanan, *Macroenvironmental Analysis*, p. 39.
34. H. E. Klein and R. E. Linneman, "Environmental Assessment: An International Study of Corporate Practice," *Journal of Business Strategy* 5 (1984), pp. 66–75.
35. David O. Weber, "The Working Uninsured: A Lucrative Market for Innovative Providers," *Healthcare Growth Strategies 2001* (Santa Barbara, CA: COR Health LLC, 2000), pp. 115–121. For details see the SimpleCare website at www.simplecare.com.
36. James L. Webster, William E. Reif, and Jeffery S. Bracker, "The Manager's Guide to Strategic Planning Tools and Techniques," *Planning Review* 17, no. 6 (1989), pp. 4–13 and Pamela Tierney and Steven M. Farmer, "The Pygmalion Process and Employee Creativity," *Journal of Management* 30, no. 3 (2004), pp. 413–432.
37. S. C. Jain, "Environmental Scanning in US Corporations," *Long Range Planning* 17 (1984), p. 125.
38. B. Thompson, D. MacAuley, O. McNally, and S. O'Neill, "Defining Sports Medicine Specialist in the United Kingdom: A Delphi Study," *British Journal of Sports Medicine* 38, no. 2 (2004), pp. 14–18.
39. Ricky W. Griffin and Gregory Moorhead, *Organizational Behavior* (Boston: Houghton Mifflin, 1986), pp. 496–497 and Lucy L. Gilson and Christina E. Shalley, "A Little Creativity Goes A Long Way: An Examination of Teams' Engagement in Creative Processes," *Journal of Management* 30, no. 4 (2004), pp. 453–470.
40. Ibid., pp. 495–496.
41. "CMS Provides Details on Specialty Hospital Moratorium," *Healthcare Financial Management* 58, no. 5 (2004), pp. 12–14.
42. Barbara Karmel, *Point and Counterpoint in Organizational Behavior* (Hinsdale, IL: Dryden Press, 1980), p. 11.
43. Webster, Reif, and Bracker, "The Manager's Guide," p. 13.
44. Ibid.
45. Myron D. Fottler, John D. Blair, Carlton J. Whitehead, Michael D. Laus, and G. T. Savage, "Assessing Key Stakeholders: Who Matters to Hospitals and Why?" *Hospital and Health Services Administration* 34, no. 4 (1989), p. 527.
46. Marco Iansiti and Roy Levien, "Strategy as Ecology," *Harvard Business Review* 82, no. 3 (2004), pp. 68–78.
47. Fottler, Blair, Whitehead, Laus, and Savage, "Assessing Key Stakeholders," p. 532.
48. John D. Blair and J. A. Buesseler, "Competitive Forces in the Medical Group Industry: A Stakeholder Analysis," *Health Care Management Review* 23, no. 2 (1998), pp. 7–27.
49. Don Daake and William P. Anthony, "Understanding Stakeholder Power and Influence Gaps in a Health Care Organization: An Empirical Study," *Health Care Management Review* 25, no. 3 (2000), pp. 94–106.
50. Stuart L. Hart and Sanjay Sharma, "Engaging Fringe Stakeholders for Competitive Imagination," *The Academy of Management Executive* 18, no. 1 (2004), pp. 7–18.
51. Ibid.
52. William E. Halal, "Corporate Community: A Theory of the Firm Uniting Profitability and Responsibility," *Strategy & Leadership* 28, no. 2 (2000), pp. 10–16.
53. Audrey Schriefer, "Getting the Most Out of Scenarios: Advice from the Experts," *Planning Review* 23, no. 5 (1995), pp. 33–35 and J. Alberto Aragón-Correa and Sanjay Sharma, "The Social Side of Creativity: A Static and Dynamic Social Network Perspective," *Academy of Management Review* 28, no. 1 (2003), pp. 89–106.
54. P. Leemhuis, "Using Scenarios to Develop Strategies," *Long Range Planning* 18 (1985), pp. 30–37.

ADDITIONAL READINGS

Capper, Stuart A., Peter M. Ginter, and Linda E. Swayne (eds) *Public Health Management and Leadership: Cases and Context* (Thousand Oaks, CA: Sage Publications, 2002). Two comprehensive industry notes and four chapters provide the context for the 15 public health cases. One industry note profiles the US health care system and the other focuses on the US public health system. The chapters cover case analysis, health care information sources, oral presentations, and health care finance. The 15 cases deal with a variety of community health issues for leaders in public health.

Enthoven, Alain C. and Laura A. Tollen, *Toward the 21st Century Health System* (Indianapolis, IN: Jossey-Bass, 2004). New and significant research is provided in this book that argues pre-paid group practices are a cost-efficient, high-quality alternative to HMOs. Topics include integrated health care systems, quality of care, working with physicians, and financing physician practices.

Kovner, Anthony R. and Steven Jonas, *Jonas & Kovner's Health Care Delivery in the United States,* 7th edn (New York: Springer Publishing, 2004). The authors address emergent and recurring issues such as national and local health care reform, primary care and prevention, alternative medicine, multicultural issues, hospital organization, ethics, physician-assisted suicide, and so on. The book attempts to answer several key questions: How do we assess and understand the health care sector of our economy? Where is health care provided? What are the characteristics of those institutions that provide it? How are the changes in health care systems affecting the health of the population, the cost, and access to care?

Mahoney, Joseph T., *Economic Foundations of Strategy* (Thousand Oaks, CA: Sage Publishing, 2004). This book looks at the essential concepts of business strategy and integrates them with five major theories of the firm. These theories have stood the test of time and provide important insights into the nature of strategy formulation. Applications of the theories of the firm, strategy, and organization are made to management practice.

McGee, Kenneth G., *Heads Up: How to Anticipate Business Surprises and Seize Opportunities First* (Boston, MA: Harvard Business School Press, 2004). Even the worst business crises rarely happen without some warning. Leaders in organizations can minimize the surprises that are too often followed by desperate reactions. The author argues that leaders need to master understanding the present, what is happening now, and develop methods for understanding how current events will affect the future. Potential disasters can be turned into opportunities.

Mitchell, Donald and Carol Coles, *The Ultimate Competitive Advantage* (New York: Berrett-Koehler, 2003). Continuous business model innovation is the key to improving organizational performance. Do not focus solely on doing better what you did poorly yesterday. Instead, find better ways to prepare for unexpected events in the future. It is important to deliver value by developing and implementing a superior management process and fairly reward all stakeholders.

Robinson, Alan G. and Dean M. Schroeder, *Ideas Are Free: How the Idea Revolution Is Liberating People and Transforming Organizations* (Williston, VT: BK Publishers, 2004). People working in the trenches of factories, hospitals, and other organizations often see opportunities and challenges that those managing them miss. Unfortunately, very few organizations take advantage of the revenue-enhancing and cost-reducing knowledge that exists among rank-and-file employees. This book provides recommendations for tapping into this virtually free and perpetually renewable source of ideas and innovations.

3

CHAPTER

Service Area Competitor Analysis

"The competition will bite you if you keep running; if you stand still, they will swallow you."

William Knudsen, Jr.

Introductory Incident

Competition Revs Up in the Indianapolis Service Area

A heart-care building boom is occurring in many cities, although the volume for open heart surgery seems to be declining. Critics believe that over-building may split up heart surgery volume enough that many facilities will not meet Leapfrog-recommended volume standards just at a time when consumers are becoming much more aware of them (see Perspective 6–1 on the Leapfrog Group). For example, in Milwaukee, 13 cardiology programs serve a population of 1.6 million, whereas Cleveland has five open-heart centers for a metropolitan statistical area (MSA) of 2.7 million and Rochester has two programs for a population of 1.1 million.

In the Indianapolis service area, cardiac capacity increased 15–20 percent in the past three years. The reason? MedCath, the for-profit corporation

that built and was operating 13 free-standing heart hospitals, began having discussions with local cardiologists. MedCath partnered with cardiologists, cardiovascular surgeons, and other physicians to deliver patient-focused health care to those with cardiovascular disease. MedCath enabled physicians to be involved in the design and planning of the facility as well as managing its operations. Often physicians were involved in ownership, enabling them to enhance stagnant incomes. MedCath targeted states, such as Indiana, that did not have certificate of need (CON) laws.

As a defensive ploy, and to avoid the potential loss of physicians (and through them, their patients), Indianapolis service area hospitals forged partnerships with physicians to consolidate or expand ▶

heart surgery programs. Each of the four hospital systems – Clarian Health Partners, Community Hospitals of Indianapolis, St. Vincent Hospitals, and Wishard Health Services – built free-standing heart hospitals and two of them – Clarian and St. Vincent – were built as joint ventures with physicians.

Population for Marion County (which includes Indianapolis) is 1.62 million. The Indianapolis MSA includes nine counties with a population of more than 1.8 million. The MSA has more than 3,600 physicians (1.9 per 1,000 population) and 15,800 registered nurses. Although the MSA has 2.5 staffed hospital beds per 1,000 population, the city of Indianapolis has 3.0 staffed beds per 1,000 population.

HMO penetration is low in the city (21 percent and declining); most of the 22 major employers (including Eli Lilly, Anthem, Inc., and Conseco, Inc. on the Fortune 500 list) offer PPOs. About 12 percent of the population is without health insurance (13 percent in the county). In both the city and the county 11 percent of the population is over 65 years of age (compared with an average of 15 percent for the United States).

Indianapolis had been a city where health care was described as "genteel competition" but that is no longer the case. Competition among the hospitals has intensified as several of the systems have built new hospitals or significantly renovated older facilities in what has traditionally been others' geographic market areas. Some of the construction is designed to move services of flagship hospitals to more lucrative, faster growing areas (outside the city limits of Indianapolis). In addition, St. Vincent's Hospital opened a children's hospital to compete with Clarian's Riley Children's Hospital (affiliated with Indiana University and historically the only children's hospital in the region). Orthopedics groups were announcing plans to open orthopedic hospitals and oncologists were in discussions with a for-profit national company, spurring hospitals to build additional outpatient cancer facilities.

In addition, there has been friction among the physicians at Indiana University and Methodist Hospital (merged in 1997 to become Clarian Health Partners) such that many physicians affiliated with Methodist have left to go to competing hospitals, undermining Clarian's dominant market position.

Health and medical care in the Indianapolis service area is very competitive. With population growth, will demand for cardiac services increase 20 percent over the next few years to utilize the new facilities? Will each of the heart centers perform sufficient numbers of surgeries to remain competitive? Which of the systems will be survivors in such a competitive market?

Source: Aaron Katz, Robert E. Hurley, Kelly Devers, Leslie Jackson Conwell, Bradley C. Strunk, Andrea Staiti, J. Lee Hargraves, and Robert A. Bereson, "Competition Revs Up the Indianapolis Health Care Market," *Community Report No. 1: Indianapolis* (Washington, DC: Center for Studying Health System Change, Winter 2003) and Michelle Rogers, "Cardiovascular Services: Heart Race," *HealthLeaders* (January 28, 2004) at http://www.healthleaders.com/magazine/cover.

Learning Objectives

After completing this chapter the student should be able to:

1. Understand the importance of service area competitor analysis as well as its purpose.

2. Understand the relationship between general and health care environmental issue identification and analysis and service area competitor analysis.

3. Define and analyze the service area for a health care organization or specific health service.

4. Conduct a service area structure analysis for a health care organization.

5. Understand strategic groups and be able to map competitors' strategies along important service and market dimensions.

6. Understand the elements of service area competitor analysis and assess likely competitor strategies.

7. Aggregate general environmental and health care industry issues with service area and competitor issues and synthesize specific strategy implications.

8. Suggest several questions to initiate strategic thinking concerning the service area and competitors as a part of managing the strategic momentum.

Further Focus in External Environmental Analysis

Environmental analysis involves strategic thinking and strategic planning, focusing on increasingly more specific issues. Chapter 2, "Understanding and Analyzing the General Environment and the Health Care Environment," provided the fundamental approach and strategic thinking frameworks for scanning, monitoring, forecasting, and assessing trends and issues in the environment. However, once the general and industry trends and issues in the external environment have been identified and assessed, a more specific analysis is required. As shown in Exhibit 2–1, service area competitor analysis is the third part of a comprehensive environmental analysis. *Service area competitor analysis* attempts to further define and understand an organization's environment through identifying specific service area/service category issues, identifying its competitors, determining the strengths and weaknesses of these rivals, and anticipating their strategic moves. It involves collecting data concerning the service area and rivals to analyze and interpret the data for strategic decision making.[1]

The Service Area

The *service area* is considered to be the geographic area surrounding the health care provider from which it pulls the majority of its customers/patients. It is usually limited by fairly well-defined geographic borders. Beyond these borders, services may be difficult to render because of distance, cost, time, and so on. Therefore, a health care organization must not only define its service area but must also analyze in detail all relevant and important aspects of the service area, including economic, demographic, psychographic (lifestyle), and disease pattern characteristics.[2]

The service area is defined by customers' preferences and the health care providers that are available. Certainly, the consumer has become empowered by the amount of information available concerning disease conditions and providers (see Perspective 3–1). Exhibit 3–1 shows the determinants of a service area

Perspective 3–1
The Empowered Patient – Challenge and Opportunity

The empowered patient has become a significant presence in the health care environment and a challenge for health care organizations. With confidence gained from Internet access and media exposure, the patient often has an opinion and may not appreciate the paternalistic style of health care delivery, no matter how well-intentioned. "Informed" consumers expect to be participating partners in their own health care and when their families need care.

There is an upside to this challenge. Fully informed patients who participate in the decision process are more likely to be satisfied with their care and to adhere to the treatment advice.[1] Treatments will reflect patient preferences and values. Patient expectations will be knowledge-based. The challenge is to make sure that the patient's information is based on good evidence.

To become a fully informed and participating partner, a patient must experience the following process: (1) The patient must obtain an accurate understanding of the risks or seriousness of the condition. (2) The patient must understand the risks, benefits, and uncertainties of the treatment under consideration and the alternatives. (3) The patient must have weighed his or her values as they relate to the potential harm and benefit of the treatment. (4) The patient must have had the opportunity to participate in the decisionmaking process at whatever level he or she desires.[2]

Health care providers may see this task as unreasonable in the face of reduced reimbursements and the pressure to streamline care. However, failure to ensure that the patient is fully informed will leave a void to be filled by other suppliers of information. Such information may be poorly researched or subtly biased to serve ulterior motives. Providers who succeed in this educational endeavor will gain their patient's trust and loyalty. The power of this approach can be seen on the web page of Cancer Treatment Centers of America. Their message presents their model of "Patient Empowered Medicine" as an argument for choosing their centers over the more traditional medical center.

As patients are asked to face higher deductibles and cost sharing of premiums, this empowerment phenomenon seems even more appropriate. Providers need patients to be active partners in the redesign of a delivery system that is more efficient and is available to everyone. The empowered patient should fit well into the health care system of tomorrow.

Notes
1. R. Grol, "Improving the Quality of Medical Care: Building Bridges Among Professional Pride, Payer Profit, and Patient Satisfaction," *JAMA* 286, no. 20 (2001), pp. 2578–2586.
2. S. Sheridan, R. Harris, and S. Woolf, "Shared Decision Making About Screening and Chemoprevention," *American Journal of Preventive Medicine* 26, no. 1 (2004), pp. 56–66.

Source: Edmond F. Tipton, MD, MBA, and PhD student, University of Alabama at Birmingham.

Exhibit 3–1: Service Area Determinants

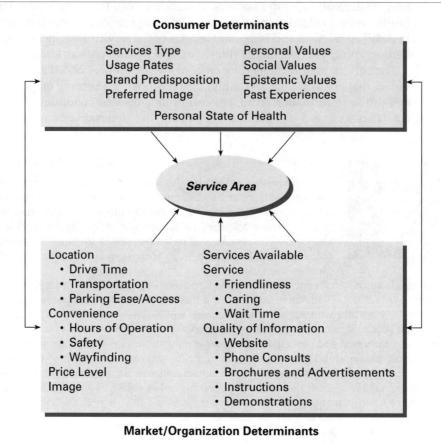

Consumer Determinants

Services Type   Personal Values
Usage Rates   Social Values
Brand Predisposition   Epistemic Values
Preferred Image   Past Experiences
Personal State of Health

Service Area

Location
- Drive Time
- Transportation
- Parking Ease/Access

Convenience
- Hours of Operation
- Safety
- Wayfinding

Price Level
Image

Services Available
Service
- Friendliness
- Caring
- Wait Time

Quality of Information
- Website
- Phone Consults
- Brochures and Advertisements
- Instructions
- Demonstrations

Market/Organization Determinants

including the consumer variables and the market (provider) variables. For the consumer, the services need could include health care that is preventive, diagnostic, alternative, routine, episodic, acute, or chronic. Usage rate would be related to a variety of economic, demographic, psychographic, and disease pattern variables. Brand predisposition indicates the consumer has a preference for some health care providers over others. For example, if there is only one hospital in town, and the consumer does not like its "looks," location, or perceived quality of care, he or she may prefer to drive to the nearest larger city. For routine medical care, some consumers prefer to go to specialists; others prefer a primary care doctor; still others prefer clinics that have primary care physicians and specialists; and, finally, some consumers prefer physician assistants or nurse practitioners. These different consumer preferences will be determinants in defining the service area.

Another group of consumer determinants will be related to personal factors such as personal and social values, epistemic (knowledge) values, past experiences, and the individual's personal state of health. In concert, these variables develop the individual's preferences for health care providers. However, if providers are not available in that there are limited or no options in the immediate area, the consumer will travel greater distances to gain the desired care.

Options or choices are controlled by the health care structure. The market and organizations within it determine what will be offered or made available to the consumer. The "market" contains health care providers in a variety of locations that bear on convenience and image. Location includes drive time from home (or, increasingly, work), availability of transportation, as well as access and parking ease. Convenience may be hours of operation, safety, availability of food, signs to assist in finding the way, and so on. Image for the market entails positioning among the various providers. The health care provider might have the image of being more caring, friendlier, or more high-tech; or it may be perceived as attracting desirable or undesirable demographic, socioeconomic, or ethnic groups. The organization itself has an image of the services (health care provided) as well as the service and the quality of information provided. Location, convenience, and image are all in relationship to the other providers in the area, including those within driving distance and those that are remote but perceived as providing better quality, further services, or other desirable characteristics. Health care providers make these decisions, in part, based on their understanding of consumers' needs and wants.

Managed care interrupts the normal decision making by consumers. An employed individual today usually has some choice in health care insurance. The employer may offer one or more different health plans. However, once the consumer has selected a managed care plan, the ability to choose providers – both hospitals and physicians – becomes more restrictive. And, in fact, the more the HMO attempts to control health care costs by further structuring health care delivery, the more restricted the choice becomes for consumers. Restricted choice is not favored by most Americans and they have been quite vocal about it with their employers. The result is that many employers are only willing to commit to a health plan that offers choice (and thereby removes the quantity discounts previously offered) and, hence, organizations have seen health care cost increases in double digits again.

Competitor Analysis

In addition to the trends and issues associated with the service area, health care organizations must focus specifically on service area competitors. Business organizations have long engaged in competitor analysis, viewing it as an essential part of environmental analysis. These companies have learned that focusing on competitor analysis aids in the identification of new business opportunities, the clarification of emerging ideas, improved ability to anticipate surprises, and the development of market penetration and market share growth strategies.[3] As a matter of fact, one well-documented reason Japanese automobile firms were able to penetrate the US market successfully, especially during the 1970s, was that they were much better at doing competitor analysis than US firms.[4] For business organizations the task of understanding the industry and specific competitors is a challenge; it is far more difficult for health care organizations because consumers will travel great distances for some kinds of care. For example, people from around the world travel to the Mayo Clinic in Rochester, Minnesota for care.

In the past, general environmental and industry analysis were sufficient for most health care organizations. General and health care industry technological, social, political, regulatory, economic, and competitive issues provided enough information to make most strategic decisions. Service area competitor moves and countermoves were not that important. However, during the past decade, because of fundamental changes within the industry brought about by the influences of managed care, efforts to reduce costs and increase efficiency, and the increased presence of for-profit health care organizations, every segment of the industry has become highly competitive. Certainly, as suggested in the Introductory Incident, aggressive competition has entered the health care market in Indianapolis.

CHALLENGES FOR THE HEALTH CARE MARKET

Analyzing this new competitive environment is difficult for health care organizations for a variety of reasons. Perhaps most obvious is that in the recent past very few health care organizations were concerned with competition. In fact, those in the "helping professions" believed there was no need to compete. Hospitals, long-term care facilities, and physicians were more concerned with trying to meet the demand for their services. This history of noncompetition changed when legislation led to an increased number of hospital beds and an increased number of physicians (particularly within certain specialties). Eventually, the oversupply led to a more competitive environment. As discussed in Perspective 3–2, in health care, competition has occurred between health plans, health care networks, and hospital systems when perhaps health care organizations should instead compete on specific disease treatment and outcomes.

Another major reason for the lack of competitor analysis within health care is that the separation of consumers of health services (patients) from payors (insurance companies and employers) provided few checks on the system. When all the health care providers in a service area were well paid by insured patients, increasingly higher costs for more and more services provided to insured as well as uninsured patients were passed on to the insured patients. This "cost shifting" became a major concern in the tight economy of the early 1990s, and again in the first years of the twenty-first century, because employers paid for most insurance coverage for their employees. When US companies felt they could no longer be competitive in world markets because of high health care costs, they began searching for ways to decrease the burden. They brought pressure on health care providers to reduce costs and began focusing on price competition. Employers began requiring employees to pay a higher portion of the health care costs (higher premiums, co-pays, and then higher co-pays) and businesses became increasingly interested in "managing health care."

The philosophy of managed care was that by controlling consumer choice to a limited number of providers, greater buying power was achieved through economies of scale. When patients' choices of hospitals or physicians were

Perspective 3–2

Redefining Competition in Health Care

According to Michael Porter and Elizabeth Teisberg, in healthy competition: ongoing improvements in processes and methods drive down costs; product/service quality improves; innovation leads to improvements which are quickly adopted; uncompetitive producers go out of business; value-adjusted prices fall; and the market expands. However, in health care: costs are high and rising, despite efforts to reduce them; rising costs are not the direct result of improvements in quality; medical services are restricted (rationed to those who can pay); patients receive care that is not the current accepted practice; and high rates of medical error continue. In addition, considerable variation in cost and quality occurs among providers and across geographic areas. Diffusion of best practices takes, on average, 17 years to become standard practice.

Clearly the health care system is broken but the authors do not advocate that government takes over and "solves" the problem. Rather, they suggest that business could cause changes to occur if employers were to insist on competition occurring at the right level. For Porter and Teisberg, problems in health care occur because the competition is at the level of health plans, networks, and hospital systems whereas the "right level" is competition to care for the various health conditions or diseases. If providers competed directly across a broad geographic area for cardiac patients, for example, businesses would pay a premium for best results. The provider with the best results would attract patients and would be imitated quickly or the other providers (who did not achieve good results) would end up with no patients. Currently, hospitals and physicians are paid to provide care for the citizens in a service area regardless of the quality of outcomes.

According to the authors, wrong forms of competition include:

- Annual competition among health plans to sign subscribers (effectively blocking competition at the disease level);
- Deep discounting to payors/employers with large patient populations (it does not cost less to treat a patient employed by a large business versus a small one);
- Provider concentration that does not create patient value but boosts bargaining power;
- Cost shifting that creates no patient value;
- Local competition insulating mediocre providers and inhibiting the use of best practices;
- Suppressing information that would enable patients to choose the best provider (many providers do not even make available how many patients they have treated for a specific disease/condition);
- Incentives for payors to enroll healthy people and deny coverage to sick people (and complicate the billing process); and
- Not referring to other providers with more experience.

Porter and Teisberg believe positive competition occurs when:

- Providers develop distinctivenesses (create unique value);
- No restrictions are placed on patients' selection of providers;
- Pricing is transparent;
- Billing is simplified;
- Information is easily accessible and comparable;
- Non-discriminatory insurance underwriting is available (large risk pools for small businesses);
- Fewer lawsuits reduce defensive medicine; and
- Minimum levels of coverage are offered.

Companies have purchased health care on the basis of cost not quality. If employers were to refocus their goals to have healthy employees, they would buy health care differently. Competition would be efficient – the best providers would thrive and those delivering inferior service would go out of business.

Source: Michael E. Porter and Elizabeth O. Teisberg, "Redefining Competition in Health Care," *Harvard Business Review* 82, no. 6 (June 2004), pp. 65–76.

limited, strong competition emerged among health care providers for the managed care organization's insured group. Physicians, notably primary care physicians, became "gatekeepers" into the system and attempted to direct patients to only one hospital to obtain the best possible rates. Hospitals "competed" for these desirable contracts.

In the first decade of the twenty-first century, managed care has produced considerable backlash from physicians, who do not want managed care "bureaucrats" telling them how they should practice medicine, and from consumers, who want choices. Some state legislatures have enacted laws dictating to HMOs the minimum length of stay for various diseases and conditions. The federal government and several state legislatures are investigating a patient's bill of rights. Exclusive contracts have been replaced by greater choice for employees by employers – multiple health plans to choose from – and greater choice within a specific plan – the option to go outside the plan to seek care from a specific physician who might not be a member of that particular plan. The result, according to the *Interstudy Competitive Edge Report 4.0*, is that HMO enrollment has declined from around 80 million in 1999 to less than 72 million in 2003.[5]

STRATEGIC SIGNIFICANCE OF COMPETITOR ANALYSIS

Within the health care community there is a growing understanding that health care organizations must be positioned effectively vis-à-vis their competitors. Competitor information is essential for selecting viable strategies that position the organization strongly within the market. Many health care managers agree that an organized competitor intelligence system is necessary for survival. The system acts like an interlinked radar grid constantly monitoring competitor activity, filtering the raw information picked up by external and internal sources, processing it for strategic significance, and efficiently communicating actionable intelligence to those who need it.[6]

The pharmaceutical industry makes extensive use of competitive intelligence gathering – estimates are that more than $20 billion per year is used on government filings, trade news, and market research. A number of services, such as DRUGLAUNCH, DRUGNL, and DRUGUPDATES provide information on R&D activities, new product launches, and patent analysis for the US market as well as around the globe.[7] Others, such as PHAR (Pharmaprojects) and PHIN (Pharmaceutical and Healthcare Industry News), provide information on new product development in major markets worldwide through publications and prepublication news. A relatively new competitive intelligence company, Skila (named after Dustin Hoffman's secret agent brother in *Marathon Man*), goes beyond data gathering to information analysis (see Perspective 3–3).

The Focus of Competitor Analysis

An organization engages in *competitor analysis* to gain a general understanding of the competitors in the service area, identify any vulnerabilities of the competitors,

Perspective 3–3

Skila Is a Secret Weapon

Skila is an information services company that operates as a virtual intelligence officer by improving decision making in the pharmaceutical, medical device, and biotechnology industries. Its Internet-based information system combines all the pieces of data, sifts and sorts them, and then selects just the information that clients need to make decisions about their products and markets. Leveraging its proprietary Intelligration® technology, services, and methodology, Skila integrates all relevant information and people into a *Single Touch Point* (Skila's term for a sophisticated database accessible by all members of a team, department, group, or organization) to deliver the right information, to the right people, at the right time, for commercialization processes. By providing fast and easy access to up-to-date, dynamic, and relevant knowledge to brand management (improving the coordination across subteams), alliance management (enabling alliance partners to function as a single fast, agile, and effective team), medical teams (helping build and maintain the support of opinion-leading physicians with local, regional, national, and global influence), and managed markets (creating access and coordinating pull-through), Skila offers technology that rapidly brings together a variety of information and people relevant to the achievement of the organization's objectives.

Skila's strategic advantage is well-packaged information and a delivery system full of "bells and whistles" to create its Intelligration® platform. The system seeks and automatically integrates information from Skila's proprietary research, a client's own databases and computer banks, and third-party sources such as Lexis/Nexis, Edgar, and Medline. Intelligration® summarizes huge amounts of data and then consolidates, categorizes, and organizes all relevant information based on the client's requirements. The client's team is able to find the precise information needed to make effective business decisions by aligning objectives and increasing the speed of access to relevant knowledge. The system sends the data through various tags, filters, and matching programs to develop what lands on the client's desk – a comprehensive but tightly focused report on, for example, treating psoriasis, that is delivered electronically in the morning and added to or updated daily until the decision maker feels that he or she can develop closure.

Skila's service offers three benefits:

1. One-stop shopping for information;
2. Content determined by the client's business needs; and
3. Information delivered directly to decision makers.

Skila's service offers time and money savings as well as better intelligence to provide "knowledge for the business of health care."

Source: Company sources.

assess the impact of its own strategic actions against specific competitors, and identify potential moves that a competitor might make that would endanger the organization's position in the market. Analyzing competitors assists organizations in identifying a clear *competitive advantage* – some basis on which they are willing to compete with anyone. Competitive advantage is the means by which the organization seeks to develop cost advantage or to differentiate itself from other organizations. Organizations constantly take offensive and defensive actions in their quests for competitive advantage vis-à-vis competitors.[8] Competitive advantage might be centered on image, high-quality services, an excellent and widely recognized staff, or efficiency and low cost, among others.

It is useful to classify competitor information as general, offensive, and defensive. This classification system will aid in strategy development.

General competitor information is important for an organization to:

- avoid surprises in the marketplace;
- provide a forum for leaders to discuss and evaluate their assumptions about the organization's capabilities, market position, and competition;
- make everyone aware of significant and formidable competitors to whom the organization must respond;
- help the organization learn from rivals through benchmarking (specific measures comparing the organization with its competitors on a set of key variables);
- build consensus among executives on the organization's goals and capabilities, thus increasing their commitment to the chosen strategy; and
- foster strategic thinking throughout the organization.

Offensive competitor information is helpful to:

- identify market niches and discontinuities,
- select a viable strategy, and
- contribute to the successful implementation of the strategy.

Defensive competitor information will aid in:

- anticipating competitors' moves, and
- shortening the time required to respond (countermoves) to a competitor's moves.

Depending on the intent of the competitor analysis, an organization might use all of these categories or just one or two. For example, in the early stages of competitor analysis, the organization may seek only general information. As an organization plans to enter new markets, offensive information may be the primary focus of the competitor analysis. In the face of strategic moves by a powerful competitor, defensive information may take precedence. In large, complex markets, all of these information categories are appropriate and essential for positioning the organization.

Impediments to Effective Competitor Analysis

Monitoring the actions and understanding the intentions of competitors is often difficult. Health care executives agree that it is necessary and growing in importance, yet they are still not doing effective competitor analysis. Six common impediments or "blind spots" have been identified that slow an organization's response to its competitors' moves or even cause the selection of the wrong competitive approach. Flawed competitor analysis, resulting from these blind spots, weakens an organization's capacity to seize opportunities or interact effectively with its rivals, ultimately leading to an erosion in the organization's market position and profitability.[9] The six impediments to effective competitor analysis include:

- misjudging industry and service area boundaries,
- poor identification of the competition,
- overemphasis on competitors' visible competence,
- overemphasis on where, rather than how, to compete,
- faulty assumptions about the competition, and
- paralysis by analysis.[10]

CLEARLY DEFINED SERVICE AREA

A major contribution of competitor analysis is the development of a clear defini-tion of the industry, industry segment, or service area. To avoid a focus that is too narrow, the industry, industry segment, and service area must be defined in the broadest terms that are useful. In today's health care environment, competition may come from very nontraditional competitors (outside the health care industry). For instance, based on their experience in the hotel business, the Marriott Cor-poration entered the long-term care and retirement center markets. Utilizing its expertise in accommodations management, Marriott created Senior Living Services in 1984. In 2000, the corporation had 144 senior living communities in 29 states with others under development. Marriott's mission statement for its Senior Living Centers is summed up in two words: "We Care." Accommodations for independent and assisted living, Alzheimer's and other memory loss disorders, and nursing care were provided.[11] However, by mid-2003, Marriott had concluded that even inde-pendent senior living centers were not part of its core competency and sold Senior Living Services to Sunrise Senior Living and a number of its properties to CNL Retirement Properties, Inc. The total sale amounted to almost $350 million. In the past, multihospital systems and nursing home chains dominated this industry seg-ment. As competition increases from nontraditional competitors, social activities, décor, meals, and housekeeping may become more important competitive factors.

Typically, health care managers have focused their analysis on locally served markets. Patients were treated by the local doctor, in a local hospital (or the closest one available). There was little travel for medical or health care. Thus, doctors and hospitals were insulated from other health care organizations outside their geographic service area; however, that is no longer the case. Market entry by com-petitors from outside the metropolitan area, the region, or the state is now quite common. For example, expansion by multihospital for-profit systems such as HCA–The Healthcare Company (formerly Columbia/HCA) and Tenet represent serious new competitive challenges in many markets. MedCath has built specialty hospitals in a number of markets for cardiac care. Nationally recognized clinics, such as the Mayo Clinic and the Cleveland Clinic, have expanded to locations in Florida and Arizona. A health care organization that maintains a local or regional focus may be delayed in recognizing changes in the service area boundaries.

COMPETITOR IDENTIFICATION

Often, only cursory attention is given to other segments of the health care industry. Hospitals traditionally focused on acute care. They were not concerned with intermediate care or home care as a competing segment. Yet, because of length-of-stay issues, patients have been sent to an intermediate care or home care situation outside the hospital's purview, which increased revenues to those organizations and decreased the hospital's revenues. For hospitals to survive, integrated delivery systems, seamless care, and continuum of care emerged. As a result there are fewer but more direct competitors in many market areas today. Clearly, misjudging how the industry, industry segments, or service area is defined will lead to poor competitor analysis.

Another possible flaw of competitor analysis is the improper or poor identification of precisely which organizations are the competitors. In many cases, health care executives focus on a single established major competitor and ignore emerging or lesser-known potential competitors. This is especially true when the perceived strengths of competitor organizations do not fit traditional measures or there is an inflexible commitment to historical critical success factors (traditional inpatient services instead of outpatient approaches). Academic medical centers, with their focus on research, have traditionally viewed only other academic medical centers as competitors. However, with the impact of managed care and lowered reimbursements, some of them are in real danger of having to close.

INFORMATION ABOUT COMPETITORS

Another problem in performing competitor analysis is the tendency to be concerned only with the visible activities of competitors. Less visible attributes and capabilities such as organizational structure, culture, human resources, service features, intellectual capital, management acumen, and strategy may cause misinterpretation of a competitor's strengths or strategic intent. Certainly the Mayo Clinic's strong culture of excellence has played an important role in shaping its strategic decisions. Similarly, in an environment of rapid change, intellectual capital represents a primary value creation asset of the organization.[12] In addition, effective competitor analysis requires predicting how competitors plan to position themselves. Although often difficult, determining competitors' strategic intent is at the heart of competitor analysis. An effective competitor analysis should focus on what rivals can do with their resources, capabilities, and competencies – an extension of what competitors are currently doing – and include possible radical departures from existing strategies.[13]

Accurate and timely information concerning competitors is extremely important in competitor analysis. Misjudging or underestimating competitors' resources, capabilities, or competencies is a serious misstep. Faulty assumptions can suggest inappropriate strategies for an organization. Poor environmental scanning perpetuates faulty assumptions.

Because of the sheer volume of data that can be collected concerning the external environment and competition, paralysis by analysis can occur. In environments undergoing profound change, huge quantities of data are generated and access to it becomes easier. Under such conditions, information overload is possible and separating the essential from the nonessential is often difficult. As a result, it should be emphasized that the intent of competitor analysis is to support strategic decision making; overanalysis or "endless" analysis should be avoided. Competitor information must be focused and contribute to strategy formulation.

A Process for Service Area Competitor Analysis

Service area competitor analysis is a process of understanding the market and identifying and evaluating competitors. Together with the general and health care trends and issues, service area competitor analysis must be synthesized into the strategic issues facing the organization. The synthesis will be an explicit input into the formulation of the organization's strategy.

As illustrated in the strategic thinking map in Exhibit 3–2, service area competitor analysis begins with an understanding and specification of services or service categories the organization provides to its customers. Next, the service area must be specified for the various services or service categories. Then the service area structure or competitive dynamics should be assessed. Competitors providing services in the same category in and around the service area must be analyzed. Each of the organizations can be positioned against the important dimensions of the market and assessed as to their likely strategic moves. Finally, the results of the analysis must be synthesized and implications drawn. These conclusions will provide important information for strategy formulation.

Exhibit 3–2: Service Area Competitor Analysis

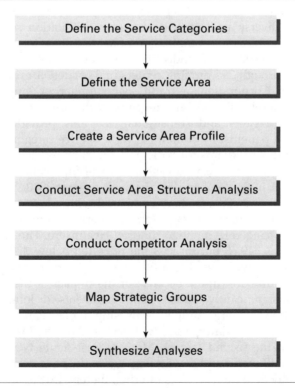

Defining the Service Categories

The first step in service area competitor analysis is to specify the *service category* to be analyzed. Many health care organizations have several service categories or products, and each may have different geographic and demographic service areas. For a multihospital chain deciding to enter a new market, the service category may be defined as acute hospital care, but for a rehabilitation hospital, the service category might be defined as physical therapy or occupational therapy or orthopedic surgery. In addition, because many health care services can be broken down into more specific subservices, the level of service category specificity should be agreed on before analysis begins. For example, pediatric care may be broken down into well-baby care, infectious diseases, developmental pediatrics, pediatric hematology-oncology, and so on. Certainly pediatric hematology-oncology as a service category would have a far larger service area than well-baby care. A parent with a child who has cancer would travel farther for care from a specialist than a parent who sought well-baby care available from nurse practitioners.

Another example of a service that requires a clear definition is the subacute care segment. Subacute care, sometimes termed the middle ground of health care, provides services for those patients who no longer require inpatient acute care, but need a higher level of care than can be provided in a skilled-nursing facility or through home care. There are multiple ways to segment this market that includes diverse post-acute care and rehabilitation services. An organization could select one or a combination of services to offer within subacute care. For example, Vencor, Inc., founded in 1985, provides long-term care and rehabilitation services through 295 nursing centers in 31 states. It grew rapidly by purchasing Hillhaven Corporation, a traditional supplier of long-term care; TheraTx, a provider of rehabilitation and respiratory therapy program management services to nursing centers; and Transitional Hospitals, providers of care for ventilator-dependent patients. By combining these service categories the company focused on treatment programs for patients with complex medical conditions. However, its strategy was not very successful: Vencor filed voluntary reorganization under Chapter 11 in September 1999. In third quarter 2000, Vencor reported a loss of $27 million or $0.38 per share compared with a loss of $42 million or $0.61 per share in third quarter 1999.[14] Vencor emerged from the reorganization in April 2001 and changed its name to Kindred Healthcare. The 52-week high for its stock in 2002 was $49.78 but in 2003 the price fell below $20 per share. By mid-2004 the stock had rebounded to a little over $25 per share. Many long-term care facilities are in bankruptcy because of the impact of the Balanced Budget Act of 1997 that significantly reduced reimbursements for long-term care.

In addition, several competitor nursing home chains, such as the largest in the industry, Beverly Enterprises, with 550 facilities in 30 states and 62,878 licensed beds, and the second largest, Mariner Post-Acute Network, with over 430 facilities in 40 states and 50,686 licensed beds, have added subacute care for the chronically ill to their services offering, thereby further increasing competition for

Vencor. On the other hand, the number of seniors requiring care is projected to rise drastically in the near future. Thus, to have a clear idea of what is to be accomplished by the service area competitor analysis, it is important to first understand and define the service category, starting narrowly with direct competitors, but then expanding the category to include more indirect competitors.

Plastic surgery is a medical specialty that can be defined as a service category. However, there are additional service categories that need to be explored to determine direct and indirect competitors. For instance, reconstructive plastic surgeons often specialize on the face, dealing with congenital deformities and injuries due to trauma. Eye, ear, nose, and throat physicians as well as oral surgeons are performing some of the same procedures. Cosmetic plastic surgeons may offer a full range of services including reconstructive surgery, or they may specialize on the face, breast, or other body parts. Furthermore, they may specialize on the basis of procedures they use, such as laser or liposuction. Thus, to understand how customers perceive the organization's service category is an important determination for a beneficial service area competitor analysis.

Determining Service Area Boundaries

Understanding the geographic boundaries is important in defining the service area, but is often difficult because of the variety of services offered. In an acute care hospital, the service area for cardiac services may be the entire state or region, whereas the service area for the emergency room might be only a few blocks. Thus, for a health care organization that offers several service categories, it may be necessary to conduct several service area analyses. For example, the Des Moines, Iowa, market has two geographic components: the metropolitan area of the city as well as the suburbs of Polk County (population approximately 350,000) and the 43 primarily rural counties of central Iowa that surround the capital (population about 1 million). The opportunities and threats for each of these multiple service areas may be quite different; therefore, considerable effort is directed toward understanding and analyzing the nature of the health care organization's various service areas. At the same time, for some organizations, defining only one service category may suffice (such as in the case of a long-term care facility).

Service areas will be different for different organizations. A national for-profit hospital chain may define its service area quite generally, but even then there may be different strategies in place. For example, HCA–The Healthcare Company's strategy is to become a major health care presence in highly concentrated markets, whereas Health Management Associates' strategy is to only enter nonurban markets. An individual hospital, home health care organization, or HMO may define its service area much more specifically. In general, health services are provided and received within a well-defined service area, where the competition is clearly identified and critical forces for the survival of the organization originate. For instance, hospitals in rural areas have well-defined service areas for their particular services. These hospitals must be familiar with the needs of the population and with other organizations providing competing services. Some of the competitive

Perspective 3–4
Small Community Hospitals Can Compete

Small community hospitals face a number of challenges. They cannot offer the depth and breadth of physician subspecialties and clinical professionals as academic medical centers and integrated health care systems. They face considerable patient out-migration to larger competitors in nearby or distant markets, especially when consumers with the desire and means to shop around perceive that the local provider offers low quality. In addition, small community hospitals often are weaker financially because they have limited access to capital, they have a larger proportion of underinsured and uninsured to treat, and they encounter diseconomies of scale because of lower patient volumes. Yet small community hospitals do have their own strengths and can compete effectively with academic health centers and larger health care networks for services that are appropriately delivered in the community hospital setting. Bigger is not always better.

Today, there is considerable evidence that the customer is beginning to drive health care. Customers are exercising considerable influence over the selection, purchase, and use of health care products and services. Forces contributing to consumer-directed health care include the number of baby boomers aging into retirement, higher education levels and greater access to medical and health care information through the Internet, advances in technology and science (accompanied by consumer expectation to access the latest innovations in pharmaceuticals and treatments), public pressure to scrutinize provider quality and patient safety, and the shifting of more of the risk and burden for health care to consumers through higher co-pays, defined contribution plans, and other financial incentive plans. In addition, pay-for-performance initiatives are developing among government, employers, and insurors. Measures of quality performance are required for many of these initiatives and provider "scorecards" are increasingly available.

All hospitals are facing increased expectations to deliver quality care. Quality is definitely an issue given:

- According to the Institute of Medicine reports, between 44,000 and 98,000 Americans die annually from medical error;[1]
- Only 55 percent of patients sampled from 12 metropolitan areas received recommended care, whether for acute episodes, chronic conditions, or prevention;[2]
- The lag between the discovery of more effective treatment and incorporation into routine patient care is 17 years;[3]
- The Institute of Medicine reports that 18,000 Americans die each year from heart attacks because they did not receive preventative medications for which they were eligible;[4]
- The Institute of Health reports that more than 50 percent of patients with diabetes, hypertension, tobacco addiction, hyperlipidemia, congestive heart failure, asthma, depression, and chronic fibrillation are currently managed inadequately.[5]

According to consultants with The Strategy Group (TSG), "Academic medical centers and large clinically advanced hospital systems often draw headlines and build brand reputations with miraculous medical breakthroughs that most health care consumers are fortunate enough to never need. This is not the arena in which community and rural hospitals should, or can, compete." They point out that the health care needs and illnesses of many consumers can be treated and managed in the small community hospital. For example, diabetes, pneumonia, heart attack, and heart failure can be treated locally through the adoption and application of evidence-based standards of medicine. A smaller facility that adheres to standards and objective measures of performance can stand up against a larger competitor.

For the most part, the standards of care reporting requirements are not focused on rare or complex surgeries and procedures; nor do they require extensive investment in staff and technology. For instance, evidence-based protocols for acute myocardial infarction include aspirin on arrival, aspirin prescribed at ▶

discharge, beta-blocker on arrival, beta-blocker prescribed at discharge, and ACE inhibitor for left ventricular systolic dys-function. Over time, a small community or rural hospital can adhere to the standards and objective measures and perform better than many larger competitors. In this situation, a smaller hospital is not necessarily at a disadvantage because a larger hospital with "failing grades" will struggle more to turn it around than a small hospital that is quick to grasp the opportunity to do what it does very well.

The authors conclude, "Embracing targeted clinical excellence is likely to be the most important initiative of the decade for community hospitals. Success will be defined by the speed and scope of clinical improvement, physician participation/commitment to the strategy, and then the organization's ability to create customer preference for superior care." A community hospital will need to achieve clinical excellence and then market it to an ever more educated health care consumer. Consumers want quality care and prefer to stay in their community if they can receive it there.

Notes

1. Linda Kohn, Janet M. Corrigan, and Molla S. Donaldson (eds) *To Err is Human: Building a Safer Health System* (Washington, DC: Committee on Quality of Health Care in America, Institute of Medicine, 2000).
2. Elizabeth McGlynn, Steven M. Asch, John Adams, Joan Keesey, Jennifer Hicks, Alison DeCristofaro, and Eve A. Kerr, "The Quality of Health Care Delivered to Adults in the United States," *New England Journal of Medicine* 348, no. 26 (June 26, 2003), pp. 2635–2646.
3. E. Andrew Balas, "Information Systems Can Prevent Errors and Improve Quality," *Journal of the American Informatics Association* 8, no. 4 (July–August 2001), pp. 398–399.
4. Karen Adams and Janet M. Corrigan (eds) *Priority Areas for National Action: Transforming Health Care Quality* (Washington, DC: Committee on Identifying Priority Areas for Quality Improvement, Institute of Medicine, 2003).
5. Institute of Health 2003 and *Sixth Report of the Joint National Committee on Prevention, Detection, Evaluation, and Treatment of High Blood Pressure* (Washington, DC: National Institutes of Health, November 1997).

Source: Karen V. Corrigan and Robert H. Ryan, MD, "Community Hospitals Can Leverage Unique Strengths to 'Raise the Quality Bar' in their Market," *COR Healthcare Market Strategist* 5, no. 8 (August 2004), pp. 1, 21–24.

challenges of small community hospitals are discussed in Perspective 3–4. Similarly, the service areas for public health departments vary within a state, depending on whether they are metropolitan or rural, and may suggest quite different opportunities and threats.[15]

Determining the geographic boundaries of the service area may be highly subjective and is usually based on patient histories, the reputation of the organization, available technology, physician recognition, and so on. In addition, geographic impediments such as a river, mountains, and limited access highways can influence how the service area is defined. The definition of communities (see Perspective 3–5) is often helpful in determining a service area.

SERVICE AREA PROFILE

Once the geographic boundaries of the service area have been defined, a general service area profile should be developed. Capturing the dimensions of a service area requires tapping and synthesizing information from various sources:

- both quantitative and qualitative data for framing and understanding a service area;

- population-based health status data (specifics of the various health dimensions of an entire population and its subgroups); and
- health services utilization data (specifics on the patterns and frequency of health service use for various health conditions by different groups of individuals in the population).[16]

Perspective 3–5
What Is a Community?

Community is a very important concept in public health as well as health care policy, planning, and management. In general parlance, a community refers to a group of people living together in a defined place; the place could be a neighborhood, a rural village, an urban area or an entire country. In addition, community implies a collective group of individuals who share some feature in common, be it a profession (the scientific community), a religion (the Jewish community), or some other characteristic (the gay community; the Hispanic community).

The public health community (a group of professionals who share a common purpose) spends considerable effort monitoring the health of communities (groups of people living together in geographic communities within states and nations) because of its interest in promoting and preserving the health of entire populations. Within the health care community, issues relating to the larger community within which health care organizations do business must be critically examined and either accommodated or exploited to promote successful health care outcomes.

In this context, the community represents the competitive environment within which health care organizations function, while also representing a set of community factors – values, needs, resources, and constraints – that may suggest modifications to a typical health care structure or a usual set of services arranged and delivered. The *competitive environment* as community would include such factors as availability of and access to care, available financing strategies, the ways in which resources are allocated, and systems of accountability.

Examples of *community factors* that can affect health care organizations include:

1. The level (federal, state, local) and scope of governmental entities that regulate the health system and the extent of regulation directed at health care organizations;
2. The nature and scope of professional organizations that set standards, accredit or otherwise engage in accountability functions for health care organizations;
3. The nature and scope of health care financing agencies, including purchasers and private and public insurors, that participate in the health care marketplace in the community;
4. The availability of health care providers, facilities, supplies, and ancillary services across the community; and
5. The characteristics of the populations ultimately paying for and receiving health care services. These characteristics could include socioeconomic status (education, occupation and income), race and ethnicity, family structure, health status, health risk, and health seeking behaviors.

A community, then, in this context, can refer to the health care community, the community of individuals served by a health care system, the physical community within which the individuals reside and the health system functions, and the competitive environment within which any given health care organization operates. Identifying and considering the community of interest (service area) facilitates strategic planning and strategic management of health care organizations.

Source: Donna J. Petersen, MHS, ScD, Dean, College of Public Health, University of South Florida.

The *service area profile* includes key competitively relevant economic, demographic, psychographic (lifestyle), and community health status indicators. Relevant economic information may include income distribution, major industries and employers, types of businesses and institutions, economic growth rate, seasonality of businesses, unemployment statistics, and so on. Demographic variables most commonly used in describing the service area include age, gender, race, marital status, education level, mobility, religious affiliation, and occupation.

Psychographic variables are often better predictors of consumer behavior than demographic variables and include values, attitudes, lifestyle, social class, or personality. For example, consumers in the service area might be classified as medically conservative or medically innovative. Medical conservatives are only interested in traditional health care – drugs, therapies, and diagnostics they are familiar with – whereas medically innovative individuals are willing (often eager) to try new alternative drugs, therapies, or diagnostics. Although medically independent individuals are high in self-esteem and assertiveness, often questioning one physician's diagnosis and seeking a second opinion, medically dependent individuals follow what the doctor prescribes exactly and would never think of questioning "doctor's orders."

Health status of the service area is also important in considering its viability, as disease may be related to age, occupation, environment, or economics. Health status includes all types of data normally considered to represent the physical and mental well-being of a population. Demographic, psychographic, and health status information should be included in the analysis only if it is competitively relevant. Possible variables in developing a service area profile are summarized in Exhibit 3–3.[17] These variables produce issues that must be integrated and considered in conjunction with the general and health care environmental issues.

Service Area Structural Analysis

Harvard's Michael E. Porter developed a five forces framework for analyzing the external environment through an examination of the competitive nature of the industry. *Service area structural analysis* provides considerable insight into the attractiveness of an industry and provides a framework for understanding the competitive dynamics (the future viability of an industry). Porter's five forces framework has been applied to industry analysis for many industries – however, because of the nature of competition in health care, it is more appropriate to apply the framework to the service category/service area. Use of Porter's five forces in health care can be referred to as service area structural analysis.

Porter suggested that the level of competitive intensity within the industry is the most critical factor in an organization's environment. In Porter's model, intensity is a function of the threat of new entrants to the market, the level of rivalry among existing organizations, the threat of substitute products and services, the bargaining power of buyers (customers), and the bargaining power of suppliers.[18] The strength and impact of these five forces must be carefully monitored and assessed to determine the viability of the service category today

Exhibit 3–3: Service Area Profile Variables

Economic
• Income Distribution
• Foundation of the Economy
• Major Employers
• Types of Businesses
• Growth Rate
• Seasonality
• Unemployment

Demographic
• Age Profile
• Gender Distribution
• Average Income
• Race Distribution
• Marital Status
• Education Level
• Religious Affiliation
• Population Mobility
• Stage in Family Life Cycle
• Occupational Mix
• Residence Locations

Psychographic
• Medical Conservatives
• Medical Innovators
• Medical Dependents
• Personal Health Controllers
• Youthfulness
• Sociability

Health Status Indicators
• Mortality
• Deaths from all causes per 100,000 population

• Motor vehicle crash deaths per 100,000 population
• Suicides per 100,000 population
• Female breast cancer deaths per 100,000 population
• Stroke deaths per 100,000 population
• Cardiovascular deaths per 100,000 population
• Work-related injury/deaths per 100,000 population
• Lung cancer deaths per 100,000 population
• Heart disease deaths per 100,000 population
• Homicides per 100,000 population
• Infant deaths per 1,000 live births

Notifiable Disease Incidence
• AIDS incidence per 100,000 population
• Tuberculosis incidence per 100,000 population
• Measles incidence per 100,000 population
• STD incidence per 100,000 population

Risk Indicators
• Percentage of live-born infants weighing under 2,500 g at birth
• Births to adolescents as a percentage of live births
• Percentage of mothers delivering infants who received no prenatal care in first trimester of pregnancy
• Percentage of children under 15 years of age living in families at or below the poverty level
• Percentage of children under 15 years of age without all childhood inoculations
• Percentage of women over 50 without a mammogram
• Percentage of population more than 50 pounds overweight
• Percentage of persons living in areas exceeding the US EPA air quality standards
• Percentage of persons who do not wear seatbelts

and may be used to assess the changes likely to occur in the future. As illustrated in Exhibit 3–4, Porter's industry structural analysis may be adapted to service areas to understand the competitive forces for health care organizations.

THREAT OF NEW ENTRANTS

New entrants into a market are typically a threat to existing organizations because they increase the intensity of competition. New entrants may have substantial resources and often attempt to rapidly gain market share. Such actions may force prices and profits down. The threat of a new competitor entering into

Exhibit 3–4: Service Area Structural Analysis: Forces Driving Service Area Competition

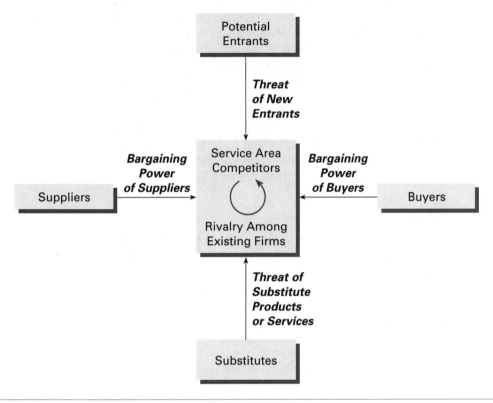

Source: Michael E. Porter, *Competitive Strategy: Techniques for Analyzing Industries and Competitors.* Copyright © 1980 by the Free Press. All rights Reserved. Adapted with the permission of The Free Press, a division of Simon & Schuster Adult Publishing Group.

a market depends on the industry or service area barriers. If the barriers are substantial, the threat of entry is low. Porter identified several barriers to entry that may protect organizations already serving a market:

- Existing organizations' economies of scale;
- Existing product or service differentiation;
- Capital requirements needed to compete;
- Switching costs – the one-time costs for buyers to switch from one provider to another;
- Access to distribution channels;
- Cost advantages (independent of scale) of established competitors; and
- Government and legal constraints.

These barriers may be assessed to determine the current or expected level of competition within an industry or service area. In health care markets, the barriers to entry for new "players" may be substantial. Consolidation (creation of large health care systems) and system integration (control of physicians and insurors) may make entry into a particular service area difficult because of economies and cost advantages. In an effort to create cost efficiencies, managed care has had the effect of limiting the ease of entry into markets. Where managed care penetration is high, market entry by new competitors will be more difficult because switching costs for some populations are high. However, the difficulty of adding new service categories for existing organizations in a managed care market may be lessened. Service categories may be added to better serve a captured (managed care) market.

Certificate of need, or CON, laws and regulations can present significant barriers to entry in those states that have them. CON is the reason that MedCath, based in the southeast, started building heart hospitals in states in the southwestern US and Midwest, where there are no CON barriers.

INTENSITY OF RIVALRY AMONG EXISTING ORGANIZATIONS

Organizations within an industry are mutually dependent because the strategy of one organization affects the others. Rivalry occurs because competitors attempt to improve their position. Typically, actions by one competitor foster reactions by others. Intense rivalry is the result of the following factors:

- Numerous or equally balanced competitors;
- Slow industry (service area) growth;
- High fixed or storage costs;
- A lack of differentiation or switching costs;
- Capacity augmented in large increments;
- Diverse competitors – diverse objectives, personalities, strategies, and so on;
- High strategic stakes – competitors place great importance on achieving success within the industry; and
- High exit barriers.

Often consolidation has created several balanced large health care systems in a service area. For example, in the Cleveland market, consolidation has resulted in two large integrated systems with high fixed costs and extremely high strategic stakes. For some markets, consolidation has resulted in competition between large for-profit and not-for-profit systems. Additionally, because of managed care, switching costs for consumers are high. Because many markets have supported too many providers in the past, the strategic stakes are extremely high. Most experts agree that further consolidations are likely, rivalry will intensify, and still more providers will not survive.

THREAT OF SUBSTITUTE PRODUCTS AND SERVICES

For many products and services there are various substitutes that perform the same function as the established products. Substitute products limit returns to an industry because at some price point consumers will switch to alternative products and services. Usually, the more diverse the industry, the more likely there will be substitute products and services. A major substitution taking place in health care has been the switch from inpatient care to outpatient alternatives. In addition, alternative therapies such as chiropractic, massage therapy, acupuncture, biofeedback, and so on, are increasingly substituted for traditional health care (see Perspective 3–6).

BARGAINING POWER OF CUSTOMERS

Buyers of products and services attempt to obtain the lowest price possible while demanding high quality and better service. If buyers are powerful, then the competitive rivalry will be high. A buyer group is powerful if it:

- purchases large volumes;
- concentrates purchases in an industry (service area);
- purchases products that are standard or undifferentiated;
- has low switching costs;
- earns low profits (low profits force lower purchasing costs);
- poses a threat of backward integration;
- has low quality requirements (the quality of the products purchased by the buyer is unimportant to the final product's quality); and
- has enough information to gain bargaining leverage.

Perspective 3–6

Complementary and Alternative Medicine: Moved to Integrative Medicine?

Americans are frustrated with the inability of traditional medicine to meet their expectations and needs. In addition, US society has a growing interest in generally better health and wellness. Further, individuals have access to more health care information than ever before through the Internet. Discontent and the search for "more" have led many Americans to explore complementary and alternative medicine (CAM).

The five domains of CAM used in the United States include alternative medical systems built on complete systems of theory and practice separate from conventional medical approaches, including homeopathy and naturopathy; biologically based therapies that use substances found in nature, such as herbs, special diets, or vitamins (in doses outside those used in conventional medicine); energy therapies that involve the use of energy fields, such as magnetic fields or biofields (energy fields that some believe surround and penetrate the human body); manipulative and body-based methods including massage therapy, chiropractic, and osteopathy; and mind–body medicine that uses a variety of techniques designed to enhance the mind's ability to affect bodily function and symptoms (yoga, spirituality, and relaxation therapy).

According to the CDC Advance Data Report more than 36 percent of adults are using some form of CAM. (When megavitamin therapy and prayer specifically for health reasons are included in the definition of CAM, that number rises to 62 percent.) CAM use spans people of all backgrounds, although, according to the survey, some people are more likely than others to use CAM. Overall, CAM use is greater by women than men; people with higher educational levels; people who have been hospitalized in the past year; and former smokers, compared with current smokers or those who have never smoked. ▶

According to a 2004 American Hospital Association Health Forum survey, about 16.6 percent of US hospitals provided CAM services (up from 7.9 percent in 1998). The most frequently provided services by those hospitals that offer CAM include massage therapy (78 percent), pastoral counseling (62 percent), stress management (61 percent), and yoga (58 percent).

Consumers are somewhat wary of untested CAM therapies. A possible threat to CAM potential is that some complementary therapies interfere with effective conventional treatments and cause unintended but harmful side effects. Although the threat exists, the majority of patients integrate both conventional care and CAM interventions into their health care and wellness programs instead of viewing the two entities as substitutes.

In 1998, cognizant of society's changing perspectives on health care and well-being, Congress expanded the Office of Alternative Medicine (started in 1993) by creating the National Center for Complementary and Alternative Medicine (NCCAM). NCCAM is one of the 27 institutes and centers that make up the National Institutes of Health (NIH). The NIH is one of eight agencies under the Public Health Service (PHS) in the Department of Health and Human Services (DHHS). According to the "NCCAM Strategic Plan: 2005–2009," it has four primary areas of focus:

1. *Research.* We support clinical and basic science research projects in CAM by awarding grants across the country and around the world; we also design, study, and analyze clinical and laboratory-based studies on the NIH campus in Bethesda, Maryland.
2. *Research training and career development.* We award grants that provide training and career development opportunities for predoctoral, postdoctoral, and career researchers.
3. *Outreach.* We sponsor conferences, educational programs, and exhibits; operate an information clearinghouse to answer inquiries and requests for information; provide a website and printed publications; and hold town meetings at selected locations in the United States.
4. *Integration.* To integrate scientifically proven CAM practices into conventional medicine, we announce published research results; study ways to integrate evidence-based CAM practices into conventional medical practice; and support programs to develop models for incorporating CAM into the curriculum of medical, dental, and nursing schools.

With a budget of $117.8 million in 2004, its mission states: "NCCAM is dedicated to exploring complementary and alternative healing practices in the context of rigorous science, training complementary and alternative medicine researchers, and disseminating authoritative information to the public and professionals." Its vision includes: "NCCAM will advance research to yield insights and tools derived from complementary and alternative medicine to benefit the health and well-being of the public, while enabling an informed public to reject ineffective or unsafe practices."

As stated by Dr. Stephen E. Straus, the first and current Director of NCCAM, "As CAM interventions are incorporated into conventional medical education and practice, the exclusionary terms 'complementary and alternative medicine,' will be superseded by the more inclusive, 'integrative medicine.' Integrative medicine will be seen as providing novel insights and tools for human health, practiced by health care providers skilled and knowledgeable in the multiple traditions and disciplines that contribute to the healing arts."

Source: Originally written by Meredith Willard Luber, UNC Charlotte MBA, from the National Center for Complementary and Alternative Medicine website (http://nccam.nih.gov/) and its strategic plan, *Expanding Horizons of Healthcare 2001 to 2005*; updated from the website and P. Barnes, E. Powell-Griner, K. McFann, and R. Nahin, "Complementary and Alternative Medicine Use Among Adults: United States, 2002," *CDC Advance Data Report #343* (Washington, DC: May 27, 2004); and "Hospital Trends," *Marketing Healthcare Services* 24, no. 2 (Summer 2004), p. 9.

Perhaps the greatest change in the nature of the health care industry in the past decade has been the growing power of the buyers. Managed care organizations purchase services in large volume and control provider choices. The increasing power of the buyers has fueled system integration as well as blurring of providers and insurors. Large employers as buyers have power over managed care organizations, because they determine whether the MCO will be on the list that employees have to choose from for their health care. The poor economy, resulting in lowered profits during the period between 2000 and 2004 has pushed employers to find ways to lower their health care costs.

BARGAINING POWER OF SUPPLIERS

Much like the power of buyers, suppliers can affect the intensity of competition through their ability to control prices and the quality of materials they supply. Through these mechanisms, suppliers can exert considerable pressure on an industry. Factors that make suppliers powerful tend to mirror those making buyers powerful. Suppliers tend to be powerful if:

- there are few suppliers;
- there are few substitutes;
- the suppliers' products are differentiated;
- the product or service supplied is important to the buyer's business;
- the buyer's industry is not considered an important customer; and
- the suppliers pose a threat of forward integration (entering the industry).

Traditionally, physicians and other health care professionals have been important and powerful "suppliers" to the industry because of their importance to health care institutions. Because of the nature of managed care, the physician remains the "gatekeeper" to the system and plays a crucial role in controlling consumer choice. This supplier power has added pressure to include physicians in system integration through the purchase of primary care individual and group practices by hospital systems. Other suppliers, such as those who supply general medical needs such as bandages, suture materials, thermometers, and so on, have tended not to exercise a great deal of control over the industry.

Concluding Structural Analysis

Porter's approach is a powerful tool for assessing the level of competitive intensity within the health care service area. Porter's framework for analyzing the external environment is applied to a nursing home in Exhibit 3–5. Competitive intensity and ultimately the profitability of the service category in the service area is determined by the number of favorable factors. In Exhibit 3–5, the threat of entry is low which is favorable to the existing skilled-nursing facilities. Similarly the intensity of rivalry among existing organizations is low, the threat of substitutes is relatively low, and suppliers (labor) have not been powerful players. All these factors are favorable. However, the bargaining power of the buyer is high

Exhibit 3–5: Using Porter's Industry Structure Analysis

The Hanover House Nursing Home, a skilled-nursing facility, used differentiation as its major competitive advantage. In its early years, in a less regulated environment, the home was very profitable. As the facility began to age, and with increasingly stricter regulations for long-term care, profit margins began to deteriorate. The administrators of Hanover House used Porter's Industry Structure Analysis to better understand the forces in their external environment. The following is a summary of their analysis.

Threat of New Entrants
The supply of nursing homes and other long-term care facilities is currently limited because there is a moratorium on additional beds within the geographic area. Competition is based on process or quality. If the moratorium is lifted, it will remain costly to enter the market because it is highly regulated. The greatest threat as a new entrant (when the moratorium is lifted) will be hospitals attempting to compensate for decreasing occupancy rates. Switching costs are low for hospitals (the same bed can be used for acute care or long-term care). Access to the distribution channel is high as hospitals have many of the required resources, including access to nurses, familiarity with the regulations, and capability to enter quickly (by converting acute care beds to long-term care).

Intensity of Rivalry Among Existing Organizations
Although there is competition, the long-term care industry is not fiercely competitive. Hanover House has six competitors – Mary Lewis Convalescence Center, Hillhaven, Altamont Retirement Community, St. Martins in the Pines, Lake Villa, and Kirkwood – that have relatively stable market shares. Because the service has both quality and dollar value, there is the opportunity to differentiate, and switching costs are high for the consumer. It is a highly regulated area and, therefore, not a great deal of diversity among competitors is apparent. The long-term care industry is maturing but remains a rapid-growth industry driven by demographic and social trends (the graying of America and the deterioration of the extended family). The most significant factor creating rivalry is the high fixed assets, which make exit difficult and success important.

Threat of Substitute Products and Services
There are few substitute products for nursing home care. Home care is a substitute but an increasingly less available alternative because of the mobility and dissolution of the family unit. Other alternatives include nonskilled homes, retirement housing, and domiciliaries. Increased costs and DRGs have virtually eliminated hospitals as an alternative. On balance, substitutes do not appear to be a strong force in the nursing home industry.

Bargaining Power of Customers
The power of the customer in the industry is generally high. The major consumer, the government, purchases over 45 percent of nursing home care and regulates reimbursement procedures as well as the industry. Therefore, significant levels of information are available. In addition, for private-pay customers, the purchase represents a significant investment and comparison shopping is prevalent. Product differentiation tends to reduce buying power but relatively low switching costs and government involvement make nursing home care a buyers' market.

Bargaining Power of Suppliers
Because the product is simultaneously produced and consumed in service industries, labor is the major supplier in the nursing home industry. Although Hanover House is unionized, it has maintained good labor relations, and the union is not particularly powerful. Most who work in long-term care have selected the field to satisfy their need to care for others or make a contribution rather than to earn large salaries. Suppliers are not a dominant force in the nursing home industry.

Source: Elaine Asper, "Hanover House Nursing Home," an unpublished case study.

and thus unfavorable to the service category. As a result, four factors are favorable and one is unfavorable. Competitive intensity for this service category in this service area is relatively low, leading to favorable returns. Four or five unfavorable factors make competition intense and will lower profitability.

Conducting Competitor Analysis and Mapping Strategic Groups

The next step in service area competitor analysis (refer back to Exhibit 3–2) is to evaluate the strengths and weakness of competitors, characterize their strategies, group competitors by the types of strategies they have exhibited, and predict competitive future moves or likely responses to strategic issues and initiatives by other organizations.

COMPETITOR STRENGTHS, WEAKNESSES, AND STRATEGY

In assessing the rivalry of the service area, the competitors are identified. Next, the strengths and weaknesses of each competitor should be specified and evaluated. Organizations have a unique resource endowment and a comparison with a given competitor will help to illuminate the relationship between them and to predict how they compete with (or respond to) each other in the market.[19] Evaluation of competitors' strengths and weaknesses provides clues as to their future strategies and to areas where competitive advantage might be achieved.

Both quantitative and qualitative information may be used to identify strengths and weaknesses. Competitor information is not always easy to obtain, and it is often necessary to draw conclusions from sketchy information. A list of possible competitor strengths and weaknesses is presented in Exhibit 3–6

Exhibit 3–6: Potential Competitor Strengths and Weaknesses

Potential Strengths	Potential Weaknesses
• Distinctive competence	• Lack of clear strategic direction
• Financial resources	• Deteriorating competitive position
• Good competitive skills	• Obsolete facilities
• Positive image	• Subpar profitability
• Acknowledged market leader	• Lack of managerial depth and talent
• Well-conceived functional area strategies	• Missing key skills or competencies
• Achievement of economies of scale	• Poor track record in implementing strategies
• Insulated from strong competitive pressures	• Plagued with internal operating problems
• Proprietary technology	• Vulnerable to competitive pressures
• Cost advantages	• Falling behind in R&D
• Competitive advantages	• Too narrow a product/service line
• Product/service innovation abilities	• Weak market image
• Proven management	• Below-average marketing skills
• Ahead on experience curve	• Unable to finance needed changes in strategy
	• Higher overall costs relative to key competitors

Such information may be obtained through local newspapers, trade journals, websites, focus groups with customers and stakeholders, consultants who specialize in the industry, securities analysts, outside health care professionals, and so on. Identification of competitor strengths and weaknesses will aid in speculating on competitor strategic moves. The range of possible competitive actions available to organizations varies from tactical moves, such as price cuts, promotions, and service improvements that require few resources, to strategic moves, such as service category/area changes, facilities expansions, strategic alliances, and new product or service introductions that require more substantial commitments of resources and are more difficult to reverse. Such competitive actions represent clear, offensive challenges that invite competitor responses.[20]

SERVICE CATEGORY CRITICAL SUCCESS FACTOR ANALYSIS

Critical success factor analysis involves the identification of a limited number of activities for a service category within a service area for which the organization must achieve a high level of performance if it is to be successful. The rationale behind critical success factor analysis is that there are five or six areas in which the organization must perform well and that it is possible to identify them through careful analysis of the environment. In addition, critical success factor analysis may be used to examine new market opportunities by matching an organization's strengths with critical success factors.

Typically, once the service category critical success factors have been identified, several goals may be developed for each success factor. At that point, a strategy may be developed around the goals. Important in critical success factor analysis is the establishment of linkages among the environment, the critical success factors, the goals, and the strategy. In addition, it is important to evaluate competitors on these critical success factors. Indeed, excellence in any (or several) of these factors may be the basis of competitive advantage. Further, these factors form the fundamental dimensions of strategy.

Organizational strategies may differ in a wide variety of ways. Michael Porter identified several strategic dimensions that capture the possible differences among an organization's strategic options in a given service area:

- *Specialization*: the degree to which the organization focuses its efforts in terms of the number of product categories, the target market, and size of its service area.
- *Reputation*: the degree to which it seeks name recognition rather than competition based on other variables.
- *Service/product quality*: the level of emphasis on the quality of its offering to the marketplace.
- *Technological leadership*: the degree to which it seeks superiority in diagnostic and therapeutic equipment and procedures.
- *Vertical integration*: the extent of value added as reflected in the level of forward and backward integration.
- *Cost position*: the extent to which it seeks the low-cost position through efficiency programs and cost-minimizing facilities and equipment.

- *Service*: the degree to which it provides ancillary services in addition to its main services.
- *Price policy*: its relative price position in the market (although price positioning will usually be related to other variables such as cost position and product quality, price is a distinct strategic variable that must be treated separately).
- *Relationship with the parent company*: requirements concerning the behavior of the unit based on the relationship between a unit and its parent company. (The nature of the relationship with the parent will influence the objectives by which the organization is managed, the resources available to it, and perhaps determine some operations or functions that it shares with other units.)[21]

The organization can determine the strategic dimension or dimensions that it will use to compete – however, these decisions cannot be made in a vacuum. Consideration must be given to which of the dimensions competitors have selected and how well they are meeting the needs of customers.

STRATEGIC GROUPS

Service area analysis concentrates on the characteristics of the specific geographic market whereas strategic group analysis concentrates on the characteristics of the strategies of the organizations competing within a given service area. Strategic groups have been studied in many different industries and there are often several strategic groups within a service area. A *strategic group* is a number of organizations within the same service category making similar strategic decisions. Members of a strategic group have similar "recipes" for success or core strategies.[22] Therefore, members of a strategic group primarily compete with each other and do not compete with organizations outside their strategic group – even though there are other competitors outside the group that may offer similar products or services.

External stakeholders have an image of the strategic group and develop an idea of the group's reputation. The reputation of each strategic group differs because the identity and strategy of each group differ.[23] Organizations within a strategic group use similar resources to serve similar markets. However, leadership in an individual organization must find ways (sometimes subtle) to have its organization stand out from the group (differentiation) to develop competitive advantage over other group members.[24]

Reputation has been defined as an organization's true character and the emotions toward the organization held by its stakeholders. Strategic group reputation may be a mobility barrier leading to increased performance. If reputation does lead to increased performance, individual organizations within the strategic group may need to consider the impact of their actions on the collective reputation of the group.[25] Thus, if several managed care organizations in a service area are in the same strategic group, the actions of one influence the reputation of them all. The grouping of organizations according to strategic similarities and differences among competitors can aid in understanding the nature of competition and facilitate strategic decision making. There are four major implications for the strategic group concept:

1. Organizations pursue different strategies within service categories and service areas. Creating competitive advantage is often a matter of selecting an appropriate basis on which to compete.
2. Organizations within a strategic group are each other's primary or direct competitors. As Bruce Henderson, founder of Boston Consulting Group, has noted, "Organizations most like yours are the most dangerous."
3. Strategic group analysis can indicate other formulas for success for a service category. Such insight may broaden a manager's view of important market needs.
4. Strategic group analysis may indicate important market dimensions or niches that are not being capitalized on by the existing competitors. Lack of attention to critical success factors by other competitive organizations offering the same or a similar service may provide an opportunity for management to differentiate its services.

Organizations within a group follow the same or similar strategy along the strategic dimensions. Group membership defines the essential characteristics of an organization's strategy. Within a service category or service area there may be only one strategic group (if all the organizations follow the same strategy) or there may be many different groups. Usually, however, there are a small number of strategic groups that capture the essential strategic differences among organizations in the service area.[26]

The analysis of competitors along key strategic dimensions can provide considerable insight into the nature of competition within the service area. Such an analysis complements Porter's structural analysis but provides some additional insights. As a means of gaining a broad picture of the types of organizations within a service area and the kinds of strategies that have proven viable, strategic group analysis can contribute to understanding the structure, competitive dynamics, and evolution of a service area as well as the issues of strategic management within it.[27] More specifically, the usefulness of strategic group analysis is that it:

- can be used to preserve information characterizing individual competitors that may be lost in studies using averaged and aggregated data;
- allows for the investigation of multiple competitors concurrently;
- allows assessment of the effectiveness of competitors' strategies over a wider range of variation than a single organization's experience affords; and
- captures the intuitive notion that "within-group" rivalry and "between-group" rivalry differ.[28]

When analyzing strategic groups, care must be taken to ensure that they are engaging in market-based competition. Many organizations may not be direct or primary competitors because of a different market focus. Organizations will have little motivation to engage each other competitively if they have limited markets in common. It is not unusual for organizations that serve completely different markets yet have similar strategic postures to be grouped together and assumed by analysts to be direct competitors when in fact they are not.[29] For example, a pediatric group practice affiliated with a children's hospital and a community health clinic emphasizing preventive and well care may serve the same population but not be direct competitors because of a different market focus.

Exhibit 3–7: Service Area Assisted-Living Competitors

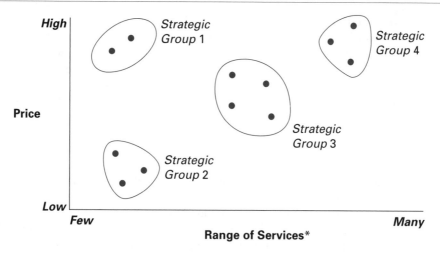

For this service area, assisted living organizations are pursuing four basic strategies:
high price with highly specialized services (*Strategic Group* 1), low price with few ancillary services (*Strategic Group* 2), medium price with some (selected) services (*Strategic Group* 3), and high price with many services (*Strategic Group* 4). The primary (direct) competitors for these organizations are other organizations within their own strategic group. Customers who seek the attributes of one strategic group, such as highly specialized rehabilitation services, are unlikely to be attracted to another strategic group. These assisted-living organizations should change strategy cautiously as a decision to add services may move an organization to a new strategic group and therefore a new set of competitors. Note that in this example there may be an opportunity to enter or move toward a medium-cost, many services niche and become a strategic group of one.

---

*Range of services includes skilled nursing, organized social activities, outings, physical therapy, education, rehabilitation, speech therapy, Alzheimer's care, nutritional services, infusion, pharmacy, homemaker services, live-ins, companions, and so on.

MAPPING COMPETITORS

Mapping competitors for any service category (broadly or narrowly defined) within a service area may be based on the critical success factors or important strategy dimensions. Exhibit 3–7 shows strategic groups of assisted-living organizations within a service area. Several strategic maps may be constructed demonstrating different strategic views of the service area. In addition, a single dimension may be so important as a critical factor for success that it may appear on several strategic maps.

Likely Competitor Actions or Responses

Strategy formulation is future oriented, requiring that management anticipate the next strategic moves of competitors. These moves may be projected through an evaluation of competitor strengths and weaknesses, membership in strategic groups, and the characterization of past strategies. In many cases competitor strategic goals are not difficult to project, given past behaviors of the organization. Strategic thinking is a matter of anticipating what is next in a stream of consistent decisions. Strategic behavior is the result of consistency in decision making, and decision consistency is central to strategy. Therefore, in determining competitors' future strategies, strategic managers must look for the behavioral patterns that emerge from a stream of consistent decisions concerning the positioning of the organization in the past. A thorough analysis of the key strategic decisions of competitors may reveal their strategic intent. A strategic decision timeline can be helpful in showing the stream of decisions. *Strategic response* includes the likely strategic objectives and next strategic moves of competitors. These may be anticipated because of their perceived strengths and weaknesses, past strategies, or strategic group membership. If an organization is planning an offensive move within a service area, an evaluation of competitor strengths and weaknesses, past strategies, strategic group membership, and assumed strategic objectives can anticipate the likely strategic response. For example, HCA–The Healthcare Company's analysis of the strategic response of competitors for a new market they are considering is an important variable in their expansion strategy.

Synthesizing the Analyses

To be useful for strategy formulation, general and health care external environmental analysis (see Chapter 2) and service area competitor analysis (as covered in this chapter) must be synthesized and then conclusions drawn. It is easy for strategic decision makers to be overwhelmed by information. To avoid paralysis by analysis, external environmental analysis should be summarized into key issues and trends, including their likely impact, and then service area competitor analysis summarized.

Example of a Service Area Competitor Analysis

Service area competitor analysis is increasingly important for health care organizations. For-profit as well as not-for-profit health care organizations will have to understand the competitive dynamics of service categories and service areas. For example, ophthalmologists are in a medical specialty that is quite competitive, not only because there are typically a number of them in a given service area but also because there are licensed optometrists that deliver some of the same services and at a lower price to the consumer. If an ophthalmologist were to consider entering the refractive surgery market in Charlotte, North Carolina, the service area competitor analysis is a systematic method to evaluate whether the area represents a potentially profitable opportunity. Refractive surgery is a surgical procedure aimed at improving the focusing power of the eye. Perspective 3–7 provides an overview of the nature of eye care and serves as background for a service area competitor analysis.

Perspective 3–7
Eye Care

Three different types of health care professionals provide care of the eye: ophthalmologists, optometrists, and opticians. Ophthalmologists are medical doctors (MDs) who specialize in the medical and surgical care of the eyes and visual system and in the prevention of eye disease. They are trained to diagnose, treat, and manage all eye and visual systems and licensed by a state to practice medicine and surgery. In addition, they can deliver total eye care including vision services, contact lenses, and eye exams.

Optometrists have attended a four-year course in optometry but not medical school. They are state licensed to examine the eyes and to determine the presence of vision problems. They prescribe spectacles, contact lenses, and eye exercises. In some states they are permitted to prescribe pharmaceuticals for some eye conditions.

Opticians are technicians who make, verify, and deliver lenses, frames, and other specialty fabricated optical devices or contact lenses. They provide the product prescribed by the ophthalmologist or the optometrist.

Service categories for care of the eye include the following:

- *General services* – eye chart exams, pupil exams, optometric eye exams, vision therapy, low-vision aids, prescription contact lenses, prescription eyeglass lenses, prescription eye drop solutions and ointments, custom contact and eyeglass fittings, eye dilation.
- *Specialized services* – glaucoma, cataracts, legally defined blindness protocols, pediatric ophthalmology, geriatric ophthalmology, eye disease, and eye injury.
- *Surgery* – radial keratotomy (RK); corrective laser surgery: photorefractive keratectomy (PRK), laser in-situ keratomileusis (LASIK), laser thermokeratoplasty (LTK); NearVision CK (for presbyopia); corneal rings, implantable contact lenses (ICLs), and transplants; reconstructive and plastic surgery; and catarectomy (removal of cataracts).
- *Retail services* – glasses and sunglasses, nonprescription eye drop solutions, carrying cases, frames, eyeglass straps, designer frames, and so on.

In the example marketplace discussed in the text – Charlotte, North Carolina – all eye care services are offered. Analysis and a strategic group map in Exhibits 3–8 to 3–11 illustrate the major competitive groups.

Corrective refractive surgery is an elective surgery performed on the eye to improve focus and lessen dependence on glasses and contact lenses. Treated primarily as cosmetic surgery by insurance companies, consumers are paying out of pocket for this surgery because it offers freedom from dependency on glasses or contact lenses. Many consumers are tired of the inconvenience of contacts, the discomfort of glasses, the limitations of glasses or contacts while playing sports (comfort and safety), and the insecurity of knowing that they are helpless without their corrective lenses (such as felt by mothers of young children). Some consumers will choose surgery for occupational enhancement (fire fighters, airline pilots, police officers, professional athletes, and so on), and frequent travelers want to be less dependent on corrective eye wear for safety and convenience. Others choose surgery simply to improve their looks or self-image. It is an expensive choice – the average was $1,700 per eye in 2004, up from the lower average of $1,590 in 2002. The increase was primarily because of new technology that allows for greater accuracy in vision correction. The total value of the surgery includes: direct out-of-pocket cost, long- and short-term effects of the surgery (no need to buy glasses or contact lenses times the number of years), experience of the surgeon, risk versus benefits, and recovery time from the surgery (time away from work). In addition, consumers have to understand what the price of the surgery does and does not include and that prices charged can vary tremendously. Many ads tout $299 per eye for LASIK, but that "price" is available only to those who need minimal vision correction and have no astigmatism (uneven cornea). Factors affecting price include:

▶

1. Severity of vision correction required and presence or absence of astigmatism;
2. Expertise of the physician performing the surgery;
3. Pre-operative and post-operative visits (included in the price or extra?);
4. Surgeon performing the surgery (customer choice or assigned the day of surgery?);
5. Post-operative care (surgeon or optometrist?);
6. Complications (if they occur, who will provide care and cover the cost?);
7. Enhancements (provided as part of the initial procedure price, or, if extra, how much – full price or reduced price?) and for how long after the initial procedure (specified time period or lifetime?).

Research on the excimer laser began in the 1970s. Its use in ophthalmology was introduced in the 1980s. In 1995 the FDA granted approval to use excimer lasers for photorefractive keratectomy (PRK) in the United States. Analysts predicted that there would be as many as 1.4 million surgeries to correct myopia by 1998. There were actually about 250 thousand, translating into an $840 million business. The excimer laser brought more accuracy to refractive surgery, less discomfort, and faster healing. The newest technology, wavefront guided laser surgery, was approved by the FDA in 2003.

During 2003, global demand for refractive surgery was 3.02 million procedures, up from 2.87 million procedures in 2002. The increase resulted primarily from rapid growth in China, India, and other developing countries. In the United States, the number of procedures was flat (attributable to the generally poor economy during 2000 through 2003, uncertainty in the economy between 2004 and 2005, and unemployment figures that persistently remained higher than desired over the same period). Consumers who are uncertain about their future job prospects are hesitant to spend on discretionary items such as LASIK. During 2001, 1.31 million refractive procedures were performed in the United States, but the number declined to 1.15 million in 2002. For 2003 the number performed was 1.3 million and estimates were that the number of surgeries in 2004 would be improved, assuming the economy strengthened and unemployment declined.

Over 4,500 US ophthalmologists are trained to perform laser vision correction. Vision may need to be corrected for myopia (nearsightedness), hyperopia (farsightedness), astigmatism (uneven corneas, resulting in impaired sight), or presbyopia (aging eye syndrome). Over 162 million people in the United States need corrected vision; 150 million use corrective eyewear; over 70 million are nearsighted. Americans spend approximately $18 billion each year on corrective eyewear.

LASIK surgery provides the greatest range of correction, is the least painful, has the quickest recovery time, and incurs the fewest infections of any of the current vision correcting surgeries. According to the American Society for Cataract and Refractive Surgery, 56 percent of consumers who undergo LASIK surgery achieve vision of 20/20 or better and 90 percent achieve 20/40 or better (the minimum requirement for driving without corrective lenses). Between 8 and 17 percent of patients require enhancements (undergoing further surgery in the attempt to improve vision or correct for errors). Some enhancements are deliberate, as when the patient has severe myopia and the surgeon proceeds cautiously, allowing several months to pass to see how much further correction is necessary. With LASIK procedures, vision can continue to improve up to six months for some patients (three months is typical). Recently approved by the FDA, wavefront "custom" LASIK uses sophisticated measuring technology with a guided laser to improve correction and eliminate some of the problems such as nightblindness, haloing, and so on with traditional LASIK.

Service Category and Service Area

The analysis would begin by identifying the service category – refractive eye surgery – and investigating the service area – Charlotte, North Carolina – as in Exhibit 3–8. All analyses of the service area should be related to the identified service category. The "comments" column is used to indicate the applicability.

Service Area Structural Analysis

To assess the viability of the market, Michael Porter's five forces analysis is used to evaluate the service area. As described in Exhibit 3–9, the five forces suggest that it would be challenging to enter this market, but opportunities do exist. Barriers to entry for new competitors are somewhat high and the other forces suggest that this is a difficult market in which to compete – rivalry is high, consumers (buyers) wield a great deal of power, there are substitutes (which continue to increase), and suppliers of laser equipment (required to do refractive surgery) have increased to five in number and they have had to become somewhat more competitive: however, not all lasers are the same and the best technology is still tightly controlled. One of the manufacturers (Bausch & Lomb) is rumored to be thinking of withdrawing from the market in the near future. Thus, the power of suppliers has decreased somewhat but remains powerful for those physicians who want to use the very best equipment. In the future, the five forces for this service category, in this service area, are not likely to change dramatically. Barriers to entry for new competitors may decrease somewhat, rivalry will remain high, the consumer will be able to shop on price and defer purchase, and substitutes will likely increase. The number of suppliers of the technology may decrease from the current five major suppliers.

Strengths and Weaknesses

Next, the strengths and weaknesses (see Exhibit 3–10) should be assessed for providers of refractive surgery. Assessing strengths and weaknesses of competitors is often difficult for outsiders. However, careful observation and data gathering through websites and media can make this somewhat speculative process fairly accurate. In addition, over time the understanding of competitors' strengths and weaknesses can be refined and improved.

Critical Success Factors

From the preceding analysis the critical success factors for this service category in this service area may be surmised. The critical success factors for refractive eye surgery in Charlotte include the following:

Exhibit 3–8: Analysis of the Charlotte, North Carolina, Eye Care Market

| Service Category | Eye Care Services, Refractive Surgery |

Service Category   Eye Care Services, Refractive Surgery

Service Area   Charlotte, Mecklenburg County, North Carolina

I. Service Area – General

Competitively Relevant Issues	Comments
• The largest city in either of the Carolinas, located on the border. The nearest city, Winston-Salem, is more than 90 miles away • Many people come to Charlotte for their health care. People travel to Duke University for extraordinary care (no medical school in Charlotte) • Insurance covers injury to the eye, diseases of the eye, and malfunctions of the eye, but does not typically cover correcting vision (although it may be covered and some employers offer flexible spending accounts that can be used to cover the cost of refractive surgery so that it is at least pretax dollars that are spent) • Nearly 60 percent of all Americans need corrective lenses, 30 percent have myopia • Cataracts and glaucoma are eye diseases that occur with aging	• Not much need to travel outside of Charlotte for health care, especially routine care • Physicians who have pursued corneal fellowships after ophthalmology residency practice in Charlotte • There are few employers that offer eye care insurance for routine care in the Charlotte area. Flexible spending accounts are common among the major employers, but uncommon among small businesses • 60 percent in a growing market represents an opportunity • Laser surgery has been used for cataracts

II. Service Area – Economic

Competitively Relevant Issues	Comments
• Median household income in Charlotte is $48,975 (compared with $38,204 in NC and $43,057 in US) • Percentage below poverty at 10.6% is less than the state and nation (NC: 12.3%; US: 12.4%) • Retail sales per capita $13,867 (NC: $9,740; US: $9,190) • Economy improving and number of jobs increasing – however, unemployment is still considerably higher than pre-9/11/01, at 5.6% for Charlotte (NC: 6.3%; US: 6.0%) • Identified as one of the top cities for entrepreneurs • Nearly 80 percent of residents work in businesses of less than 100 employees	• Charlotte has a population that can afford the procedure • People with a higher standard of living are interested in LASIK • People in Charlotte spend 39.5% of the money they earn at retail (27.5% in NC; 24.8% in the US) • Unemployed postpone the purchase because it is an out-of-pocket expense (not covered by insurance) • Entrepreneurs are often innovators and early adopters • Big business tends to require the corporate "look"

Exhibit 3–8: (cont'd)

III. Service Area – Demographic

Competitively Relevant Issues

- More than 620,000 people live within Charlotte's city limits; 800,000 in Mecklenburg County; 1.5 million in the Charlotte MSA; Mecklenburg County is expected to grow by 3.6% in 2005
- Population over 65 at 7.6% is lower than the state and nation (11.6% in NC; 11.9% in US); median age in Charlotte is 32.7 years (NC: 35.3 years; US: 35.3)
- Population over 25 with college degree in Charlotte: 36.4% (NC: 22.5%; US: 24.4%)
- Ethnic mix is 58.3% white (NC: 72.1%; US: 75.1%), black 32.7% (NC: 21.6%; US: 12.3%), Native American 0.3% (NC: 1.2%; US 0.9%), Asian 3.4% (NC: 1.4%; US: 3.6%), Hispanic 7.4% (NC: 4.7%; US: 12.5%)

Comments

- A growing population may mean there is more room for a new provider using LASIK surgery
- A younger population is more likely to adopt the new surgery
- Better educated consumers are more likely to pay for the surgery
- The black population has been slower to adopt the new surgery, but as more experience occurs, it presents an expanding market

IV. Service Area – Psychographic

Competitively Relevant Issues

- Younger, upwardly mobile population; youthful orientation
- Business-oriented community: second largest banking center, sixth largest in wholesaling, sixth in number of Fortune 500 company headquarters
- Bible belt – 73% church or synagogue members
- Outdoor activities at the beach or mountains; both in easy driving distance

Comments

- LASIK is generally surgery for lifestyle and cosmetic reasons
- Population wants to "look" successful and not be hindered by glasses or wearing contacts
- Religious question: is surgery for cosmetic reasons the right thing to do?
- Outdoor activities are easier without having to keep up with glasses or search for a lost contact

V. Service Area – Health Status

Competitively Relevant Issues

- Generally healthy population
- NC is in the middle range of numbers of the population that requires vision correction
- Diabetes occurs more frequently in the South and contributes to problems with the eyes often leading to blindness

Comments

- Healthy candidates required for this elective procedure
- Sufficient market size
- Refractive surgery is *not* recommended for anyone with diabetes or the possibility of developing diabetes, although the new technologies are enabling many diabetics to have LASIK if they choose to

Exhibit 3–9: Service Area Structural Analysis

Five Forces	Forces Driving Service Area Competition	Conclusion
Threat of New Entrants	• Existing providers have already climbed the learning curve – experience level is important in successful surgeries (need more than 500 performed to be "experienced") and establishment of economies of scale • Capital requirements are high – the laser equipment costs $200,000 to $800,000 to buy, requires frequent and costly upgrades as well as maintenance, and a $150/eye to $500/eye royalty fee • Barriers to entry – only ophthalmologists (MD degree) who have been trained on the laser equipment and have access to it can perform the procedure • Existing service differentiation – perceived differentiation (high image) for Christenbury Eye Center as the first provider of LASIK and Dr. Christenbury performs the most procedures each month	*Medium* Threat of new entrants into market is presently medium, primarily because of the increase in the number of providers (new graduates with the ophthalmology specialty have learned to use the equipment) Economies of scale and the high equipment costs are still barriers but more options exist and equipment costs have declined somewhat, although new technology (wavefront custom) has raised the cost of equipment
Intensity of Rivalry	• Thirteen practices have physicians who perform laser eye surgery • Capacity is augmented in large increments – a laser costs between $200,000 and $800,000 • Diverse competitors – competitors employ distinctly different strategies (also diverse personalities) • High strategic stakes – focusing primarily on refractive surgery increases risks (narrow product line) • High exit barriers – once the equipment commitment is made, it is difficult to alter strategy or move in new direction	*High* Rivalry is likely to remain intense in this market as the competitors are well balanced, strategic stakes are high, and it is difficult to exit the market
Threat of Substitutes	• Do not bother to correct vision that is worse than 20/20 • Nonsurgical vision correction – contacts and glasses • Orthokeratology – use of specially designed rigid contact lenses that progressively reshape the curvature of the cornea over time (nonsurgical) • Older methods: RK – the oldest surgical procedure; PRK – older laser surgery; LASIK (without wavefront custom) • Implantable corneal rings and contact lenses • Cornea replacements	*High* Currently there are a number of low-cost, nonsurgical substitutes Older surgical methods are less expensive
Bargaining Power of Customers	• Elective surgery – rarely covered by insurance and consumer can easily defer procedure to later time • Can obtain enough information to gain bargaining leverage – some customers are traveling to Canada where the procedure is as much as $1,200 per eye less expensive	*High* Consumers have high bargaining power because of elective nature of the procedure and its out-of-pocket cost

Exhibit 3–9: (cont'd)

Five Forces	Forces Driving Service Area Competition	Conclusion
	• Consumers can "shop" for price and service (low switching costs before procedure) • Word-of-mouth is powerful	Consumers can opt for a much less expensive substitute, shop price, or wait for prices to decline

Bargaining Power of Suppliers	• Few suppliers of equipment:
	  – Alcon, Inc. manufactures the LADARVision System
	  – Bausch & Lomb manufactures the Technolas 217Z
	  – INTRALASE manufactures the INTRALASE FS
	  – NIDEK manufactures the NIDEK EC-5000
	  – VISX manufactures the VISX Star S3
	• Equipment substitutes are not expected in the near future
	• Equipment is essential to the business
		Medium
		Currently there are five suppliers, all have FDA approval as of 2005

1. Expertise in number of procedures performed. Number of procedures has to be more than 80 procedures per month to break even because of high fixed costs: $200,000 to $800,000 to buy a laser with all the various components to perform LASIK or custom LASIK surgery and $150 to $500/eye royalty depending on volume, surgeons' fees, and referral fees.
   • Experience and reputation of the surgeon.
   • Price.
   • Service – pre-op, post-op, and billing.
2. By 2004, low rate of complications: < 3 percent generally, < 1 percent for experienced surgeons. (Many consumers believe that even 1 percent of complications is high for elective surgery.)
   • Success with achieving 20/20 vision.
   • Number of enhancements (additional surgeries required to fine tune and improve vision).
   • Lifetime guarantee.
3. Positive word-of-mouth (estimates are that a satisfied patient refers on average five others); 55 to 75 percent of new patients are referrals.
   • Satisfaction of the clients.
   • Latest technology.
4. Offer complementary consultations (all current practices offer free consultations although what is included in the consultation may vary considerably from a simple eye check and discussion with an aide to a full work-up and discussion with the surgeon).

Exhibit 3–10: Competitor Strengths and Weaknesses

Competitor	Strengths	Weaknesses
Carolinas Eye Center	• Owned by local ophthalmologist and does only refractive surgery • Performed more than 25,000 surgeries; 200/month • Less than 4% enhancements required • $299/eye to $1,500/eye • Uses Bausch&Lomb Technolas 217Z wavefront custom laser • Extensive payment plans offered	• Dr. Clement is the sole provider of the procedure • No lifetime program; however, enhancement discount offered • Pre-op and post-op handled by another physician
Charlotte Eye, Ear, Nose, and Throat	• A large, comprehensive practice with 20 physicians who specialize in treatment of the eye • Ophthalmologist has done more than 5,000 procedures • Handles all care, pre-op and post-op, unless the patient prefers to use their own optometrist • Payment plan is handled through TLC, although Charlotte EENT offers a discount with some insurance companies • Cost/eye is $2,450 to $2,750	• Although six MDs were doing LASIK surgery, there is now one physician in the practice that performs laser surgery • Performs 50 surgeries per month (two Fridays/month) • No laser on site; uses TLC Laser Center
Christenbury Eye Center	• Personality and energy of Dr. Christenbury • First to do LASIK surgery and first to perform Wavefront Custom IntraLASIK in Charlotte; completed more than 50,000 procedures • General manager who's responsible for strategic planning • Extensive marketing by a marketing manager and Dr. Christenbury • Business development director makes sales calls on companies to speak to corporate discounts and flexible spending accounts • Systematic marketing research • Skilled staff of 45 • Number of procedures done per month: 600 to 800, all by Dr. Christenbury • Offers five machines: IntraLASIK FS, LADARVision 4000, LaserSight LSX, Nidek EC-5000, or Bausch & Lomb Technolas 217Z	• Dr. Christenbury is the sole provider of the procedure • Clients feel "herded" to "keep the doctor on schedule" • So much advertising that it diminishes the image • Very fast-paced, sometimes stressful work environment • Minimal discounts (special promotional discount for teachers in the month of August)

Exhibit 3–10: (cont'd)

Competitor	Strengths	Weaknesses
	• Cost based on severity of impairment from $595/eye to $2,195/eye; financing available • Ad agency that creates and places ads in TV, radio, direct mail, newspaper, magazines, Yellow Pages, and Internet • Good information systems, budgeting, and billing procedures • Locally owned	
Horizon Eye Care	• "Charlotte's Leader in Refractive Surgery" because seven MDs of thirteen in the clinic perform refractive surgery • One price, $1,799/eye, complete package (all services covered, enhancements for two years, any prescription, no extra charge for astigmatism) • Financing payment plan options available through The Vision Fee Plan (custom plan), assistance with flexible spending accounts • Chosen surgeon provides all patient services • Locally owned; five locations • Uses VISX Star S4 wavefront custom system – FDA approved • Website excellent	• Variability in physician experience: Ugland & Galentine more than 3,000 procedures each; others "several hundred" to "less than a hundred;" the group performs about 10,000 in a year • They "do not keep numbers" of individual doctors' procedures • No numbers on frequency of "enhancements;" enhancements are "done for those who have higher prescriptions to fine tune" • Between 5 and 10% are not candidates for LASIK (these numbers have fallen as the use of wavefront custom lasers allows for greater correction)
LASIKPlus Center	• National organization, headquartered in Cincinnati, Ohio; 39 centers in major markets in the US, plus four centers in Canada and Finland • Four employees operate the Center along with one ophthalmologist (Selkin) who has had a corneal fellowship after residency, is certified on four different lasers, and has performed more than 40,000 procedures • All employees are cross-trained and can substitute for each other • Number of procedures is 200/month	• Less "local" orientation • Dr. Selkin rotates between centers in North Carolina, Tennessee, and Texas. He spends about six to eight days (occasionally up to ten days) a month in Charlotte • Pre-op and post-op is done by the patient's own ophthalmologist • Ophthalmologists generally have older patients

Exhibit 3–10: (cont'd)

Competitor	Strengths	Weaknesses
	• Area ophthalmologists are invited to use the facilities • Cost $299/eye to $2,200/eye, one seminar attendee will be given a free procedure (drawn from a hat) • Three different payment plan options available; assistance with flexible spending accounts • Lifetime Continuous Care Program (no additional charges) • Good information systems, budgeting, and billing procedures • Surgery is done on one Saturday per month with day-after follow-up done at 8:00 A.M. on Sunday morning	• LCA does little marketing for the Center; rather it expects physicians to market themselves and use the Center • General manager often has to make appointments and handle phones • Scheduling of independent physicians to perform the procedure on their clients • Employees are consistently asked to work overtime • Only a moderately helpful website
TLC Laser Center	• National organization, headquartered in Canada; 50 centers in the US, seven in Canada, two in Mexico, and one in London • Six employees plus two local ophthalmologists on staff (Jaben has performed over 4,900 surgeries and Tate has performed over 15,000 surgeries) • Performs 176 procedures per month • Advertises in radio, magazines, Yellow Pages, and Internet with personal calls on local optometrists • Customer satisfaction: 93% satisfied or very satisfied; 99% would recommend TLC to family/friends; enhancements at no charge for up to two years • Tiger Woods is a well-known and credible spokesperson • Lifetime Commitment Program (for additional fee and required annual visits with a TLC-affiliate doctor; no charge for additional myopic procedures forever) • Developed a network of 45 physicians and optometrists who use or refer to the Center (of 92 ophthalmologists and 180 optometrists in the Charlotte area)	• Less "local" orientation • Marketing handled by corporate, with local coordinator • Near capacity at current location • Referrals usually from optometrists who will be responsible for follow-up and are owed $400/eye for referral • Tate performs surgeries every other Thursday and Jaben performs surgeries three Tuesdays and two Fridays per month • Website only moderately helpful. Refers to telephone numbers often

Exhibit 3–10: (cont'd)

Competitor	Strengths	Weaknesses
	• Payment plan financing available, negotiated contracts with some insurance plans for reduced rates, assists with flexible spending accounts; $250/eye discount if procedure can be watched by others, $100/eye discount if attended a seminar prior to surgery • VISX Star3 laser used • Good information systems, budgeting, and billing procedures	
Mecklenburg Eye Associates	• One ophthalmologist has performed several hundred procedures • Uses custom LASIK and IntraLase lasers • Full service eye care (three physicians) • Cost $1,000/eye to $2,000/eye	• Dr. Blotnick is the sole provider of the procedure • Uses TLC Center for surgeries • Difficult to get through on the phone • Website only moderately helpful
Providence Eye & Laser Specialists	• One ophthalmologist who has performed more than 10,000 procedures; corneal fellowship after residency • Doctor works with the patient from pre-op through post-operative care • Three different lasers • Cost is $1,200/eye to $1,800/eye • Excellent website • Extensive newspaper advertising	• Dr. Mozayeni is the sole provider of the procedure

Competitor Analysis – Strategic Groups

There are many opticians located in the offices of ophthalmologists as well as offices of optometrists. Many opticians work in nationally owned vision center chains where customers seek retail purchase of eye wear. They may receive referral fees for recommending a particular practice, but they do not otherwise participate in refractive surgery.

There are 92 optometrists in the Charlotte/Mecklenburg area, with estimates of another 200 in the service area. Younger, healthier clients who simply need periodic eye exams for glasses or contacts typically go to optometrists because the average price for an eye exam by an optometrist is between $80 and $90 in the Charlotte area. (Contact lens exams/fittings are nearly twice that amount.)

Older patients are advised to see an ophthalmologist because of their increased risk of eye diseases such as cataracts and glaucoma. The average price for an eye exam performed by an ophthalmologist in the Charlotte area is between $160 and $180. (Some physicians charge as high as $250.)

Prior to 1998, most of the ophthalmologists in Charlotte were in solo practices although there were several practices of three or four. As managed care became more of a market force in North Carolina, a number of mergers occurred. In 2004, 57 ophthalmologists practiced in the Charlotte market area and more than half work in two large practices: Horizon Eye Care has 13 eye care physicians (seven perform refractive surgery) and Charlotte Eye, Ear, Nose, and Throat has 20 physicians who specialize in eye care (six performed refractive surgery but did not perform enough to include it in their practice long-term; now just one physician performs the procedure routinely and the others in the practice refer to him).

There are three practices that have three physicians. In each of these smaller practices, there is one physician who performs refractive surgery (Childers/*Cook*/ Woody, *Christenbury*/Gross/Santander, and Adair/Bedrick/*Blotnick*). There are three partnerships. In one partnership, both partners perform refractive surgery (*Mundorf/Renaldo*); in the other two partnerships, none of the partners performs refractive surgery (Greenman/Greenman and Tillett/Tillett). The nine remaining ophthalmologists are solo practitioners. Seven of the nine solo practitioners perform refractive surgery in their own practice (*Grayson, Mozoyeni, Reeves*, and *Titone*) or as employees of one of the surgery centers (*Clement, Selkin*, and *Tate*). A total of 18 physicians from 13 different practices in the Charlotte area have training and expertise in laser surgery. However, only eight locations have the laser equipment necessary to perform the procedures; consequently, those without equipment on site use LASIKPlus or TLC Laser Centers.

In Charlotte's eye care market, four providers – Carolinas Eye Center, LASIKPlus, and TLC Laser Eye Center, and Providence Eye & Laser Specialists – are surgery centers that offer only or primarily LASIK surgery. Several local ophthalmologists focus on LASIK surgery but their practices offer other aspects of eye care in addition to the LASIK – Charlotte Ophthalmology Clinic, Christenbury Eye Center, Eye Care Clinic Vision & Laser Center, Genesis Eye Center, Mecklenburg Eye Associates, Mundorf & Renaldo, and Reeves Eye Clinic. Charlotte EENT (Eye, Ear, Nose, and Throat) and Horizon Eye Care are large practices that provide comprehensive, full-service eye care from routine eye exams to treatment of complex disease and surgery on the eye. Therefore, at the beginning of 2005, three strategic groups existed for the service category, each one having emerged using a different strategy.

Competitor Analysis – Mapping Competitors

Exhibit 3–11 shows a map of the strategic groups for refractive surgery in the Charlotte eye care market. In 2000, there was just one strategic group for refractive surgery. By the beginning of 2005, three distinct groups had emerged – the laser centers that only provide refractive surgery, the large group practices that

Exhibit 3–11: Competitor Analysis – Mapping Competitors

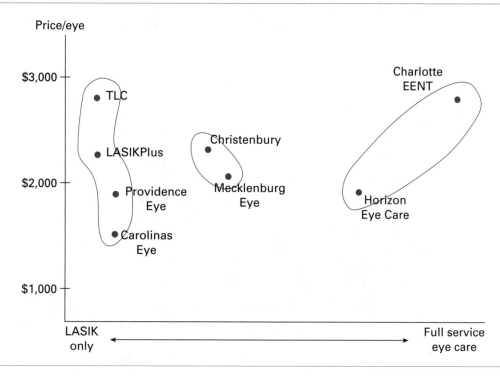

provide comprehensive care plus refractive surgery, and the very small group practice/solo practitioners who provide eye care and refractive surgery. The competitors will likely attempt to maintain the positioning that they have already established – or attempt to differentiate. The providers are somewhat different in their prices, equipment, the number of refractive procedures they perform in a month, and the comprehensiveness of the practice.

Competitor Analysis – Likely Response

A new competitor or any of the existing competitors have to realize the following:

- Any price decrease will likely be matched.
- Dr. Christenbury was the first to perform refractive eye surgery in the city. He owns more equipment than the other practitioners and continues to perform a high number of surgeries. More than likely he will continue to be at the fore-front of any new technology.
- Competition is intense and the entrance of a new provider will be met with considerable resistance.

- Preemptive strategies – more advertising, reduced prices, and so on – by current competitors are highly likely if they have any indication that a new competitor may enter the market, thereby increasing the difficulty of entering the market.

Synthesis

Surgery to correct vision problems moved into maturity between 2002 and 2005 in the Charlotte market; the number of providers, the price competition, and the amount of advertising have all increased substantially. Consumer demand is increasing as the surgery is being performed with less pain and more accurate results. Providers who perform the surgery must gain enough experience to avoid complications and gain positive word of mouth. Until costs begin to decline as the laser technology moves through the product life cycle, providers need to perform more than 80 surgeries per month to surpass break even.

The four laser centers are in a strategic group; they are mutually dependent because the strategy of one affects the others. Intense rivalry exists as they attempt to improve their position in the market. Carolinas Eye Center is owned by a local ophthalmologist who has performed more than 25,000 procedures (200 procedures per month). Providence Eye & Laser Specialists is also owned by a local ophthalmologist who had a corneal fellowship after residency and has performed more than 10,000 procedures. Both of these locally owned centers focus exclusively on corrective vision surgery.

LASIKPlus Center's strategy is to develop relationships with ophthalmologists in the area and offer the Center for them to use to perform the LASIK surgery. LASIKPlus benefits from having many ophthalmologists in the area learn the LASIK surgery techniques and use its facilities to perform the surgery on their patients. Preemptive discounting to local ophthalmologists could wrap up its referral base.

TLC's strategy is to develop relationships with the many optometrists in the area to gain referrals. Again, preemptive discounting could wrap up the optometrists' referral base for TLC. Because younger consumers tend to use optometrists more, and optometrists cannot perform surgery, TLC provides staff surgeons. The younger population (but over eighteen with no change in eye prescription in the past two years) offers better candidates for LASIK as they do not have the problem of presbyopia (aging eye).

All four in this strategic group have to be aware of and ready for any of the new technologies that may receive FDA approval at any time. The introduction of a new technology would be the best chance to enter the market as a new provider.

Among the local ophthalmologists, Dr. Christenbury has positioned his practice as the best value, himself as the most experienced in performing the surgery (50,000 at the beginning of 2005), and he owns six laser machines. He has the legitimate claim of being the first to do LASIK surgery in Charlotte and his continued referrals and full waiting room attest to the investment he has made in developing the first-mover advantage. The other partnerships and smaller group practices offer refractive surgery as part of comprehensive care.

In conclusion, a new provider entering the market would have significant challenges and would need deep pockets. Certainly the provider would have to be experienced in the procedure, willing to invest heavily in advertising to develop a position in the market, use the latest technology, and be willing (and able) to have low volume for some time. Given the risks, high barriers to entry, competitive rivalry, and so on, it appears that Charlotte would not be a new ophthalmologist's first choice location for setting up a practice to start refractive surgery. An established ophthalmologist in the Charlotte area would have a better opportunity to seek additional training and certifications on equipment and begin offering refractive surgery to his or her own patients rather than referring them to other physicians. On the other hand, for either the new-to-the-Charlotte-market or the new-to-refractive-surgery physician, the Charlotte market is growing, its population is younger than average, and it possesses higher discretionary spending ability.

This analysis reveals that a provider who is new to the service area or the service category would have to develop some competitive advantage not currently offered to be successful. Given deep pockets and excellent surgical results (no complications to achieve effective word of mouth), it is possible.

Strategic Momentum – Validating the Strategic Assumptions

As with the general and health care environments, the initial analysis of the service area provides the basic beliefs or assumptions underlying the strategy. Once the strategic plan has been developed, managers will attempt to carry it out. However, as implementation proceeds, new insights will emerge and new understanding of the competitive services will become apparent. Changes in the service area or new competitor strategies will directly affect performance of the organization and therefore must be monitored and understood. Competitive awareness and analysis are ongoing activities. The strategic thinking map presented in Exhibit 3–12 provides a series of questions designed to surface signals of new perspectives regarding the service area assumptions.

The Use of General Environmental and Competitor Analysis

In health care organizations today there is a real understanding that not every organization will survive; that no one health care organization can be "everything to everybody." Understanding the external environment – including the general, health care, and service area/competitor environments – is fundamental to strategic management and survival. A comprehensive general and health care environmental analysis and service area competitor analysis combined with an assessment of competitive advantages and disadvantages (Chapter 4) and establishment of the directional strategies (Chapter 5) provide the basis for strategy formulation.

Exhibit 3–12: Strategic Thinking Questions Validating the Strategic Assumptions

1. Is the strategy consonant with the competitive environment?
2. Do we have an honest and accurate appraisal of the competition?
3. Have we underestimated the competition?
4. Has the rivalry in the service category/service area changed?
5. Have the barriers to entering the service category/service area changed?
6. Does the strategy leave us vulnerable to the power of a few major customers?
7. Has there been any change in the number or attractiveness of substitute products or services?
8. Is the strategy vulnerable to a successful strategic counterattack by competitors?
9. Does the strategy follow that of a strong competitor?
10. Does the strategy pit us against a powerful competitor?
11. Is our market share sufficient to be competitive and generate an acceptable profit?

Summary and Conclusions

Service area competitor analysis is the third element of environmental analysis and increases the focus. Service area competitor analysis is an increasingly important aspect of environmental analysis because of the changes that have taken place in the health care industry throughout the past decade. Specifically, service area competitor analysis is the process of assessing service category/service area issues, identifying competitors, determining the strengths and weaknesses of rivals, and anticipating their moves. It provides a foundation for determining competitive advantage and subsequent strategy formulation.

Health care organizations engage in service area competitor analysis to obtain competitor information and for offensive and defensive reasons. However, analysts must be careful not to misjudge the service area boundaries, do a poor job of competitor identification, overemphasize visible competence, overemphasize where rather than how to compete, create faulty assumptions, or be paralyzed by analysis.

The process of service area competitor analysis includes an identification of the service category for analysis, assessment of the service area conditions, service area structure analysis, competitor analysis, and a synthesis of the information collected and analyzed. Identification of the service category provides the basis for the analysis. Service categories may be defined very broadly or quite specifically and will vary with the intent of the analysis. An identification of the service area will include establishing geographic boundaries and developing a service area profile that might include economic, demographic, psychographic, and disease pattern information.

Service area structural analysis may be accomplished through a Porter five forces analysis: evaluating the threat of new entrants into the market, the service area rivalry, the power of the buyers, the power of the suppliers, and the threat of substitute products or services. Next, competitor analysis should be undertaken. Comprehensive competitor analysis would include an identification and evaluation of competitor strengths and weaknesses, competitor strategy, strategic groups, critical success factors, and likely competitor actions and responses. Finally, service area and competitor information should be synthesized and strategic conclusions drawn to allow recommendations to be made.

Chapter 4 will explore how an organization examines its own strengths and weaknesses to understand competitive advantages and disadvantages as a basis for strategy formulation.

Key Terms and Concepts in Strategic Management

Competitive Advantage
Competitor Analysis
Critical Success Factor Analysis
Mapping Competitors

Service Area
Service Area Competitor
  Analysis
Service Area Profile

Service Area Structural Analysis
Service Category
Strategic Group
Strategic Response

QUESTIONS FOR CLASS DISCUSSION

1. What is entailed in service area competitor analysis? Why should health care organizations engage in competitor analysis? Should not-for-profit organizations perform competitor analysis?
2. What is the relationship between general and health care environmental analysis and service area competitor analysis?
3. What competitor information categories are useful in competitor analysis? Are these categories appropriate for health care organizations? How can these information categories provide a focus for information gathering and strategic decision making?
4. What are some impediments to effective competitor analysis? How may these impediments be overcome?
5. Explain the steps or logic of service area competitor analysis.
6. Why must the service categories be defined first in service area competitor analysis for health care organizations?
7. Why is it important to clearly define the service area? How does managed care penetration affect service area definition?
8. How does the use of Porter's five forces framework help identify the major competitive forces in the service area?
9. Why is an identification and evaluation of competitor strengths and weaknesses and the determination of strategy essential in service area competitor analysis?
10. What are the benefits of strategic group analysis and strategic mapping?
11. Why should a health care organization attempt to determine competitors' strategies and likely strategic responses?
12. What is the purpose of the synthesis stage of service area competitor analysis?
13. Conduct a service area competitor analysis for a health care service with which you are familiar.

NOTES

1. Shaker A. Zahra and Sherry S. Chaples, "Blind Spots in Competitive Analysis," *Academy of Management Executive* 7, no. 2 (1993), pp. 7–28 and Witold J. Henisz and Bennet A. Zelner, "The Strategic Organization of Political Risks and Opportunities," *Strategic Organization* 1, no. 4 (2003), pp. 451–460.

2. Carl Pegels and Kenneth A. Rogers, *Strategic Management of Hospitals and Health Care Facilities* (Rockville, MD: Aspen Publishers, 1988), pp. 35–36.

3. John E. Prescott and Daniel C. Smith, "The Largest Survey of 'Leading-Edge' Competitor Intelligence Managers," *Planning Review* 17, no. 3 (1989), p. 12.

4. David Halberstam, *The Reckoning* (New York: William Morrow, 1986), p. 310.

5. Interstudy: A Division of Decision Resources, Inc., *Interstudy Competitive Edge Report 4.0* (St. Paul, MN: Interstudy, 2003).

6. Sumantra Ghoshal and D. Eleanor Westney, "Organizing Competitor Analysis Systems," *Strategic Management Journal* 12, no. 1 (1991), pp. 17–31.

7. Chemical Abstract Service (CAS), a division of the American Chemical Society, website: http://www.cas.org.

8. Joel A. C. Baum and Helaine J. Korn, "Competitive Dynamics of Interfirm Rivalry," *Academy of Management Journal* 39, no. 2 (1996), p. 256.

9. Zahra and Chaples, "Blind Spots in Competitive Analysis," p. 9.

10. Ibid.

11. http://www.marriott.com/senior/about.asp.

12. Hubert Saint-Onge, "Tacit Knowledge: The Key to the Strategic Alignment of Intellectual Capital," *Strategy & Leadership* 24, no. 2 (1996), pp. 10–14.

13. Zahra and Chaples, "Blind Spots in Competitive Analysis," pp. 19–20.

14. http://marketguide.com/MGI/home.asp.

15. Joseph P. Peters, *A Strategic Planning Process for Hospitals* (Chicago: American Hospital Publishing, 1985), pp. 71–73 and Stephen Cummings and Duncan Angwin, "The Future Shape of Strategy: Lemmings and Chimeras," *Academy of Management Executive* 18, no. 2 (2004), pp. 21–36.

16. Voluntary Hospitals of America, Inc., *Community Health Assessment: A Process for Positive Change* (Irving, TX: Voluntary Hospitals of America, Inc., 1993), p. 49.

17. There are several community assessment approaches available such as *Advancing Community Public Health Systems in the Twenty-First Century* (Washington, DC: National Association of County and City Health Officials, 2001); Voluntary Hospitals of America, Inc., *Community Health Assessment: A Process for Positive Change* (Irving, TX: Voluntary Hospitals of America, Inc., 1993); The Hospital Association of Pennsylvania, *A Guide for Assessing and Improving Health Status: Community . . . Planting the Seeds for Good Health* (The Hospital Association of Pennsylvania, 1993); and James A. Rice, *Community Health Assessment: The First Step in Community Health Planning* (Chicago: American Hospital Association Technology Series, 1993). Perhaps the best known is *Assessment Protocol for Excellence in Public Health (APEX PH)*, a collaborative project of the American Public Health Association, the Association of Schools of Public Health, the Association of State and Territorial Health Officials, the Centers for Disease Control and Prevention, the National Association of County Health Officials, and the United States Conference of Local Health Officers funded through a cooperative agreement between the Centers for Disease Control and Prevention and the National Association of County Health Officials, 1991.

18. Michael E. Porter, *Competitive Strategy: Techniques for Analyzing Industries and Competitors* (New York: Free Press, 1980), pp. 3–33 and Benoit Mandelbrot and Richard L. Hudson, *The (Mis) Behavior of Markets* (New York: Basic Books, 2004).

19. Ming-Jer Chen, "Competitor Analysis and Interfirm Rivalry: Toward a Theoretical Integration," *Academy of Management Review* 21, no. 1 (1996), p. 101.

20. Baum and Korn, "Competitive Dynamics of Interfirm Rivalry," p. 257.

21. Adapted from Porter, *Competitive Strategy*, pp. 127–128.

22. R. K. Reger and A. S. Huff, "Strategic Groups: A Cognitive Perspective," *Strategic Management Journal* 14, no. 2 (1993), pp. 103–123.

23. Tamela D. Ferguson, David L. Deephouse, and William L. Ferguson, "Do Strategic Groups Differ in Reputation?" *Strategic Management Journal* 21, no. 12 (December 2000), pp. 1195–1214.

24. M. Peteraf and M. Shanley, "Getting to Know You: A Theory of Strategic Group Identity," *Strategic Management Journal* 18, Special Summer Issue (1997), pp. 165–186.

25. C. J. Fombrun, *Reputation* (Boston, MA: Harvard Business School Press, 1997).

26. Porter, *Competitive Strategy*, p. 129.
27. Robert M. Grant, *Contemporary Strategy Analysis*, 5th edn (Malden, MA: Blackwell Publishing, 2005), pp. 124–126.

28. Karel Cool and Ingemar Dierickx, "Rivalry, Strategic Groups and Firm Profitability," *Strategic Management Journal* 14, no. 1 (1993), pp. 47–59.
29. Chen, "Competitor Analysis and Interfirm Rivalry," p. 102.

ADDITIONAL READINGS

Cummings, Stephen and David Wilson (eds) *Images of Strategy* (Malden, MA: Blackwell Publishing, 2003). This book develops an approach to strategic management that is based on analysis and integration. It attempts to look outward at strategy from inside the organization rather than from the outside in. Readers are exposed to the way in which strategic choices are made and how these choices result in actions that shape the business and organizational world.

Institute for the Future, *Health and Health Care 2010*, 2nd edn (Indianapolis, IN: Jossey-Bass Publishing, 2003). This is the second edition of a comprehensive review of the technological and diagnostic advances of today's health care system. The book provides an overview of a number of areas critical to an understanding of the US health care system. Some of the important topics include demographic trends, managed care, health care customers and competitors, public health services, and a variety of other important topics.

Morley, David and Scott Miller, *The Underdog Advantage: Using the Power of Insurgent Strategy to Put Your Business on Top* (New York: McGraw-Hill, 2004). The underdog advantage is a set of principles that have been proven successful over time. The advantage of the incumbent has diminished over time and may have disappeared completely. According to these authors, today is the day of the underdog. Since today's customers are empowered with instant information they often feel overloaded and many traditional approaches to marketing are no longer effective. This book provides a strategy for the insurgent that is designed to overcome established competitors.

Porter, Michael E., *Competitive Strategy: Techniques for Analyzing Industries and Competitors* (Boston: The Free Press, 1998). In this classic work, Porter reviews competitive structure and the generic strategies in the first chapter – vintage Porter. The third chapter provides a detailed approach and framework for competitive analysis. He goes on to address competition in various types of industries. The discussion of industries that are fragmented, those in transition, and those with vertical integration are particularly pertinent for health care leaders.

Salaman, Graeme and David Asch, *Strategy and Capability: Sustaining Organizational Change* (Malden, MA: Blackwell Publishing, 2003). Virtually every writer has a formula for changing complex organizations in a way that will improve their effectiveness. This book also looks at how to effect organizational change in a fast-paced world. The major approaches to organizational improvement are identified, analyzed, assessed, and evaluated. The sometimes subtle relationships between strategy and capabilities are highlighted.

Tsoukas, Haridimos and Jill Shepherd (eds) *Managing the Future: Strategic Foresight in the Knowledge Economy* (Malden, MA: Blackwell Publishing, 2004). A set of ten papers by leading authorities on strategy and organizational learning. The papers address questions such as how organizational foresight can be conceptualized, how organizations make sense of their environments, how foresight can be developed, and similar issues. The book is a valuable source of information on strategic management in the knowledge-based society of today.

Zook, Chris, *Beyond the Core: Expand Your Market Without Abandoning Your Roots* (Boston, MA: Harvard Business School Press, 2004). Growth is an imperative. Growth, however, involves risks. Only about one fourth of growth initiatives succeed. Most of the business disasters of the past five years were growth initiatives gone bad. Most enduring performers succeeded by focusing on one or two well-defined dominant cores. Many organizations fail because they prematurely abandon their core to chase after a hot topic or fad.

Internal Environmental Analysis and Competitive Advantage

"An organization is assured of a competitive advantage only after others' efforts to duplicate its strategy have ceased or failed."

Robert E. Hoskisson, Michael A. Hitt, and R. Duane Ireland,
Competing for Advantage

Introductory Incident

Adding Value at York Hospital

York Hospital is a not-for-profit 79-bed hospital located on the southern coast of Maine. The hospital was incorporated on September 17, 1904 when a certificate of organization prepared by seven local physicians was signed. The doors opened for patient services on July 22, 1906. Begun in a cottage as a small hospital designed to accommodate the summer community, York Hospital has grown as residents from York as well as Portsmouth to Kennebunk began using the facility. Nearly a century later, the hospital provides medical/surgical care; an emergency center; maternity care through its family-oriented birthing center; cardiology, oncology, and respiratory centers; an intensive care unit; radiology/imaging using the latest technology; laboratory; home care; a sleep lab; wellness center; and wound healing.

York Hospital's vision is "Caring, Listening, Satisfying . . . One by One." Its mission is as follows:

At York Hospital, each one of us is devoted to satisfying the needs and expectations of every patient by:

- Deeply caring about and understanding each patient's unique needs and concerns.
- Meeting each patient's expectations by providing value through their eyes.
- Responding to each patient with clear information, personal attention, and respect.
- Allowing patients to make their own decisions about their treatment and care.
- Nurturing an enduring relationship with each patient and their family that begins prior to their hospital experience and continues after they return home.
- Our unique spirit of dedication to patient satisfaction sets us apart. It is the promise on which our current patients rely, to which new patients are attracted, and by which each one of us lives.

Beginning in 1995, York Hospital focused on providing outstanding patient care – starting before the patient arrives at the hospital and extending to after they return home. The PATH program (patient approach to health) initially focused on maternity patients but was so successful in developing patient loyalty that it was expanded to all patients.

The hospital assigns nursing and support staff to learn about the communities where its patients live and about the physicians and support services in those communities. Before a hospital admission, nurses that are familiar with the particular community visit the patient to get to know him or her personally. These are the same nurses that will care for the patient at admission and during the inpatient stay because patients are assigned to community-based units. (The hospital's primary service area covers four main communities where its patients live.)

York nurses prepare patients for their upcoming hospitalization by performing pre-registration activities to speed admission, describing the procedures to help patients know what to expect, and making sure their questions are answered. In addition, the staff begins developing plans for the patient's stay, for discharge, and post-discharge follow-up.

Based on what the nurses learn about a patient's home and family situation, they may offer to make arrangements for delivery of meals to a disabled family member who normally depends on the patient for such support. Or they might make arrangements for child care at home while "mom" is in the hospital with the new baby brother or sister or they may find a volunteer to care for a pet.

At discharge, the patient who needs it will have transportation home provided. In addition, if it benefits the patients' care, home visits are conducted by the same nurses who cared for them when they were inpatients. Even up to a year after discharge, patients may receive follow-up phone calls from the same staff members who cared for them to see if there are any questions, concerns, or problems.

The PATH program is not limited just to the services that York Hospital provides. If discharged patients would benefit from local community services to complete their recovery and adjust to life changes caused by their condition, the staff makes arrangements or helps with referrals to programs with which they are personally familiar.

Both physicians and employees have embraced the PATH program, believing it to be a better way to organize and deliver optimal value to patients from each inpatient experience. The hospital averages 90 percent of its patients rating it "exceptional" on satisfaction surveys.

Source: Scott MacStravic, "Make It Personal," *Marketing Health Services* 24, no. 3 (Fall 2004), pp. 21–25 and the York Hospital website: www.yorkhospital.com.

Learning Objectives

After completing this chapter the student should be able to:

1. Understand the role of internal environmental analysis in identifying the basis for sustained competitive advantage.

2. Describe the organizational value chain, including the components of the service delivery and support activities.

3. Understand the ways in which value can be created at various places in the organization with the aid of the value chain.

4. Use the value chain to identify organizational strengths and weaknesses.

5. Determine the competitive relevance of each strength and weakness with the aid of a series of carefully formulated questions.

6. Describe how competitively relevant strengths and weaknesses can be used to suggest appropriate strategic actions.

Identifying Competitive Advantage

To this point, situational analysis has concentrated on factors in the external environment of the health care organization in an attempt to answer the first of three strategic questions concerning situational analysis – "What *should* the organization do?" (refer to Exhibit 1–5). Because the rules of success are written outside the organization in the environment, it is appropriate that health care organizations attempt to first understand the context within which they operate. After assessing the opportunities, threats, and nature of its strategic competitors, the emphasis of situational analysis shifts to the organization itself and the ways in which competitive advantage may be established. For example, as described in the Introductory Incident, York Hospital had created competitive advantage by increasing patient satisfaction. The creation of some type of competitive advantage is essential. Experts writing on competitive advantage have suggested that successful organizations "focus relentlessly on competitive advantage . . . [they] strive to widen the performance gap between themselves and competitors. They are not satisfied with today's competitive advantage – they want tomorrow's."[1] As suggested in Perspective 4–1, health care strategists must sometimes think like an MBA.

The task of establishing competitive advantage is sometimes perplexing, and not always successful. Developing a better product, charging a lower price, or delivering a better service does not guarantee success. Competitive advantage requires an organization to develop a distinctiveness that competitors do not have and cannot easily imitate. Identifying this distinctiveness requires a shift in focus

Perspective 4–1
Think Like an MBA

Medicine is not a business. It follows a higher standard and doctors have to choose between high quality medicine and running a business. Right? Not necessarily. Physicians can practice good medicine and make a profit but they have to think as a business person to accomplish both of these goals. At the American Urogynecologic Society, Dr. Neeraj Kohli shared the lessons he learned while earning an MBA. His ten important tips for doctors who want to be good business people include:

1. Develop a strategic edge. Differentiate yourself from your competitors. Find a niche and do it immediately.
2. Create a competitive advantage. A competitive advantage can be developed in a number of ways – promoting product excellence, customer service, or streamlining operations could be examples. Dr. Kohli recommends developing customer intimacy by understanding and responding to the needs of patients.
3. Know your customer. Survey patients. Patients like being asked their opinions. Because needs change and patients come and go, survey them regularly.
4. Market yourself. Even if you do not attract patients, marketing may increase payors and increase revenue, reduce competition, and establish a brand image.
5. Perform a business analysis at regular intervals. Financial accounting is crucial to success. Study and understand your primary and ancillary revenues, as well as office expenses and methods to control expenses.
6. Base decisions on quantitative factors not just qualitative assessments. Before you bring in a partner, hire a nurse practitioner or a physician's assistant. Use available spreadsheet programs for modeling, forecasting, and scenario development.
7. Use activity-based costing. With the help of an accountant, a physician can determine the best way to allocate resources and generate revenues.
8. Design your practice around your strategic vision.
9. Establish an integrated team approach. Demonstrate leadership and establish rewards that are consistent with the goals of the practice.
10. Manage change. Practice change management. Lead the team and continually assess the costs and benefits of proposed changes.

Source: Sherry Boschert, "Think Like an MBA to Make Practice Profitable," *Internal Medicine News* 36, no. 6 (March 15, 2003), pp. 44–45.

to the internal environment and an introspective view that allows the organization to answer the second strategically relevant question of situational analysis – "What *can* the organization do?"

Analyzing the Internal Environment

Internal environmental analysis is sometimes accomplished by evaluating functional areas such as clinical operations, information systems, marketing, clinical support, human resources, financial administration, and so on. With such an approach, each function or organizational subsystem is carefully analyzed and a list of strengths and weaknesses is developed and evaluated. Although this approach has been successful in some instances, by itself it does not adequately address strategic issues. A better approach is to evaluate the various ways that organizations create value for present and prospective customers (patients) and other stakeholders. The organizational value chain is a useful tool for identifying and assessing how health care organizations create value.

Value Creation in Health Care Organizations

Organizations are successful when they create value for their customers. Similarly health care organizations are successful to the extent that they create value for the patients, physicians, and other stakeholders that rely on their services. *Value* is defined as the amount of satisfaction received relative to the price paid for a health care service.[2] For example, a patient may go to a cosmetic surgeon and pay an extremely high price. Despite the high price, the perception of social acceptance, increased feeling of self-esteem, and improved self-confidence may provide so much satisfaction that the patient believes a very high value was received. By contrast, patients may go to a family practice clinic where services are provided in a rude and disrespectful manner and perceive that they have received little or no value. Value is the perceived relationship between satisfaction and price, not price alone.[3]

Organizational Value Chain

Health care organizations have numerous opportunities to create value for patients and other stakeholders.[4] For example, efficient appointment systems, courteous doctors and nurses, "patient friendly" billing systems, easy-to-navigate physical facilities, and the absence of bureaucratic red tape can greatly increase the ratio of satisfaction to price.[5] As discussed in Perspective 4–2 even an organization's culture – "how we do things" – can create value. The organizational value chain is an effective means of illustrating how and where value may be created.[6]

The value chain illustrated in Exhibit 4–1 has been adapted from the value chain used in industrial organizations to more closely reflect the value adding components for health care organizations. The *value chain* utilizes a systems approach; value may be created in the *service delivery* subsystem (upper portion of the value chain) and by effective use of the support subsystem (lower portion). Service delivery activities (pre-service, point-of-service, and after-service) are placed above the support activities as they are the fundamental value creation activities but they are buttressed by, or "supported" by, activities that facilitate and improve service delivery. The three elements of service delivery – pre-service, point-of-service, and after-service – incorporate the production or creation of the service (product) of health care and include primarily operational processes and marketing activities. Organizational culture, organizational structure, and strategic resources are the

Perspective 4–2

A Constructive Culture Adds Value for Patients and Employees

An organizational culture is a shared value system that defines how people in the organization succeed. The culture of a health care organization not only influences its ability to manage employees and serve patients, but also is an important factor in building and sustaining a competitive advantage.

Health care organizations with constructive cultures put people first. When Baptist Hospital in Pensacola, Florida developed its vision to become "the best health care system in America," the CEO began with the organizational culture. Constructive relationships between patients and employees became the top priority. When Griffin Hospital in Derby, Connecticut transformed itself from a bureaucratic culture to a caring culture, patient satisfaction soared 96 percent, nursing turnover decreased, and the hospital was in a better strategic position to compete against neighboring hospitals.

Some of the things necessary for a constructive organizational culture include:

- A sense of collectivity to build teamwork. Teamwork facilitates coordination of efforts and builds consensus among group members.
- Human values are emphasized in every aspect of work. Effective human resource management is a top priority.

Building constructive cultures in health care requires leaders who look beyond the professional training of a prospective employee and use the recruitment process to identify individuals whose values are consistent with the organization's culture.

Constructive cultures are patient-centered cultures. If the "right" people are hired and socialized into a constructive culture, everyone will be more involved in creating value through patient service. Constructive cultures promote an inherent value of delivering quality patient service by encouraging and rewarding people for service excellence.

Developing and maintaining a constructive culture requires that leaders and employees work together to create a culture that balances human values, organizational goals, and patient advocacy. The first step in achieving this goal requires leaders to recognize the importance of organizational culture because it explains how people relate to one another at work.

Leaders have to take on the responsibility of "culture gatekeeper." They must become accessible and visible to the staff. The role of culture gatekeeper requires leaders to confront, control, and change behaviors that violate the values of a constructive culture.

Source: Adapted from Lynn Perry Wooten and Patricia Crane, "Nurses as Implementers of Organizational Culture," *Nursing Economics* 26, no. 6 (2003), pp. 275–280.

subsystems that support service delivery by ensuring an inviting and supportive atmosphere, an effective organization, and sufficient resources such as finances, highly qualified staff, information systems, and appropriate facilities and equipment. Although not always apparent, such support systems are critical for an effective and efficient organization.

The value chain as a strategic thinking map provides the health care strategist with a framework for assessing the internal environment of the organization (see Exhibit 4–2). The value chain and its use in developing implementation strategies will be discussed in Chapters 8 through 10.

Exhibit 4–1: The Value Chain

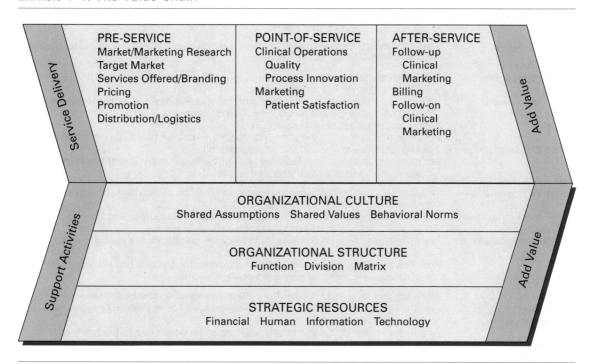

Source: Adapted from Michael E. Porter, *Competitive Advantage: Creating and Sustaining Superior Performance* (New York: Free Press, 1985), p. 37.

SERVICE DELIVERY ACTIVITIES

Health care organizations can create value and significant advantages over competitors in all three of the service delivery subsystems. For example, in late summer and early fall, public health officials begin to remind citizens that it is time for immunization against influenza. It is possible for a health care provider that views administering flu shots as an effective way to build a caring, quality image in the minds of potential patients to do considerable research to determine which patients need flu shots (or would benefit from having flu shots); where those patients live or work and where they might find it convenient to go for flu shots; how much they might be willing to pay; and how they might best find out about the benefits, convenience, and affordability. The research and promotion activities undertaken by this provider are part of the pre-service subsystem. In deciding where to go, those consumers who feel they could benefit from a flu shot might scan the local newspaper and discover one provider that is offering flu shots at the shopping mall. The provider has done research to discover that consumers want to get flu shots, but making an appointment, waiting, and so on, is too inconvenient. Thus, the provider rented space at the mall to enable consumers to receive shots easily. Additional information may be sought on the price of the shot at the mall

Exhibit 4-2: Description of Value Chain Components

Value Chain Component	Description
Service Delivery	The activities in the value chain that are directly involved in ensuring access to, provision of, and follow-up for health services
Pre-Service	
• Market/Marketing Research	Determine the services that create value prior to the actual delivery of health services, determine appropriate target market
• Services offered/ Branding	Information dissemination to present and prospective patients and other stakeholders regarding the range and location of available services
• Pricing	Charge schedule for available services
• Promotion	Activities that ensure all the elements needed to deliver health services are available at the appropriate place at the appropriate time
• Distribution/Logistics	Activities and systems that facilitate patient/customer entry into the service delivery system, including appointments and registration
Point-of-Service	
• Clinical Operations Quality	Those service delivery activities that create value at the point where services are actually delivered
Process Innovation	The activities that convert the human and nonhuman resources into health services
• Marketing	Actual provision of health services to the individual patient
Patient Satisfaction	Activities and groups of activities that are designed specifically to improve the quality and quantity of health services
	Activities to offer new products, seek new customers, provide better services delivery, and cause services to be perceived as higher value
After-Service	
• Follow-up	Activities that create value after the patient has received the health services
Clinical Marketing	Activities designed to determine the effectiveness of or the patient's satisfaction with health services received
• Billing	Activities that assist in determining what other services need to be delivered
• Follow-on Clinical	Value creating activities that ensure more understandable and efficient billing procedures
Marketing	Activities that facilitate entry into another value chain (from hospital to home care, etc.)
Support Activities	The activities in the value chain that are designed to aid in the efficient and effective delivery of health services
Organizational Culture	
• Shared Assumptions	The overarching environment within which the health services organization operates
• Shared Values	The assumptions employees and others share in the organization regarding all aspects of service delivery (e.g., needs of patients, goals of the organization)
• Behavioral Norms	The guiding principles of the organization and its employees. The understandings people in the organization have regarding excellence, risk taking, etc.
	Understandings about behavior in the organization that can create value for patients
Organizational Structure	Those aspects of the organization structure that are capable of creating value for customers/patients
• Function	Structure based on process or activities used by employees (e.g., surgery, finance, human resources)
• Division	Major units operate relatively autonomously subject to overarching policy guidelines (e.g., hospital division; outpatient division; northwest division)
• Matrix	Two-dimensional structure where more than a single authority structure operates simultaneously (e.g., interdisciplinary team with representatives from medicine, nursing, administration)
Strategic Resources	
• Financial	Value creating financial, human, information resources, and technology necessary for the delivery of health services
• Human	Financial resources required to provide the facilities, equipment, and specialized competencies demanded by the delivery of health services
• Information	Individuals with the specialized skills and commitment to deliver health services
• Technology	Hardware, software, and information processing systems needed to support the delivery of health services
	The facilities and equipment required to provide health services

---

Perspective 4–3
Guarantees in
Health Care

Oakwood Healthcare System in Michigan has gained attention and improved customer satisfaction with a series of brand guarantees. In 1999 when a task force investigated consumer waits in the emergency room of one of its hospitals, the hospital streamlined its procedures and reduced the wait time to 15 minutes. The marketing department then advertised a 30-minute guarantee – ER patients would see a physician within 30 minutes of arrival or they would receive a letter of apology and two movie tickets. Fewer than 1 percent of Oakwood's ER patients since 2000 have received a letter and tickets. Patient volume and satisfaction increased and Oakwood extended the guarantee to three other hospitals in its system.

The ER guarantee was so successful that other areas of the hospital have developed similar guarantees to distinguish its customer service from that of its competition. Oakwood's ambulatory centers now promise patients who call in to schedule a sick visit that they will be able to schedule an appointment either the same day or by the end of the next business day.

Oakwood developed a successful ad campaign for the system with the theme "Designed Around You" that showcases many of the improvements that Oakwood's facilities have made to benefit the consumer. Additional departments within the facilities are working at identifying other guarantees that might be offered.

Source: Darla Dernovsek, "Improving Operations Delivers Marketing Clout," *Healthcare Marketing Report* (October 2003), pp. 12–14.

---

compared with the health department (promotion/pricing). These decisions relate to *pre-service* activities, providing numerous opportunities to create value before the patient arrives.

Once the patient arrives, *point-of-service* activities take place. The environment is clean and attractive. There is no waiting time. The nurse is courteous, provides information about possible side effects, and the injection is painless. Perspective 4–3 demonstrates how one health care organization "guaranteed" value and created competitive advantage by reducing waiting time.

Further, value can be created through effective *after-service* activities, such as providing assistance in filing the necessary insurance papers or ensuring credit cards are accepted as a payment alternative in addition to cash or personal checks. Finally, a friendly call (follow-up) from someone the next day to check that there were no adverse side effects is a thoughtful gesture and can create considerable satisfaction for the consumer. Patient satisfaction studies at a later date can serve to remind the consumer of the outstanding care received or, if the consumer was not delighted with the care, the study can identify areas that need improvement.

SUPPORT ACTIVITIES

Value creation in service delivery can be greatly enhanced by *support activities*. If the organizational culture is service oriented, patients can feel it when they walk in the door.[7] The organizational structure increases patient satisfaction by effectively and efficiently facilitating the service delivery. The structure should have enough standardization to ensure consistent quality but enough flexibility to allow for responding to special needs. Strategic resources are important to the overall perception of value received at the health care organization. Employees with the proper skills, an up-to-date information system, an accessible parking lot, well-maintained buildings and grounds, and up-to-date diagnostic and treatment equipment will have a positive impact on a patient's satisfaction with the visit. A lost patient record may imply that the entire clinic is disorganized and an inefficient billing system suggests that the technology is out of date (see Perspective 4–4).

Perspective 4–4

E-Billing Comes of Age

Who understands the typical health care organization's billing system? Probably very few people really understand what they are being charged for when they receive a bill from a physician or hospital. Humana decided to change its paper and snail mail billing system to offer its employer-group customers a more user-friendly e-billing alternative.

In 1999, Humana, Inc. implemented an e-business strategy designed to provide better customer satisfaction across all its business lines. It updated the core billing processes by converting its outdated mainframe system to a relational database with a client/server environment. But even after massive expenditures, employer groups could only view invoices on the computer screen. They could not add or remove employees from coverage or even sort the bills. In some cases employers had to scroll through 1,000 to 2,000 names just to verify whether a new employee had health coverage. Customers began to demand a web-enabled e-billing system. Eventually, Humana was able to use features of a system marketed by edocs, Inc. and provide the services customers were demanding.

Historically, when a bill was incorrect, employer groups either asked the insuror to correct the bill before they paid it or they made corrections on the bill and submitted the revised amount they had calculated. In either case, reconciliation was a nightmare and payment was delayed. Now, for those customers participating in the e-billing program, invoices are available one day after the billing date on the computer screen. Customers can sort, store, analyze, and adjust bills themselves and a significant amount of unnecessary work is eliminated. Humana's customers can make real-time changes to their invoices online and arrange for electronic funds transfers without time consuming back-and-forth haggling over bills.

Since the program has been implemented, there has been a significant drop in retroactive premium adjustments. The number of employer groups using the web-enabled billing system is increasing. In terms of its overall web-enabled self-service system, Humana customer service representatives answered two-thirds of all inbound calls and one-third were handled over the web or through interactive voice systems in September 2001. By April 2002 inbound calls answered by customer service representatives equaled those handled by the web or interactive voice response systems. By the end of 2003, service representatives were handling only 39 percent of inbound calls. The web-enabled self-service system allowed Humana to increase customer satisfaction and reduce its customer service staff, with corresponding labor cost savings.

Source: Adapted from Brian S. Moskal, "Just What the Doctor Ordered: Humana, Inc. Implements Electronic Billing System," *Insurance Networking News: Executive Strategies for Technology Management* 6, no. 12 (2003), pp. 1–3.

As this example of the value chain illustrates, there are a number of opportunities for health care organizations to create value when patients come for a service as simple as a flu shot. It is important to recognize that opportunities for value creation may be lost or value destroyed within each subsystem just as it can be created.[8] Therefore, the goals, values, and behaviors of all employees must be integrated toward the common objective of patient satisfaction and service.

Identifying Current and Potential Competitive Advantage

Ascertaining and assessing an organization's current and potential competitively relevant strengths and weaknesses is the goal of internal environmental analysis. Competitively relevant strengths are the pathways to sustained competitive advantage.[9] *Competitive advantage* is created within the organization in the form of strengths that relate to important aspects of the external environment. The strategic thinking map shown in Exhibit 4–3 illustrates the process involved in determining an organization's sources of competitive advantage. The first step is to carefully assess the activities that the organization does well and the activities it does not do as well for each component of the value chain. After the organization's strengths and weaknesses have been identified, each one is assessed to determine whether it is – or could become – a competitive advantage or competitive

Exhibit 4–3: Strategic Thinking Map for Discovering Competitive Advantages and Disadvantages

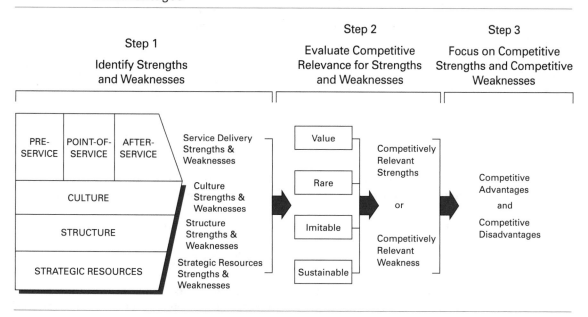

Perspective 4–5

Alternative Views
of Competitive
Advantage

Achieving and maintaining a competitive advantage is the goal of strategy. This is no less true in health care than in other industries. Organizations try different strategies for achieving advantage over competitors depending on what they perceive to be their competitively relevant strengths and weaknesses.

In the management literature, competitive advantage is discussed at three levels – global, industry, and firm. For health care strategists, the firm level is the most important. Firm level competitive advantage is the ability of an organization to design, produce, and market products/services that are superior to those offered by competitors, considering price and nonprice qualities. Sources of competitive advantage are those tangible and intangible assets (resources and competencies) and processes (capabilities) in the organization that provide an advantage over competitors in the mind of customers.

Traditionally in health care, factors such as location and facilities have been thought of as the primary sources of competitive advantage. Competitiveness has been associated with an organization's resource base which is, no doubt, an important factor in firm-level competitiveness. Unfortunately, focusing on resources alone may overlook important factors – such as patient orientation and positioning in the marketplace – and certainly has a "large organization bias." In the dynamic environment of health care today, capabilities such as flexibility, agility, speed, and adaptability may be even more important than resources in achieving and maintaining competitive advantage.

Perhaps the most promising views of competitiveness are those that integrate the importance of resources and capabilities in achieving competitive advantage. These approaches are sometimes referred to as APP (asset–process–performance) models. Consideration of how all the tangible and intangible assets of the organization are combined through the application of capabilities and processes to achieve desired outcomes (performance) has the potential for greatly assisting health care leaders in thinking about competitive advantage. Perhaps most important, it discourages functional-centric silo thinking and encourages strategists to think in terms of the entire organizational system. A wider net is cast in the search for competitively relevant strengths and advantages are found that do not reside within a single organizational subsystem. This should be particularly valuable for health care organizations that have often relied on a single area (e.g. clinical excellence) to achieve competitive advantage only to discover that excellence in a single area of the value chain is not sufficient to overcome weaknesses such as lack of accessibility, stubbornness of bureaucracy, and reluctance to change.

Source: Ajitabh Ambastha and K. Momaya, "Competitiveness of Firms: Review of Theory, Frameworks, and Models," *Singapore Management Review* 26, no. 1 (2004), pp. 45–56.

disadvantage. As illustrated in Perspective 4–5, there are a variety of ways competitively relevant strengths can affect an organization's ability to build and sustain a competitive advantage.

Step 1. Identifying Strengths and Weaknesses

Identifying an organization's internal strengths and internal weaknesses is a challenging yet essential task of health care strategists as they assess the internal environment. However, organizational characteristics that appear to represent key strengths to strategists may have little importance to patients and other stakeholders or may be strengths of competitors.

In the past, a stable environment allowed static strategies based on one or two strengths to be successful for years, particularly for large, dominant organizations. Thus, competitive advantage for many health care organizations was primarily a matter of "position" where the physician's office, hospital, or sales office occupied a well-defined competitive niche.[10] In today's changing environment, strengths can quickly become weaknesses as successful strategies are challenged by competitors. A critical component of strategic momentum is continuous evaluation of the organization's strengths and weaknesses relative to the changing environment.

Some strengths that health care organizations possess are clear and easily recognizable (objective strengths). For example, a particular location may be a strategic strength because it prohibits other organizations from occupying that specific location. Weaknesses may be easy to recognize as well. For example, when an organization assumes excessive debt financing for its facilities, it may not be able to finance a new emerging technology (objective weakness). Other strengths are subjective in that they represent the opinions of the people who are doing the evaluating. For example, employees stating that the long-term care facility offers a caring environment would be a subjective strength. Employees may believe they provide a caring environment, but do the patients?

Still other strengths and weaknesses are not so obvious and can only be determined in relationship to the strengths and weaknesses of primary competitors (relative strength or weakness). For example, a world-renowned academic health center may lose a famous surgeon to a local hospital that is attempting to build more strength in the clinical area of the surgeon's specialty. The health center may remain very strong in terms of the services it provides but have a relative weakness with regard to the facility where the surgeon is now located.

Competitive advantages of an organization may be based on having rare or abundant resources, special competencies or skills, or management or logistical capabilities. Similarly, competitive disadvantages may result from a lack of resources, competencies, or capabilities. Therefore, strengths and weaknesses are easier to identify if one thinks in terms of organizational resources, competencies, and capabilities.[11]

RESOURCES

The *resource-based view* of strategy argues that valuable, expensive or difficult-to-copy resources provide a key to sustainable competitive advantage.[12] The basic assumption is that "resource bundles" used by health care organizations to create and distribute services are unevenly developed and distributed, explaining – at least to some extent – the ability of each organization to compete effectively. Organizations with marginal resources may break even; those with inferior resources might disappear; and those with superior resources typically generate profits.[13] Perspective 4–6 illustrates how one hospital effectively leveraged its resources by selectively divesting or outsourcing certain services.

Perspective 4–6

Resourcing Facilities Management

Sometimes you have to change even when things are going well. Several years ago the William Beaumont Hospital (Royal Oak, Michigan) decided that even though it had an excellent facilities management department, others might be able to do an even better job. The hospital was a health care organization, not a facilities management company, so it decided to look outside for new ideas. With the assistance of PricewaterhouseCoopers in Chicago and Jacobs Engineering in Pasadena, a new company, Beaumont Services Company, was formed. PricewaterhouseCoopers and Jacobs Engineering, through a partnership called ReSourcing Services Company, had assisted another client in outsourcing its real estate, design, and construction functions.

Beaumont Services Company (BSC) enabled the hospital to outsource its facilities management function without downsizing. The results have been impressive. BSC has saved Beaumont Hospital an estimated $6 million since its formation. Maintenance costs are down by $500,000. In addition to the tangible savings, BSC has generated much goodwill among workers at the hospital because there were no lay-offs. A spokesperson at Pricewaterhouse Coopers stated that the "fundamental premise of resouing is that the best people to do the work tomorrow are the people doing it today." The 300-person facilities management personnel who once planned, designed, constructed, and maintained facilities as well as performed the biomedical engineering function as employees of the hospital, now work on site and share their talents but are employed by Beaumont Services.

Resourcing has transformed the workforce, which is comprised of two-thirds skilled trades and one-third office workers, from a hospital facilities management group to a facility-focused company. Many observers believe this resourcing concept will grow in popularity in the future and be extended to many functions presently performed by health care organizations.

Source: Diana Mosher, "Resourcing Revitalizes the Bottom Line," *Facilities Design & Management* 19, no. 5 (2000), pp. 46–49.

"Basing strategy on the [resource] differences between firms should be automatic rather than noteworthy."[14] However, the argument is far from evident, especially in light of the overwhelming attention given to the external environment in strategy formulation. In addition, there are many different types of resources.

Resources are the stocks of human and nonhuman factors that are available for use in producing goods and services. Resources may be tangible, as in the case of land, labor, and capital, or they may be intangible, as in the case of intellectual property, reputation, and goodwill.[15] The importance of intangible resources should not be underestimated. Robert Kaplan and David Norton point out that unlike financial and physical ones, intangible resources are hard for competitors to imitate, making them a powerful source of sustainable competitive advantage.[16] Furthermore, according to a Harris Interactive Health Care Poll, a good reputation and a trusted physician's recommendation are two of the most important indicators of the quality of medical care. These factors ranked above more tangible indicators of resources, including location, appearance, and condition of physical plant.[17]

COMPETENCIES

The collective knowledge and skills possessed by individuals, called competencies, may be a source of sustained competitive advantage for the organization. In the pharmaceutical industry, for example, strategically important competency is acquired by developing disciplinary expertise (such as medicinal chemistry or crystallography) or expertise in a particular disease category (cancer or heart disease, for instance).[18]

Competency is knowledge and skill based and, therefore, inherently human; in many cases, it is socially complex and requires large numbers of people engaged in coordinated activities.[19] To enter a particular market or offer specific services the organization must possess, at a minimum, threshold competencies – the minimally required knowledge and skills necessary to compete in a particular area. To offer cardiac services, an acute care hospital must have a minimum number of clinical personnel with specific knowledge and skill in cardiac care. Although all organizations offering cardiac services presumably possess threshold competencies, only one or two will develop the knowledge and skills to the point that it becomes a distinctive competency. This type of competency is a highly developed strength that can be critical in developing a sustained competitive advantage.

CAPABILITIES

A health care organization's ability to deploy resources and competencies, usually in combination, to produce desired services is known as its *capability*. The purposeful coordination of resources and competencies is another potential source of sustained competitive advantage.[20] The ability to effectively and efficiently coordinate resources and competencies to achieve integrative synergies through leadership and management represents strategic capability.[21] For example, some assets almost never create value by themselves, they need to be combined with other assets – investments in IT (a resource) have little value unless complemented with effective HR training (competencies). Conversely, many HR training programs have little value unless complemented with modern technology and managerial tools.[22] As discussed in Perspective 4–7, one managerial tool to better utilize resources and competencies to reduce errors in health care is Six Sigma.

Capabilities fall into one of the two following categories:

1. The ability to make dynamic improvements to the organization's activities through learning, renewal, and change over time; or
2. The ability to develop strategic insights and recognize and arrange resources and competencies to develop novel strategies before or better than competitors.[23]

Capabilities are architectural[24] or bonding mechanisms whereby leaders make use of resources and competencies and integrate them in new and flexible ways to develop new resources and competencies as they learn, change, and continually renew themselves and their organizations.[25] Capabilities, therefore, are integrative and coordinating abilities of managers and leaders that bring

Perspective 4–7
Six Sigma

Errors lurk in all facets of organizations and, in 2002, the seven-hospital Fairview Health System in Minneapolis turned to the techniques of Six Sigma to find them. Developed in the 1980s by Motorola to define, identify, and control defects, Six Sigma has since been used with great success by manufacturing companies such as General Electric, Honeywell, and 3M.

A sigma is a notation employed by statisticians to represent one standard deviation from the mean (a measure of variation). A key goal of Six Sigma is to virtually eliminate variation or defects. Although most companies are estimated to be operating at the four sigma level – tolerating 6,210 defects per million units – the goal of Six Sigma is to reduce defects to only 3.4 defects per million units. This aggressive, but attainable, goal is accomplished through a five-phased approach: defining goals, measuring current performance, determining root causes of defects, improving processes to eliminate defects, and controlling ongoing performance.

Six Sigma is a process heavily focused on data, not opinions or anecdotal evidence, that aims to improve both financial performance and customer satisfaction. A basic premise of Six Sigma is that even the most complex processes can be broken down into a relatively small number of key factors that are responsible for the majority of defects.

The executives of the Fairview Health System recognized that Six Sigma methods provided a means to both understand and manage the complexities within a large hospital system. Management initially set out to improve three key processes by:

1. reducing the time delay in a physician's office between patient check-in and the doctor entering the exam room,
2. increasing the rate of patient encounters that are free of medication-related harm from 80 percent (2.3 sigma) to 98 percent (3.5 sigma), and
3. decreasing the percentage of orthopedic patients with DRG 209 that stay longer than four days from 42 percent to 7 percent.

All improvements were to be accomplished without diminishing the quality of patient care.

Today, the growing popularity of Six Sigma techniques suggests that many executives have found in it a way to manage processes once believed to be unmanageable.

Source: Written by Nelson Weichold, PhD student, Health Services Administration, University of Alabama at Birmingham. Adapted from Greg Brue, *Six Sigma for Managers* (New York: McGraw-Hill, 2002), pp. 1–20, and Center for the Study of Healthcare Management, Publication Series 2: *Deploying Six Sigma in a Healthcare System.* Carlson School of Management, University of Minnesota.

together resources and competencies in ways that are superior to those of competitors.[26] Sustained competitive advantage is based on resources, competencies, and capabilities that possess important relationships to key factors in the external environment.

The stock of resources, knowledge, and integrative skills contained in a health care organization may not be sufficient to ensure a sustained competitive advantage. It is likely that two or more organizations competing in the same health care market could have essentially the same resources and similar competencies. Yet, one of the organizations may be more effective or efficient. When this is the case, the competitive advantage is likely to be the result of different capabilities – a unique culture, strategic leadership, or a set of business processes strategically understood.[27] In other words, capabilities are best thought of as processes or ways of bringing together and organizing competencies and resources so as to obtain competitive advantage. Capabilities represent an ability to muster resources, skills, and knowledge in unique ways, coordinate diverse operational skills, and integrate multiple streams of technologies.[28]

Health care organizations that do not have superior resources or unique competencies may still develop sustainable competitive advantages if they are extraordinarily competent at converting ordinary resources and skills into genuine strategic assets.[29] For example, effective management of technology is more important than new computers and software. This results in services that respond uniquely to customer needs and, thereby, provide a competitive advantage. The development of this type of capability is based on four interrelated principles:

1. The building blocks of strategy may be processes as well as people, products, services, and markets.
2. Competitive success depends on transforming an organization's key processes into services that consistently provide superior value to customers.
3. Organizations create these capabilities by making strategic investments in a support infrastructure that link together and transcend traditional functions and any single component of the value chain.
4. Because capabilities necessarily cross functions and value chain components, the champion of capabilities-based strategy must be the chief executive.[30]

THE IMPORTANCE OF CONTEXT

In today's more competitive and dynamic environment, the ability to develop a sustained competitive advantage is increasingly more difficult. A health care organization enjoys a sustained competitive advantage only so long as the services it delivers have attributes that correspond to the key "buying criteria" of a substantial number of customers in the target market. *Sustained competitive advantage* is the result of an enduring value differential between the services of one organization and that of its competitors in the minds of patients, physicians, and so on. This makes an understanding of internal factors extremely important. Health care organizations must consider more than the fit between the external environment and the present internal characteristics. They must also consider how their own strengths and weaknesses with regard to resources, competencies, and capabilities relate to those of competitors.[31] Exhibit 4–4 illustrates some important value creating strengths and value reducing weaknesses of a particular health care organization – American Healthways, Inc.

Step 1. An Example: American Healthways, Inc. "Improved health is the outcome"

Founded in 1981, American Healthways, Inc. provides care enhancement and disease management services to patients in all 50 states, the District of Columbia,

Exhibit 4–4: Value Creating Strengths and Value Reducing Weaknesses for American Healthways, Inc.

Value Chain Component	Value Creating Strength	Value Reducing Weakness
Service Delivery, Pre-Service	• Customer benefit: care enhancement/disease management concept (attractive to health plans, hospitals, physicians, patients) • Customer benefit developed: geographical coverage (attractive to large health plans) • Six care enhancement centers	• Limited brand identity • Disease management and care enhancement contracts require extensive selling because of lack of knowledge of key benefits • Revenues subject to seasonal pressures from enrollment processes of contracted health plans
Service Delivery, Point-of-Service	• Successful management of diseases leading to reduced costs and increased customer satisfaction • Company employees highly experienced in implementing care enhancement programs in certain areas, such as diabetes • Integrated care product line attracts broad range of patients • Number of covered lives increasing making economies of scale possible	• Company/employees have less experience in care enhancement programs in expanded product line areas such as end-state renal disease, fibromyalgia, etc. • A majority of company's revenues accounted for by three health plans
Service Delivery, After-Service	• Alliance with Johns Hopkins Health System to independently evaluate effectiveness of clinical interventions	• Incomplete or inaccurate data could render independent evaluation of clinical interventions useless
Support Activities, Culture	• First disease management and care enhancement provider in nation accredited by all three accrediting agencies • Highly professionalized culture • Experienced management team of individuals with extensive health care experience and longevity with the company • Conservative fiscal management philosophy: retain earnings for future growth and development	• Acquisition of StatusOne Health System with different culture • Company's reluctance to declare cash dividend may discourage some classes of investors
Support Activities, Strategic Resources	• Company has state-of-the-art medical information technology • Company has sound financial position: cash, working capital, stockholder equity increasing over past year • Earnings per share of common stock has increased despite 3:2 stock split in 2001 and 2:1 stock split in 2003	• Hospital contracts decreasing • Cost to maintain IT for compliance with federal and state regulations • High labor costs from competition for staff • Volatility of stock price and trading volume

Puerto Rico, and Guam through contracts with health plans and integrated systems (hospitals). The company's integrated care enhancement programs serve entire health plan populations through member and physician care support interventions, advanced neural network predictive modeling, and confidential, secure Internet-based applications that provide patients and physicians with individualized health information and data. Each subsystem of the value chain (areas that create value for health care organizations) may be examined to identify American Healthways' competitive strengths and weaknesses.[32]

SERVICE DELIVERY ACTIVITIES

American Healthways, Inc. possesses important value creating strengths and value reducing weaknesses in service delivery. During pre-service, the company's customer awareness and its marketing research determined that geographical coverage of all 50 states and the geographic placement of its six care centers represent important strengths. However, disease management and care enhancement is a relatively new and somewhat unproven concept requiring significant promotional efforts. The growth stage of the product life cycle suggests that personal selling would be an important promotional effort. Selling to health plans is somewhat seasonally directed; most plans have a specific enrollment period. In addition, because the benefits of care enhancement and disease management are only recently being documented – especially the financial benefits for health plans – a great deal of customer education is required through multiple levels of management. Because of the severe cost pressures they face, hospitals in particular are difficult to convince that the benefits of disease management are greater than the costs. During 2004 the company targeted health plans as hospitals are likely to continue facing increasing cost pressures and are less likely to contract for services. The contract period of between three and seven years slows the deal making as well.

American Healthways has had difficulty building brand identity in part because the sales cycle is long and because few health plans subscribe to the philosophy of comprehensive care and disease management enough to purchase the service. A majority of the company's revenues are generated from three major health plans.

A major strength of American Healthway's service delivery is the integrated product line that serves a wide range of patients and many different diseases. However, the diversity of the product line places pressure on the organization to perform equally well for all diseases to maintain its high-quality image and accreditation status. The company has had a declining number of hospitals under contract (55 in 2001 and 49 in 2003), hospitals as a percentage of its business has declined (26 percent in 2001 to 9 percent in 2003), and the average revenue per hospital contract declined by 11 percent in the past fiscal year. However, American Healthways has 23 health plans under contract, covering 838,000 enrollees. The increasing number of lives covered is making economies of scale possible. The company is highly experienced in disease management and care enhancement for its traditional product lines, such as diabetes, but has had less experience in newer areas that it has introduced, such as end-stage renal disease and fibromyalgia.

In the area of after-service, American Healthways, Inc. formed an affiliation with the Johns Hopkins University Medical System to independently evaluate the effectiveness of the company's services. This independent evaluation requires timely and accurate data collection and analysis. With validation from a highly recognized brand (Johns Hopkins), American Healthways improves its ability to build its own brand identity.

SUPPORT ACTIVITIES

American Healthways has a strong corporate culture based on quality service delivery. It is the first company in its industry to be accredited by all three relevant accrediting agencies (National Committee on Quality Assurance, American Accreditation Health Care Commission, and Joint Commission on Accreditation of Health Care Organizations), thereby providing tangible evidence of a commitment to quality and professionalism. More than 90 percent of its employees have achieved professional qualifications (degrees, licensures, or certifications).

American Healthways has attracted and retained a highly qualified management team comprised of individuals with extensive health care experience and longevity with the company. The leadership of the company has followed a conservative philosophy of reinvesting earnings to fuel future growth. The company's acquisition of StatusOne Health Systems (the leading provider of health management services for high-risk populations) has provided coverage for additional diseases/conditions but at the same time has created challenges relating to the merging of two different corporate cultures.

In the area of strategic resources, American Healthways, Inc. has built six state-of-the-art care enhancement centers. The company has created or purchased state-of-the-art medical information technologies that are absolutely necessary to the effective management of its diverse product line. There are a number of cost pressures that impact the company's bottom line. There is a constant need to invest in expensive information technology to be current in delivering its products. Compliance with any new federal and state regulations will likely add to the cost for IT. Shortages of qualified staff increase the cost of labor – American Healthways faces fierce competition in the market for qualified professionals.

The company is in a sound financial position. Cash, working capital, and stockholders' equity have increased over the past year. Earnings per share have increased despite a 3:2 stock split in 2001 and a 2:1 stock split in 2003.

After carefully searching through the value chain of an organization and reflecting on its resources, competencies, and capabilities in developing value, it is possible to move to Step 2 and evaluate the competitive relevance of the strengths and weaknesses discovered in Step 1 (see Exhibit 4–3).

Step 2. Evaluating Competitive Relevance

Identification of the strengths and weaknesses in the various components of the value chain inevitably results in a lengthy list of things "we do pretty well" and "things we do not do so well." However, not all of the strengths will necessarily be sources of competitive advantage for the organization. For example, executives often believe that "our reputation is our greatest asset." However, if all competitors in the industry have excellent reputations, then reputation is not a significant source of competitive advantage for any of the organizations. Similarly, an identified weakness may not necessarily be a competitive disadvantage if it is not competitively relevant or all competitors have the same weakness (such as a shortage of nurses).

ORGANIZATIONAL STRENGTHS

Strengths must have value, be rare, be difficult to imitate, and be sustainable in order to create competitive advantage.[33] Strengths that are merely present do not represent competitive advantages in themselves. To be competitively significant, the specialized resources and competencies must be marshaled in a way that allows them to become genuine strategic assets, resulting in the accumulation of economic returns greater than could be achieved in any alternative use.[34]

The competitive relevance is determined by critically considering four important questions.[35]

1. *Question of Value.* Is the resource, competency, or capability of value to customers?
2. *Question of Rareness.* Is this organization the only one that possesses the resource, competency, or capability or do many or all of its competitors possess it?
3. *Question of Imitability.* Is it easy or difficult to duplicate the resource, competency, or capability?
4. *Question of Sustainability.* Can the resource, competency, or capability be maintained over time?

A judgment must be made as to whether the strength is of high (H) or low (L) value in the marketplace. This is a critically important question because if a strength does not have high value in the marketplace there is no reason to ask the other three questions. A strength that does not have value is simply not relevant in a competitive sense.

The second question requires that a judgment be made as to whether the strength is rare or commonly found among competitors. If the strength is rare, an answer of "yes" (Y) is appropriate. If it is possessed by many or all competitors, the answer is "no" (N). Combined with value, the relative rareness of a strength is key to competitive advantage. Even critically valuable strengths that are not rare among competitors do not create a competitive advantage.

Question 3 attempts to determine whether it would be difficult (D) or easy (E) for competitors to obtain or imitate the strength. The rareness of a strength becomes even more important the more difficult the strength is to imitate. If a valuable and rare strength is easy to imitate, it may be the basis for a competitive advantage in the short run but is not a good bet for long-term strategy formulation.

Competitors will likely imitate any resource, competency, or capability that is valuable and rare as soon as possible.

Finally, the fourth question involves a judgment as to whether the organization can sustain the resource, competency, or capability. A "yes" (Y) or "no" (N) answer is required to this question. If the strength cannot be sustained it will provide, at best, only a short-term advantage over competitors. Strengths are competitively relevant if they are valuable to customers and rare in the marketplace. The difficulty or ease with which competitors can imitate the strengths and the organization's ability to sustain them determines the extent of its long-term or short-term advantage.

To further illustrate how this process may be used, the strengths of American Healthways, Inc. (identified in Step 1) are evaluated with regard to the four questions (Exhibit 4–5). From the initial assessment, American Healthways, Inc. appears to have 11 potentially important strengths (those strengths that have a high value in the marketplace). These are: (1) geographical service throughout the 50 United States, Puerto Rico, and Guam; (2) broad range of integrated services; (3) large base and increasing number of lives covered; (4) employees experienced at enhancing care with regard to specific diseases; (5) alliance with Johns Hopkins to evaluate outcomes of services; (6) highly professional culture; (7) accreditation; (8) experienced management team; (9) fiscally responsible leadership; (10) state-of-the-art information system; and (11) financially sound condition. One resource – six comprehensive care centers – although perhaps considered a strength by the company (subjective strength) may not have high value when considered by customers; most customers in the 50 states do not have physical access to the six centers (plus the company's services are conveniently delivered electronically).

Consider, for example, the profiles of various combinations of strengths listed in Exhibit 4–5. The high value strengths are examined relative to the three additional questions. Strengths such as "employees experienced with care enhancement for certain diseases" and "an experienced management team" that are valuable but are not rare, are easy to imitate, and can be sustained (HNEY) require a maintenance strategy. If the organization does not maintain them, it will be at a disadvantage relative to competitors. Strengths such as "highly liquid financial condition" that are valuable but not rare, are easy to imitate, and cannot be sustained (HNEN) provide no advantage. Few resources should be devoted to trying to maintain these strengths. Although a liquid financial condition is beneficial, the demands placed on financial resources for continued growth will likely require less liquidity. Further, more productive uses will be found for the funds currently held in the cash account. Strengths, such as "professional culture" that are valuable but not rare, are difficult to imitate, yet can be sustained (HNDY) should be maintained. Valuable strengths that are not rare, are difficult to imitate, and cannot be sustained (HNDN) provide little advantage and the organization should be cautious in devoting resources to maintain this type of strength.

Strengths such as the "alliance with Johns Hopkins" and the "state-of-the-art information system" that are valuable and rare, are easy to imitate, and can be

Exhibit 4–5: Competitive Relevance of the Strengths of American Healthways, Inc.

Strengths	Is Strength of *Value?* (High/Low)	Is Strength *Rare?* (Yes/No)	Ease of *Imitation?* (Easy/Difficult)	Can Strength Be *Sustained?* (Yes/No)
Service Delivery				
Geographical presence	H	Y	D	Y
Broad range of services in integrated service line	H	Y	D	Y
Number of lives covered increasing	H	Y	D	N
Company and employees experienced at enhancing care with respect to certain diseases	H	N	E	Y
Six care enhancement centers	L	–	–	–
Alliance with Johns Hopkins to evaluate effectiveness of services	H	Y	E	Y
Culture				
Highly professionalized culture	H	N	D	Y
Quality culture – Accreditation	H	Y	D	Y
Organizational Structure				
Experienced management team	H	N	E	Y
Fiscally responsible management team	H	N	E	Y
Strategic Resources				
State-of-the-art information system	H	Y	E	Y
Liquid financial condition	H	N	E	N

sustained (HYEY) may be a source of a short-term advantage and should be exploited for as long as possible. One effort to create competitive advantage by building a state-of-the-art information system is discussed in Perspective 4–8. However, strategies should not be based on this type of strength. Highly valued, rare, easily imitated, and nonsustainable strengths (HYEN) may provide a short-term advantage but, again, developing strategies around such strengths would not be recommended. Highly valued strengths such as the "large number of lives covered" that are rare, difficult to imitate, yet cannot be sustained (HYDN) only provide the possibility of a short-term advantage. Finally, highly valued strengths that are rare, difficult to imitate, and are sustainable (HYDY) provide the basis for a long-term competitive advantage and should be developed as much as possible. In the case of American Healthways, the company's "extensive geographical presence," "broad range of integrated services," and "comprehensive accreditation" represent possibilities for long-term competitive advantage. Exhibit 4–6 provides a strategic thinking map for the possible combinations of the four questions regarding strengths and the implications for strategic leaders.

When Bruce Morin accepted the title of Chief Information Officer at Jackson Hospital, he faced an information systems crisis of gargantuan proportions. Rather than attempting to resolve individual issues with existing systems and vendors, Morin and the executive leadership team determined to seek an integrated information system solution that would better serve the clinical and administrative needs of the hospital. Four strategic issues were identified:

1. They acknowledged the continuing financial pressure from Medicare and other payors. Maintaining financial viability under the current and evolving payment structure would require both improved productivity and decreased resource consumption. Morin believed that automating key processes to provide real-time information to physicians and to reduce redundancy in staff tasks was essential.
2. Patient safety could be enhanced by reducing medication errors that placed the patient at health risk and the hospital at financial risk. Again, automation was an intuitive key to control errors.
3. Staff shortages in selected specialty areas such as nursing and pharmacy placed additional stress on the efficiency of clinical operations. To the extent that automation could substitute for personnel, the technology solution they sought would have to address these key shortage areas as well.
4. Because the requirements for reporting to government/regulatory agencies were expected to increase, the new information system should produce the information required for reporting without redundant manipulation.

Once the executive team reached agreement that these business pressures would drive the design of the information system, they looked to the information industry to identify a partner for the venture that was likely to carry a $50–60 million price tag. For Jackson's management team, the "best of breed" model would not only allow for maximizing functionality in individual applications, but also would disperse the risk of vendor failure and lower switching costs. However, for a total system solution, a single vendor would eliminate the need to manage multiple vendors (each with its own business practices and requirements). Morin believed that a partnership, where risks were shared and each partner realized important benefits, would be pivotal to the success of the venture.

As the health care industry becomes more integrated, most of the larger information system vendors are consolidating and offering full-service suites of applications. No vendors have dominant market share in community hospitals. Through Jackson's due diligence process, eight vendors were narrowed to two. Each of the two finalist vendors made 20 to 30 on-site demonstrations of various applications to key user groups at Jackson, and coordinated site visits for Jackson users to observe live system operations at other client sites. Price quotes were similar, but the final choice of McKesson Corporation was based on its geographic proximity and its scope of products and services that would achieve a fully integrated system, thus maximizing Jackson's return on investment.

Extensive information sharing and negotiation among executives established a high level of trust between McKesson and Jackson Hospital. The implementation plan established an aggressive roll-out of all major applications within a 12-month period; enhancements and minor applications would be installed within a second 12-month period. The plan was validated during the first application installation at 10 weeks and at 13 weeks was in full operation/ongoing support mode.

Partnership benefits for Jackson Hospital included price considerations and an integrated business solution that will address its identified strategic issues as a system. McKesson's primary benefit accrues from successfully installing a fully integrated system in a community hospital. As most fully integrated systems currently are installed in hospital systems or networks, McKesson stands to gain considerable market advantage in sales to community hospitals.

Source: Donna Slovensky, PhD, School of Health Related Professions, University of Alabama at Birmingham.

Exhibit 4–6: Strategic Thinking Map of Competitive Advantages Relative to Strengths in General

Is the *Value* of the Strength High or Low? (High/Low?)	Is the Strength *Rare*? (Yes/No)	Is the Strength Easy or Difficult to *Imitate*? (Easy/Difficult)	Can the Strength Be *Sustained*? (Yes/No)	Implications
H	N	E	Y	No competitive advantage. Most competitors have the strength and those that do not can develop it easily. All can sustain it. Maintenance strategy.
H	N	E	N	No competitive advantage. All competitors have the strength which is easy to develop. Strength is not sustainable so it represents only a short-term advantage.
H	N	D	Y	No competitive advantage. Many competitors possess the strength but it is difficult to develop, so care should be taken to maintain this strength.
H	N	D	N	No competitive advantage. Many competitors possess the strength but it is difficult to develop, and those who do possess it will not be able to sustain the strength. Only a short-term advantage.
H	Y	E	Y	Not a source of long-term competitive advantage. Because it is valuable and rare, competitors will do what is necessary to develop this easy-to-imitate strength. Short-term advantage. Should not base strategy on this type of strength but should obtain benefits of short-term advantage.
H	Y	E	N	Not a source of competitive advantage. The strength is easy to imitate and cannot be sustained. Short-term advantage. Do not base strategy on this type of strength but obtain benefits of short-term advantage.
H	Y	D	Y	Source of long-term competitive advantage. If value is very high, it may be worth "betting the organization" on this strength.
H	Y	D	N	Possible source of short-term competitive advantage but not a strength that can be sustained over the long run.

Organizational Weaknesses

The strategic relevancy of each weakness can be determined by asking similar questions used to evaluate strengths. *Weaknesses,* as illustrated in Exhibit 4–7, are serious competitive disadvantages if the criteria they represent have high value to patients and other stakeholders (H), are not possessed by competitors (N), cannot be easily eliminated or corrected (D), and competitors can sustain their strengths (Y).

An assessment of the value chain in Step 1 for American Healthways, Inc. revealed 13 weaknesses. These are: (1) long sales cycle; (2) large portion of revenue from

Exhibit 4–7: Competitive Relevance of the Weaknesses of American Healthways, Inc.

Weaknesses	Is Weakness of High or Low *Value?* (High/Low)	Is Weakness *Common* (Not Rare) Among Competitors? (Yes/No)	Is it Easy or Difficult to *Correct* the Weakness? (Easy/Difficult)	Can Competitors *Sustain* Their Advantage? (Yes/No)
Service Delivery				
Contracts have long sales cycle	H	Y	D	N
Large percent of revenues generated from three contracts	H	Y	D	N
Less experience/success with some diseases and programs	H	N	D	Y
Data dependency to independently evaluate effectiveness of services	H	N	D	N
Operating contracts have to be carefully serviced for retention	H	Y	D	N
Culture				
Integrating corporate culture of StatusOne	H	N	D	N
Management's overly conservative fiscal philosophy	H	Y	E	Y
Strategic Resources				
Hospital contracts decreasing	H	Y	D	N
Average revenue per hospital contract decreasing by 11 percent	H	Y	D	N
Cost to maintain IT for compliance with Federal and state regulations	H	Y	D	N
Ability to compete in tight labor market	H	Y	D	N
Failure of IT materially affects business	H	Y	D	N
Volatility of stock price and volume	H	N	D	N

three health plans; (3) employees' inexperience with some diseases in the service line; (4) data dependency for evaluation of outcomes; (5) contract renewal requires careful servicing; (6) integration of StatusOne culture; (7) management's overly conservative fiscal philosophy; (8) hospital contracts decreasing; (9) average revenue per hospital contract decreasing; (10) cost to maintain IT for compliance with Federal and state regulations; (11) ability to compete in a tight labor market for skilled professionals; (12) failure of IT adversely affects business; and (13) volatile stock price.

American Healthways, Inc. possesses one serious strategic weakness (HNDY) that could represent a long-term competitive disadvantage – "less experience and success with some diseases and programs." This factor is valuable to customers, most competitors do not possess the weakness (it is rare because they perform well in very specific areas), it is difficult to correct, and competitors that do not have this weakness can sustain their advantage. Attention must be given to correcting this weakness.

The company faces some serious short-term disadvantages such as "data dependency for outcome evaluation," "integrating culture of StatusOne," and "volatility of stock price." These criteria – which are valuable to customers, most competitors do not possess them (they are rare), they are difficult to correct, and competitors may not be able to sustain their advantage (HNDN) – require attention to prevent competitors from obtaining a longer term advantage.

Most of American Healthways' weaknesses, "long sales cycle," "large portion of revenue obtained from three contracts," "need to carefully service existing contracts," "decreasing hospital contracts," "hospital contract revenues decreasing because of cost containment pressures," "cost to maintain IT for compliance with Federal and state regulations," "labor market competition," and "adverse effect of IT failure," are issues that, although valuable to customers, are common weaknesses for all competitors, difficult to correct, and competitors are not able to sustain advantage (HYDN). Therefore, they represent no serious competitive disadvantage to the company at this time. However, a competitor may attempt to overcome one or more of these weaknesses to create competitive advantage for its organization. "Management's overly conservative fiscal philosophy" is a weakness because an aggressive fiscal policy is valued in this industry; competitors are aggressive; it is relatively easy to correct; and competitors are not able to sustain their advantage (HYEY). It is one weakness that could be corrected more easily than others. Exhibit 4–8 provides a strategic thinking map listing the suggested actions of strategic leaders relative to possible combinations of weaknesses.

Step 3. Focusing on Competitive Advantage

As illustrated in Exhibit 4–3, the final step in exploiting competitive advantage is to determine how each competitively relevant strength and weakness is likely to affect an organization's ability to compete in the marketplace. *Competitively relevant strengths* are those that are valued in the marketplace, are rare, are difficult to imitate, and can be sustained. *Competitively relevant weaknesses* relate to

Exhibit 4–8: Strategic Thinking Map of Competitive Disadvantages Relative to Weaknesses

Is this Characteristic of High or Low *Value*? (High/Low)	Is this Weakness *Common* (Not Rare) Among Competitors? (Yes/No)	Is it Easy or Difficult to *Correct* this Weakness? (Easy/ Difficult)	Can Competitors Sustain Their *Advantage*? (Yes/No)	Implications
H	Y	E	Y	No competitive disadvantage in short run. Weakness of our organization but others are also weak. Weakness is easy to correct. Competitors will work to correct weakness. If we fail to correct, competitors could achieve an advantage
H	Y	E	N	No competitive disadvantage. Weakness of our organization but also a weakness of competitors. Easy to correct weakness and competitors are not able to sustain their advantage
H	Y	D	Y	No short-term competitive disadvantage. Competitors also possess the weakness, but it is a dangerous situation that must be addressed to ensure competitors do not overcome this difficulty and correct it first. Competitors' ability to sustain advantage could become long-term competitive disadvantage
H	Y	D	N	No competitive disadvantage. Weakness is common and is difficult to correct. Competitors cannot sustain any advantage represented by this weakness
H	N	E	Y	Short-term competitive disadvantage. Competitors are not weak in this area but the weakness is easy to correct. The organization should move quickly to correct this type of weakness
H	N	E	N	Not a competitive disadvantage. Competitors are not weak in this area but the weakness is easy to correct. Competitors cannot sustain any advantage provided by our weakness. Should correct even though any advantage will be short term
H	N	D	Y	Weakness represents a serious competitive disadvantage. The weakness is valuable, most competitors do not have it, it is difficult for us to correct, and competitors can sustain their advantage. Attention is demanded
H	N	D	N	A serious competitive disadvantage in the short term. Attention directed toward difficulty of overcoming weakness relative to the ability of competitors to retain the advantage

Exhibit 4–9: Strategic Implications of Competitively Relevant Strengths and Weaknesses

Competitively Relevant Strength or Weakness	Basis of Competitive Advantage or Disadvantage	Strategic Implications
Strengths		
Geographical presence in all 50 states	Cost Driver	Meet the need for national health plans to serve all enrollees through one program leading to economies of scale
Broad range of services in integrated service line	Uniqueness Driver	Few disease management and care enhancement firms have such a broad service line. This makes the company more attractive to managed care plans
Accreditation by all three relevant accrediting agencies	Uniqueness Driver	Provides company with a perceived quality advantage relative to competitors
Weaknesses Less experience/success with some diseases and programs	Uniqueness Driver	The breadth of the service line makes it difficult to be equally efficient and effective in all areas of disease management and could hurt company reputation for high-quality services

areas that are valued in the marketplace, are not common weaknesses attributed to competitors, are difficult for the organization to correct, and offer advantages that can be sustained by others. Exhibit 4–9 lists each of the competitively relevant strengths and weaknesses that have been identified (those displaying the pattern HYDY for strengths and HNDY for weaknesses from Exhibit 4–5 and Exhibit 4–7) and speculates as to whether or not American Healthways has the potential to differentiate itself from its competitors or provide a cost advantage over its competitors. A strength that provides the organization with a differentiated service is referred to as a *uniqueness driver*. It has the potential to make the organization different from competitors and may lead to a positioning strategy of differentiation (discussed in Chapter 6). The same is true for a weakness if it enables competitors to differentiate their services.

Some competitively relevant strengths may not enable an organization to differentiate its services but may provide it with the ability to offer services at a lower cost. These strengths are *cost drivers* and may lead to a positioning strategy of cost leadership (discussed in Chapter 6). If competitors have the ability to offer comparable services at a lower cost, they may develop cost advantage.

Note that the assessment indicates that American Healthway's strategic leadership has the ability to differentiate the organization and its services through the breadth of its service line and quality image as supported by its comprehensive accreditation (accredited by all relevant agencies). In other words, the organization has the potential to create a value added image in the minds of patients and other stakeholders. Leaders must be careful, however, because competitors have an advantage in that they have fewer services in their service line and may be able to maintain more consistent quality with a more narrow focus.

This careful analysis of the internal environment provides a better understanding of where strategic leaders should focus their efforts to compete effectively and where they should be careful to avoid vulnerability relative to competitors. It is not possible to be everything to everyone; an organization must focus its efforts on what it does best.

A Final Challenge

The basic endowment of resources, competencies, and capabilities in a health care organization and the way they are allocated are critical determinants of the organization's ability to compete effectively. American Healthways, Inc. has invested extensively in state-of-the-art care centers, information systems, accreditation, and a broad service line and is using these strengths to enhance its positioning of differentiation through geographic availability and high-quality care. However, the organization must remain proactive to new and challenging opportunities if it is to remain competitive. In fact, it has been argued that the essential character of strategic thinking is the acceptance of "an aspiration that creates, by design, a chasm between ambitions and resources." It is further argued that spanning the chasm and encouraging stretch "is the single most important task senior management faces."[36]

Stretch is accomplished through resource leveraging or systematically achieving the most possible from the available resources. Stretch enables smaller health care organizations that are less rich in resources, competencies, and capabilities to compete against large, powerful, national and regional health networks and managed care organizations. Leveraging is usually thought of in terms of financial leveraging through the use of debt; however, other resources may be leveraged as well.

Leveraging may be accomplished by concentrating, accumulating, complementing, conserving, and recovering resources.[37] Resources, competencies, and capabilities are more effectively directed toward strategic goals when they are concentrated. Prioritizing goals and focusing on relatively few things at one time aids the concentration of limited resources. Successful concentration of resources, competencies, and capabilities requires not only focusing on relatively few things but also focusing on the right things – those activities that make the greatest impact on patients' perceived value. Nurses, receptionists, therapists, maintenance employees, and others come into contact with patients and observe organizational realities in ways that are different from physicians, CEOs, and management personnel. The stockpiles of experience accumulated by the individuals with extensive patient contact are valuable competitive resources if properly mined and extracted.

Complementary resources, competencies, and capabilities can be combined to create synergy or higher order value. In the value chain, linking activities will provide unique opportunities to integrate functions such as service delivery, organizational culture, and strategic resources. In other words, there is a creative interweaving of different types of skills that assists in creating competitive advantage.

The more often that a particular resource, competency, or capability is used, the greater the potential for leveraging. The ability to quickly switch hard-won knowledge from delivering one service to another conserves service development resources and reduces the learning curve in introducing and perfecting service delivery. Conserving and recovering resources by restricting their exposure to unnecessary risks is essential to the conservation of limited resources. An aspiring competitor in a health care market should think carefully before attacking the dominant player at the point of the competitor's greatest strength. To do so would be to subject limited resources, competencies, and capabilities to excessive risks and would likely be unsuccessful. Challenging a stronger competitor requires creativity and innovation.

Expediting success – increasing the resource multiplier by reducing the time between expenditure of resources and their recovery through revenue generation – is an important means to leverage resources. Reducing the payback period of technological improvements in health care organizations is a substantial resource recovery challenge. On one hand, high-quality service delivery depends on state-of-the-art technology. On the other hand, this type of technology is expensive and usually has a relatively short economic life. Careful planning is required to ensure that paybacks are evaluated and accelerated in every possible way.

Interestingly, a great deal of resource leveraging is a matter of attitude and willingness to take reasonable risks, to do things in new and innovative ways, to learn from the experiences of others, and generally pursue excellence in all aspects of organizational performance. In fact, Hamel and Prahalad note that traditional strategic as well as behavioral factors may lead to competitive advantage: "Cross-functioning teams, focusing on a few core competencies, strategic alliances, programs of employee involvement, and consensus are all parts of stretch."[38] In the end, determination of competitive advantage requires an integration of what health care strategists know about the external environment with a sophisticated understanding of competitively relevant strengths and weaknesses.

Managing Strategic Momentum

For sustained competitive advantage, strategic momentum must be maintained. After the strategy has been initiated, the internal environment must be continuously evaluated to stay informed and current about the organization's competitively relevant strengths and weaknesses. Sustaining a competitive advantage is difficult in a dynamic market and what might be a competitive advantage today may not be an advantage tomorrow. Carefully evaluating the strengths and weaknesses relative to the four critical questions allows the strategist to focus on the relatively few aspects of the value chain that have the potential for building and sustaining competitive advantage. Care must be exercised, however, to ensure that new and emerging strengths or weaknesses are adequately considered in the continuous assessment of the internal environment. The questions presented in Exhibit 4–10 provide for such an ongoing evaluation of the effectiveness of the internal environmental assessment. Ensuring appropriate strategic fit requires that the internal as well as the external environments be continuously assessed and evaluated.

Exhibit 4–10: Questions for Evaluating the Internal Strategic Assumptions

1. Have the strengths and weaknesses been correctly identified?
2. Is there a clear basis on which to compete?
3. Does the strategy exploit the strengths and avoid the major weaknesses of the organization?
4. Are the competitive advantages related to the critical success factors in the service area?
5. Have we protected our short- and long-term competitive advantages?
6. Has the competition made strategic moves that have weakened our competitive advantages?
7. Are we creating new competitive advantages?

Summary and Conclusions

In this chapter the orientation shifted from factors outside the organization to an introspective view. Competitive advantage resides within the organization, whether it be a hospital, physician's office, or health maintenance organization.

Understanding competitive advantage requires a careful analysis of the internal organizational environment. In this chapter the value chain was used as a guide to this internal assessment. The value chain is a useful tool for focusing on those areas in a health care organization where value can be added. The value chain is divided into two major components. The first relates to the delivery of health services and includes pre-service activities, point-of-service activities, and afterservice activities. The second major component consists of support activities that include organizational culture, organizational structure, and strategic resources.

By investigating all systems and subsystems of the value chain and questioning the various resources, competencies, and capabilities that might or might not be used to create value, strategic thinkers are better able to identify possible strengths and weaknesses. Once each strength and weakness is evaluated in terms of its value, rareness, imitability, and sustainability, a basis is established for determining the strengths and weaknesses that are competitively relevant. Competitively relevant strengths and weaknesses provide the bases for developing strategies that capitalize on strengths and avoid weaknesses and establish competitive advantage.

Understanding competitive advantage is important to health care strategists but often more is required of successful organizations. Successful health care organizations must always insist on stretching their resources, competencies, and capabilities to the limit while creatively looking for new opportunities. Sustained competitive advantage, therefore, requires that leaders understand what the environment demands of successful health care organizations, configure competitively relevant strengths to the organization's greatest advantage, eliminate or minimize the adverse effects of competitively relevant weaknesses, and establish demanding aspirations that require strategic assets to be pushed to their limits while constantly searching for new opportunities.

Key Terms and Concepts in Strategic Management

After-Service
Capability
Competency
Competitive Advantage
Competitively Relevant
    Strength
Competitively Relevant
    Weakness

Cost Driver
Point-of-Service
Pre-Service
Resources
Resource-Based View
Service Delivery
Strength
Stretch

Support Activities
Sustained Competitive
    Advantage
Uniqueness Driver
Value
Value Chain
Weakness

QUESTIONS FOR CLASS DISCUSSION

1. It has been said that the rules for success are written outside the organization but competitive advantage must be found within the organization. Explain this statement.
2. Why is value creation an important concept to health care organizations? Is value creation more or less important in health care than in other industries?
3. Which activities, service delivery or support, are more important in the organizational value chain? Explain your answer.
4. Why is the value chain consistent with total systems concepts discussed in Chapter 1? Why is a systems approach to internal environmental analysis important?
5. Why is the concept of competitively relevant strengths and weaknesses so important to internal environmental analysis?
6. What is the difference between an objective and subjective strength and weakness? Give examples of each type of strength and weakness in a health care organization.
7. Discuss the resource-based view of competitive advantage. Why is it important to understand organizational differences in order to use this approach?
8. Briefly define what is meant by competitive advantage. Are competitive advantage and sustained competitive advantage identical concepts? Why or why not?
9. What are the differences between capabilities and competencies? How are capabilities related to both resources and competencies?
10. Why are capabilities referred to as architectural competencies? Would you consider management a capability or a competency? Explain your answer.
11. When searching for competitive advantage, which characteristic of a strength or weakness (value, rareness, imitability, sustainability) is the most important in health care organizations? Discuss your response.
12. Why are some strengths and weaknesses that are not competitively relevant deserving of attention by health care strategists? Provide one example of a strength and weakness that are not competitively relevant but deserving of attention.
13. Why is resource leveraging an important concept in internal environmental analysis?

NOTES

1. George Stalk, Jr. and Rob Lachenauer, "Hardball: Five Killer Strategies for Trouncing the Competition," *Harvard Business Review* 82, no. 4 (2004), p. 64.

2. David Bovet and Joseph Martha, *Value Nets: Breaking the Supply Chain to Unlock Profits* (New York: John Wiley & Sons, 2000).

3. Stuart L. Hart and Mark B. Milstein, "Creating Sustainable Value," *Academy of Management Executive* 17, no. 2 (2003), pp. 56–69.

4. Dennis Gioia, Majken Schultz, and Kevin C. Corley, "Organizational Identity, Image, and Adaptive Strategy," *Academy of Management Review* 25, no. 1 (2000), pp. 63–81.

5. Stephen D. Mallard, Terri Leakeas, W. Jack Duncan, Michael E. Fleenor, and Richard J. Sinsky, "Same-Day Scheduling in A Public Health Clinic: A Pilot Study," *Journal of Public Health Management and Practice* 10, no. 2 (2004), pp. 152–157.

6. Michael E. Porter, *Competitive Advantage: Creating and Sustaining Superior Performance* (New York: Free Press, 1985), ch. 2. See also Michael E. Porter, "Toward a Dynamic Theory of Strategy," *Strategic Management Journal* 12, no. 1 (1991), pp. 95–117.

7. Laurence D. Ackerman, *Identity Is Destiny: Leadership and the Roots of Value Creation* (San Francisco: Berrett-Koehler Publishing, 2000).

8. Melissa A. Schilling, "Toward a General Modular Systems Theory and Its Application to Interfirm Product Modularity," *Academy of Management Review* 25, no. 2 (2000), pp. 312–334.

9. T. Russell Crook, David J. Ketchen, Jr., and Charles C. Snow, "Competitive Edge: A Strategic Management Model," *Cornell Hotel and Restaurant Administration Quarterly* 44, no. 3 (2003), pp. 44–56.

10. George Stalk, Philip Evans, and Lawrence Shulman, "Competing on Capabilities: The New Rules of Corporate Strategy," *Harvard Business Review* 70, no. 2 (March–April 1992), p. 62.

11. William Boulding and Markus Christen, "Sustainable Pioneering Advantage? Profit Implications of Market Entry Order," *Marketing Science* 22, no. 3 (2003), pp. 371–383.

12. Glen R. Carroll, "A Sociological View on Why Firms Differ," *Strategic Management Journal* 14, no. 4 (1993), pp. 237–249; Giovanni Azzone and Umberto Bertele, "Measuring Resources for Supporting Resource-Based Competencies," *Management Decision* 33, no. 9 (1995), pp. 57–58; and Richard L. Priem and John E. Butler, "Is the Resource-Based 'View' a Useful Perspective for Strategic Management Research?" *Academy of Management Review* 26, no. 1 (2001), pp. 22–40.

13. Richard Hall, "A Framework for Linking Intangible Resources and Capabilities to Sustainable Competitive Advantage," *Strategic Management Journal* 14, no. 6 (1993), pp. 607–618. See also T. K. Das and Bing-Sheng Teng, "A Resource-Based Theory of Strategic Alliances," *Journal of Management* 26, no. 1 (2000), pp. 31–62.

14. Birger Wernerfelt, "The Resource-Based View of the Firm: Ten Years After," *Strategic Management Journal* 16, no. 3 (1995), p. 173. Insert added. See also Yasemin Y. Kor and Joseph T. Mahoney, "Edith Penrose's (1959) Contributions to the Resource-Based View of Strategic Management," *Journal of Management Studies* 41, no. 1 (2004), pp. 183–190 and Andy Lockett and Steve Thompson, "Edith Penrose's Contributions to the Resource-Based View: An Alternative Perspective," *Journal of Management Studies* 41, no. 1 (2004), pp. 193–198.

15. J. H. Davis, F. D. Schoorman, R. C. Mayer, and H. H. Tan, "The Trusted General Manager and Business Unit Performance: Empirical Evidence of a Competitive Advantage," *Strategic Management Journal* 21, no. 5 (2000), pp. 563–576.

16. Robert S. Kaplan and David P. Norton, "Measuring the Strategic Readiness of Intangible Assets," *Harvard Business Review* 82, no. 2 (2004), pp. 52–64.

17. Anonymous, "Americans Rank Good Reputation, Doctor's Recommendation as Top Indicators of Quality Care," *Health Care Strategic Management* 21, no. 11 (2003), p. 8.

18. Jörgen Sandbert, "Understanding Human Competence at Work: An Integrative Approach," *Academy of Management Journal* 43, no. 1 (2000), pp. 9–25; Maurice Penner, "Administrative Competencies for Physicians with Capitation," *Journal of Healthcare Management* 44, no. 3 (1999), pp. 26–34; and Kurt Haanes and Øystein Fjeldstad, "Linking Intangible Resources and Competition," *European Management Journal* 18, no. 1 (2000), pp. 52–62.

19. Raphael Amit and Paul J. H. Schoemaker, "Strategic Assets and Organizational Rent," *Strategic Management Journal* 14, no. 1 (1993), pp. 33–46 and Juan Florin, Michael Lubatkin, and William Schulze, "A Social Capital Model of High-Growth Firms," *Academy of Management Journal* 46, no. 3 (2003), pp. 374–386.

20. Stuart L. Hart, "A Natural-Resource-Based View of the Firm," *Academy of Management Review* 20, no. 4 (1995), pp. 986–1014.

21. Richard Makadok, "Doing the Right Thing and Knowing the Right Thing to Do: Why the Whole Is Greater than the Sum of the Parts," *Academy of Management Journal* 24, no. 10 (2003), pp. 1043–1052.

22. Kaplan and Norton, "Measuring the Strategic Readiness," p. 54.

23. Dave Ulrich and Dale Lake, "Organizational Capability: Creating Competitive Advantage," *Academy of Management Executive* 5, no. 1 (1991), pp. 77–85.

24. David J. Collis, "Research Note: How Valuable Are Organizational Capabilities?" *Strategic Management Journal* 15, no. 2 (1994), pp. 143–152.

25. Jill Irvin, Laura Pedro, and Paul Gennaro, "Strategy from the Inside Out: Lessons in Creating Organic Growth," *Journal of Business Strategy* 24, no. 5 (2003), pp. 10–15.

26. Isabelle Bouty, "Interpersonal and Interaction Influences on Informal Resource Exchanges Between R&D Researchers Across Organizational Boundaries," *Academy of Management Journal* 43, no. 1 (2000), pp. 50–65.

27. Stalk, Evans, and Shulman, "Competing on Capabilities," p. 62.

28. C. K. Prahalad and Gary Hamel, "The Core Competency of the Corporation," *Harvard Business Review* 68, no. 3 (May–June 1990), p. 82; David Lei, John W. Slocum, and Robert A. Pitts, "Designing Organizations for Competitive Advantage: The Power of Unlearning and Learning," *Organizational Dynamics* 27, no. 3 (1999), pp. 24–38; and Ali Khatibi, Ahasanul Haque, and Hishamudin Ismail, "Gaining A Competitive Advantage from Advertising," *Journal of Academy of Business* 4, no. 1 (2004), pp. 302–312.

29. Constantinos C. Markides and Peter J. Williamson, "Related Diversification, Core Competencies, and Corporate Performance," *Strategic Management Journal* 15, no. 3 (1994), pp. 149–165 and Ray Gautam, Jay B. Barney, and Waleed A. Muhanna, "Capabilities, Business Processes, and Competitive Advantage: Choosing the Dependent Variable in Empirical Tests of the Resource-Based View," *Strategic Management Journal* 25, no. 1 (2004), pp. 23–31.

30. Stalk, Evans, and Shulman, "Competing on Capabilities," p. 62.

31. Richard M. Hodgetts, Fred Luthans, and John W. Slocum, "Redefining Roles and Boundaries, Linking Competencies and Resources," *Organizational Dynamics* 28, no. 2 (1999), pp. 7–21.

32. Descriptive and financial information on American Healthways, Inc. were taken from the company's form 10-K filed with the United States Securities and Exchange Commission for fiscal year ended August 31, 2003 and *Reaching Critical Mass*, American Healthways Annual Report, 2003.

33. Amit and Schoemaker, "Strategic Assets and Organizational Rent," p. 35. See also Danny Miller, "An Asymmetry-Based View of Advantage: Towards an Attainable Sustainability," *Strategic Management Journal* 24, no. 10 (2003), pp. 961–972 and Margaret A. Peteraf and Mark E. Bergen, "Scanning Dynamic Competitive Landscapes: A Market-Based and Resource-Based Framework," *Strategic Management Journal* 24, no. 10 (2003), pp. 1027–1035.

34. Amit and Schoemaker, ibid., p. 37. See in addition Constantine Kontoghiorghes, "Identification of Key Predictors of Organizational Competitiveness in a Service Organization," *Organizational Development Journal* 21, no. 2 (2003), pp. 28–36.

35. Jay B. Barney, "Looking Inside for Competitive Advantage," *Academy of Management Executive* 9, no. 4 (1995), pp. 49–61. Note that Barney added an additional question, that of organization, that was not included in this discussion.

36. Gary Hamel and C. K. Prahalad, "Strategy as Stretch and Leverage," *Harvard Business Review* 71, no. 3 (1993), pp. 75–84.

37. This discussion has been adapted from Gary Hamel and C. K. Prahalad, *Competing for the Future* (Boston, MA: Harvard Business School Press, 1994), ch. 7.

38. Gary Hamel and C. K. Prahalad, "Competing in the New Economy: Managing Out of Bounds," *Strategic Management Journal* 17, no. 1 (1996), pp. 237–242.

ADDITIONAL READINGS

Allard, Kenneth, *Business as War: Battling for Competitive Advantage* (New York: John Wiley & Sons, Inc., 2004). The author, a retired colonel and military analyst for *NBC News*, attempts to apply lessons learned by the military to business strategy. This book is added to the growing list of books that attempt to exploit an exaggerated analogy equating business and war. Although the book provides an interesting and important perspective on competitive advantage, it is more military and political in its orientation than strategic.

Hoskisson, Robert E., Michael A. Hitt, and R. Duane Ireland, *Competing for Advantage* (Mason, OH: Thomson-Southwestern, 2004). A comprehensive yet concise description of the core concepts of strategic management with an emphasis on gaining and maintaining competitive advantage. The book is thoroughly documented and summarizes the latest academic research. Directed primarily toward graduate management programs, *Competing for Advantage* will be useful to practicing managers as well.

Mitchell, Donald and Carol Coles, *The Ultimate Competitive Advantage* (San Francisco: Berrett-Koehler, 2003). Organizations should stop trying to get better at what they did poorly yesterday and focus on doing things that will contribute to the interests of various stakeholders. This book includes analyses of companies such as Dell, Paycheck, Tellabs, and others, concluding that organizations should study customer and stakeholder needs rather than simply copying strategic practices of other organizations. Organizations become vulnerable to competitors when they stop improving their business model.

Paine, Lynn Sharp, *Value Shift: Why Companies Must Merge Social and Financial Imperatives to Achieve Superior Performance* (New York: McGraw-Hill, 2003). If organizations want to be considered as superior performing corporations they must behave in ways that are morally as well as financially responsible. The author develops a comprehensive argument regarding shareholder responsibility for the behavior of managers based on agency theory.

Peters, Tom, *Re-Imagine: Business Excellence in A Disruptive Age* (New York: Dorling Kindersley, 2003). Organizations are at their best when they deliver exciting services to their customers and provide opportunities for employees. A convincing argument is made that complacent bureaucracies are becoming increasingly obsolete. Organizations that succeed in the future will have to give up their devotion to order and efficiency and create a culture that encourages creativity and innovation. Peters maintains that it is time to destroy and discard the old myths of business and make re-imagination the order of the day.

Stead, W. Edward and Jean Garner Stead, *Sustainable Strategic Management* (Armonk, NY: M. E. Sharpe, Inc., 2004). Primarily a supplemental text, *Sustainable Strategic Management* looks at competitive advantages that are consistent with environmental sustainability. Organizations are recognized as social institutions that play a key role in the ecology of modern civilization.

CHAPTER

Directional Strategies

Introductory Incident

The Value of Loyalty

In today's health care environment, with its emphasis on cost reduction, consumer loyalty assumes strategic importance because loyal customers enable the organization to make more money, save money, and save time. Placing the customer first is an organizational value that must permeate the entire staff from administrators to physicians to housekeepers. Yet, placing the customer first to achieve customer loyalty cannot be realized without also having the organization value employee loyalty – customer loyalty starts with employee loyalty.

Employee loyalty starts with hiring the right people who are truly oriented to delivering "service from the heart with consistency and a smile." Loyal employees are fundamental to delivering differentiated customer service with consistency. If employees do not have the right attitude, they should never have been hired; and if they are currently with the organization, they should be fired because employees with a poor attitude will not deliver exemplary service and will spread an "anti-attitude virus" that infects customer loyalty one customer at a time. The organization must value

its customers and its employees for customer and employee loyalty to flourish.

To determine whether an organization values loyalty for patients, start with an assessment of employee loyalty. If employees report that they plan to continue working for the organization, feel part of the team, and are proud of where they work, they are more likely to be loyal. If they believe that the organization values them and that customers can rely on outstanding quality in service delivery – and the employees' role in delivering it – the employees are more likely to be loyal. If the organization's leaders value the employees' loyalty and reward it and the employees feel that the organization deserves their loyalty, they are more likely to be loyal. An organization's employees can be its greatest asset – if they value the development of loyal customers and if management values the loyalty of employees who deliver it.

Loyalty is a long-term commitment and is dependent on an organization's ability to consistently deliver a memorable customer experience that leaves them with an ongoing favorable image, feeling,

▶

and union with the provider. A memorable customer experience is not a single event but includes many differentiating service encounters that are delivered across a wide spectrum of employee–customer interactions. The customers' experiences should be synergistic – greater than the sum of the specific service opportunity parts. Although customer satisfaction is often used as a measure of success, satisfaction is more short term in nature and has only a small amount to do with customer delight. Being satisfied does not necessarily depict anything more than a customer feels that he or she received the service for which they paid. Customer satisfaction and customer loyalty are actually very different.

Loyal customers generate word-of-mouth advertising (the best kind), reduce the chance of litigation, and are more apt to volunteer, refer others to the organization, and make financial donations. In addition, greater customer loyalty encourages greater customer cooperation that may lead to better clinical outcomes. Thus, loyal customers can enable the organization to achieve greater rev-

enues because they continue to use the provider's services and refer others. In addition, they save money because they do not require the costs associated with gaining a new customer, they do not bring lawsuits, and they volunteer their time. Loyal customers save time for the health care organization because they try to conform to treatment plans and more readily adopt new offerings from the organization that has their trust.

Establishing customer loyalty is critical in highly competitive markets (such as health care). Most health care organizations measure customer satisfaction and have some form of customer service program. Very few measure customer loyalty or have a loyalty program in place. The organization that has a value to place customers first and values employees who achieve customer loyalty will have value itself.

Source: John O'Malley, "The Caring Before the Care," *Marketing Health Services* 24, no. 2 (Summer 2004), pp. 12–13.

Learning Objectives

After completing this chapter the student should be able to:

1. Understand the roles and relationships among organizational mission, vision, values, and strategic goals and why they are called directional strategies.

2. Recognize the important characteristics and components of organizational mission statements and be able to write a mission statement.

3. Recognize the important characteristics and components of vision and be able to write an organizational vision statement.

4. Recognize the important characteristics and components and be able to write values statements.

5. Recognize the important characteristics and components and be able to write strategic goals.

6. Identify service category critical success factors.

7. Develop a set of strategic goals that contribute to the mission, move the organization toward the realization of its vision, and are consistent with the organization's values.

8. Recognize the important issues in the governance of health care organizations and the role of the board of directors in maintaining policy-making direction.

Directional Strategies

Mission, vision, values, and strategic goals are appropriately called directional strategies because they guide strategists when they make key organizational decisions. The *mission* attempts to capture the organization's distinctive purpose or reason for being. The *vision* creates a mental image of what the managers, employees, physicians, patients, and other stakeholders want the organization to be when it is accomplishing its purpose or mission. It is the organization's hope for the future. *Values* are the principles that are held dear by members of the organization. These are guiding principles the managers and employees will not compromise while they are in the process of achieving the mission and pursuing the vision and strategic goals. *Strategic goals* are those overarching end results that the organization pursues to accomplish its mission and achieve its vision. As discussed in Perspective 5–1 vision, mission, values, and even goals have a good dose of intuition and judgment.

Perspective 5–1

The Heart, Head, and Gut of Strategic Planning

There are a number of ways to get a weather forecast. We can rely on hard data regarding humidity, temperature, radar scans, and wind velocity. Or, we can walk outside, look at the sky, think back on our experiences with the weather and make our own forecast. Each approach appears equally accurate.

Some people think of strategic planning the same way they think about forecasting the weather. Sometimes health care strategists get so consumed by databases, models, and financial analysis that they forget to step out on the porch and look up into the sky and apply a good dose of intuition and judgment. Sometimes health care strategists neglect the facts and rely too much on experience and intuition.

There are three elements to strategic planning – the heart, the head, and the gut. Each is critical to success and each plays an important role in the organization's ultimate course of action. The *heart* of strategic planning involves the mission, vision, and values of the organization and testing actions against these important directional strategies. This has been called the "motherhood and apple pie" check. If the strategy does not pass this test, find another strategy.

The *head* of strategic planning is the analytical aspect of the process. Assessments, strategic goals, and competitive analysis are important parts of strategic analysis, as are financial and marketing data. This can be thought of as everything that can be put on the table and passed out. It is similar to going to the weather channel to hear the facts and the forecast.

The strategic planning *gut* utilizes the collective experience and intuition of as many people as possible in the organization. It is the organization's ability to predict and interpret the changing winds. Successful prediction involves internalization of the concerns of doctors, nurses, patients, and community leaders. It is taking intangible intelligence and putting it to practical use.

It is critically important that the heart remain a part of strategic planning because it provides inspiration and commitment. The head is important because without strategic goals and outcomes, little focus can be obtained; and without focus, progress is virtually impossible. Gut and intuition are important because a great deal of strategic intelligence resides in health care organizations and should be integrated into all strategic thinking processes.

Source: Adapted from Alden Solovy, "Strategy for the Porch," *Hospitals and Health Networks* 74, no. 9 (2000), p. 32.

Organizational Purpose and Mission

Chester Barnard, in *The Functions of the Executive*, stated that only three things are needed to have an organization: (1) communication, (2) a willingness to serve, and (3) a common purpose. The inculcation of the "belief in the real existence of a common purpose" is, according to Barnard, "the essential executive function."[1] This purpose, among other things, helps managers make sense of the environment. When the purpose of an organization is clearly understood, the complexity of the environment can be reduced and organized in a way that can be analyzed in light of the goals the organization wishes to achieve. The complex environment is no longer a "mere mess of things."[2] As a statement of purpose, the mission plays an important role in focusing strategists' attention on relevant aspects of the environment.

For example, if the CEO of a long-term care facility simultaneously considers all the turbulence in the organization's environment, the environment will appear confusing and overwhelming. Can anyone effectively track all of the changes taking place in biotechnology, cultural values, demographics, and politics? However, if the CEO were to focus on only those aspects of the environment that related to the elderly (such as the aging trend of the population and the increased financial well-being of this group of aging people) from the perspective of the mission of the long-term care organization, the task becomes more manageable.

The common purpose (mission) to which Barnard referred is the reason that organizations exist. Some organizations exist to make money for the owners; some are founded to provide health care to indigent patients; others are started to deliver health services in as convenient a way as possible or to provide the care needed by groups of individuals who belong to the same managed care plan.

Mission: A Statement of Distinctiveness

In the hierarchy of goals (end results and organizational plans to accomplish them), the mission captures the organization's distinctive character. Although a well-conceived mission is general, it is more concrete than vision. An organizational mission is not an expression of hope. On the contrary, it is an attempt to capture the essence of the organizational purpose and commit it to writing. Amedisys, a provider of home health nursing services, states that its purpose is to "assist patients in maintaining and improving their quality of life."[3] This is the company's purpose – the reason it exists.

An organizational mission is a broadly defined and enduring statement of purpose that distinguishes a health care organization from other organizations of its type and identifies the scope of its operations in product, service, and market (competitive) terms.[4] The mission statement of the University of Texas M. D. Anderson Cancer Center in Exhibit 5–1, for example, distinguishes the Center from other health care organizations in the service area by its relationship with the University of Texas; its emphasis on a specific disease (cancer); and its commitment

Exhibit 5–1: Mission of the University of Texas M. D. Anderson Cancer Center

The mission of The University of Texas M. D. Anderson Cancer Center is to eliminate cancer in Texas, the nation and the world through outstanding integrated programs in patient care, research, education and prevention.

Source: University of Texas M. D. Anderson Cancer Center.

to the integration of patient care, research, education, and prevention. Although mission statements are relatively enduring, they must be flexible in light of changing conditions. The changes facing academic medicine will continue to impose pressures on specialized centers of excellence such as M. D. Anderson because of the substantial costs involved in integrating patient care with the teaching and research mission and the increasing reluctance of payors to reimburse for educational costs.

Mission statements are sometimes not the true "living documents" that are capable of encouraging high performance. Studies of mission statements confirm that the full potential of this directional strategy is rarely achieved.[5] To be effective, service delivery and support strategies must be designed to contribute to mission accomplishment.

One study of hospital mission statements found that almost 85 percent of the respondents had mission statements.[6] However, some of the executives who completed the survey did not perceive a high level of commitment to the statement by employees or that specific actions were influenced very much by the mission. Another study of state-level departments of public health indicated that more than 90 percent had formal, written mission statements. Despite the frequency with which formal mission statements are encountered, a great deal of disagreement exists regarding their value and the influence that these statements actually have on behavior within organizations. This is unfortunate because the mission statement is a crucially important part of strategic goal setting. It is the superordinate goal that stands the test of time and assists top management in navigating through periods of turbulence and change. It is, in other words, the "stake in the ground" that provides the anchor for strategic planning. It must be emphasized, however, that mission statements, even at their best, can never be substitutes for well-conceived and carefully formulated strategies.[7] Moreover, a sense of mission is not a guarantee of success. As illustrated in Perspective 5–2, a nice sounding mission statement is not enough. The organization has to adhere to the mission and regularly review it to be sure it remains relevant in changing times.

Mission statements remind managers in health care organizations to ask a series of questions.[8] The answers radically affect how the organization performs. These questions include:

1. *Are we not doing some things now that we should be doing?* A rehabilitative medicine center, after analyzing the environment and studying its own referral patterns, might determine that it should enter a joint venture with a group of surgeons to provide outpatient surgery services. This particular

Perspective 5–2

Do Mission
Statements Matter?

Prominent displays of mission statements by the elevator and placement on employees' name badges and business cards are not enough to ensure that the message is taken to heart. Informed people often wonder why organizations spend so much time talking about mission statements when they are often not taken seriously. Do organizations actually plan their future based on the mission (directional strategy) or do they simply respond to changing conditions?

Undoubtedly, some mission statements are not very good. They may sound fine and even have been crafted by an astute consultant or flashy public relations firm; however, if they do not speak the language of employees and stakeholders they will not have much influence on behavior or performance. Organizations must think seriously about the future of their industry and their unique role in capitalizing on the opportunities created by changing times. This distinctiveness must then be captured in the mission statement.

Mission statements often suffer from the following problems:

1. Many organizations write the mission statement for public relations value.
2. Many organizations write mission statements that essentially describe the mission of any organization in their service category. Mission statements should capture the uniqueness of the organization and not just be a generic statement that could be adapted to any competitor.
3. Many organizations spend more time crafting a "good" mission statement than trying to implement and follow it. People need to see words in action!

Mission statements, if they are to be useful, must state the purpose of the organization and provide a good sense of what the organization is devoted to achieve. A mission statement should help the organization focus on its uniqueness. Writing a mission statement is important; however, living it is more important. Whatever is incorporated into the mission statement must be credible, realistic, attainable, and assist in differentiating the organization from all its competitors.

Source: Greg Kitzmiller, "Do Mission Statements Matter? Reviewing the Importance of a Mission Statement and, More Importantly, Sticking to It," *Nutraceuticals World* 6, no. 10 (October 2003), p. 22.

rehabilitative medicine center, located in a professional building adjacent to an acute care hospital, had simply referred patients requiring surgery to the hospital. However, insurance company policies and patient preferences suggested that the majority of surgeries could be performed on an outpatient basis.

2. *Are we doing some things now that we should not be doing?* The same rehabilitative medicine center, after extensive analysis, concluded that it should divest its rehabilitative equipment business and contract with medical and sports equipment suppliers for needed services.

3. *Are we doing some things now that we should be doing, but in a different way?* Throughout its history the rehabilitative medicine center required patients to come to the facility for services. For many patients, particularly those with sports injuries, travel to the facility was difficult and often impossible. Recently, the center purchased a mobile trailer with a fully equipped diagnostic and treatment facility that can transport services to local high schools and industrial locations.

Exhibit 5–2: Mission Statement of Medtronic

Mission:

- To contribute to human welfare by application of biomedical engineering in the research, design, manufacture, and sale of instruments or appliances that alleviate pain, restore health, and extend life.
- To direct our growth in areas of biomedical engineering where we display maximum strength and ability; to gather people and facilities that tend to augment these areas; to continually build on these areas through education and knowledge assimilation; to avoid participation in areas where we cannot make unique and worthy contributions.
- To strive without reserve for the greatest possible reliability and quality of our products; to be the unsurpassed standard of comparison and to be recognized as a company of dedication, honesty, integrity, and service.
- To make a fair profit on current operations to meet our obligations, sustain our growth, and reach our goals.
- To recognize the personal worth of employees by providing an employment framework that allows personal satisfaction in work accomplishment, security, advancement opportunity, and means to share in the company's success.
- To maintain good citizenship as a company.

Source: Medtronic, Inc.

An organization should carefully evaluate strategic decisions with the use of its mission statement. When new opportunities are presented it can use the three key questions "Are we not doing some things we should be doing? Are we doing some things we should not be doing? Are we doing some things we should continue to do but in a fundamentally different way?" to determine whether or not the new opportunity is consistent with its essential distinctiveness. As an example, Medtronic's mission statement (see Exhibit 5–2) provides guidance for its strategic leaders to determine whether new opportunities should be pursued. To be consistent with the mission, opportunities need to be in the area of biomedical engineering. More specifically, they need to be in areas of biomedical engineering that build on Medtronic's strengths by augmenting areas of expertise while avoiding areas where unique and worthy contributions cannot be made.

Characteristics of Mission Statements

The definition presented previously highlights several important characteristics of effective mission statements. (The mission statement of Triad Hospitals illustrates some of these characteristics – see Exhibit 5–3.)

1. Missions are broadly defined statements of purpose. Well-formulated mission statements are written and communicated to those involved in doing the work of the organization. They are broad but also, in a sense, specific. That is, mission statements should be general enough to allow for innovation and expansion into new activities when advisable, yet narrow enough to provide direction.[9]

Exhibit 5–3: Mission Statement of Triad Hospitals

To continuously improve the quality of healthcare services provided to the communities we serve by creating an environment that fosters physician participation, recognizes the value and contributions of our employees, and strives to meet the unique healthcare needs of our local communities.

Source: Triad Hospitals.

2. Mission statements are enduring. The purpose, and consequently the mission, of an organization does not change often and should be enduring. People are committed to ideas and causes that remain relatively stable over time. Triad Hospitals, Inc. owns and manages hospitals and ambulatory surgery centers in small cities and selected larger urban markets. Through a subsidiary, Triad provides hospital management, consulting, and advisory services to independent community hospitals and health systems throughout the United States. The enduring nature of the mission statement has allowed Triad to expand its size and diversity of operations without violating the spirit of the mission statement – serving local communities.

3. Mission statements should underscore the uniqueness of the organization. Good mission statements distinguish the organization from all others of its type. One of the important uniqueness features of Triad is its commitment to small cities and a few urban centers. This distinguishes Triad from many health systems.

4. Mission statements should identify the scope of operations in terms of service and market. It is important for the mission statement to specify what business the organization is in (health care) and who it believes are the primary stakeholders. Note that Triad is specific in its commitment to assisting in the health care needs of local communities. It does not attempt to address needs outside its area of primary expertise even though local communities may need things other than health care.

Although missions are enduring, this should not imply that the mission will never, or should never, change. New technologies, demographic trends, and so on might be very good reasons to rethink the mission of an organization. For example, a number of hospitals have incorporated the desire to be an "independent provider of health care" in their statement of mission. In today's managed-care-oriented health care environment, that aspect of mission may need to be revisited. In some markets, alignment with managed care organizations might become a necessity for survival and the mission statement should not stand in the way.

These characteristics illustrate the essential properties of well-conceived and communicated mission statements.[10] They outline worthy ideals that are always in the process of being achieved by strategic leaders in health care institutions. The mission provides direction. Good mission statements are not easy to write, but fortunately there is general agreement on what they should include.

Components of Mission Statements

There is no single way to develop and write mission statements. In fact, studies of Canadian not-for-profit hospitals indicate that they emphasize a variety of factors in their mission statements.[11] To define the distinctiveness of an organization, mission statements must highlight those things that constitute uniqueness. Some of the more important components of a mission are discussed and illustrated with the use of mission statements from a variety of health care institutions.[12]

1. Mission statements target customers and markets. Frequently the mission statement provides evidence of the kind of customers or patients the organization seeks to serve and the markets where it intends to compete. The mission statement of Renal Care Group, Inc., for example, makes explicit the organization's intent to improve the quality of life and to care for patients with chronic and acute renal disease. Exhibit 5–4 provides an illustration of the mission statement of MedCath, Inc. that focuses all of its services on cardiac patients.
2. Mission statements indicate the principal services delivered or products provided by the organization. A specialized health care organization might highlight the special services it provides in its mission statement. The mission statement of Advanced Medical Optics illustrates a statement built around primary products provided (see Exhibit 5–5). Note that the products produced relate specifically to eye care.
3. Mission statements specify the geographical area within which the organization intends to concentrate. This element is most frequently included when there is a local, state, or regional aspect to the organization's service delivery. The Arkansas Department of Health mission statement specifies the geographical areas within which it offers its services (see Exhibit 5–6).
4. Mission statements identify the organization's philosophy. Frequently the mission of an organization will include statements about unique beliefs,

Exhibit 5–4: Mission Statement of MedCath, Inc.

Improve clinical outcomes for cardiac patients through a physician driven, patient focused approach.

Source: MedCath, Inc.

Exhibit 5–5: Mission Statement of Advanced Medical Optics

Advanced Medical Optics is a trusted global leader in providing high quality products and services to eye care professionals, patients and consumers. AMO is dedicated to advancing the science of eye care through the development of new innovations and technologies designed to achieve better patient outcomes and increased practitioner productivity. AMO delivers results which benefit customers, patients, employees and shareholders.

Source: Advanced Medical Optics.

Exhibit 5–6: Mission Statement of Arkansas Department of Health

The mission of the Arkansas Department of Health is to assure conditions which encourage a healthier quality of life for the people of the state. We ensure compliance with public health laws and regulations. Our colleagues are committed to providing leadership to help individuals, communities, and institutions meet their needs for disease prevention, community health assessment, health promotion, and service delivery. Our guiding efforts result in the development of sound public health policy for Arkansas.

Source: Arkansas Department of Health.

Exhibit 5–7: Mission Statement of the Saint Louis University Hospital

Saint Louis University Hospital exists for the glory of God and the health of God's people, in the Judeo-Christian and Jesuit traditions of service to others. We are an academic community dedicated to healing, teaching, and research with a commitment to quality and innovative care.

Saint Louis University Hospital is a regional leader providing tertiary-quaternary healthcare in the Tenet Healthcare Network, in partnership with the physicians of the Saint Louis University School of Medicine. We are the primary teaching site for health professions' education for the University, training tomorrow's health care leaders. We engage the passion of our people and partners in holistic care, respectful and inclusive of the uniqueness of each person.

Source: Saint Louis University Hospital.

Exhibit 5–8: Mission Statement of Genesis Health Care

We improve the lives we touch through the delivery of high quality health care and everyday compassion.

Source: Genesis Health Care.

values, aspirations, and priorities. This is particularly true for health facilities operated by religious denominations. The mission statement of the Saint Louis University Hospital in Exhibit 5–7 illustrates the faith-based philosophy as well as a commitment to educating health professionals.

5. Mission statements include confirmation of the organization's preferred self-image. The manner in which a health care organization views itself may constitute a uniqueness that should be included in the mission. The Genesis Health Care mission statement reinforces that organization's commitment to compassionate and high-quality health care (see Exhibit 5–8).

6. Mission statements specify the organization's desired public image. This customarily manifests itself in statements such as the organization's desire to be a "good citizen" or a leader in the communities where its operations are located or a similar concern. However, organizations may have a unique approach or focus that they want to communicate to the public. The mission statement of the Mayo Clinic underscores its desire to continue its reputation as the provider of "the best" medical service to its patients (see Exhibit 5–9).

Exhibit 5-9: Mission Statement of Mayo Clinic

Mayo will provide the best care to every patient every day through integrated clinical practice, education, and research.

Source: Mayo Clinic.

Not every one of the characteristics can or should be included in the mission statement. Any particular statement will likely include one or several of these characteristics but seldom will all of the components be included. The organization must decide which of these or some other characteristics really account for its distinctiveness and emphasize them in the mission statement. Interestingly, studies have found that higher performing organizations generally have more comprehensive mission statements. Moreover, it seemed that components such as organizational philosophy, self-concept, and desired public image were particularly associated with higher performing organizations in the sample studied.[13]

Building a Mission Statement

For a mission statement to be useful there has to be a leader who begins the discussion concerning the need to examine or reexamine the organization's mission to clearly state its purpose. This statement helps all employees focus their efforts on the most important priorities. One process that has been useful in building mission statements is to convene a group of interested personnel (administrative and nonadministrative) to begin the task of developing or rethinking a mission statement. This group should be composed of individuals who understand the issues facing the health care industry as well as the strengths and weaknesses of the organization.

Prior to actually writing the mission statement, a series of meetings should be held to ensure that there is a desire for a well-understood and widely communicated statement of organizational distinctiveness. Once commitment has been established, assessments should be made of what makes the organization successful from the perspectives of employees and other key stakeholders. Further, consideration should be given to what these perceptions of success would likely be in the future.

After the group has been given time to think about the organization, its distinctiveness in its environment, and the likely future it will face, the group may meet in a planning retreat. Often it is useful to remove the participants from the office, phones, and beepers to have the opportunity to truly focus on the organization's mission. To stimulate strategic thinking, each person should be asked to reflect on the mission statement components listed in Exhibit 5-10. Recognizing that some members may not have been previously involved in writing a mission statement, this exhibit was developed to encourage initial thought without introducing too much structure into the process. Group members should be asked to present key words relative to each of the components. The key words should be recorded and eventually used as the raw material for the mission statement.

Exhibit 5–10: Strategic Thinking Map for Writing a Mission Statement

Component:	Key Words Reflecting Component		
1. Target customers and clients: *"The individuals and groups we attempt to serve are . . ."* Do not be limited to only the obvious.			
2. Principal services delivered: *"The specific services or range of services we will provide to our customers are . . ."*			
3. Geographical domain of the services delivered: *"The geographical boundaries within which we will deliver our services to our customers are . . ."*			
4. Specific *values*: *"Specific values that constitute our distinctiveness in the delivery of our services to customers are . . ."*			
5. Explicit philosophy: *"The explicit philosophy that makes us distinctive in our industry is . . ."*			
6. Other important aspects of distinctiveness: *"Any other factors that make us unique among competitors are . . ."*			

Participants are encouraged to generate the key words through a series of questions listed under each mission statement component.

After discussion and fine-tuning the language, a draft of the mission statement can be developed. The draft should be refined and rewritten by the group until there is consensus on the wording and meaning of the mission statement. Once the group is satisfied with the statement, it should be circulated among key individuals to gain their input and eventually their support for the mission.

Top-Level Leadership: A Must for Mission Development

For a mission statement to be a living document, employees must develop a sense of ownership and commitment to the mission of the organization. For this reason, employees should be involved in the development and communication of the mission. However, top-level leadership must be committed if the process is to actually begin. Developing a mission statement is a challenging task. Frequently, attempts are made to formulate "blue sky" statements of environmental and competitive constraints and little more. More often mission statements are public relations documents formulated by advertising and consulting firms. For example, it is of little real value to state that a health care organization is devoted to being a good citizen in the community and to paying wages and benefits comparable to those of other organizations in the area. Realistically, the organization must be a good citizen and, if it wants employees, its wages and benefits must be competitive.

The role of the chief executive officer in formulating the mission should not be underestimated. Mission statement development is not a task that should be delegated to a planning staff. The CEO, selected line officers, and other key individuals who will be instrumental in accomplishing the mission should have input into the document. Perspective 5–3 illustrates the importance of ensuring

---

Perspective 5–3

Redefining the Organization's Purpose

Threats often create opportunities and sometimes the greater the threat, the greater the opportunity. Some people believe that the recent corporate scandals, although a threat to the competitive enterprise system, create the opportunity to carefully reevaluate and redefine the purpose of the corporation. An important competitive advantage may be gained for those who redefine themselves and become more responsive to the environment. Self-reform is almost certain to effect more fundamental change than externally imposed regulations. The agenda for self-reform consists of five important actions.

1. Develop consensus on a revised statement of corporate purpose and values. The terms "profit making" and "creating shareholder value" do not reflect the reality of today's environment. The function of the profit-oriented concern is economic but its purpose is social. Profit-oriented firms in health care or any other industry exist at the discretion of society and must serve society's needs.
2. Clarify the true role of profit. Corporations must have profits. If they do not generate a profit, they cease to exist (over the long run). Profit is a means, a motivator, and a measure of corporate performance. Moreover, profit is an important incentive for entrepreneurial action and innovation. It provides the reward for taking the risks that are critical to success.
3. Articulate and communicate the distinctions between the old purpose, values, and behaviors, and the new. Once the new mission and values are crafted, they require a cheerleader and advocate to emphasize the importance of the value shift. Strategic leaders must use every opportunity to explain and, if need be, defend the importance of the culture and value shifts.
4. Set a strong personal example. Changing a culture from one that is purely profit focused to one that balances the interests of employees, customers, the community, and other relevant stakeholders requires that leaders embody in action – as well as in pronouncements – the qualities of the new culture.
5. Revise the management measurement and reward system. If an organization only measures and rewards profitability, that is all it will receive. If, however, the purpose is defined more broadly and responsibly, broader measures have to be refined and utilized. The triple bottom line approach – focusing on economic performance as well as social and environmental outcomes – is a step in the right direction.

George Merck, founder of the pharmaceutical giant stated, "We try never to forget that medicine is for people. It is not for profits. The profits follow, and we have to remember that they have never failed to appear. The better we have remembered that, the larger they have been." David Packard, co-founder of Hewlett-Packard, made a similar point: "Profit is not the proper end and aim of management – it is what makes all of the proper ends and aims possible." To retain the public trust, corporations – including health care organizations – must engage in radical rethinking about their role in society.

Source: Ian Wilson, "The Agenda for Redefining Corporate Purpose: Five Key Executive Actions," *Strategy & Leadership* 32, no. 1 (2004), pp. 21–27.

that top management is committed to the mission and that all areas of the organization plan and coordinate their actions in such a way as to reinforce the organizational mission.

Although the process appears to be simple, the actual work of writing a mission statement is time consuming and complex, with many "drafts" before the final document is produced. A strategic thinking map (refer to Exhibit 5–10) is a useful aid to thinking about clients, services, and domain; however, the development and communication of a well-conceived mission statement requires use of the compass (leadership) as well. Although developing a mission statement is not an easy task, it is a necessary one. Missions must be relevant not only to the present but also to the future.

Vision: Hope for the Future

The mission is developed from the needs of all the stakeholders – groups who have a vested interest in the success and survival of the organization. Vision, on the other hand, is an expression of hope. It is a description of what the organization will be like and look like when it is fulfilling its purpose.[14]

Effective visions possess four important attributes: idealism, uniqueness, future orientation, and imagery.[15] Visions are about ideals, standards, and desired future states. The focus on ideals encourages everyone in the organization to think about possibilities. Vision communicates what the organization could be if everyone worked diligently to realize the potential. Health care organizations need leaders who are forward looking. Effective visions are statements of destination that provide a compass heading to where the organization's leadership collectively wants to go. Finally, visions are built on images of the future. When people are asked to describe a desirable place or thing they almost always do so in terms of images. Rarely do they focus on tangible outcomes. Images motivate people to pursue the seemingly impossible.

Origins of Vision

Health care leaders acquire vision from an appreciation of the history of the organization, a perception of the opportunities present in the environment, and an understanding of the strategic capacity of the organization to take advantage of these opportunities. All of these factors work together to form an organization's hope for the future.

HISTORY AND VISION

An organization's history is made up of a variety of events and activities that affect the development of vision. The founder's philosophy is important if the organization's inception is sufficiently recent to recall who actually started the hospital, clinic, long-term care facility, or home care agency. Consider, for example, the

Mayo Clinic in Rochester, Minnesota, an organization that is rich in history and tradition. Children's books tell successive generations how a destructive tornado in Rochester one night caused the Sisters of Saint Francis to aid the elder Dr. Mayo in caring for storm victims and encouraged his two sons, Will and Charlie, to follow in their father's footsteps. The result is a world-famous research, teaching, and patient care facility that continues to thrive and expand far beyond the boundaries of Minnesota. Anyone who hopes to succeed at the Mayo Clinic and understand its unique vision must be aware of the founders and the past. The history of an organization is instrumental in the formation of its image and its vision or hope for what it is capable of becoming.[16]

VISION AND THE ENVIRONMENT

Another important determinant of an organization's vision is the leader's view of the environment. Some organizations have negative experiences with environmental forces such as the government. Many private physicians and health care managers look at attempts by the government to get involved in setting rates, regulating quality, and so on as unnecessary and unwarranted interventions in private enterprise. When this view is adopted, enemies are seen "out there" in the environment and the vision becomes altered accordingly.[17] The vision is compromised and lack of accomplishment is blamed on these external forces. Sometimes the past experiences of organizations and the uncontrollable nature of environmental forces cause managers to engage in strategies that either over- or underreact to crises.

VISION AND INTERNAL CAPACITY

A leader's vision is related to the perceived strengths and weaknesses of the organization. The challenge to reconcile vision with internal capacity is illustrated by Senge's integrative principle of creative tension.[18] Creative tension comes into play when leaders develop a view of where they want to be in the future (vision) and tell the truth about where they are now or understand the current reality. The current reality is heavily determined by the organization's present internal capacity and how this capacity relates to its aspirations.

Organizations deal with this creative tension in different ways. If the organization has been successful in the past, it may be aggressive about the future and raise its current aspirations in pursuit of the vision. If it has experienced failure, limited success, or merely has a cautious philosophy, management may choose instead to revise and reduce the vision to bring it more in line with current reality.

Leaders have visions; organizations gain and lose competitive advantage based on how the vision fits the environment and the strategic capability of the organization to capitalize on opportunities. However, developing a vision is "messy work," and for this reason it is necessary to examine more closely what organizational vision actually means.[19] Perspective 5–4 provides some important considerations when thinking of vision statements.

Perspective 5–4

Creating Meaningful Vision Statements

The advice of corporate communication experts: do not allow an organization's vision to take on a self-centered tone. Vision should "reach out" to clients and stakeholders and underline the organization's appreciation for their concerns. Too often sentences in vision statements begin with "we" or "our." However, an organization's vision should not be about "us" but about "them."

Careful reading of organizational vision statements frequently uncovers an uncanny sameness and vagueness. Often organizations appear to be unprepared to commit to anything that is not safe and relatively certain. Vision statements are most effective when they highlight the ways that the organization can assist stakeholders in doing a better job at what they do, contribute to more satis-fied employees, increase profits or market share, or decrease costs.

The purpose of a vision statement is to provide a group with a shared image of its direction over the long term. It catalyzes a group's efforts and focuses decisions. Vision statements should:

- describe an organization's big picture and project its future,
- be grounded in sound knowledge of the business,
- be concrete and as specific as practical,
- contrast the present and the future,
- stretch the imaginations and creative energies of people in the organization,
- have a sense of significance, and
- matter.

Source: Harriet Lemer, "Vision Statements," *Beyond Numbers* (November, 2003), p. 9 and "Vision Statements," *Principal's Report* 3, no. 12 (2003), p. 2.

Health Care Strategists as Pathfinders

The job of building a vision for an organization is frequently referred to as pathfinding.[20] When the leader of a health care organization functions as a pathfinder, the focus is on the long run. The goal of the pathfinder is to provide a vision, find the paths the organization should pursue, and provide a clearly marked trail for those who will follow. As Senge notes, pathfinders have an ability to create a natural energy for changing reality by "holding a picture of what might be that is more important to people than what is."[21]

Strategic leaders are the key to establishing a vision for an organization. A vision-led organization is guided by a philosophy to which leaders are committed but that has not yet become obvious in the daily life of the organization. The *vision-led approach* hopes for higher levels of performance that are inspiring although they cannot yet be achieved.[22] A primary role of management under this approach is to clarify goals and priorities and to ensure that they are understood and accepted by employees.[23]

The role of the strategic leader, however, is more than pathfinding. As Barnard noted, because executives are responsible for inculcating the purpose into every employee, the leader must also be the *keeper of the vision* – a cheerleader who holds on to the vision even when others lose hope. Employees want to believe that what they are doing is important, and nothing convinces employees of the importance of their jobs more than a leader who keeps the inspirational vision before them (especially when things are not going well).

Strategic leadership has traditionally focused on top management, particularly the CEO. This individual is considered the person most responsible for scanning and influencing the environment, developing adaptive strategies, and managing key constituencies.[24] Unfortunately, the exclusive focus on the CEO's role in strategic leadership has implied that middle management has little or no involvement in determining the strategic direction of the organization. Admittedly, the primary responsibility of middle management is strategy implementation; however, certain strategic directions require middle-management involvement. The increasing importance of quality as a strategic objective and middle management's role in keeping this objective before all employees is a good example.[25] Quality has become an important value to which employees at all levels can be committed; middle managers are in the best position to encourage and reinforce this commitment.

Another important area in which middle management should be involved is in the redefinition of organizational vision. Grand strategies and futuristic visions are important for health care organizations. If the vision is to become meaningful to nurses, pharmacists, medical laboratory technicians, and others, middle- and first-line managers must take the lead in redefining the organizational vision in terms that are meaningful to departments and work groups. Finally, with regard to building involvement and commitment to service and quality, middle managers are in the best position to appeal to the social and economic motives important to health care employees.

Characteristics of Effective Vision

If vision is based on hope, it is – in reality – a snapshot of the future that the health care manager wants to create. It has been said that for an organizational vision to be successful it must be clear, coherent, consistent, have communicative power, and be flexible.[26]

A clear vision is simple. Basic directions and commitments should be the driving forces of a vision, not complex analysis beyond the understanding of most employees.[27] A vision is coherent when it "fits" with other statements, including the mission and values. It is consistent when it is reflected in decision-making behavior throughout the organization.[28] A vision "communicates" when it is shared and people believe in the importance of cooperation in creating the future that managers, employees, and other stakeholders desire. Finally, to be meaningful, a vision must be flexible. The future, by definition, is uncertain. Therefore, an effective vision must remain open to change as the picture of the future changes and as the strategic capabilities of the organization evolve over time.

According to Tom Peters, to effectively outline the future and facilitate the pursuit of organizational and individual excellence, visions should possess certain characteristics:[29]

1. Visions should be inspiring, not merely quantitative goals to be achieved in the next performance evaluation period. In fact, visions are rarely stated in quantitative terms. They are, however, nothing less than revolutionary in character and in terms of their potential impact on behavior. The vision of HCA for example, states the lofty goal of improving human life (see Exhibit 5–11).

2. Visions should be clear, challenging, and about excellence. There must be no doubt in the manager's mind about the importance of the vision. If the "keeper of the vision" has doubts, those who follow will have even more. The vision statement of Coventry Health Care expresses its intention to revolutionize the health care industry, improve the quality of life for all people the company serves, conduct its business ethically, and set the standard for all others to achieve (see Exhibit 5–12).

3. Visions must make sense in the relevant community, be flexible, and stand the test of time. If the vision is pragmatically irrelevant, it will not inspire high performance.

4. Visions must be stable, but constantly challenged and changed when necessary. The vision statement of Advanced Medical Optics illustrates the manner in which a vision can be formulated so as to provide focus (improving eye care) but remain broad enough to allow for changing conditions and developments (see Exhibit 5–13). Future advances in eye care can be easily accommodated with only minor changes in the vision statement.

5. Visions are beacons and controls when everything else seems up for grabs. A vision is important to provide interested people with a sense of direction.

Exhibit 5–11: Vision of HCA

Above all else, we are committed to the care and improvement of human life.

Source: HCA.

Exhibit 5–12: Vision Statement of Coventry Health Care

We intend to revolutionize the health care industry in our markets through innovation, technology, quality performance, and commitment to our customers and constituents. Our aim is to offer products and services that will responsibly improve the quality of life for all we serve. We will conduct our business affairs in an ethical and financially prudent manner through employee development, involvement and empowerment, while demonstrating compassion to our members and setting the standard for all others to achieve.

Source: Coventry Health Care.

Exhibit 5–13: Vision Statement of Advanced Medical Optics

Advanced Medical Optics is a leader and trusted partner in helping the world achieve the best possible vision. We are dedicated to delivering innovative technologies that provide eye care professionals and patients with superior technology and the highest quality products and services. We will create *The Future in Sight*™

Source: Advanced Medical Optics.

A well-formulated vision statement guides decision making because it provides inspiration for success in the future. The founders of the Cleveland Clinic Foundation, more than three-quarters of a century ago, set out to develop an institution where diverse specialists would be able to think and act as a unit. This can only be realized when everyone understands the vision and accepts the legitimacy of the direction it offers.

6. Visions empower employees (the organization's own people) first and then the clients, patients, or others to be served. Because visions are about inspiration and excellence, it is critical to recognize that employees are the ones who must be inspired first. Employees must ultimately be inspired to achieve excellence. Many health care organizations make a mistake by devoting resources to pre-service promotion programs designed to enhance potential patients' image of the organization only to disappoint them when they arrive and are greeted by the same lack of service they experienced before the advertising campaign.

7. Visions prepare for the future while honoring the past. Although vision is the hope an organization has for the future, it is important to always acknowledge and honor a history of distinction and service. The University of Texas M. D. Anderson Cancer Center acknowledges its commitment to making history using a great play on words: "We shall be the premier cancer center in the world, based on the excellence of our people, our research-driven patient care, and our science. We are Making Cancer History." Not only is Anderson making history through its continued commitment to cancer research, the center also expects to eliminate cancer.

8. Visions come alive in details, not in broad generalities. Although inspirational visions are generally unconcerned with details, the accomplishment of the vision eventually has to lead to tangible results, whether in health care, business, government, or education. Although visions are futuristic and based on hope, they require strategic leaders who can articulate the vision and translate it into terms that everyone in the organization understands and accepts. Details should be provided in words that relevant parties understand.

In the past decade more and more attention has been given to written vision statements. Vision statements are difficult to write because they require insights into the future. However, there are some useful aids that can assist managers in thinking about their vision and the direction they desire for the future. Exhibit 5–14 provides a strategic thinking map to assist in developing a vision statement. As with Exhibit 5–10 used for mission statement development, Exhibit 5–14 provides a series of questions that are useful to aid in thinking about the vision statement. Planning retreats can be used as effective forums for gaining insights into the thinking of organization members regarding their hopes for the future.

A Cautionary Note: The Problem of Newness

Strategic leaders are one of the most important elements in the strategically managed organization. Visionary leaders provide their greatest service by making the

Exhibit 5–14: Strategic Thinking Map for Writing a Vision Statement

Component:	Key Words Reflecting Component		
1. Clear hope for the future: *"If everything went as we would like it to go, what would our organization look like five years from now? How would we be different/better than today?"*			
2. Challenging and about excellence: *"When stakeholders (patients, employees, owners) describe our organization, what terms would we like for them to use?"*			
3. Inspirational and emotional: *"When we think about the kind of organization we could be if we all contributed our best, what terms would describe our collective contributions?"*			
4. Empower employees first: *"How can we ensure that employees understand and are committed to the vision? What needs to be done to get everyone's buy in?"*			
5. Memorable and provides guidance: *"What types of words should be included to ensure all organizational members remember and behave in accordance with the vision?"*			

organization flexible and able to enter new markets, disengage from old ones, and experiment with new ideas. By entering into a new market first, organizations can obtain certain *first-mover advantages. Pioneering* organizations seek first-mover advantages. A reputation for pioneering can be generated and market position can be more easily established when there are no, or only a few, competitors. Sometimes it is expensive (monetarily and emotionally) for clients and patients to switch to other providers once loyalty and mutual trust have been developed.

However, visionary change when directed toward early entry into markets has its disadvantages. This has been referred to as the *liability of newness*.[30] Innovators often experience pioneering costs. Pioneers make mistakes that others learn from and eventually correct. First movers face greater uncertainty because the demand for the service has not been proven. Patient and client needs may change and, particularly when large technological investments are required, the first mover may be left with expensive equipment and little demand. Therefore, it is important that the demand for visionary management be tempered with realistic knowledge of the market, consumers, and other factors that will affect the organization. The rewards often go to the first mover, but the risks are greater.

Research confirms some of the dangers of being the first mover. Studies of companies that were first in their markets exclude those firms that failed by focusing only on those that survived, prospered, and eventually dominated their markets.[31]

However, in reality, it is argued, market pioneers rarely endure as market leaders. Market leadership has less to do with when an organization enters the market and more to do with will and vision. Enduring leaders seem to have inspiring visions and the will to realize the vision. These enduring leaders are persistent in the pursuit of their vision, innovative, committed financially to the vision, and leverage their assets.

Values as Guiding Principles

Values are the fundamental principles that organizations and people stand for – along with the mission and vision, they make an organization unique. Most often, discussions of organizational values relate to ethical behavior and socially responsible decision making. Ethical and social responsibility values are extremely important, not just to a single hospital, HMO, or long-term care facility, but to all citizens. There are, however, other values that are very specific to a particular organization and the conduct that has either characterized its members' behavior in the past or the behavior to which members collectively aspire in the future. Total quality management or continuous improvement is in this sense a value, as is entrepreneurial spirit, teamwork, innovation, and so on.[32] It is important that managers, employees, and key stakeholders understand the values that are expected to drive an organization.

Core values, beliefs, and philosophy seem to be clear during the early stages of an organization's development but become less clear as the organization matures.[33] The values of Genesis Healthcare begin with a statement of the company's core belief in its employees and expands into the core values of the organization (see Exhibit 5–15).

Exhibit 5–15: Core Belief and Values of Genesis Healthcare

Core Belief:

Patients and residents are the center of our work. Our employees are the vital link between Genesis Healthcare and our patients and residents. They are the service we provide, the product we deliver – they are our most valuable resource. Achievement of our vision comes only through the talents and extraordinary dedication employees bring with them every day of the year.

Core Values:

- *Care & Compassion* for every life we touch.
- *Respect & Appreciation* for each other.
- *Teamwork & Enjoyment* in working together.
- *Focus & Discipline* on improving the quality of care.
- *Creativity & Innovation* to develop effective solutions.
- *Honesty & Integrity* in all dealings.

Source: Genesis Healthcare.

Exhibit 5–16 illustrates American Dental Partners' well-developed and articulated set of organizational values. Note that these values focus on what the organization believes are its key responsibilities to people, communities, shareholders, and so on. Throughout the value statement are references to ideals such as honesty, respect, dignity, and excellence. Anyone reading this set of guiding principles can understand the motivational force such a statement of values might have on employees and the comfort it might give consumers.

Not all statements of values or guiding principles are as elaborate as that of American Dental Partners. However, they need to be as well conceived. Value statements can be useful in clarifying to employees the specific behavioral norms that are expected of them as a member of the organization. This clarification is effectively accomplished in the values of HCA (see Exhibit 5–17).

Mission, vision, and value statements are tools for "getting better at what we do." The usefulness of any of these statements is the ownership developed on the part of employees and the commitments observed by stakeholders. Framed mission, vision, values, and slogans are merely exercises – and futile ones at that – if they are not made real by commitment and action.[34] See Perspective 5–5 for a discussion of why it is important to carefully think about the substance of directional strategies – especially values. The point is to motivate and guide all employees, managerial and nonmanagerial; provide high-quality care and respond to external as well as internal customers; to distinguish the organization

Exhibit 5–16: Core Values of American Dental Partners

American Dental Partners believes in five core values which provide the foundation on which our Company is built. These values represent the way we intend to do business, and we endeavor to uphold them at all times.

Ethical – A promise to conduct business in an honest, fair, manner and with the utmost integrity.

Relationship – Put people first. A commitment to treat all people with respect and human decency.

Social Responsibility – A commitment to act in a responsible manner with total regard for our families, communities, and environment.

Fiscal Responsibility – An obligation to act in a financially prudent manner for the benefit of our patients, shareholders, affiliates, and employees.

Excellence – In all we do, commitment to achieving the best results.

Source: American Dental Partners.

Exhibit 5–17: Values of HCA

In pursuit of our mission, we believe the following value statements are essential and timeless.

We recognize and affirm the unique and intrinsic worth of each individual.

We treat all those we serve with compassion and kindness.

We act with absolute honesty, integrity, and fairness in the way we conduct our business and the way we live our lives.

We trust our colleagues as valuable members of our healthcare team and pledge to treat one another with loyalty, respect, and dignity.

Source: HCA.

Leaders set the climate for the health care organization. Effective strategic leaders inspire employees to achieve the organizational mission and pursue the vision. They excite people by practicing the language of leadership. This language elevates the ordinary to the extraordinary. Leaders, for example, show how critically important everyone's performance is to the welfare of the community, the healing of patients, and the comfort of families. These tasks are not unimportant and ordinary. Strategic leaders are masters at making everyone feel important.

Strategic leaders make hard decisions when they are necessary to move the health care organization forward. They are diplomatic when they deal with external constituencies and forge community and organizational partnerships. They know when to delegate and get out of the way and how to stay informed in order to avoid surprises.

Strategic leaders are rare individuals who possess three important competencies. These competencies are (1) capacity for strategic thinking – understanding strategic issues, appreciating organizational strengths and weaknesses and those of competitors, and the ability to translate a coherent vision into strategic goals and eventually timelines and assessments of outcomes; (2) organizational savviness – awareness of nuances of prestige, status, and power relationships in the organization; and (3) decisiveness – ability to make tough and timely decisions.

Source: Michael Zwell and James L. Lubawski, "Hiring the Right Management Team," *Trustee* 53, no. 2 (2000), pp. 24–28.

from others in the perceptions of key stakeholders; and to let everyone know the organization stands for something important.

These statements and beliefs, as mentioned in Chapter 1, are directional strategies that provide the focus and parameters for the strategic goals. In addition, directional strategies provide a means of determining the essentials that must be accomplished if the organization is to be effective.

From Mission, Vision, and Values to Strategic Goals

Once strategic leaders are confident that the mission, vision, and values are well formulated, understood, communicated, and expressed in writing, they have to focus on the activities that will make the most progress toward accomplishing the mission and moving the organization toward a realization of its vision. Strategic leaders with knowledge of the service category and service area, appreciation for the organizational values, commitment to the mission, and passion for the vision can focus on a series of critical success factors that must be accomplished if the organization is to succeed and if momentum is to build toward the realization of the vision. Well-written mission statements are the beginning point for strategic goal setting. Goal setting should be focused on those areas that are critical to mission accomplishment. Steven Hillestad and Eric Berkowitz recommend the following questions when attempting to ensure that mission statements and strategic goals are consistent.

1. Does the mission of the organization reflect a broad enough orientation and provide flexibility to make required changes?
2. Did all important constituencies have an opportunity to provide input or comment on the mission?
3. Did the organization work through possible alternative operation scenarios to see how the mission might be applied?
4. Does the mission provide for the formulation of a set of goals that are specific enough to give guidance to the organization yet are broad enough to provide for the necessary flexibility?[35]

The critical success factors are the foundations for strategic goal setting. The strategic goals, in turn, become the anchors for objectives and action plans.

Critical Success Factors for the Service Category

Critical success factors are those things that organizations must do in order for the organization to achieve high performance.[36] Critical success factors for the service category, as the term implies, are similar for all members of a strategic group; however, the factors will vary from one service category to another and one strategic group to another. The critical factors for success in a medical practice are not the same as critical success factors in acute care hospitals.

Alex. Brown, & Sons, Inc., an investment research service, indicated that there are five keys to success for providers of health care services: (1) ability to serve a market; (2) strong information systems; (3) lowest cost structure; (4) ability to replicate its services in other geographical markets; and (5) ability to accept near-term risks. The critical success factors for the service category provide an important bridge between external and internal environmental analysis.[37] Strategic leaders must continually ask themselves whether the mission, vision, and values of the organization are compatible with the critical success factors. Once compatibility is ensured, leaders must identify a relatively small number of activities that are absolutely essential to accomplish the mission and build momentum to realize the vision. See Perspective 5–6 for an illustration of the factors that are critical to reducing medical errors in hospitals.

MedCath is a provider of cardiology and cardiovascular services through the development, operation, and management of heart hospitals and other specialized cardiac care facilities. The five critical success factors (as identified by Alex. Brown & Sons, Inc.) for MedCath's service category are presented in the left-hand column of Exhibit 5–18. The application of the critical success factors relative to MedCath is briefly noted in the second column. Strategic leaders need to ensure that they address the factors that lead to success in the service category.

Strategic Goals

Strategic goals should relate to critical success factor activities, providing more specific direction in accomplishing the mission and vision. At the same time,

Perspective 5–6
Critical Success
Factors for Reducing
Medical Errors

The Institute of Medicine estimates that medical errors account for more than one million injuries and 98,000 deaths annually. Medical error is the eighth leading cause of death in the United States, ahead of highway accidents, breast cancer, and AIDS. Moreover, the Institute estimates that medical errors cost the United States $37.6 billion per year. A study of four hospitals identified seven critical success factors (CSFs) that appear to reduce the likelihood of medical errors or minimize the effects of medical errors:

1. *Partner with stakeholders to reduce errors.* An error management system generally requires a change in the organizational structure and some of the processes for a hospital. Stakeholders, including the medical staff, patients, hospital management, and trustees/directors, must be supportive if the changes are to be successful.
2. *Eliminate the placing of blame.* An important factor in reducing the incidence of errors is an effective system for reporting errors without blame. Placing blame will almost surely result in a system failure. Attention should be on the overall process, not on the person reporting or making the error.
3. *Ensure open communication.* One approach is the use of small groups to encourage discussion of relevant issues.
4. *Change the culture.* Preventing medical error requires a change in the organizational culture. Culture changes are often a prerequisite for effective error management.
5. *Educate and train.* Implementing actions to reduce errors is usually focused on people providing or supporting medical care in the hospital or medical office. These individuals need education and training in error management techniques.
6. *Analyze error data.* Data collection and analysis are essential to determine the sources of poor quality and the best approaches to reduce problems. Error management is no exception.
7. *Redesign the system.* The final factor is the redesign of the system or process. The extent of system redesign can focus primarily on one part of the system or take a much broader perspective.

These seven critical factors must be considered in any attempt to reduce medical errors. Focusing on this limited number of factors improves the likelihood of being successful in developing error management programs.

Source: Kathleen L. McFadden, Elizabeth R. Towell, and Gregory N. Stock, "Critical Success Factors for Controlling and Managing Hospital Errors," *Quality Management Journal* 11, no. 1 (2004), pp. 61–64.

strategic goals should be broad enough to allow considerable discretion for managers to formulate their objectives for individual units.[38] The most appropriate strategic goals possess the following characteristics:

1. Strategic goals should relate specifically to activities that are critical to accomplish the mission. Strategic goals that focus on activities that are not mission critical have the potential to divert leadership attention and employee energy.
2. Strategic goals should be the link between critical success factors and strategic momentum (carrying out unit objectives).
3. Strategic goals should be limited in number. When too many goals are pursued, the "trivial many" rather than the "critical few" activities are accomplished.
4. Strategic goals should be formulated by leaders but should be stated in terms that can be easily understood and appreciated by everyone in the organization.

Exhibit 5–18: Critical Success Factors related to MedCath

Critical Success Factors	Related to MedCath
Ability to serve entire market	Complete range of heart-related services including outpatient (angiogram and related diagnostic testing), inpatient (angioplasty, open heart surgery, etc.), fixed-site and nuclear laboratories, mobile catheterization services for hospital networks, and cardiology consulting and management services
Strong information systems	State-of-the-art, integrated administrative and clinical information systems required to manage a national network of heart hospitals
Lowest cost structure	Because of horizontal integration (focused factory) strategy, cost structure is extremely low. Despite MedCath hospitals having higher cardiac case mix severity, the hospitals are able to obtain lower mortality rates with shorter lengths of stay
Ability to replicate services in other geographical markets	MedCath presently has ownership interest in and operates 12 hospitals in 8 states, is engaged in 9 cardiology joint ventures, 11 managed ventures, and three professional service agreements
Ability to accept near-term risks	Financially conservative leadership that maintains liquidity and allows for resources to pursue opportunities

American Dental Partners developed a set of seven strategic goals that address the company's mission and are consistent with its core values. These goals concern partnerships in management, operating excellence, integration of technology, continuous growth, financial performance, quality of work life, and quality of care and service. More specifically, American Dental Partners' goals are as follows:

1. To ensure the appropriate sharing of operating governance and financial risk and reward in the organization and operation of each ADP affiliate;
2. To pursue aggressively continuous and progressive improvement in the productivity and profitability of each ADP affiliate;
3. To optimize the provision of dental care and service through the integration of leading-edge information technology;
4. To increase progressively the market share and geographic diversity of each ADP affiliate;
5. To ensure levels of return on investment that are highly competitive in the dental industry and highly valued by the public market;
6. To create an environment in which each ADP affiliate is the employer of choice in its market; and
7. To ensure the provision of high-quality, high-value dental care and service in all ADP affiliates.

American Dental Partners has maintained its strategic focus through its goals. Perspective 5–7 provides practical guidelines for achieving and maintaining focus.

Perspective 5–7 Getting out of the Mud	To be effective a sports car has to have speed and performance. However, if it gets stuck in the mud, it cannot go very fast or perform very well. Sometimes the reason a CEO finds it difficult to get out of the mud is that there is little or no strategic focus. How does the leader and the organization achieve a better focus?

- Place the customer/patient at the center of strategic thinking. Ask four questions:
  1. What are our most profitable customer relationships?
  2. How did these relationships originate and develop?
  3. Why did our customers/patients come to us initially and why do they continue to return?
  4. What value do they see in their relationship with us?
- Talk to customers/patients face-to-face and determine ways to make the organization better by being different from competitors.
- Ask frame-breaking questions:
  1. What business are we in?
  2. At what business can we be world class?
  3. What is our passion?
  4. Which characteristics of our business should be eliminated and which should be retained?
- Refine and validate the strategy with customers/patients and key stakeholders. Everyone has to "buy it" for a strategy to be successful. Alignment of strategic understanding aids greatly in success.
- Establish a methodology for executing the strategy. There must be a clear focus, accountability, and a commitment to strategic results. If an organization has a disciplined methodology, it can avoid the hazards of strategy – distraction and compromise. The rule becomes, "If it does not fit the strategy, we do not do it."
- Focus on achieving early wins to build momentum. Nothing encourages success like success. Strategy is not a once a year activity; it is an everyday priority. Strategy is not a plan but a mindset. In the most effective organizations, opportunism is replaced with strategy.

Smart people realize that if you keep spinning the wheels you will only sink deeper and become more stuck in the mud. To get out of the mud, you must have traction. Merely exploiting an occasional opportunity is a reactive rather than a strategic mindset. To be successful in a strategic sense, being proactive rather than reactive is required.

Source: Bob Hogan, "Stuck in the Mud," *Executive Excellence* 20, no. 8 (2003), p. 15.

Governing Boards and Directional Strategies

The discussion of directional strategies has emphasized the importance of the involvement and participation of as many people as practical. The governing board is an important group that should be involved in the development of the strategic direction of the health care organization. The board members should be regularly informed about the strategic goals and the progress being made in their accomplishment. Governing boards have taken on particular importance in the past several years as ehtical issues have escalated. Health care has not been exempt, as evidenced by major corporate scandals involving companies such as HEALTHSOUTH. Increasingly the question of the role and responsibility of governing boards is discussed in health care management.

Boards of directors or boards of trustees are responsible for making policies – providing general guidelines under which the organization will operate. Therefore, boards are important in formulating the mission, vision, and value statements of the organization. It is not likely that board members will be directly involved in the process although in some cases members do participate. However, board members are often interviewed during the formulation of the mission, vision, and values and their input incorporated into the statements. It is important that the board is informed about the statements and involved in the strategic thinking that results in their formulation. Therefore the selection and composition of board members is a critical strategic decision.[39]

Health Care Performance and the Usual Suspects

Much of the discussion regarding governing boards has related to issues that have been referred to as the "usual suspects."[40] Primary attention has been given to questioning how these usual suspects influence the financial performance of an organization. Some usual suspects are the number of outsiders on the board, shareholdings of board members, board size, and CEO duality (CEO simultaneously functioning as the chief executive and board chair).[41] Of particular interest has been board size.

For health care organizations there are generally two different types of governing boards – *philanthropic governing boards* (those that are service oriented and concerned primarily with fundraising) and *corporate governing boards* (those that are more involved in strategic planning as well as policy making). Philanthropic boards are larger and more diverse to gain as much community representation as possible. The inclusion of different types of stakeholders is important and requires that board members be selected from among business leaders, physicians, local politicians, consumers of health care services, and so on. The corporate board is smaller and composed of individuals who possess expertise that will aid the organization in accomplishing its strategic goals.[42] Membership diversity is important, but less so than the actual skills or expertise possessed by the members.

The current trend in health care organizations is toward the corporate board. To a great extent, this is the result of the increasingly competitive environment facing health care organizations and the need for expertise in dealing with the complexities of the economic environment.[43] However, it should be noted that virtually no research confirms any positive relationship between the size and nature of board membership and organizational financial performance.[44]

Research findings on boards of directors suggest that when profound or radical organizational change confronts a health care organization, the corporate board is more likely to propose effective, positive responses. Philanthropic boards, on the other hand, are more likely to be associated with either no change or negative responses to profound change.[45] Boards of directors in health care organizations undergoing corporate restructuring (defined as the segmentation of the organization's assets and functions into separate corporations to reflect specific profit, regulatory, or market objectives) tended to become less philanthropic and more corporate, not only in composition but also in the way they operated.[46]

Other research provides additional information about various types of governing boards in health care organizations. When compared with boards of directors of successful high-technology firms, for example, governing boards in a sample of multihospital health care systems were almost twice as large (11–15 members).[47] In fact, boards are frequently too large to be effective aids in decision making, and where the goal is stakeholder representation, board members often know so little about health care that CEOs are forced to spend a great deal of their time informing and educating lay members.

Another study examined the issue of outside directors in large investor-owned health care organizations. Four major subsamples were examined, including hospitals, elder care organizations, HMOs, and alternative care facilities such as psychiatric clinics and ambulatory care centers.[48] This study found that, in general, governing boards of health care organizations were composed of more members from outside, rather than inside, the organization. Outside representatives were primarily physicians, financial professionals, attorneys, and academics. The inclusion of physicians was found to be particularly significant in terms of bottom-line performance. The presence of physicians on governing boards enhanced the support of the medical community, improving the organization's market share and quality.

The evidence to date is underwhelming with regard to the usual topics of board independence (percentage of outside members), board size, CEO duality, and so on. There is virtually no evidence to indicate that these factors consistently influence the financial performance of organizations.[49]

Although it is dangerous to generalize, some inferences can be drawn from the research on governing boards in health care organizations. In not-for-profit health care organizations, governing boards are more in line with the philanthropic model. They are generally large (in fact, too large to be effective aids in strategic decision making), do not compensate members, select members primarily as stakeholder representatives, and do not hold the CEO formally accountable for performance. In this case, the primary motivation for board membership is service and recognition. When health care organizations are profit oriented, their boards take on more corporate characteristics. They tend to be smaller, compensate members for service, select members for specific expertise, involve the CEO as a voting member, make him or her formally accountable to the board, and require the participation of board members in strategic decision making. From the perspective of the individual board member, the motivation to be on the hospital's board may be to provide a valuable service to the community, but board membership may be an important source of income as well.

Because of the extensive amount of research and the inconclusive nature of the findings, the search has shifted from type of governing board (philanthropic or corporate) to other aspects of board functioning that might be more influential on performance.

Board Process: Missing Link?

The lack of consistent association between factors such as board size, independence, CEO duality, member expertise, and organizational performance on financial measures has encouraged researchers to look at different variables. Of particular interest is the board process – the means by which boards of directors do their work.[50]

Interviews with experienced board members indicate that there are several factors that lead to more effective boards. They:

1. *Engage in constructive conflicts (especially with the CEO).* It is important that board members hold and debate diverse views among themselves and with the CEO. An overabundance of insiders on a board may diminish the presence of constructive conflict since debate with the CEO amounts to debate with the boss.
2. *Avoid destructive conflict.* Personal friction and tension in the boardroom should be minimized. There must be a clear distinction between constructive debate and destructive conflict.
3. *Work together as a team.* The most important component of board process is teamwork. The development of strong team norms, however, is hard to accomplish since board members spend little time together. Board members are busy and do not have time to spend together; thus, it is critical to make the most of the limited time available for board member interaction.
4. *Know the appropriate level of strategic involvement.* Board members should limit their involvement to major strategic decisions. They should be very careful not to become too involved in the day-to-day management of the firm (see Perspective 5–8).
5. *Address decisions comprehensively.* Board members should consciously attempt to address issues with sufficient depth to make sound decisions. Too often, time demands and conflicting priorities tempt boards to deal superficially with important issues. Effective boards find the time needed for important strategic decisions.[51]

The work of boards of directors is extremely important. Boards are created to ensure that strategic leaders have additional expertise available to them for making policy decisions that provide direction to the organization. The effectiveness of the board is a key factor in the effectiveness of the organization.

Managing Strategic Momentum – Evaluating Directional Strategies

As part of managing strategic momentum, managers assess the performance of the organization and try to determine whether the mission, vision, values, and goals are – and continue to be – appropriate. To illustrate, hospices today reap more than $3 billion annually in Medicare reimbursement. In just two decades since hospices began receiving reimbursement for their services, end-of-life care has emerged as an integral part of the health care system. Palliative care (end-of-life and comfort care) has become so important that hospitals and other providers have seized opportunities in this area. One hospice states that its

Perspective 5–8

CEO Succession
Planning and Boards
of Directors in
Health Care

A survey of public corporation CEOs conducted by the National Association of Corporate Directors found that CEO succession is number two on the list of the most important issues facing corporate boards of directors. The top five issues were: (1) corporate performance, (2) CEO succession, (3) strategic planning, (4) corporate governance, and (5) board–CEO relations.

Interestingly, CEO succession does not even appear in the top five most important issues facing not-for-profit health care boards. A randomly selected sample of not-for-profit health care CEOs listed their most important issues as: (1) financial survival, (2) strategic planning, (3) conflict of interest among board members, (4) quality of care oversight, and (5) board evaluation and education. This brings up an interesting question. Why do the not-for-profit health care executives not rank CEO succession as being as important as their corporate counterparts? There are a variety of possibilities. Perhaps health care executives assume a program of CEO succession is too expensive, or that no one would dare raid their CEO, or that no one wants to think about replacing the CEO, and, therefore, they just ignore the issue of succession.

Regardless of the economic sector (private, not-for-profit, health care, nonhealth care, etc.), CEO succession is a critically important issue for boards of directors to consider. Ensuring continuity of operations with a minimum of disruption should the chief executive leave is an essential part of good governance. Some organizations just assume that the search will focus on outsiders so there is no reason to develop a plan of succession involving insiders. However, it was noted in the popular book *Good to Great* that of the eleven companies that made it from good to great, ten relied on internal candidates to succeed the current CEO.

The primary responsibilities of the board of directors relative to CEO succession are as follows:

1. The board should ensure that succession planning is being done somewhere in the organization. If nothing else, it will move the current CEO off the mark to plan for his or her successor if succession is known to be a topic on the board agenda.
2. The board should sign off on any candidate identified as a possible successor and should be involved in the succession plan.
3. The board should be sure any commitment it makes relative to succession is communicated to future board members.
4. The board should always reserve the right to go outside for successors if for no other reason than to validate its plan.

Source: Errol L. Biggs, "CEO Succession Planning: An Emerging Challenge for Boards of Directors," *Academy of Management Executive* 18, no. 1 (2004), pp. 105–107.

mission is to provide care for dying patients and their families in their homes. The second hospice, aware of the changes in the environment and concerned with managing strategic momentum, has slightly revised its mission to reflect the change in the competitive environment. The new mission is to provide end-of-life and palliative care services. If both organizations should decide to offer services to Alzheimer's patients living in nursing homes, only the second hospice would be acting in accordance with its mission.[52]

Decisions to change an organization's mission, vision, values, and goals are complex and involve many variables. To manage strategic momentum, questions

Exhibit 5–19: Managing Strategic Momentum – Evaluating Directional Strategies

1. Are we not doing some things now that we should be doing?
2. Are we doing some things now that we should not be doing?
3. Are we doing some things now we should do but do in a different way?
4. Are our organization's mission and vision unique in some way?
5. Is our mission relatively enduring?
6. Do our mission and vision allow for innovation?
7. Do our mission and vision allow for expansion?
8. Is our scope of operations clear (market, products/services, customers, geographic coverage)?
9. Do our mission, vision, and values fit the needs of our stakeholders?
10. Do our fundamental values make sense?
11. Are our strategic goals moving us toward achievement of our mission?
12. Are our strategic goals moving us toward achievement of our vision?
13. Have we addressed the critical success factors?
14. Is the image of the organization what it should be?

should be asked that concern the fundamental activities and direction of the organization. Exhibit 5–19 provides guidance through several questions that will aid managers in their strategic thinking concerning the appropriateness of the organization's directional strategies. Perhaps the best approach for managing the directional strategies is to place the vision for the future, the existing mission statement, statement of values, and the organization's goals next to the questions in Exhibit 5–19 and ask the board of directors/trustees and the strategic management team to freely discuss and reach a consensus on each question. This process will either validate the existing mission, vision, values, and goals or indicate that there should be changes to maintain strategic momentum. This process invites clarification, understanding, and reinforcement of exactly "what this organization is all about" or "what this organization should be about."

Summary and Conclusions

Directional strategies allow leaders to state what they believe the organization should be doing and make explicit how they intend to conduct their business. Every attempt should be made to develop and communicate well-conceived and written statements of the organization's mission, vision, values, and strategic goals.

The topics in this chapter relate to the superordinate goals or outcomes that health care organizations plan to accomplish. Strategic leaders should recognize that strategic planning is a logical process. The progression of directional strategies discussed in this chapter illustrates the importance of logic. The mission of the organization drives decision making because it is the organization's reason for existing. The vision provides hope for the future and values tell everyone – employees, stakeholders, patients, and so on – how the organization will operate. The strategic goals specify what the leaders believe is required to achieve the mission.

A mission alone is not enough. The mission, as a statement of purpose that distinguishes the organization from all others of its type, such as the care given to patients, physical location of the facility, the unusual commitment of physicians to research as well as to healing, or any other factor that is important in the minds of those served, is only the first step. The mission may motivate a few physicians and department managers, but real motivation comes from visionary leadership. The vision is a hope that says what key stakeholders think the organization should look and be like when the mission is being achieved. Values, as guiding principles, can be powerful motivating forces, as well.

Even a well-developed and communicated mission is likely to leave the health care strategist with far too many areas of responsibility, resulting in an impossible task. For this reason, critical success factors for the service category must be identified and strategic goals must be set to accomplish the mission. This helps make the strategist's job feasible. It is likely that most strategic leaders attempt to manage far too many aspects of the business. The logic of this chapter should help health care strategists focus more effectively on those tasks that really make a difference with respect to organizational success.

Management research shows that the existence of goals can be extremely motivating. Clearly stated and communicated strategic goals provide a sense of direction – they specify what leaders are expected to accomplish and remove anxiety from those who want to succeed. Formulating mission, vision, values, and strategic goals and identifying critical success factors are often "messy" and unappreciated. In the end, however, setting directional strategies is a major responsibility for all strategic leaders.

Engaging as many groups as practical in the process of developing directional strategies is important. The board of directors should be involved in the thinking that ultimately results in the mission, vision, and value statements. In addition, board members should be regularly informed about the strategic goals of the organization and the progress being made in their accomplishment. Most importantly, the board should engage in a process that contributes to organizational effectiveness. Research confirms that merely electing or selecting a board of directors/trustees comprised of an appropriate percentage of outsiders, of individuals with the appropriate expertise, and small enough to be manageable, will not ensure its effectiveness. The board must also be willing to engage in constructive conflict, minimize destructive interpersonal tensions, avoid micromanagement, and devote the time required to make important strategic decisions.

Key Terms and Concepts in Strategic Management

Corporate Governing Boards	Liability of Newness	Strategic Goals
Critical Success Factor	Mission	Values
First-Mover Advantage	Philanthropic Governing Boards	Vision
Keeper of the Vision	Pioneering	Vision-Led Approach

QUESTIONS FOR CLASS DISCUSSION

1. Is it necessary for organizational mission statements to include all the components discussed in this chapter? How do you decide what components to include?

2. Think of an organization that you know relatively well and attempt to construct a mission statement in light of the components of missions discussed in this chapter. What components did you choose to emphasize in the statement? Why? What component do you think really embodies the distinctiveness of the organization?

3. Where do organizational missions originate? How do you explain the evolution of organizational missions as the organization grows and matures? If mission statements are "relatively enduring," how often should they be changed?

4. Indicate two ways in which an organizational vision is different from other types of directional strategies.

5. It has been said that vision is necessarily a responsibility of leaders. Why is it important for health care organizations to have keepers of the vision?

6. Who determines the values of the health care organization? What values do you think should be shared by all health care organizations? Why?

7. Why are values referred to as an organization's guiding principles? In what sense do values constitute a directional strategy for the organization?

8. How many strategic goals should a health care organization develop?

9. How can health care managers more effectively use directional strategies to stimulate higher levels of performance among all personnel?

10. Why is the board of directors an important group to include in the formulation of directional strategies? What is the board's proper role in formulating these strategies?

11. What is the best way to involve the board in the development of directional strategies? Explain your answer.

12. What are the important elements of an effective board process? Why do you think board process is more important than board composition and size?

13. List three reasons why boards of directors or trustees have become increasingly important factors in the effectiveness of health care organizations.

NOTES

1. Chester I. Barnard, *Functions of the Executive* (Cambridge, MA: Harvard University Press, 1938), p. 87.

2. W. Jack Duncan, *Management: Ideas and Actions* (New York: Oxford University Press, 1999), pp. 122–123.

3. Website of Amedisys, Inc.

4. Perry Pascarella and Mark A. Frohman, *The Purpose Driven Organization* (San Francisco: Jossey-Bass Publishers, 1989), p. 23.

5. Forest R. David and Fred R. David, "It's Time to Redraft Your Mission Statement," *Journal of Business Strategy* 24, no. 1 (2003), pp. 11–14.

6. C. Kendrick Gibson, David J. Newton, and Dennis S. Cochran, "An Empirical Investigation of the Nature of Hospital Mission Statements," *Health Care Management Review* 15, no. 3 (1990), pp. 35–46.

7. Thomas T. Brown, "Noble Purpose," *Executive Excellence* 21, no. 1 (January 2004), p. 7.

8. R. Duane Ireland and Michael A. Hitt, "Mission Statements: Importance, Challenge, and Recommendations," *Business Horizons* 35, no. 3 (1992), pp. 34–42.

9. Darrell Rigby, "Management Tools Survey 2003: Usage Up As Companies Strive to Make Headway

in Tough Times," *Strategy & Leadership* 31, no. 5 (2003), pp. 4–7.

10. Aimee Forehand, "Mission and Organizational Performance in the Healthcare Industry," *Journal of Healthcare Management* 45, no. 4 (2000), pp. 267–275.

11. Christopher K. Bart and John C. Tabone, "Mission Statement Content and Hospital Performance in the Canadian Not-for-Profit Health Care Sector," *Health Care Management Review* 24, no. 2 (1999), pp. 18–26; and Christopher K. Bart and J. C. Tabone, "Mission Statement Rationales and Organizational Alignment in the Not-for-Profit Health Care Sector," *Health Care Management Review* 23, no. 1 (1998), pp. 54–70.

12. These components adapted from John A. Pearce, II and Fred David, "Corporate Mission Statements and the Bottom Line," *Academy of Management Executive* 1, no. 1 (1987), pp. 109–116.

13. Ibid.

14. Cecilia Falbe, Mark Driger, Lauri Larwood, and Paul Miesing, "Structure and Meaning of Organizational Vision," *Academy of Management Journal* 38, no. 3 (1995), pp. 740–767.

15. James M. Kouzes and Barry Z. Posner, "Envisioning Your Future: Imagining Ideal Scenarios," *Futurist* 30, no. 3 (1996), pp. 14–19. See also Shelley A. Kirkpatrick, J. C. Wofford, and J. Robert Baum, "Measuring Motive Imagery Contained in the Vision Statement," *Leadership Quarterly* 13, no. 2 (2002), pp. 139–151.

16. See Alan M. Zuckerman, "Creating a Vision for the Twenty-First Century Health Care Organization," *Journal of Healthcare Management* 45, no. 5 (2000), pp. 294–306; Stanley Harris, Kevin W. Mossholder, and Sharon Oswald, "Vision Salience and Strategic Involvement: Implications for Psychological Attachment to Organization and Job," *Strategic Management Journal* 15, no. 3 (1994), pp. 477–489; Terrence Femsler, "Build Mission and Vision Statements Step by Step: Book Review," *Nonprofit World* 21, no. 2 (2003), p. 32; and Anonymous, "Preparing A Vision Statement: Book Review," *Futurist* 36, no. 4 (2002), p. 59.

17. Manfred F. R. Kets de Vries, "The Leadership Mystique," *Academy of Management Executive* 8, no. 3 (1994), pp. 73–83. See also T. C. Reeves, W. J. Duncan, and P. M. Ginter, "Leading Change by Managing Paradoxes," *Journal of Leadership Studies* 7, no. 1 (2000), pp. 13–30.

18. Peter M. Senge, "The Leader's New Work: Building Learning Organizations," *Sloan Management Review* 31, no. 1 (1990), pp. 13–14.

19. Montgomery Van Wart, "The First Step in the Reinvention Process: Assessment," *Public Administration Review* 55, no. 5 (1995), pp. 429–438.

20. G. B. Morris, "The Executive: A Pathfinder," *Organizational Dynamics* 16, no. 2 (1988), pp. 62–77.

21. Senge, "The Leader's New Work," p. 8.

22. James C. Collins and Jerry I. Porras, "Organizational Vision and Visionary Organizations," *California Management Review* 34, no. 1 (1991), pp. 30–52.

23. Timothy W. Coombs and Sherry J. Holladay, "Speaking of Visions and Visions Being Spoken," *Management Communication Quarterly* 8, no. 2 (1994), pp. 165–189.

24. Howard S. Zuckerman, "Redefining the Role of the CEO: Challenges and Conflicts," *Hospital & Health Services Administration* 34, no. 1 (1989), pp. 25–38. See also Stephen C. Harper, "The Challenges Facing CEOs: Past, Present, and Future," *Academy of Management Executive* 6, no. 3 (1992), pp. 7–25.

25. Arnold D. Kaluzny, "Revitalizing Decision Making at the Middle Management Level," *Hospital & Health Services Administration* 34, no. 1 (1989), pp. 39–51. See also S. W. Floyd and Bill Wooldridge, "Dinosaurs or Dynamos? Recognizing Middle Management's Strategic Role," *Academy of Management Executive* 8, no. 4 (1994), pp. 47–57.

26. Ian Wilson, "Realizing the Power of Strategic Vision," *Long Range Planning* 25, no. 5 (1992), pp. 18–28.

27. James R. Lucas, "Anatomy of a Vision Statement," *Management Review* 87, no. 2 (1998), pp. 22–26.

28. David Silvers, "Vision – Not Just for CEOs," *Management Quarterly* 35, no. 2 (1994), pp. 10–15.

29. Tom Peters, *Thriving on Chaos* (New York: Alfred A Knopf, 1988), pp. 401–404.

30. The term "liability of newness" was suggested by James March. However, the most extensive treatment of "first-mover" advantages and disadvantages is presented in Michael E. Porter, *Competitive Advantage* (New York: Free Press, 1986), pp. 186–191.

31. Gerald J. Tellis and Peter N. Golder, *Will and Vision: How Latecomers Grow to Dominate Markets* (New York: McGraw-Hill Companies, Inc., 2002).

32. L. D. DeSimone, "How Can Big Companies Keep the Entrepreneurial Spirit Alive?" *Harvard Business Review* 73, no. 5 (1995), pp. 183–186 and I. Morrison, "Creating a Vision from Our Values," *Modern Healthcare* 29, no. 39 (2000), p. 30.

33. Gerald E. Ledford, James T. Strahley, and Jon R. Wendenhof, "Realizing a Corporate Philosophy," *Organizational Dynamics* 23, no. 3 (1995), pp. 4–19. See

also D. P. Ashmos and Dennis Duchon, "Spirituality at Work: A Conceptualization and Measure," *Journal of Management Inquiry* 9, no. 2 (2000), pp. 134–145 and Susan Taft, Katherine Hawn, Jane Barber, and Jamie Bidwell, "The Creation of a Value Driven Culture," *Health Care Management Review* 24, no. 1 (1999), pp. 17–32.

34. For some criticisms of these tools see Colin Coulson-Thomas, "Strategic Vision or Strategic Con: Rhetoric or Reality," *Long Range Planning* 25, no. 1 (1992), pp. 81–89 and Lee D. Parker, "Financial Management Strategy in A Community Welfare Organization: A Boardroom Perspective," *Financial Accountability and Management* 19, no. 4 (2003), pp. 341–374.

35. Steven G. Hillestad and Eric N. Berkowitz, *Health Care Marketing Strategy: From Planning to Action* (Boston: Jones and Bartlett Publishers, 2004) quoted in "Mission Statement Is Key to a Good Marketing Plan: Goals Should Be Tied to Statement," *Hospice Management Advisor* 8, no. 2 (2003), p. 17.

36. M. E. Freisen and J. A. Johnson, *The Success Paradigm: Creating Organizational Effectiveness through Quality and Strategy* (Westport, CT: Quorum Books, 1995), p. 3. Also see Robert S. Kaplan and David P. Norton, "How Strategy Maps Frame An Organization's Objectives," *Financial Executive* 20, no. 2 (2004), pp. 40–46.

37. Jeffery K. Pinto and John E. Prescott, "Variations in Critical Success Factors over the Stages in the Product Life Cycle," *Journal of Management* 14, no. 1 (1988), pp. 5–18.

38. John Karlewski, "Profit Versus Public Welfare Goals in Investor-Owned and Not-for-Profit Hospitals," *Hospital & Health Services Administration* 33, no. 3 (1988), pp. 312–329. See also David P. Tarantino, "Using Simple Rules to Achieve Strategic Objectives," *Physician Executive* 29, no. 3 (May 2003), pp. 56–57 and Fabrizio Cesaroni, Alberto DiMinin, and Andrea Piccaluga, "New Strategic Goals and Organizational Solutions in Large R&D Labs: Lessons from Centro Ricerche Fiat and Telecom Italia Lab," *R & D Management* 34, no. 1 (2004), pp. 45–57. The discussion of American Dental Partners' goals is adapted from information on the ADP website.

39. P. Michel Maher, Malcolm C. Munro, and Flora L. Stromer, "Building a Better Board: Six Keys to Enhancing Corporate Director Performance," *Strategy & Leadership* 28, no. 5 (2000), pp. 31–32.

40. Sydney Finkelstein and Ann C. Mooney, "Not the Usual Suspects: How to Use Board Process to Make Boards Better," *Academy of Management Executive* 17, no. 2 (2003), pp. 101–113.

41. Wayne F. Cascio, "Board Governance: A Social Systems Perspective," *Academy of Management Executive* 18, no. 1 (2004), pp. 97–100.

42. J. A. Alexander, L. L. Morlock, and B. D. Gifford, "The Effects of Corporate Restructuring on Hospital Policymaking," *Health Services Research* 23, no. 2 (1988), pp. 311–338 and A. R. Kovner, "Improving Hospital Board Effectiveness: An Update," *Frontiers in Health Services Management* 6, no. 2 (1990), pp. 3–27.

43. S. M. Shortell, "New Directions in Hospital Governance," *Hospital & Health Services Administration* 34, no. 1 (1989), pp. 7–23. See also M. J. Conyon and Simon I. Peck, "Board Control, Remuneration Committees, and Top Management Compensation," *Academy of Management Journal* 41, no. 2 (1998), pp. 158–178.

44. Catherine M. Daily, Dan R. Dalton, and Nandini Rajagopalan, "Governance through Ownership: Centuries of Practice, Decades of Research," *Academy of Management Journal* 46, no. 2 (2003), pp. 151–158.

45. M. L. Fennell and J. A. Alexander, "Governing Boards and Profound Organizational Change," *Medical Care Review* 46, no. 2 (1989), pp. 157–187.

46. J. A. Alexander and L. L. Morlock, "CEO–Board Relations Under Hospital Corporate Restructuring," *Hospital & Health Services Administration* 33, no. 3 (1988), p. 436.

47. A. L. Delbecq and S. L. Gill, "Developing Strategic Direction for Governing Boards," *Hospital & Health Services Administration* 33, no. 1 (1988), pp. 25–35.

48. R. A. McLean, "Outside Directors: Stakeholder Representation in Investor-Owned Health Care Organizations," *Hospital & Health Services Administration* 34, no. 1 (1989), pp. 25–38.

49. Catherine M. Daily, Dan R. Dalton, and Albert A. Cannella, Jr., "Corporate Governance: Decades of Dialogue and Data," *Academy of Management Review* 28, no. 3 (2003), pp. 371–382 and Matthew D. Lynall, Brian R. Golden, and Amy J. Hillman, "Board Composition from Adolescence to Maturity: A Multitheoretic View," *Academy of Management Review* 28, no. 3 (2003), pp. 416–431.

50. See Jeffrey Sonnenfeld, "Good Governance and the Misleading Myths of Bad Metrics," *Academy of Management Executive* 18, no. 1 (2004), pp. 108–113 and Jeffrey Sonnenfeld, "What Makes Great Boards Great?" *Harvard Business Review* 80, no. 9 (2002), pp. 106–113.

51. Finkelstein and Mooney, "Not the Usual Suspects," pp. 103–106.

52. "Mission Statement is Key to a Good Marketing Plan," *Hospice Management Advisor*, pp. 18–19.

**ADDITIONAL
READINGS**

Biggs, Errol, *The Governance Factor: 33 Keys to Success in Healthcare* (Chicago: Health Administration Press, 2003). An easy-to-read and understand guidebook that answers questions commonly asked about organizational governance. Issues such as board structure, responsibility, board member job descriptions, and the relationship of the board to the CEO are examined. The increasingly popular topic of board performance appraisals is included.

Bornstein, David, *How to Change the World: Social Entrepreneurs and the Power of New Ideas* (New York: Oxford University Press, 2004). What entrepreneurs are to business, social entrepreneurs are to social change. The social entrepreneurs are the driven and creative people who question things as they are and exploit new opportunities. Social entrepreneurs are more committed to making the world a better place than making money.

Carter, Colin B. and Jay W. Lorsch, *Back to the Drawing Board* (Boston: Harvard Business School Press, 2004). Corporate boards are not working. According to the authors, the theory was great but the practice has proven to be flawed. They argue that boards of directors require major redesign. Reflections from their actual experiences serving on corporate boards provide the foundation for their suggestions. A description of how a board's role should be defined and a clear approach to board design is provided to help organizations develop and maintain effective boards.

Hendry, John, *Between Enterprise and Ethics: Management in a Bimoral Society* (New York: Oxford University Press, 2004). The author notes that we live in a bimoral society. On one hand there are principles associated with traditional morality. On the other hand, there are the principles associated with entrepreneurial self-interest. These value systems have always been present but in recent years, the author argues, traditional morality has lost much to the principles of self-interest. A key role for management has become determining purposes and priorities, reconciling divergent interests, and nurturing trust in interpersonal relationships.

Klein, Merom and Rod Napier, *The Courage to Act: 5 Factors of Courage to Transform Business* (Palo Alto, CA: Davies-Black Publishing, 2003). This book offers suggestions on how to survive and prosper in this age of uncertainty. The five factors that can lead to business transformation are discussed throughout the book. Candor is the courage to speak and hear the truth. Purpose is courage to pursue audacious goals. Will is the courage to inspire optimism. Rigor is the courage to create new disciplines. Risk is the courage to empower others. The authors effectively use brief case studies of actual experiences and carefully blend this practical knowledge with a minimum of theory. The book contains many interesting company stories that are used to effectively make and reinforce key points.

6

CHAPTER

Developing Strategic Alternatives

"The understanding that underlies the right decision grows out of the clash and conflict of divergent opinions and out of the serious consideration of competing alternatives. . . . Unless one has considered alternatives, one has a closed mind."

Peter F. Drucker

Introductory Incident

Responding to the Leapfrog Group's *Hospital Quality and Safety Survey*: A Strategic Choice?

The Leapfrog Group publishes the results of its *Hospital Quality and Safety Survey* in a comparative fashion on a market-by-market basis. It is intended to aid consumers in selecting a provider and employers in designing health plans that ensure the highest quality of care (see Perspective 6–1). For a hospital's leaders, adopting any of the Leaps, if not already undertaken, represents a major strategic choice that invariably precludes pursuing other strategic alternatives. Further, even within the general realm of patient safety and quality, each of the Leaps has other alternatives available that address the same patient safety issue – potentially more effectively.

Overall, choosing to adopt all or part of the Leapfrog agenda represents a major strategic choice and the success of the strategy is far from

guaranteed. However, choosing not to adopt any of the standards potentially signals to a hospital's market that quality and safety are not major strategic objectives for the institution.

For hospitals already meeting some or all of the Leaps being promulgated, responding to the survey may represent an opportunity to pursue a differentiation strategy emphasizing quality. However, relatively few hospitals in the United States have computerized physician order entry (CPOE), meet all the evidence-based hospital referral (EHR) volume standards, and employ ICU specialists to meet the intensive-care-unit physician staffing (IPS) requirements. For example, a preponderance of academic medical centers fail to meet a majority of the standards; in 2004 only 5.2 percent of the 497 hospitals reporting fully met the CPOE Leap.

▶

Therefore, very few facilities stand to benefit from a Leapfrog windfall without making a significant strategic choice and a commitment of resources. In fact, resistance to the Leapfrog initiative has been very strong in some markets where hospital systems with significant market share and influence viewed the survey results as a threat to the strategic advantages they had assiduously built over the years.

The St. Louis market has been among the most difficult for Leapfrog to gain a foothold. The largest system in the region – Barnes-Jewish Christian HealthCare – has successfully countered the local regional roll-out leader's attempts to have other hospitals complete the Leapfrog survey. In the first year of the regional roll-out in St. Louis, almost all hospitals declined to participate in the Leapfrog hospital survey effort. The exception was St. John's Mercy Hospital, affiliated with Sisters of Mercy Health System (SMHS). St. John's had made substantial progress on all of the Leapfrog Leaps prior to the roll-out, so it made strategic sense for it to report. In the most recent survey, the Tenet-affiliated hospitals responded because of a nation-wide policy adopted by that organization to participate.

The resistance of St. Louis hospitals to the Leapfrog roll-out in their community attracted considerable national attention. Local roll-out leaders met with each hospital CEO at least once – and met twice with the CEOs of the largest hospital systems – to encourage their participation. Mr. Steven Lipstein, President and CEO of BJC HealthCare, was adamant in his opposition to the Leapfrog effort in the initial year and was invited to a Gateway Purchasers for Health (a coalition of 30 large employers in St. Louis) board meeting to present his views. This meeting led some St. Louis employers to conclude that it would be very difficult to have a successful regional roll-out in St. Louis. In addition, some employers felt that the arguments made by BJC's CEO in opposition to the Leapfrog approach were legitimate and congruent with their own interests. A statement explaining its viewpoint was posted on the BJC website:

While BJC HealthCare and all hospitals support and strive for patient safety improvements, this recent effort is guiding the course of a very serious concern in a new and

unsettling direction. The business coalition's "Leapfrog" initiative selects three very specific metrics of comparison between hospitals, none of which measure outcomes of patient care. It risks presenting information that has the potential to mislead the very people with whom we must establish the most trust – our patients.

BJC created its own program for public disclosure called Best in Class. As BJC describes on its website:

"Best in Class" was created by BJC's Center for Health-Care Quality and Effectiveness in response to two factors. First was BJC President Steven Lipstein's focus on getting the organization to the "next level" of excellence by enhancing BJC's reputation and maintaining its leadership role. The second was the Leapfrog Group's emphasis on defining what quality means to purchasers of health care and how quality can be improved.

In essence, BJC is attempting to develop its own strategic alternative to the Leapfrog plan. Despite resisting the Leapfrog initiative, BJC did undertake the implementation of a $10 million CPOE system in 2002 and appears to be striving to meet the other Leapfrog standards. Does this represent a tacit acceptance of strategic choices being made outside the firm or is it merely a coincidence? Is the Leapfrog Group's effort a one-time and temporary phenomenon that can safely be ignored? The answer to the latter question is undoubtedly no.

References

Committee on Quality of Health Care in America, *Crossing the Quality Chasm: A New Health System for the 21st Century* (Washington, DC: National Academy Press, 2001).

S. Lipstein, *Patients Seek Medical Information from Those They Trust Most* (BJC HealthCare: St. Louis, 2004).

M. Manning, "Computers to Replace Docs' Scribbles at Barnes-Jewish," *St. Louis Business Journal* (2002), p. 7.

The Leapfrog Group, *Patient Safety* (Washington, DC: Leapfrog Group, 2004).

Source: Eric W. Ford, PhD, Tulane University; Dennis P. Scanlon, PhD, The Pennsylvania State University; and Jon B. Christianson, PhD, University of Minnesota.

Learning Objectives

After completing this chapter the student should be able to:

1. Understand the decision logic of strategy development and be able to discuss its steps.

2. Synthesize and integrate strategic thinking accomplished in situational analysis into a strategic plan for an organization.

3. Identify the hierarchy of strategies and strategic decisions required in strategic planning.

4. Understand the nature of directional strategies, adaptive strategies, market entry strategies, and competitive strategies.

5. Identify strategic alternatives available to health care organizations.

6. Provide the rationale as well as advantages and disadvantages for each of the strategic alternatives.

7. Understand that strategies may have to be used in combination to accomplish the organization's goals.

8. Map strategic decisions showing how they are linked as an *ends–means chain*.

Developing a Strategy

Strategic thinking involves an awareness of the environment; intellectual curiosity that is always gathering, organizing, and analyzing information; and a willingness to be open to creative ideas and solutions. Strategic planning concerns reaching conclusions about the information, setting a course of action, and documenting the plan. Therefore, strategic planning is essentially decision making – determining which from among the many available alternatives the organization will pursue. The strategy of an organization is the result of a series of increasingly more specific decisions. *Strategy formulation* incorporates the broadest decisions that set direction and provide the fundamental strategy for the organization.

There are many strategic alternatives available to a health care organization and a particular organization may pursue several different types of strategies simultaneously or sequentially. Therefore, a decision logic is required for strategy development. For instance, hospitals selecting to pursue various Leapfrog Leaps, as discussed in the Introductory Incident, are making strategic choices that will both limit and create opportunities to pursue several different strategies (see Perspective 6–1). In what order should strategic decisions be made? A merger or affiliation decision is part of a series of decisions rather than a single decision or an end in itself. In other words, there is a broader strategy that precipitated the

Perspective 6–1

The Leapfrog
Group

The 1999 Institute of Medicine's (IOM) report *To Err is Human: Building a Safer Health System* found widespread medical errors within America's hospitals – between 44,000 and 98,000 patients suffer death due to systemic errors, with many more suffering avoidable disabilities and other adverse events.[1] The response to the IOM report was not limited to researchers and policymakers.

Large private employers realized that at the frequency systemic errors were occurring in hospitals, a significant number of their employees were being put at risk. In addition, years of experience with total quality management gave leaders of large firms, manufacturers in particular, a strong indication that low quality and high practice variance were contributing significantly to health insurance premium inflation. Health care inflation became a major concern and limiting factor in many industries. Therefore, The Business Roundtable – an association of the CEOs of 200 of the Fortune 500 companies – decided it needed to take action and became involved in several initiatives to improve quality. In particular, it provided funding for the Leapfrog Group's start-up.

The Leapfrog Group was created as a catalyst to initiate improvements in hospitals' patient safety practices. Leapfrog sought to connect evidence-based medicine and management by promoting scientifically proven practices that can be implemented at the hospital level. Further, the organization chose to focus on "three practices that have tremendous potential to save lives by reducing preventable mistakes in hospitals."[2] The three Leaps are:

1. Computerized physician order entry (CPOE);
2. Evidence-based hospital referral (EHR); and
3. ICU physician staffing (IPS) using intensive care specialists.

CPOE systems are relatively expensive, rely on decision support software, and require extensive reengineering of units' workflows. Physicians resist using CPOE technology, viewing it as a threat to their clinical autonomy, and find reengineering of work to be an unnecessary inconvenience. The implementation of a system to increase medication safety that relies on bar coding technology to ensure that the patient receives the intended medication faces much less resistance from clinical employees. Two limitations of bar coding are that it does not attempt to reduce adverse drug interactions or prevent dosage errors. However, bar coding drugs requires a relatively low capital investment, poses no threat to physicians' autonomy, and does not disrupt existing workflows significantly.

The EHR Leap is a surgical volume standard related to specific high-risk procedures such as coronary artery bypass grafts (CABGs). To meet the Leapfrog standard, a facility must either exceed the volume expectation or discontinue providing the procedures. Despite strong research findings that higher volume levels for complex surgical procedures are positively correlated with better clinical outcomes, a hospital may feel compelled to perform lower numbers of the procedure to ensure its community has adequate and readily available access to a full array of services. In this sense, pursuing the clinical quality aspect of a hospital's mission may come directly into conflict with its mission to ensure adequate access for the community.

Lastly, IPS requires staffing a hospital's intensive care unit with physicians specifically trained for that setting. Generally, the decision to use intensive care specialists means that the hospital will have to employ those clinicians. It changes the service delivery model of a hospital by asking admitting physicians to cede control of their patients to an ICU physician. To successfully implement such a program requires a significant change in the culture of the admitting physicians. Many hospital administrators cited the unavailability of physicians with the necessary training as a barrier to pursuing this strategy for improving safety.

Notes

1. L. T. Kohn, J. M. Corrigan, and M. S. Donaldson (eds) *To Err is Human: Building a Safer Health System* (Washington, DC: National Academy Press, 2000).
2. The Leapfrog Group, *Patient Safety* (Washington, DC: The Leapfrog Group, 2004).

Source: Eric W. Ford, PhD, Tulane University; Dennis P. Scanlon, PhD, The Pennsylvania State University; and Jon B. Christianson, PhD, University of Minnesota.

merger or affiliation decision; and there will be subsequent strategic decisions that will have to be made to support the decision and make it successful.

Strategy formulation includes development of strategic alternatives, evaluation of alternatives, and strategic choice. This chapter classifies the types of strategies required to specify an organization's fundamental strategy and develops a hierarchy of strategic alternatives available to health care organizations. This hierarchy provides a strategic thinking map as guidance in decision making and strategic planning. Chapter 7 discusses strategic thinking methods for analyzing these alternatives to make a strategic choice.

Linking Strategy with Situational Analysis

The relationship of strategy formulation to situational analysis and planning the implementation may be reviewed in the strategic thinking map in Exhibit 1–3. Situational analysis provides information concerning the external and internal environments that is used in strategy formulation to develop strategic alternatives and select the strategies for the organization. External environmental analysis identifies important general and health care industry opportunities and threats, including a comprehensive service area competitor analysis. Internal environmental analysis identifies strengths and weaknesses, specifying whether they are sources of short- or long-term competitive advantages or disadvantages. Strategic thinking has led to the identification of the organization's mission, vision, values, and strategic goals that provide broad direction for the organization.

As demonstrated by the check list in Exhibit 6–1, the strategies selected by the organization should address external opportunities or threats, draw on competitive advantages or fix competitive disadvantages, keep the organization within the parameters of the mission and values, move the organization toward the vision, and make progress toward achieving one or more of the organization's strategic goals. This check-list procedure is an important part of the strategic thinking

Exhibit 6–1: Check List for Linking Strategic Alternatives with Situational Analysis

Strategic Alternative	Addresses an External Issue?	Draws On a Competitive Advantage or Fixes a Competitive Disadvantage?	Fits with Mission, Values?	Moves the Organization Toward the Vision?	Achieves One or More Goals?
Strategy 1	Yes	Yes	Yes	Yes	Yes
Strategy 2	Yes	Yes	Yes	Yes	Yes
Strategy 3	Yes	Yes	Yes	Yes	Yes

process and helps assure consistency of analysis and action. Each selected strategy should be tested against these questions. Strategies that do not have a "yes" in each column should be subject to additional scrutiny and justification.

The Decision Logic of Strategy Development

The decision logic of strategy formulation is illustrated in Exhibit 6–2. Decisions concerning the five categories of strategies – directional strategies, adaptive strategies, market entry strategies, competitive strategies, and implementation strategies – should be addressed sequentially with each subsequent decision more specifically defining the activities of the organization. The first four of these strategy types make up strategy formulation and set the fundamental direction for the organization to achieve its mission and vision. Strategic momentum includes implementation strategies and will set specific objectives for various units to accomplish the organization's strategic goals.

The strategies form an *ends–means chain*. Thus, directional strategies must be made first, followed by adaptive strategies because the adaptive strategies are the means to accomplish the directional strategies or the desired end result. Further, market entry strategies are the means to accomplish the adaptive strategies. Next, the organization's *strategic posture* and basis of competition (competitive strategies) must carry out the strategic decisions made previously. Once these strategic decisions are made, implementation strategies provide strategic momentum – the final means to accomplish all of the strategy formulation decisions.

At each stage in the ends–means decision chain, previous upstream decisions and the implications for subsequent downstream decisions must be considered and perhaps reconsidered. As strategic managers work through strategic decisions, new insights and perspectives may emerge (strategic thinking) that suggest reconsideration of previous strategic decisions. Therefore, although the decision logic for strategic decisions is generally sequential, in practice it is very much an iterative process. Nevertheless, the underlying logic is that the environment

Exhibit 6–2: The Decision Logic of Strategy Formulation

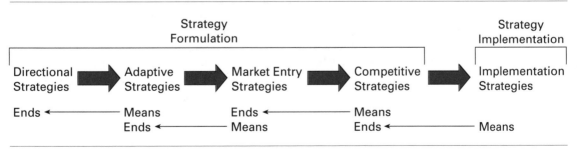

(including external, competitive, and internal), mission, and vision drive strategy. Strategy includes a plurality of inputs, a multiplicity of options, and an ability to accommodate more than one possible outcome. However, where mission and vision are ignored, or where there is no ends–means linkage between vision and strategy, strategy has no end object. In these situations, strategy suffers from being a means without an end, an end in itself, or a means of achieving an operational end, rather than being a design or plan for achieving the organization's mission and vision.[1]

Understanding the decision logic of strategy formulation presented in Exhibit 6–2 is important as each step in the process more specifically defines and articulates the strategy of the organization. The organization must first establish or reaffirm and reach consensus on its mission, vision, values, and strategic goals. These decisions set the direction for the organization and, as noted in Chapter 5, are referred to as directional strategies. Next, the adaptive strategies must be identified. *Adaptive strategies* are concerned with scope of operations and specify how the organization will expand, contract, or maintain operations. The potential adaptive strategic alternatives must be evaluated and a specific strategy or combination of strategies adopted. The adaptive strategies outline the major strategic emphasis for the organization to accomplish its vision and goals (the directional strategies). Third, market entry strategies must be identified, evaluated, and specified. *Market entry strategies* indicate how expansion or maintenance of scope strategies will be carried out. Fourth, competitive strategies must be identified, evaluated, and selected. *Competitive strategies* determine the organization's strategic posture and identify the basis for competing in the market in relation to other market "players." Finally, *implementation strategies* (value adding service delivery strategies, value adding support strategies, and action plans) must be identified, evaluated, and selected to carry out the adaptive, market entry, and competitive strategies. The scope and role of the four strategy formulation types and the implementation strategies are summarized in Exhibit 6–3.

Recall that decisions should be based on as much information and strategic thinking as possible. Sometimes this strategic thinking occurs in situational analysis and at other times it occurs when managing the strategic momentum. Before the strategic plan is adopted, it is important to remember that organization-wide understanding of, and commitment to, the strategies must be developed if they are to be managed successfully (strategic momentum). The choice of a strategic alternative creates direction for an organization and subsequently shapes its internal systems (organization, technology, information systems, culture, policies, skills, and so on). This strategic momentum is reinforced as managers understand, commit, and make decisions according to the strategy.

Exhibit 6–4 presents a comprehensive strategic thinking map of the hierarchy of strategic alternatives. The hierarchy represents a number of strategic alternatives available to health care organizations. This map not only identifies the alternatives but also the general sequential relationships among them. In this context, strategy development should be viewed as a sequential decision-making process that, at each stage, reevaluates previous decisions and considers the implications for subsequent decisions. It is a process of evaluating and selecting from various

Exhibit 6-3: Scope and Role of Strategy Types in Strategy Formulation

Strategy	Scope and Role
Directional Strategies	The broadest strategies set the fundamental direction of the organization by establishing a mission for the organization (Who are we?) and providing a vision for the future (What should we be?). In addition, directional strategies specify the organization's values and the broad goals it wants to accomplish.
Adaptive Strategies	These strategies are more specific than directional strategies and provide the primary methods for achieving the vision of the organization – adapting to the environment. These strategies determine the scope of the organization and specify how the organization will expand scope, contract scope, or maintain scope.
Market Entry Strategies	These strategies carry out the expansion of scope and the maintenance of scope strategies through purchase, cooperation, or internal development. These strategies provide methods for access or entry to the market. Market entry strategies are not used for contraction of scope strategies.
Competitive Strategies	Two types of strategies, one that determines an organization's strategic posture and one that positions the organization vis-à-vis other organizations within the market. These strategies are market oriented and best articulate the competitive advantage within the market.
Implementation Strategies	These strategies are the most specific strategies and are directed toward value added service delivery and the value added support areas such as the culture, structure, and strategic resources. In addition, individual organizational units develop action plans that carry out the value added service delivery and value added support strategies.

alternatives. Each strategy type and the available alternatives will be discussed in the remainder of this chapter.

Using an organizing framework or decision logic in strategy formulation keeps it from becoming overwhelming and focuses strategic thinking. Therefore, the decision logic is the map to initiate strategy formulation and encourage managers to start thinking strategically. However, as pointed out in Chapter 1, strategic managers may also have to use a compass and rely on intuitive thinking, leadership, and learning, especially later when they are managing strategic momentum. As strategic managers work through the strategic decisions, new understandings, insights, and strategies may (and in fact, should) emerge. Therefore, decision makers must work through the decision logic and back again, ensuring that all the proposed strategies make sense together. Strategic thinkers must always be able to see the bigger picture. Decision makers should be prepared to adjust and refine

Exhibit 6–4: Strategic Thinking Map – Hierarchy of Strategic Decisions and Alternatives

Directional Strategies ➡	Adaptive Strategies ➡	Market Entry Strategies ➡	Competitive Strategies ➡	Implementation Strategies
• Mission	***Expansion of Scope*** • Diversification • Vertical Integration • Market Development • Product Development	***Purchase*** • Acquisition • Licensing • Venture Capital Investment	***Strategic Posture*** • Defender • Prospector • Analyzer	***Service Delivery*** • Pre-service • Point-of-service • After-service
• Vision	• Penetration	***Cooperation*** • Merger	***Positioning*** Marketwide • Cost Leadership • Differentiation	***Support*** • Culture • Structure • Strategic Resources
• Values	***Contraction of Scope*** • Divestiture • Liquidation • Harvesting • Retrenchment	• Alliance • Joint Venture ***Development*** • Internal Development • Internal Venture	Market Segment • Focus/ Cost Leadership • Focus/ Differentiation	***Unit Action Plans*** • Objectives • Actions • Timelines • Responsibilities
• Goals	***Maintenance of Scope*** • Enhancement • Status Quo			

earlier decisions in the decision logic as they make "downstream" decisions. Strategy making is a two-steps-forward, one-step-back process.

How-to formulas, techniques, or a linear process, of course, can never replace strategic thinking. Many of the greatest achievements in science, law, government, medicine, or other intellectual pursuits are dependent on the development of rational, logical thinkers; however, linear thinking can limit potential.[2] That is why leadership is essential to foster creativity and innovation and allow for the reinvention of the strategy formulation process. Strategy formulation involves managing dilemmas, tolerating ambiguity, coping with contradictions, and dealing with paradox.[3] In addition, strategy development cannot ignore the entrepreneurial spirit, politics, ethical considerations (see Perspective 6–2) and culture in an organization. The strategy formulation decision logic discussed in this chapter provides a starting point. It should foster strategic thinking, not limit it. The map starts the decision makers on their journey.

Directional Strategies: Mission, Vision, Values, and Goals

Chapter 5 explored mission, vision, values, and strategic goals and indicated that these elements are part of both situational analysis and strategy formulation. They are a part of situational analysis because they describe the current state of the organization and codify its basic beliefs and philosophy. In addition, mission, vision,

Ethics are guidelines for action that are based on values, moral principles, or moral rights, and duties, such as honesty, respect, and compassion. Some ethical guidelines are reflected in laws, whereas others are norms, customs, and social expectations that develop and are maintained by mutual consent.

It is useful to distinguish two categories of ethics in the health care environment: professional ethics and applied ethics. Professional ethics are the customs, norms, expectations, values, rights, and duties that guide individuals as they carry out particular work roles in society. Professional ethics reflect the expectations that society has for people who perform specific roles. We expect physicians and nurses to help rather than harm patients. We expect administrators and business officers to accept fiduciary responsibility (act for the benefit of the organization rather than themselves) and to be accountable to stockholders or boards of trustees for their decisions.

The norms guiding professional behavior can change over time, as society's expectations change. For example, physicians' roles have evolved over the past few decades away from the expectation that doctors will make decisions on behalf of patients and for their health benefit to the expectation that they will provide all relevant information to patients and families and help them make decisions about their treatment. As another example, the implementation of the Health Insurance Portability and Accountability Act (HIPAA) in April 2003 represented the legal enforcement of a social expectation that health-related information on patients will be kept strictly confidential; some widely accepted practices of information sharing in health care organizations had to be altered under the HIPAA guidelines because they were not perceived to reflect the priority that members of society placed on confidentiality.

Health care organizations involve the interaction of many sets of health professionals who, by definition, are bound by differing sets of ethics and norms. Decisions that must be made by the organization as a whole must be negotiated across these norms. For example, the imperative to help anyone in need of medical care must be balanced with the imperative to operate organizations that are financially sound. Organizations are best served when professionals are able both to represent their own guiding values and principles and to comprehend the values and principles that guide their colleagues.

In contrast to professional ethics, applied ethics is the application of values, principles, and expectations to broader social choices, such as whether all residents of a society have a right to some basic level of health care, or whether health care is a commodity that individuals can choose to purchase or not. Some social choices have a broad consensus. In the United States the responsibility of society to cover the costs of health care for the elderly is generally accepted. Other social choices are the subject of considerable disagreement and conflict, even when one set of values or expectations has been codified into laws. The rights of individuals to have abortions or to enforce their preferences on care at the end of life are examples of areas of ethical conflict that impact health care organizations. Organizations whose decision-making processes are affected by social choices that are the basis of ethical conflicts must consider carefully the values and norms that guide their constituents and the laws that represent the current societal consensus on the issue.

All actions have an ethical component, but often the underlying values for a decision are so widely shared that we do not recognize the ethical choices that we make. For example, we do not question the principle that health care is meant to benefit those who are sick. When faced with a decision about whether to provide effective or harmful treatment to someone who is sick, we automatically make the ethical decision to help rather than to harm the person. On the other hand, we sometimes face situations where alternative courses of action reflect contrasting values. For example, we value individuals' autonomy and their right to make decisions about their own health. If an individual wants a treatment that we believe to be harmful, should we respect his or her wishes and provide the treatment, or refuse the treatment and adhere to the principle that treatment should not be provided if it is known to cause harm?

Source: Janet M. Bronstein, PhD, School of Public Health, University of Alabama at Birmingham.

values, and strategic goals are also a part of strategy formulation because they set the boundaries and indicate the broadest direction for the organization.

The directional strategies should provide a sensible and realistic planning framework for the organization. Within this planning framework, more specific strategic alternatives are selected. Therefore, it is important that environmental analysis has been used to identify the current and emerging issues (opportunities and threats) that will affect the success of the organization. Concurrently, strategic managers should have carefully analyzed the organization's strengths and weaknesses, especially in terms of its resources, competencies, and capabilities. Having assimilated and evaluated all this information, strategic managers then decide what strategic alternatives are appropriate for the organization.

Because formulation of the mission, vision, values, and strategic goals provides the broad direction for the organization, directional strategic decisions must be made first. Then the adaptive strategies provide further progression by specifying the scope of product/market expansion, contraction, or maintenance. The adaptive strategies form the core of strategy formulation and are most visible to those outside the organization. After the adaptive strategies have been selected, the directional strategies should be reevaluated. Seeing the directional strategies (ends) and the adaptive strategies (means) together may suggest refinements to either or both. This broader perspective is essential in strategic thinking.

Adaptive Strategies

From a practical standpoint, whether the organization should expand, contract, or maintain scope is the first decision that must be made once the direction of the organization has been set (or reaffirmed). As shown in Exhibit 6–5, several specific alternatives are available to expand operations, contract operations, or maintain the scope of operations. These alternatives provide the major strategic choices for the organization and may be classified as corporate- or divisional-level strategies.

Corporate-level strategies consider the best mix of semi-autonomous divisions operating in separate markets (service areas) with distinct products or services (service categories). Therefore, corporate-level strategies generally address the current viability and potential of a portfolio of separate divisions. Corporate strategies are not concerned with one market or product/service, but rather with several "businesses" assembled to fulfill the mission of the organization given the demands of the external environment. Corporate-level strategies address the question "What business(es) should we be in?" Thus, an integrated health system must consider what portfolio of businesses – acute care hospital, long-term care, home health, and so on (or businesses outside the health care industry) – best serves the mission of the system. Corporate expansion strategies increase the scope of the organization.

In contrast to corporate strategies, *divisional strategies* are concerned with a single well-defined market and with a product/service line that serves a specific market or service area. Division-level strategies deal with the question "How should

Exhibit 6–5: Strategic Thinking Map of Adaptive Strategic Alternatives

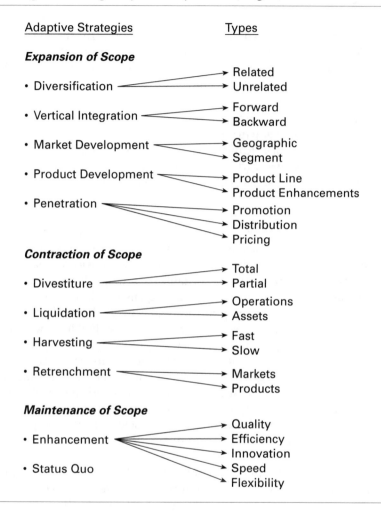

an organization compete in a given market?" Therefore, division-level strategic alternatives are concerned with an organization's current area of operations and are used by organizations such as strategic service units (SSUs), single-unit hospitals, and small group practices to compete within a service area. Zook and Allen refer to these strategies as "repeatable adjacentcy expansion." They conclude, "... profitable growth comes when a company pushes out the boundaries of its core business into adjacent space."[4] They identified several ways to grow into an adjacent space – expand along the external value chain (penetration), grow new products and services (product development), enter new geographies (market development), and address new customer segments (market development).

Expansion of Scope Strategies

If expansion is selected as the best way to perform the mission and realize the vision of the organization, several alternatives are available. Two of these alternatives are corporate-level strategies and three are division-level strategies. The *expansion of scope strategies* include:

- *diversification* (corporate level),
- *vertical integration* (corporate level),
- *market development* (divisional/SBU or SSU level),
- *product development* (divisional/SBU or SSU level), and
- *penetration* (divisional/SBU or SSU level).

DIVERSIFICATION

Diversification strategies, in many cases, are selected because markets have been identified outside of the organization's core business that offer potential for substantial growth. Often, an organization that selects a diversification strategy is not achieving its growth or revenue goals within its current market, and these new markets provide an opportunity to achieve them. There are, of course, other reasons why organizations decide to diversify. For instance, health care organizations may identify opportunities for growth in less-regulated markets such as specialty hospitals, long-term care facilities, or managed care.

Diversification is generally seen as a risky alternative because the organization is entering relatively unfamiliar markets or new businesses that are different from its current activities. Organizations have found that the risk of diversification can be reduced if markets and products are selected that complement one another. Therefore, managers engaging in diversification seek synergy between corporate divisions (SSUs).

There are two types of diversification: related (concentric) and unrelated (conglomerate) diversification. Exhibit 6–6 illustrates possible related and unrelated diversification strategies for one type of primary health care organization.

In *related diversification*, an organization chooses to enter a market that is similar or related to its present operations. This form of diversification is sometimes called *concentric diversification* because the organization develops a "circle" of related businesses (products/services). Exhibit 6–7 illustrates the circle of related products for a hospital that is interested in diversifying into another segment of the health care market, the long-term care market.

The general assumption underlying related diversification is that the organization will be able to obtain some level of synergy (a complementary relationship where the total effect is greater than the sum of its parts) between the production/delivery, marketing, or technology of the core business and the new related product or service. For hospitals, the two primary reasons for diversifying are to introduce nonacute care or subacute care services that reduce hospital costs or to offer a wider range of services to large employers and purchasing coalitions through

Exhibit 6–6: Related and Unrelated Diversification by a Primary Provider

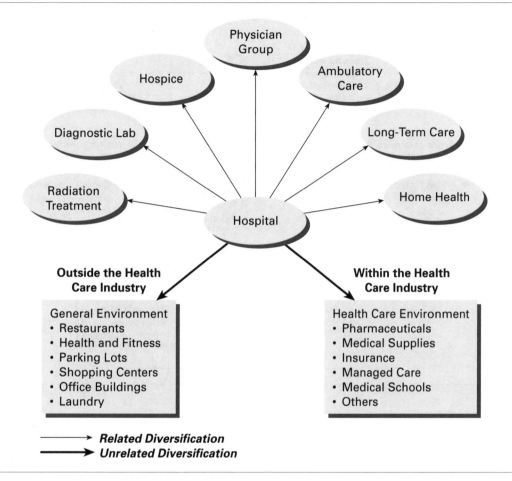

capitated contracts.[5] The movement of acute care hospitals into skilled-nursing care is an example of related diversification.

On the other hand, in *unrelated diversification*, an organization enters a market that is unlike its present operations. This action creates a "portfolio" of separate products/services. Unrelated diversification, or *conglomerate diversification*, generally involves semi-autonomous divisions or strategic service units. An example of unrelated diversification would be a hospital diversifying into the operation of a restaurant, parking lot, or medical office building. In such a case, the new business is unrelated to health care although it may be complementary (synergistic) to the provision of health services.

Research on diversification indicates that financial performance increases as organizations shift from single-business strategies to related diversification, but performance decreases as organizations change from related diversification

Exhibit 6–7: Long-Term Care Options for Hospital Diversification

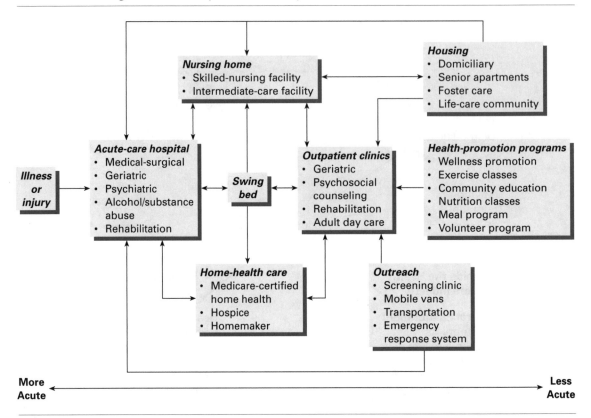

Source: Health Care Management Review 15, no. 1, p. 73. Copyright © 1990. Reprinted by permission of Aspen Publishers, Inc.

to unrelated diversification.[6] Single-business organizations may suffer from limited economies of scope whereas organizations using related diversification can convert underutilized assets and achieve economics of scope by sharing resources and combining activities along the value chain. Unrelated diversification has been found to increase strain on top management in the areas of decision making, control, and governance. In addition, unrelated diversification makes it difficult to share activities and transfer competencies between units. This has been particularly true for hospital diversification.[7] Unrelated diversification has been generally unsuccessful in generating revenue for acute care hospitals, as illustrated in Perspective 6–3.

VERTICAL INTEGRATION

A *vertical integration* strategy is a decision to grow along the channel of distribution of the core operations. Thus, a health care organization may grow toward suppliers or toward patients. When an organization grows along the channel of

Perspective 6–3

Unrelated
Diversification
Difficult for
Hospitals

In the 1980s hospitals were buying dude ranches in Montana and bottling companies in Ohio. They were expanding into janitorial services, catering firms, condominiums, travel agencies, and health clubs. Unrelated diversification was intended to spread risks or develop new sources of revenue to support acute care operations. However, many of the diversified businesses have been divested or liquidated as they were losing money or were not in the best interests of a health care organization. Some unrelated diversification businesses broke even or were marginally profitable, but they did not justify the diversion of executive time. Many hospital administrators lacked the skills to manage these nonacute care businesses. In addition, boards of trustees questioned the additional capital needed and wondered when these diversified businesses would become profitable.

In the 1990s health care organizations were more apt to employ market development (horizontal integration) or vertical integration to manage the health of a population. Simply owning an asset to increase revenue has not been an effective strategy. Often market development and vertical integration have been achieved though mergers or alliances with similar providers.

In the 2000s many hospitals have been divesting their health maintenance organizations (HMOs). Many hospitals and health systems developed (internal development) or purchased (acquisition) HMOs, but diversifying into this risk product has not been profitable for most of them. For example, in Charlotte, North Carolina there were 26 HMOs registered in the mid-1990s (3 of them were hospital owned). By the beginning of the next decade, more than half had closed or left the area or were sold (including two of the hospital-based HMOs as well as Kaiser Permanente).

distribution toward its suppliers (upstream) it is called *backward vertical integration*. When an organization grows toward the consumer or patient (downstream) it is called *forward vertical integration*.

A vertically integrated health care system offers a range of patient care and support services operated in a functionally unified manner. The expansion of services may be arranged around an acute care hospital and include pre-acute, acute, and post-acute services or might be organized around specialized services related solely to long-term care, mental health care, or some other specialized area.[8] The purpose of vertical integration is to increase the comprehensiveness and continuity of care, while simultaneously controlling the channel of demand for health care services.[9]

Vertical integration can reduce costs and thus enhance an organization's competitive position. Cost reductions may occur through lower supply costs and better integration of the "elements of production." With vertical integration, management can better ensure that supplies are of the appropriate quality and delivered at the right time. For instance, some hospitals have instituted technical educational programs because many health professionals (the major element of production in health care) are in critically short supply.

Because a decision to vertically integrate further commits an organization to a particular product or market, management must believe in the long-term viability of the product/service and market. As a result, the opportunity costs of vertical integration must be weighed against the benefits of other strategic alternatives such as diversification or product development. Examples of vertical integration would be a hospital chain acquiring one of its major medical products suppliers (backward integration) or a drug manufacturer moving into drug distribution (forward integration). An interesting form of forward vertical integration in the 1990s was hospitals opening retail operations in malls. These retail operations typically were health and information centers staffed by registered nurses. Visitors could watch videos, check out books, attend health screenings, and receive free or low-cost lessons on diabetes management, yoga, smoking cessation, and numerous other health topics. Retail business has proven to be a good strategy for some urban hospitals trying to tap the suburban market.

Whether a strategic alternative is viewed as vertical integration or related diversification may depend on the objective or intent of the alternative. For instance, when the primary intent is to enter a new market in order to grow, the decision is to diversify. However, if the intent is to control the flow of patients to various units, the decision is to vertically integrate. Thus, a decision by an acute care hospital to acquire a skilled-nursing unit may be viewed as related diversification (entering a new growth market) or vertical integration (controlling downstream patient flow). Vertical integration is the fundamental adaptive strategy for developing integrated systems of care and is central to many health care organizations' strategy.

Numerous extensive health networks are the result of integration strategies since the early 1980s. One study showed that over 70 percent of US hospitals belong to health networks or systems.[10] The major reason that hospitals join networks and systems is to help secure needed resources (financial, human, information systems, and technologies), increase capabilities (management and marketing), and gain greater bargaining power with purchasers and health plans.[11] However, it appears that the pace of integration has slowed. In fact there has been some degree of "disintegration," with health care systems divesting health plans, physician groups, home health care companies, as well as selling or closing hospitals and divesting themselves of skilled care services or facilities.[12]

To expand the supply of patients to various health care units, several patterns of vertical integration may be identified.[13] In Exhibit 6–8, an inpatient acute care facility is the strategic service unit or core technology that decides to vertically integrate. Example 1 represents a hospital that is not vertically integrated. The hospital admits and discharges patients from and to other units outside the organization. Example 2 illustrates a totally integrated system in which integration occurs both upstream and downstream. In this case, patients flow through the system from one unit to the next, and upstream units are viewed as "feeder" units to downstream units.

Example 3 represents a hospital that has vertically integrated upstream. In addition, more than one unit is involved at several stages of the integration. For instance, there are two wellness/health promotion units, three primary care units, and three urgent care units. The dashed line represents the receipt of patients via external or market transfers. Example 4 illustrates a multihospital system

Exhibit 6–8: Patterns of Vertical Integration Among Health Care Organizations

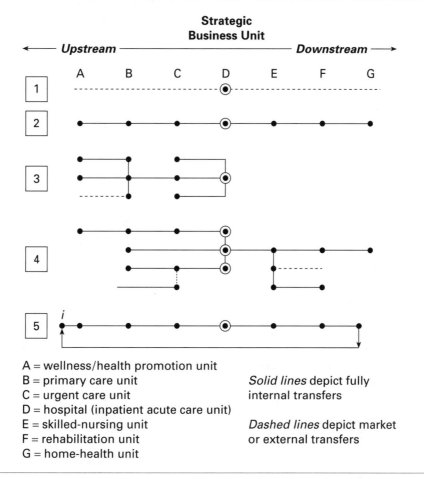

A = wellness/health promotion unit
B = primary care unit
C = urgent care unit
D = hospital (inpatient acute care unit)
E = skilled-nursing unit
F = rehabilitation unit
G = home-health unit

Solid lines depict fully internal transfers

Dashed lines depict market or external transfers

Source: Adapted in part from K. R. Harrigan, "Formulating Vertical Integration Strategies," *Academy of Management Review* 9, no. 4 (1984), pp. 638–652. Reprinted by permission of Academy of Management. And adapted in part from Stephen S. Mick and Douglas A. Conrad, "The Decision to Integrate Vertically in Health Care Organizations," *Hospital and Health Services Administration* 33, no. 3 (fall 1988), p. 351. Reprinted by permission from Health Administration Press, Chicago.

engaged in vertical integration. Three hospitals form the core of the system, which also contains three nursing homes, two rehab units, a home-health unit, three urgent care facilities, three primary care facilities, and a wellness center.

Finally, a quirk of the health care system is illustrated in Example 5. Some health care systems are closed systems with fixed patient populations entirely covered through prepayment. Thus, whereas in the second example, the health care organization is vertically integrated, in the fifth example, patients are a part of the system. This insurance function is shown as an additional unit and identified by the letter *i* in the example.

It is important to note that simply adding members to create an integrated health system is not enough. Institutions must be truly integrated and create a "seamless" system of care to achieve the desired benefits for patients (effectiveness) and cost savings (efficiency).

MARKET DEVELOPMENT

Market development is a divisional strategy used to enter new markets with present products or services. Specifically, market development is a strategy designed to achieve greater volume, through geographic (service area) expansion or by targeting new market segments within the present geographic area. Typically, market development is selected when the organization is fairly strong in the market (often with a differentiated product), the market is growing, and the prospects are good for long-term growth. A market development strategy is strongly supported by the marketing, financial, information systems, organizational, and human resources functions. An example of a market development strategy would be a chain of outpatient clinics opening a new clinic in a new geographic area (present products and services in a new market).

One type of market development is called horizontal integration. *Horizontal integration* is a method of obtaining growth across markets by acquiring or affiliating with direct competitors rather than using internal operational/functional strategies to take market share from them. Many hospitals and medical practices engaged in horizontal integration throughout the 1980s and early 1990s, creating multihospital systems. Such systems were expected to offer several advantages such as increased access to capital, reduction in duplication of services, economies of scale, improved productivity and operating efficiencies, access to management expertise, increased personnel benefits, improved patient access, improvement in quality, and increased political power.[14] However, many of these benefits did not materialize and the growth of horizontal integration strategies slowed in the latter part of the 1990s.

Another special type of market development is a market driven or focused factory strategy. The fundamental principle underlying a market driven or *focused factory* strategy is that an organization that focuses on only one function is likely to perform better. This strategy involves providing comprehensive services across multiple markets (horizontal integration) for one specific disease such as diabetes, renal disease, asthma, or cardiac disease. Such focus allows an organization to achieve very high levels of effectiveness and efficiency. Regina E. Herzlinger explains the shift as:

> . . . replacing giant providers and huge managed care networks, located in hard-to-reach sites with what I call "focused factories" (a nomenclature borrowed from the manufacturing sector) that provide convenient, specialized care for victims of a certain chronic disease, or for those who need a particular form of surgery, or for those who require a diagnosis, checkup, or treatment for a routine problem.[15]

Focused factories become so effective (high quality, convenient, and so on) and efficient (less costly) that other providers are "forced" to use their services. Thus, these other providers can obtain higher quality services at less cost by outsourcing to the focused factory. In turn, the focused factory commands a place in the payment systems. Herzlinger's focused factory tools for providers of health care services are outlined in Perspective 6–4. In health care, focused factories have not escaped criticism. The success of some focused factories (cardiac surgery and treatment) has led some states to propose legislation restricting them. The Federal Medicare Prescription Drug Improvement and Modernization Act became law on December 8, 2003. A potentially important part of the law included a moratorium that limited physician investments in specialty hospitals

---

Perspective 6–4 Focused Factory Tools for Providers of Health Care Services	The health care providers who flourish in this market-driven environment will give customers the mastery and convenience and the focused, cost-effective services they want by following the rules of successful service entrepreneurs:

- *Pay Attention to the Customer* – don't call them patients, don't fight their assertiveness, don't give them hype, give them real convenience and quality.
- *Focus, Focus, Focus* – throw out the general purpose, everything-for-everybody model: *focus* on your strengths; design the system that will lower costs and optimize quality.
- *Learn from the Rockettes* – make sure that all the elements of your operating systems are integrated, resembling a well-choreographed dance, where disparate elements have been integrated into a harmonious whole.
- *Resist the Edifice Complex* – bricks and mortar are distractions: fixed costs drag the enterprise down; many assets are really liabilities (money pits that consume your time and capital).
- *Lower Your Costs, Don't Raise Your Prices* – successful enterprises succeed by achieving more output from every unit of input, not by raising prices; enterprises that lower their costs create sustainable competitive advantage.
- *Use Technology Wisely* – use technology to enhance the productivity of the health care process, not as a marketing tool.
- *Don't Let the Dogma Grind You Down* – be open to new and different ways of thinking; don't be a prisoner of your own thinking; obtain advice from the widest possible range of sources about what works and what doesn't.
- *Be Ethical* – don't seek competitive advantage in unethical ways such as discriminating against sick or poor people or by denying people the health care services they need.
- *Breadth Beats Depth* – don't fall for the lure of vertical integration; remember all the problems you have experienced in running just your corner of the health services world; a horizontally integrated chain of focused factories will amplify your strengths in each of the separate units that comprise the chain.
- *Don't Get Big for Bigness's Sake* – don't think of horizontal integration as a way of blocking competitors; think of it as getting really good at what you do.
- *Measure Results: Your Own and Your Competitors'* – what gets measured gets done: don't ignore results you don't like and don't bury the results in a file – use them actively in continually recreating your operations; don't believe your own press – you are at your most vulnerable when your measurement results are at their most flattering.

Source: Regina E. Herzlinger, *Market-Driven Health Care: Who Wins, Who Loses in the Transformation of America's Largest Service Industry* (Reading, MA: Addison-Wesley Publishing Company, 1997), pp. 283–287.

for at least the following 18 months (to May 18, 2005; later extended to January 1, 2007). Specifically identified were cardiac, orthopedic, surgical, and "other" hospitals owned by physicians. The focused factories have targeted profitable procedures from insured patients, requiring local not-for-profits to care for less profitable diseases/treatments without being able to offset the costs through the more profitable procedures being captured by focused factories. Many politicians are opposed to specialty hospitals and advocated for the Federal legislation to become permanent.

PRODUCT DEVELOPMENT

Product development is the introduction of new products/services to present markets (geographic and segments). Typically, product development takes the form of product enhancements and product line extension. Product development should not be confused with related diversification. Related diversification introduces a new product category (though related to present operations), whereas product development may be viewed as refinements, complements, or natural extensions of present products. Product development strategies are common in large metropolitan areas where hospitals vie for increased market share within particular segments of the market, such as cancer treatment and open heart surgery. Another good example of product development is in the area of women's health. Many hospitals have opened clinics designed to serve the special needs of women in the present market area.

PENETRATION

An attempt to better serve current markets with current products or services is referred to as a *market penetration* strategy. Similar to market and product development, penetration strategies are used to increase volume and market share. A market penetration strategy is typically implemented by marketing strategies such as promotional, distribution, and pricing strategies, and often includes increasing advertising, offering sales promotions, increasing publicity efforts, or increasing the number of salespersons.

An example of a penetration strategy is Baptist Medical Center's (BMC) response to the expansion of the prestigious Mayo Clinic into the Jacksonville, Florida, area. BMC believed that it was unlikely that the Mayo Clinic would compete in pediatric care. Therefore, BMC capitalized on its major strength in pediatric care and initiated an aggressive adaptive/penetration strategy. To enhance availability to the market, BMC formed alliances (a market entry strategy) to develop a regional children's health center. BMC allied with the 450-bed University Medical Center, the University of Florida Health Science Center in Gainesville, and the Nemours Foundation of Wilmington, Delaware (a source of competition in the past). In addition, BMC opened a new $45 million children's hospital. BMC has supported this strategy with extensive promotion to inform the public of its strategic emphasis.[16]

The various expansion of scope strategies, their relative risks, and their rationales are summarized in Exhibit 6–9.

Exhibit 6–9: Rationales and Relative Risks of Expansion of Scope Strategic Alternatives

Strategy	Relative Risk	Rationale
Related Diversification	Moderate	• Pursuit of high-growth markets • Entering less-regulated segments • Cannot achieve current objectives • Synergy is possible from new business • Offset seasonal or cyclical influences
Unrelated Diversification	High	• Pursuit of high-growth markets • Entering less-regulated segments • Cannot achieve current objectives • Current markets are saturated or in decline • Organization has excess cash • Antitrust regulations prohibit expansion in current industry • Tax loss may be acquired
Backward Vertical Integration	High	• Control the flow of patients through the system • Scarcity of raw materials or essential inventory/supplies • Deliveries are unreliable • Lack of materials or supplies will shut down operations • Price or quality of materials or supplies variable • Industry/market seen as profitable for long term
Forward Vertical Integration	High	• Control the flow of patients through the system • Faster delivery required • High level of coordination required between one stage and another – secure needed resources • Industry/market seen as profitable for long term • Gain bargaining power
Market Development (geographic and segment)	Moderate	• New markets are available for present products • Provide comprehensive services across the market (focus factory) • New markets may be served efficiently • Expected high revenues • Organization has *cost leadership* advantage • Organization has *differentiation* advantage • Current market is growing
Product Development (product line and product enhancement)	Moderate	• Currently in strong market but product is weak or product line incomplete • Market tastes are changing • Product technology is changing • Maintenance or creation of differentiation advantage
Penetration (promotion, distribution, and pricing)	Moderate	• Present market is growing • Product/service innovation will extend product life cycle (PLC) • Expected revenues are high • Organization has cost leadership advantage • Organization has differentiation advantage

Contraction of Scope Strategies

Contraction of scope strategies decrease the size and scope of operations either at the corporate level or divisional level. Contraction strategies include:

- *divestiture* (corporate level),
- *liquidation* (corporate level),
- *harvesting* (divisional level), and
- *retrenchment* (divisional level).

DIVESTITURE

Divestiture is a contraction strategy in which an operating strategic service unit is sold off as a result of a decision to permanently and completely leave the market despite its current viability. Generally, the business to be divested has value and will continue to be operated by the purchasing organization.

Within the past decade, the strategy of "unbundling" (divesting by a hospital of one or more of its services) has become common. Thus, hospitals are carving out non-core services previously performed internally and divesting them. Typical services and products produced in a hospital that are not necessarily part of the core bundle of activities include laboratory, pharmacy, X-ray, physical therapy, occupational therapy, and dietary services.[17] In addition, "hotel" services (laundry, housekeeping, and so on) formerly performed by hospitals are being contracted to outsiders. Even medical services in such specialty areas as ophthalmology are increasingly being performed outside the hospital in "surgi-centers" and may be candidates for divestiture.

Divestiture decisions are made for a number of reasons. An organization may need cash to fund more important operations for long-term growth or the division/SSU may not be achieving management's goals. In some cases health care organizations are divesting services that are too far from their core business or area of management expertise. For example, many multihospital systems have divested their HMO (purchased only a few years earlier) to concentrate on care delivery. A multihospital system purchasing a managed care organization actually represents unrelated diversification. Although the strategy appears logical and synergistic, managed care businesses are difficult to manage and there is little skill transfer from managing provider organizations.

Some practical guidelines for the divestiture of services are presented in Exhibit 6–10. If eight or more responses are "No," consideration should be given to divesting the service. If the responses are relatively even, significant modifications in the service should be considered.

LIQUIDATION

Liquidation involves selling the assets of an organization. The assumption underlying a liquidation strategy is that the unit cannot be sold as a viable and

Exhibit 6–10: Guidelines for Divestiture of Services

1. Were the actual financial results equal to or better than those anticipated in the strategic plan?
2. Has the organization been in operation less than 18 months?
3. Is there at least an example of a known profitable operation of approximately the same size as your operation?
4. Have utilization targets been achieved?
5. Is your payor mix the same as or better than you expected?
6. Is this a high fixed-cost operation with excess capacity?
7. Can you quantify spin-off benefits to the system?
8. Can you identify any real competitive advantages this service has in the marketplace?
9. Can you identify specific management actions that can reverse the losses?
10. Is this an early stage in the PLC or a new market?
11. Would you use your own money to invest in this venture?

Source: Adapted from Jay Greene, "A Strategy for Cutting Back," *Modern Healthcare*, August 18, 1989, p. 29; developed by the Society for Healthcare Planning and Marketing, American Hospital Association.

ongoing operation. However, the assets of the organization (facilities, equipment, and so on) still have value and may be sold for other uses. Organizations, of course, may be partially or completely liquidated. Common reasons for pursuing a liquidation strategy include bankruptcy, the desire to dispose of nonproductive assets, and the emergence of a new technology that results in a rapid decline in the use of the old technology.

On leaving a market, an aging hospital building may be sold for its property value or an alternative use. In a declining market, a liquidation strategy may be a long-term strategy to be carried out in an orderly manner over a period of years. Recently many hospitals have been liquidating their emergency helicopter operations, which had historically been allowed to operate as loss leaders because they brought prestige and positive public relations to the hospital. However, because of increasing costs and limited reimbursements, many hospitals have shut down and liquidated such operations.

HARVESTING

A harvesting strategy is selected when the market has entered long-term decline. The reason underlying such a strategy is that the organization has a relatively strong market position but industry-wide revenues are expected to decline over the next several years. Therefore, the organization will "ride the decline," allowing the business to generate as much cash as possible. However, little in terms of new resources will be invested.

In a *harvesting* strategy, the organization attempts to reap maximum short-term benefits before the product or service is eliminated. Such a strategy allows the organization an orderly exit from a declining segment of the market by planned downsizing. Harvesting has not been widely used in health care but will be more frequently encountered in the future as markets mature and organizations exit various segments. For instance, some regional hospitals that have developed rural hospital networks have experienced difficulty in maintaining their commitment to health care in small communities. The 20-bed hospitals frequently found in rural networks tend to struggle financially because of a lack of support from specialists and primary care physicians, an aging population, and flight of the young to urban areas. Twenty-bed rural hospitals are probably in a long-term decline with little hope for survival. On the other hand, 50-bed hospitals have managed to maintain or improve their financial position because of effective physician recruitment, good community image, and the continued viability of the communities themselves. Therefore, regional hospitals with rural networks may have to employ a harvesting strategy for the 20-bed hospitals while using development or maintenance of scope strategies for the 50-bed and larger hospitals.

RETRENCHMENT

A *retrenchment* strategy is a response to declining profitability, usually brought about by increasing costs. The market is still viewed as viable, and the organization's products/services continue to have wide acceptance. However, costs are rising as a percentage of revenue, placing pressure on profitability. Retrenchment typically involves a redefinition of the target market and selective cost elimination or asset reduction. Retrenchment is directed toward reduction in personnel, the range of products/services, or the geographic market served and represents an effort to reduce the scope of operations.

Over time, organizations may find that they are overstaffed given the level of demand. As a result, their costs are higher than those of competitors. When market growth is anticipated, personnel are added to accommodate the growth, but during periods of decline, positions are seldom eliminated. A reduction in the staff members who have become superfluous or redundant is often central to a retrenchment strategy.

Similarly, in an attempt to "round out" the product or service line, products and services are added. Over time, these additional products/services may tend to add more costs than revenues. In many organizations, less than 20 percent of the products account for more than 80 percent of the revenue. Under these circumstances, retrenchment may be in order.

Finally, there are times when geographic growth is undertaken without regard for costs. Eventually, managers realize they are "spread too thin" to adequately serve the market. In addition, well-positioned competitors are able to provide quality products/services at lower costs because of their proximity. In this situation, geographic retrenchment (reducing the service area) is appropriate. In many cases, a retrenchment strategy is implemented after periods of aggressive market development or acquisition of competitors (horizontal integration).

The various contraction of scope strategies, their relative risks, and their rationales are summarized in Exhibit 6–11.

Exhibit 6-11: Rationales and Relative Risks of Contraction of Scope Strategic Alternatives

Strategy	Relative Risk	Rationale
Divestiture	Low	• Industry in long-term decline • Cash needed to enter new, higher growth area • Lack of expected synergy with core operation • Required investment in new technology seen as too high • Too much regulation • Unbundling
Liquidation	Low	• Organization can no longer operate • Bankruptcy • Trim/reduce assets • Superseded by new technology
Harvesting	Low	• Late maturity/decline of the product life cycle • Consider divestiture or downsizing • Short-term cash needed
Retrenchment (personnel, markets, products, assets)	Moderate	• Market has become too diverse • Market is too geographically spread out • Personnel costs are too high • Too many products or services • Marginal or nonproductive facilities

Maintenance of Scope Strategies

Often organizations pursue *maintenance of scope strategies* when management believes the past strategy has been appropriate and few changes are required in the target markets or the organization's products/services. Maintenance of scope does not necessarily mean that the organization will do nothing; it means that management believes the organization is progressing appropriately. There are two maintenance of scope strategies: enhancement and status quo.

ENHANCEMENT

When management believes that the organization is progressing toward its vision and goals but needs to "do things better," an *enhancement* strategy may be used; neither expansion nor contraction of operations is appropriate but "something needs to be done." Typically, enhancement strategies take the form of quality programs (CQI, TQM) directed toward improving organizational processes or cost-reduction programs designed to render the organization more efficient. In addition to quality and efficiency, enhancement strategies may be directed toward innovative management processes, speeding up the delivery of the products/services to the customer, and adding flexibility to the design of the products or services (marketwide customization).

Many times after an expansion strategy, an organization engages in maintenance/enhancement strategies. Typically after an acquisition, organizations initiate enhancement strategies directed toward upgrading facilities, reducing purchasing costs, installing new computer systems, enhancing information systems, improving the ability to evaluate clinical results, reducing overhead costs, or improving quality.

STATUS QUO

A *status quo* strategy is based on the assumption that the market has matured and periods of high growth are over. Often, the organization has secured an acceptable market share and managers believe the position can be defended against competitors.

In a status quo strategy, the goal is to maintain market share. Although the organization attempts to keep services at current levels, additional resources may be required. Management attempts to prolong the life of the product/service for as long as possible. Environmental influences affecting the decline of the products or services should be carefully analyzed to determine when decline is imminent. An example of this strategy would be a full-service hospital investing heavily in marketing to prevent market share erosion for inpatient services.[18]

Typically, organizations attempt a status quo strategy in some areas while engaging in market development, product development, or penetration in others to better utilize limited resources. For instance, a hospital may attempt to hold its market share (status quo) in slow-growth markets such as cardiac and pediatric services and attempt market development in higher growth services such as intense, shortterm rehabilitation care, renal dialysis, ophthalmology, or intravenous therapy.

In mature markets, industry consolidation occurs as firms attempt to add volume and reduce costs. Therefore, managers must be wary of the emergence of a single dominant competitor that has achieved a significant cost differential. A status quo strategy is appropriate when there are two or three dominant providers in a stable market segment because, in this situation, market development or product development may be quite difficult and extremely expensive.

The various maintenance of scope strategies, their relative risks, and their rationales are summarized in Exhibit 6–12.

Market Entry Strategies

The selection of the expansion or maintenance of scope strategies from among the adaptive strategic alternatives dictates that the next decision to be made is which of the *market entry* strategies should be used. If a contraction adaptive strategy is selected, normally there is no market entry decision and market entry

Exhibit 6–12: Rationales and Relative Risks of Maintenance of Scope Strategic Alternatives

Strategy	Relative Risk	Rationale
Enhancement *(quality, efficiency, innovation, speed, and flexibility)*	Low	• Organization has operational inefficiencies • Need to lower costs • Need to improve quality • Improve internal processes
Status quo	Low	• Maintain market share position • Maturity/late maturity stage of the product life cycle • Product/market generating cash but has little potential for future growth • Extremely competitive market

strategies are not used. The expansion strategies specify entering or gaining access to a new market, and the maintenance of scope strategies may call for obtaining new resources. Therefore, the next important decision that must be made for these strategies concerns how the organization will enter or develop the market.

There are three major methods to enter a market. As illustrated in Exhibit 6–4, an organization can use its financial resources to purchase a stake in the new market, team with other organizations and use cooperation to enter a market, or use its own resources to develop its own products and services. It is important to understand that market entry strategies are not ends in themselves but serve a broader aim – supporting the adaptive strategies. Any of the adaptive strategies may be carried out using any of the market entry strategies but each one places different demands on the organization.

Purchase Strategies

Purchase market entry strategies allow an organization to use its financial resources to enter a market quickly, thereby initiating the adaptive strategy. There are three purchase market entry strategies: acquisition, licensing, and venture capital investment.

ACQUISITION

Acquisitions are entry strategies to expand through the purchase of an existing organization, a unit of an organization, or a product/service. Thus, acquisition strategies may be used to carry out both corporate and divisional strategies such as diversification, vertical integration, market development, or product development. There are many reasons to purchase another organization, such as to obtain real estate or other facilities, to acquire brands, trademarks, or technology, and even to access employees. However, the most common reason is to acquire customers.[19]

The acquiring organization may integrate the operations of the newly acquired organization into its present operations or may run it as a separate business/service unit. Acquisitions offer a method for quickly entering a market, obtaining a technology, or gaining a needed channel member to improve or secure distribution. It is usually possible to assess the performance of an organization before purchase and thereby minimize the risks through careful analysis and selection. The "build internally" versus "acquire" decision is one where strategic leaders must determine whether the benefits of ownership justify the costs and whether the acquiring organization has the product and process knowledge to capitalize on an opportunity quickly. If the acquiring organization does not have the expertise or capability and there is an organization that provides a good strategic fit that does have such expertise then purchase may be warranted.[20] However, even a small acquired organization can be difficult to integrate into the existing culture and operations. Often it takes several years to "digest" an acquisition or to combine two organizational cultures.

Despite the difficulties of combining organizational cultures, the creation of health systems with unified ownership has been an effective strategy. Health systems have been better able than health networks (looser contractual- or alliance-based strategies) to provide needed resources, competencies, and capabilities. This may be because the direct ownership of assets enables systems to achieve greater unity of purpose and develop more focused strategies, on average, than more loosely organized networks. In addition, hospitals in health systems that have unified ownership generally have better financial performance than hospitals in contractually based health networks.[21]

Much of the growth of the for-profit hospital chains has been via a market development acquisition strategy (also called horizontal integration or buying market share). Aggressive market development through acquisition of independent hospitals has been used to build the nation's largest private for-profit hospital chains. For example, more than half of all hospitals in California in 2000 were affiliated with multisite systems; six systems operated more than one-third of the state's hospitals.[22] In the past two decades, horizontal integration and vertical integration through acquisitions and alliances have been key entry strategies for initiating rapid market growth by health care organizations.

LICENSING

Acquiring a technology or product through *licensing* may be viewed as an alternative to acquiring a complete company. License agreements obviate the need for costly and time-consuming product development and provide rapid access to proven technologies, generally with reduced financial and marketing risk to the organization. However, the licensee usually does not receive proprietary technology and is dependent on the licensor for support and upgrade. In addition, the up-front dollar costs may be high. Typical of licensing is IDX Systems that through its LastWord® products licenses operations software to hospitals for developing critical-care paths.

Another common form of licensing is a franchise – the granting of an exclusive territorial license assuring the licensee all rights that the licensor has with respect to a defined activity.[23] This practice is most commonly found in the field of trademark licensing. Franchisees benefit from exploitation of the goodwill, uniform format, and uniform quality standards symbolized by the franchisor's trademark. The license agreement by and between Blue Cross and Blue Shield Association and the various regional Blue Cross and Blue Shield Plans provides an example. It grants to Blue Shield Plans the right to use the Blue Cross and Blue Shield names and trademarks in its trade and corporate name and the right to use the licensed marks in the sale, marketing, and administration of health care plans and related services within a geographic area. In such agreements no other health insurance provider can encroach upon the Plans' license under the Blue Cross and Blue Shield name within the stated territory.[24]

VENTURE CAPITAL INVESTMENT

Venture capital investments offer an opportunity to enter or "try out" a market while keeping risks low. Typically, venture capital investments are used to become involved in the growth and development of a small organization that has the potential to develop a new or innovative technology. By making minority investments in young and growing enterprises, organizations have an opportunity to become close to and – possibly later – enter into new technologies.[25]

In addition, venture capital investments are a way for new health care organizations to grow. Venture capital investments in health care companies have grown from $547 million in 1995 to almost $2 billion in 2000. Venture capital investment in health care technology firms was strong throughout the decade of the 1990s but e-health (Internet related) companies began receiving the largest share of health care venture capital at the beginning of 2000. Start-up/seed or early-stage companies as well as later stage (expansion) companies received funding. Types of health care services businesses receiving venture capital funding in the early part of the twenty-first century were ventures such as life science portals for bioinformatics, e-commerce aimed at individuals and small business purchasers of health insurance, home-based health care services for the elderly, education and treatment services for at-risk youth, early-stage cardiac arrhythmia management companies, and online defined contribution health plans.[26]

Cooperation Strategies

Probably the most used – and certainly the most talked about – strategies of the late 1990s and early 2000s were *cooperation strategies*. Many organizations have carried out adaptive strategies – particularly diversification, vertical integration, product development, and market development strategies – through cooperation strategies. They include mergers, alliances, and joint ventures.

MERGERS

Mergers are similar to acquisitions. In mergers, however, the two organizations combine through mutual agreement to form a single new organization, often with a new name. Mergers have been used most often in the health care segment to combine two similar organizations (horizontal integration) in an effort to gain greater efficiency in the delivery of health care services, reduction in duplication of services, improved geographic dispersion, increased service scope, restraint in pricing increases, and improved financial performance.[27] The other primary use of merger strategies in health care has been to create integrated delivery systems (vertical integration). There are four motives underlying such mergers:

1. *Improve efficiency and effectiveness* – by combining available resources and operations it is possible to exploit cost-reducing synergies and to take fuller advantage of risk-spreading managed care opportunities.
2. *Enhance access* – by providing a broader range of sophisticated programs and services and offering services at a greater number of sites, quality of patient care is improved.
3. *Enhance financial position* – by gaining market share, the sole or one of the dominant providers in the region's health delivery system is able to increase total revenue.
4. *Overcome concerns about survival* – by merging, a free-standing health care organization is better able to survive in an increasingly aggressive, market-driven environment where huge and powerful networks are experiencing cutbacks in managed care, Medicare, and Medicaid reimbursement.[28]

However, managing organizations that merge to create integrated systems has been difficult. There are several reasons why integrated health systems encounter significant obstacles in realizing the proposed benefits. Among the most frequently cited relate to the difficulty of creating an effective strategic fit, giving away too much money and power with respect to governance to the local governing board, achieving operating efficiencies, and experiencing difficulties in realigning resources.[29]

As in acquisitions, a major difficulty in a merger is the integration of two separate organizational cultures. Mergers offer a more difficult problem than acquisitions because a totally new organization must be forged. In an acquisition, the dominant culture remains and subsumes the other. In a merger, a totally new organizational culture (the way we do things) must be developed. Typically there are significant changes in the organizational structure, governance, senior and middle management, service mix, product mix, and outside relationships. Therefore, merging two distinctly different corporate cultures is a challenge and a great deal of time must be spent in communications at all levels in the organization. Medical staff and employees should engage in a reformulation of the vision, mission, and statement of the shared values of the new organization. Work groups must be formed to address how to effectively and efficiently meet the needs of patients. As well as communicating internally, external communications must be given top priority. Even with such efforts, truly merging the two organizational cultures into one will take years to complete.

Although declining in the last part of the 1990s and first few years of the 2000s, mergers and acquisitions and other forms of combination continue to be important market entry strategies for health care organizations (see Perspective 6–5). An environment conducive to large health care combinations, institutional coordination, demands for efficiency, and the continuum of care (seamless care) have fostered many of these mergers and acquisitions.

ALLIANCES

Strategic *alliances* are loosely coupled arrangements among existing organizations that are designed to achieve some long-term strategic purpose not possible by any single organization. Alliances include configurations such as federations, consortiums, networks, and systems.[30] Strategic alliances are cooperative contractual agreements that go beyond normal company-to-company dealings but fall short of merger or full partnership.[31] Alliances have been used to create health networks – loosely coupled or organized delivery systems. They are an attempt to strengthen competitive position while maintaining the independence of the organizations involved.

There is research to suggest that organizations that develop these cooperative relationships are likely to have similar status in the marketplace and have complementary resources, competencies, and capabilities.[32] For example, two organizations may establish an alliance when each one possesses strength in a different stage of the service category value chain – one organization has expertise in service delivery and another controls the distribution channel. Further, organizations may form coalitions to defray costs and share risk when they undertake high-cost capital or development intensive initiatives. Finally, it has been suggested that the resources available from an alliance partner can facilitate an organization's effort to alter its strategic position.[33] For instance, research indicates that biotechnology start-up organizations could enhance their initial performance and strategic position by establishing upstream and downstream alliances.[34]

In health care, the term "alliance" is sometimes used to refer to the voluntary organization that hospitals join primarily to achieve economies of scale in purchasing. For some, this type of alliance provides the benefit of being part of a large system, yet allows them to exist as free-standing, self-governing institutions. Examples of some major hospital alliances include Premier, Voluntary Hospitals of America (VHA), and University HealthSystem Consortium. This is a different type of alliance than that based on an expansion/cooperation strategy.

Strategic alliances, although not mergers, have many of the same problems – previously unrelated cultures have to learn to cooperate rather than compete; numerous "sessions" are required to determine what will be shared and what is proprietary, and how to balance the two; and efforts must be made to maintain cooperation over time within such a "loose" cooperative effort. On the other hand, strategic alliances offer several opportunities, including shared learning, access to expertise not currently "owned" by the organization, strengthened market

Hospital mergers and acquisitions have declined significantly over the past decade. As indicated in the chart, the number of hospital merger and acquisition deals has declined by 70 percent between 1995 and 2003.

Highlights for 2003:*

- The largest multistate acquisition was between the for-profit giant HCA (Nashville, TN) and the not-for-profit Health Midwest (Kansas City, MO). The $1.1 billion transaction added nine hospitals to the HCA portfolio.
- Among the for-profits, Health Management Associates (Naples, FL) acquired five hospitals from Tenet Health Corporation (Santa Barbara, CA) valued at $515 million.
- Twelve of the 68 deals were joint ventures, compared with just 2 of 60 in 2002.
- Thirty hospitals closed in 2003 (19 not-for-profit, 6 for-profit, 4 public, 1 rehab facility), compared with 17 in 2002, 44 in 2000, and 43 in 1999.
- Thirty-one hospitals opened in 2003 (26 for-profit, 7 specialty hospitals), compared with 8 openings in 2002.

*Includes deals completed or pending in 2003. Includes mergers, acquisitions, joint ventures, long-term leases and other partnerships in which a change in control or equity stake occurred. Not included are management contracts and simple affiliations.
Source: Maziar Abdolrasulnia, PhD student, Administration-Health Services, University of Alabama at Birmingham, from Vince Galloro and Patrick Reilly, "Where Have All the Good Deals Gone?" *Modern Healthcare* 34, no. 4 (January 26, 2004), p. 34.

Hospital Merger Activity (1995–2003)

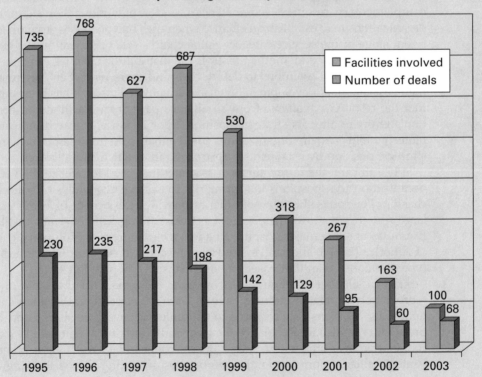

position, and direction of competitive efforts toward others instead of each other. In addition, one of the advantages of integrated networks and strategic alliances is the increased access to resources to obtain new technology or reduce the need to purchase duplicate equipment. Further, it has been suggested that these arrangements are promising mechanisms to reduce technology-driven health care cost inflation.[35] In some cases, an alliance can lead to a merger. For example, Breech Medical Center in Lebanon, Missouri, moved its affiliation agreement with St. John's Health System of Springfield, Missouri, to a full-asset merger over a several-year period.

As the environment becomes more unpredictable, a number of health care providers have been seeking strategic alliances. Many primary providers have turned to alliances as vehicles for providing services, soliciting physician loyalty, and reducing investments in operations.[36] Hospitals appear to form alliances with physicians for several reasons. Alliances serve to contract with the growing number of HMOs, to pose a countervailing bargaining force of providers in the face of HMO consolidation, and to accompany hospital downsizing and restructuring efforts.[37] However, strategic alliances between physicians and hospitals should be anchored in their common purpose – improving patient care. The physicians involved may not concur with the hospital in its management of facilities, staffing, and so forth. In addition, conflict may emerge as hospitals diversify into areas that compete more directly with the physicians' own clinics, ambulatory care centers, and diagnostic centers. Finally, although the hospital would prefer to have many qualified physicians admitted to the staff (who could refer more patients), allied physicians would prefer to limit credentialing of outside physicians (controlling competition).

JOINT VENTURES

When projects get too large, technology too expensive, internal resources, competencies or capabilities too scarce, or the costs of failure too high for a single organization, joint ventures are often used.[38] A *joint venture* (JV) is the combination of the resources of two or more separate organizations to accomplish a designated task. A joint venture may involve a pooling of assets or a combination of the specialized talents or skills of each organization. The four most common organizational forms used in health care joint ventures are:

1. *Contractual Agreements.* Two or more organizations sign a contract agreeing to work together toward a specific objective.
2. *Subsidiary Corporations.* A new corporation is formed (called an equity JV), usually to operate nonhospital activities.
3. *Partnerships.* A formal or informal arrangement in which two or more parties engage in activities of mutual benefit.
4. *Not-for-Profit Title-Holding Corporations.* Tax legislation enacted in 1986 allowed not-for-profit organizations to form tax-exempt title-holding corporations (providing significant benefits to health care organizations engaged in real estate ventures).[39]

Because of the dynamic health care environment, hospitals engage in joint ventures to lower costs and to improve and expand services. Joint ventures can be an innovative way to generate revenues, supplement operations, and remain competitive.[40] Through the first part of the 2000s, the most common joint venture was between hospitals and physicians. Hospital/physician joint ventures are popular because they allow the hospital to preempt physicians as competitors and, at the same time, stabilize the hospital's referral base. Often joint ventures with hospitals increase physicians' profitability. Physicians enter joint ventures with hospitals to protect their incomes and autonomy, whereas hospitals are motivated to form joint ventures as a means of controlling medical care costs and gaining influence over physician utilization of hospital services. Changes in third-party payments have created competition based on price – joint ventures enable hospitals to reduce costs and compete more effectively.[41]

Although there are benefits to creating joint ventures, they have their own unique set of challenges. These challenges revolve around strategy, governance, economic interdependencies, and organization. For example, the parent organizations may hold different strategic interests and maintaining strategic alignment across separate organizations with different goals, market pressures, and stakeholders can be difficult. In addition, sharing governance can complicate decision making, particularly with separate reporting systems and methods for measuring success. Further, problems develop in providing services, staffing, and other resources. Finally, building a cohesive, high-performing organization with a unique culture has proven difficult for many joint ventures.[42]

Development Strategies

Organizations may enter new markets by using internal resources in what are called *development strategies*. This entry strategy takes the form of internal development or internal ventures. Diversification and vertical integration through internal development or internal ventures usually take considerably longer to achieve than through acquisition (although the costs may be lower).

INTERNAL DEVELOPMENT

Internal development uses the existing organizational structure, personnel, and capital to generate new products/services or distribution strategies. Internal development may be most appropriate for products or services that are closely related to existing products or services. Internal development is common for growing organizations, particularly when they can exploit existing resources, competencies, and capabilities.

INTERNAL VENTURES

Internal ventures typically set up separate, relatively independent entities within the organization. Internal ventures may be most appropriate for products or services that are unrelated to the current products or services. For instance, internal ventures may be appropriate for developing vertically integrated systems. Thus, initial efforts by a hospital to develop home health care may be accomplished through an internal venture.

Market Entry Strategy Linkage

The major advantages and disadvantages of the market entry strategies are summarized in Exhibit 6–13. The adaptive and market entry strategies work in combination. The market entry strategies are the means for accomplishing the adaptive strategies. This relationship is demonstrated as organizations struggle with cost containment and their managed care strategies. Health care organizations are opting for a variety of adaptive and market entry strategies to deal with the changing health care environment. Together the adaptive (scope of the organization) and market entry strategies (means to achieve that scope) are shaping the health care landscape. Perspective 6–6 speculates on the organizational forms of care delivery for the next decade. It is the adaptive and market entry strategies of organizations that will create this future.

Competitive Strategies

Having selected the adaptive strategies and market entry strategies, managers must decide the strategic posture of the organization and how the products and services will be positioned vis-à-vis those of competitors. Strategic posture concerns the organization's fundamental behavior within the market – defending market position, prospecting for new products and markets, or balancing market defense with careful entry into selected new product areas and markets. In addition, an organization must consciously position its products and services within a market through one of the marketwide or market segment positioning strategies (generic strategies).

Strategic Posture

Organizations may be classified by how they behave within their market segments or industry – their *strategic posture*. Research by Miles, Snow, Meyer, and Coleman has shown that there are at least four typical strategic postures for organizations – defenders, prospectors, analyzers, and reactors. Defenders, prospectors, and analyzers are explicit strategies that result in a pattern of consistent and stable behavior within a market. Defender, prospector, or analyzer strategic postures may be appropriate for certain internal, market, and environmental conditions. Reactors, on the other hand, do not seem to have a strategy and demonstrate inconsistent behavior. However, unless an organization exists in a protected environment, such as a monopolistic or highly regulated market segment, it cannot

Exhibit 6–13: Advantages and Disadvantages of Market Entry Strategies

Market Entry Strategy	Major Advantages	Major Disadvantages
Acquisition	• Rapid market entry • Image already established • Performance known before purchase	• New business may be unfamiliar to parent • Takes a long time to assimilate organization's culture • New management team may be required • High initial cost
Licensing	• Rapid access to proven techology • Reduced financial exposure • Access to brand name • Exclusive territory	• Not a substitute for internal technical competence • Not proprietary technology • Dependent on licensor • Rules and regulations
Venture Capital Investment	• Can provide window on new technology or market • Low risk	• Alone, unlikely to be a major stimulus of growth • Extended time to profitability
Merger	• Uses existing resources • Retains existing markets and products • Reduces competition	• Takes a long time to merge cultures • Merger match often difficult to find
Alliance	• Fills in gaps in product line • Creates efficiencies (e.g., bargaining power) • Reduces competition in weak markets • Stabilizes referral base • Shared risk	• Potential for conflict between members • Limits potential markets/products • Difficult to align resources • Governance issues
Joint Venture	• Technological/marketing joint ventures can exploit small/large organizational synergies • Spreads distribution risks	• Potential for conflict between partners (shared vs. proprietary) • Objectives of partners may not be compatible
Internal Development	• Uses existing resources • Organization maintains a high level of control • Presents image of developing (growth) organization	• Time lag to break even • Unfamiliarity with new markets • Obtaining significant gains in market shares against strong competitors may be difficult
Internal Venture	• Uses existing resources • May enable organization to hold a talented entrepreneur • Isolates development from organization's bureaucracy	• Mixed record of success • Organization's internal climate (culture) often unsuitable

Perspective 6–6

Health Care Delivery
Organizations for the
Next Decade

No one organizational form will emerge in the next decade. Rather, to satisfy the demands of intermediaries and patients, different types of organizations will use a variety of adaptive and market entry strategies to create various organizational models. Each of these models will provide a substantial percentage of care in at least some regions of the United States. The dominant models of health care delivery will include:

- *The Hospital-Centered System* – health care systems, many built around academic health/ medical centers (AHCs), designed to provide all services in a metropolitan area across a range of facilities. The facilities include inpatient, outpatient, diagnostic, and ancillary services, as well as physician multi-specialty clinics. This approach will require market development (horizontal integration), product development, and some vertical integration adaptive strategies. To carry out these adaptive strategies the organizations will engage in acquisition, merger, alliance, and joint venture market entry strategies.
- *The Virtual Physician-Group Cooperative* – evolved from the independent practices association (IPA) and created from independent physicians with a natural set of referrals, on-call coverage, and clinical respect for each other. The virtual group cooperative's ability to use information technology and contractual flexibility to coordinate services will enable them to enter into contracts with several heath plans. Development of the virtual physician-group cooperative will require market development adaptive strategies coupled with alliance and joint venture market entry strategies.
- *The Physician Practice Management (PPM) Corporation* – represents a continuation of the development of for-profit physician management companies and will result in the accumulation of existing smaller practices. These physician practice management corporations will create administrative efficiencies through economies of scale and will mix corporate-owned and franchise-owned operations. These corporations will engage in aggressive market development adaptive strategies and acquisition and licensing (franchise) market entry strategies.
- *Single-Specialty Carve-Out* – single specialty groups and networks of specialists will market their services either directly to payors or to other providers. These networks will provide specialty disease management services for cancer, cardiovascular disease, nephrology, and AIDS, among others. Some of these organizations will provide all comprehensive specialty services, such as cancer treatment, whereas others will provide niche support services, such as patient monitoring and education. Adaptive strategies for the development of single-specialty carve-out companies incorporate market development including horizontal integration. Market entry strategies would include acquisition, alliance, and merger.
- *Remnants* – much of the present system will remain. Some independent hospitals and public hospitals will not find partners or be incorporated. In addition, many individual and small-group practices will change very little. These institutions will engage in limited market and product development, but will primarily focus on harvesting and retrenchment. In addition, many will engage in enhancement and status quo adaptive strategies.

Source: The Institute for the Future, *Health and Health Care 2010: The Forecast, The Challenge* (San Francisco: Jossey-Bass Publishers, January 2000), pp. 57–60.

continue to behave as a reactor indefinitely.[43] Furthermore, an organization's strategic posture should not be left to chance. Health care organizations are able to change their strategic postures to match the demands of their environmental context and improve their performance.[44] Therefore, strategic decision makers should examine the current market behavior, explicitly delineate the appropriate organization strategic posture, and redirect resources and competencies needed to transform themselves into a better environmentally suited posture.

DEFENDER STRATEGIC POSTURE

Stability is the chief objective of a defender strategic posture. Managers using this strategy attempt to seal off a portion of the total market to create a stable domain. A *defender posture* focuses on a narrow market with a limited number of products or services and aggressively attempts to defend this market segment through pricing or differentiation strategies.

Defenders are organizations that engage in little search for additional opportunities for growth and seldom make adjustments in existing technologies, structures, or strategies. They devote primary attention to improving the efficiencies of existing operations. Thus, cost-efficiency is central to the defender's success. In addition, defenders often engage in vertical integration to protect their market, control patient flow, and create stability. Defenders grow through penetration strategies and limited product development strategies.

PROSPECTOR STRATEGIC POSTURE

Prospectors are organizations that frequently search for new market opportunities and regularly engage in experimentation and innovation. A prospector's major capability is that of finding and exploiting new products and market opportunities. As a result the prospector's domain is usually broad and in a continuous state of development. Prospectors are typically in rapidly changing environments and frequently engage not only in diversification and product and market development expansion strategies but also divestment and retrenchment contraction strategies. One of the principal competitive advantages of a prospector strategic posture is that of creating change within the service category/service area. Defenders and prospectors are contrasted in Perspective 6–7 through a discussion of their markets.

ANALYZER STRATEGIC POSTURE

The *analyzer posture* is a combination of the prospector and defender strategic postures. The analyzer tries to balance stability and change. Analyzers are organizations that maintain stable operations in some areas, usually their core products or businesses, but also search for new opportunities and engage in market innovations. Characteristically they watch competitors and rapidly adopt those strategic ideas that appear to have the greatest potential. Analyzers tend to use penetration strategies in their stable core products and markets whereas related

Perspective 6–7

Red Defenders, Blue Prospectors

In a study of 108 companies, W. Chan Kim and Renée Mauborgne have defined two types of strategies: *blue ocean strategy* and *red ocean strategy*. Red ocean strategists compete to win market share in traditional mature markets and pursue either a differentiation or cost leader strategy. Similar to red ocean strategists, defender organizations vigorously protect their existing market share, tend to pursue strategies that create difficulties for competitors, and compete in limited "market spaces." Blue ocean strategists, on the other hand, create new environments, redefine products or services or the nature of competition, make competition irrelevant, and pursue a strategy of differentiation and low cost. The characteristics of blue ocean strategies are similar to prospectors' strategies. Prospecting organizations tend to be cutting edge, creative, seeking to differentiate themselves from competitors, and inventing or creating environments.

A good example of each strategic approach in health care can be seen in today's hospital market. General hospitals have been trying to compete and defend their market share in existing traditional markets, have focused on differentiating or lowcost strategies, and have failed to reinvent industry rules for success. In desperate times general hospitals have attempted to imitate specialty hospitals, but cannot because of the economies of scale created by specialty hospitals. As general hospitals continue to try to squeeze out pennies, specialty hospitals have been enjoying high profits – another contrast between blue prospectors and red defenders.

Specialty hospitals that focus on one service line – typically cardiac, orthopedic, or neurological services – are characterized as prospectors or blue ocean strategists. Specialty hospitals have created a new environment for specialty services; made the competition of general hospitals irrelevant; employed cutting-edge technologies to build unique, lasting brands; and have pursued both a differentiation and low-cost strategy. The lesson for the health care strategist is to be alert and think about how the market operates, how the environment is changing, and how the organization provides low-cost service and unique value to consumers. To be a prospector, an organization must think about inventing the environment while keeping in mind the value that consumers want.

Source: Maziar Abdolrasulnia, PhD student, Administration-Health Services, University of Alabama at Birmingham. From W. Chan Kim and Renée Mauborgne, "Blue Ocean Strategy," *Harvard Business Review* (October 2004), pp. 76–84 and W. Chan Kim and Renée Mauborgne, *Blue Ocean Strategy: How to Create Uncontested Market Space and Make the Competition Irrelevant* (Boston: Harvard Business School Press, 2004).

diversification, product development, and market development are used to enter new promising areas.

REACTOR STRATEGIC POSTURE

The defender, prospector, and analyzer postures are all proactive strategies. However, the *reactors* really do not have a strategy or plan and therefore such organizations are both inconsistent and unstable in their response to the environment. Reactors are organizations that perceive opportunities and turbulence but are not able to adapt effectively. They lack consistent approaches to strategy and structure and make changes primarily in response to environmental pressures. Miles, Snow, Meyer, and Coleman identified three major reasons that organizations become reactors:

1. Top management may not have clearly articulated the organization's strategy.
2. Management does not fully shape the organization's structure and processes to fit a chosen strategy.
3. Management tends to maintain the organization's current strategy–structure relationship despite overwhelming changes in environmental conditions.[45]

If the internal analysis reveals that the organization has been reactive without a clear strategy or that there is a mismatch between the strategy and implementation, changes will have to be made to move the organization toward a more effective strategic posture. There is some evidence that reactors may be able to hone their competencies and transform themselves into more viable strategic postures over time.[46]

Understanding the organization's preferred strategic posture and communicating it throughout the organization provides decision guidelines and will shape the culture of the organization. It is important that the strategic posture be consistent with the directional, adaptive, market entry, and positioning strategies. The major advantages and disadvantages of the strategic posture strategies are summarized in Exhibit 6–14.

Positioning Strategies – Marketwide or Focus

Michael Porter, a well-known strategic management writer, proposes that an organization may serve the entire market using marketwide strategies or serve a particular segment of the market using focus strategies. Porter called these *generic strategies* because they were general strategies that any organization could use to position itself in the marketplace.[47] For both marketwide and market segment focus there are two fundamental *positioning strategies* – cost leadership and differentiation.[48]

Marketwide strategies position the products/services of the organization to appeal to a broad audience (the entire market). For example, a community hospital may be positioned to serve all area residents – serve a broad market with a broad range of services. These products and services, therefore, are not tailored exclusively to the needs of any special segment of the population such as children or the aged. As shown in Exhibit 6–15, marketwide positioning strategies can be based on differentiation or cost leadership. Thus, the community hospital may try to differentiate itself from other hospitals by emphasizing quality or convenience or may compete as a low-cost provider.

Market segment strategies are directed toward the particular needs of a well-defined market segment, such as pediatric oncology or women's health, and often are called *focus strategies*. Thus, a focus strategy identifies a specific, well-defined "niche" in the total market that the organization will concentrate on or pursue. Because of its attributes, the product or service, or the organization itself, may appeal to a particular niche within the market. Similar to marketwide strategies, focus strategies may be based on cost leadership (cost/focus) or differentiation (differentiation/focus).

Exhibit 6–14: Advantages and Disadvantages of Strategic Postures

Strategic Posture	Advantages	Disadvantages
Defender	• Focus on limited set of products and services • Focus is on narrow market segment • Stable environment • Difficult for competitors to enter this segment	• Reliance on the success of narrow product line • Must have long/sustaining PLCs • Market segment must be stable – slow change • May be unable to respond to major market/industry shifts • Difficult to enter new markets or technologies
Prospector	• Always involved in "cutting-edge" developments • Organization changes with changing environment • Allows for a rapid response to a changing environment	• Organization is in constant state of change • New products and markets always being developed • Multiple technologies being employed, seldom able to achieve efficiency • Tend to have lower profits because of continuous change • Tend to overextend resources • Tend to underutilize financial, human, and physical resources
Analyzer	• Allows for the maintenance of a core of stable traditional products and services • Allows for high-risk products and services to be borne by prospectors • Lower investment in research and development	• Difficult strategy to pursue • Must respond quickly to follow lead of key prospector while maintaining efficiency in core products/services • Complex structure (matrix) • Management of both stable and dynamic products and markets • Communication is often difficult
Reactor	• Little strategic planning required (monopolistic or highly regulated environment)	• Inconsistency in response to environmental change • Instability in organization • Organization becomes both ineffective and inefficient • No effective guide for decision making

Because of the complexity of medicine and the entire health care industry, focus strategies are quite common. Just as physicians have specialized, the institutions within the field have tended to focus on specialized segments. Examples of focus strategies are rehabilitation hospitals, psychiatric hospitals, ambulatory care centers, Alzheimer's centers, and so on. These specialty organizations may be further positioned based on cost leadership or differentiation. Each of the generic

Exhibit 6–15: Porter's Matrix

		Strategic Advantage	
		Uniqueness Perceived by the Customer	***Low-Cost Position***
Strategic Target	***Marketwide (broad)***	Differentiation	Overall Cost Leadership
	Particular Segment Only (narrow)	Differentiation/Focus	Cost/Focus

Source: Michael E. Porter, *Competitive Strategy: Techniques for Analyzing Industries and Competitors.*

strategies results from an organization making consistent choices for product/services, markets (service areas), and distinctive competencies – choices that reinforce each other.

Cost Leadership

Cost leadership is a positioning strategy designed to gain an advantage over competitors by producing a product or providing a service at a lower cost than competitors' offerings. The product or service is often highly standardized to keep costs low. Cost leadership allows for more flexibility in pricing and relatively greater profit margins.

Cost leadership is based on economies of scale in operations, marketing, administration, and the use of the latest technology. Cost leadership may be used effectively as the generic strategy for any of the adaptive strategies and seems particularly applicable to the primary providers segment of the health care industry. As Porter suggests, "Cost leadership requires aggressive construction of efficient-scale facilities, vigorous pursuit of cost reduction from experience, tight cost and overhead control, avoidance of marginal customer accounts, and cost minimization in areas such as R&D, service, sales force, advertising, and so on."[49] Therefore, in order to use cost leadership effectively, an organization must be able to develop a significant cost advantage and have a reasonably large market share. This strategy must be used cautiously within health care because consumers often perceive low price as meaning low quality. However, cost leadership allows the organization the greatest flexibility in pricing.

An industry segment where cost leadership is being used successfully is in the area of long-term care. Long-term care facilities are a "thin-margin business" in which profit margins range from approximately 1.2 percent to 1.7 percent. In this industry, older facilities are at a competitive disadvantage relative to new facilities. However, long-term care facilities that have been able to drive costs down while maintaining quality have enjoyed higher margins. In addition, many of these facilities have been upgraded to be more efficient and have instituted tight cost controls. Advertising has been used to keep occupancy above 95 percent, which is often required in the industry to be profitable.

DIFFERENTIATION

Differentiation is a strategy to make the product or service different (or appear so in the mind of the buyer) from competitors' products or services. Thus, consumers see the service as unique among a group of similar competing services. Perspective 6–8 discusses how neurosciences are a service category that has great potential for differentiation.

The product or service may be differentiated by emphasizing quality, a high level of service, ease of access, convenience, reputation, and so on. There are a number of ways to differentiate a product or service, but the attributes that are to be viewed as different or unique must be valued by the consumer. Therefore, organizations using differentiation strategies rely on brand loyalty (reputation or image), distinctive products or services, and the lack of good substitutes.

The most common forms of differentiation in the health care industry have been based on quality and image. Many acute care hospitals emphasize and promote quality care as the difference between them and other hospitals in their service area. However, consumers expect to receive high quality care at every hospital, making quality a difficult differentiating factor. A "high-tech" image is another basis for differentiation among health care organizations. Affiliation with a medical school – which performs the most sophisticated procedures or uses the latest (often expensive) technology – may promote the image of "the best possible care."

Exhibit 6–16 summarizes the choices appropriate for each generic strategy. Exhibit 6–17 presents the advantages and disadvantages of each of the positioning strategies.

Combination Strategies

Combination strategies are often used, especially in larger complex organizations, because no single strategy alone may be sufficient. For example, an organization may concurrently divest itself of one of its divisions and engage in market development in another. Perhaps the most frequent combination strategy for hospital-based systems has been vertical integration through acquisition and alliances combined with market development through acquisition (horizontal integration). As conceptualized in Exhibit 6–18, the intent of these strategies has been to create regional fully integrated systems with wide market coverage and a full range of services (often referred to as providing the continuum of care).

Perspective 6–8

Neurosciences Represent Opportunities

Neurosciences are expected to change and grow drastically over the next few years, representing a potentially huge "cash cow" for hospitals as well as an opportunity for competitive differentiation and market share growth. The public does not understand this area of medicine very well. Therefore, considerable investment in communication and promotion expense is required.

Neurosurgeries require expensive equipment but can be very lucrative, although it often takes three to five years to achieve profitability. However, headache clinics, sleep centers, and epilepsy monitoring units require much less expensive equipment and can be profitable very quickly.

Spinal fusions and craniotomies are reimbursed well and predicted to be on the rise with the aging "boomers." In 2002, the average craniotomy charge was about $30,000 and the average spinal fusion was $16,000 (although an additional $10,000 was often charged for front and back hardware attached to the spine). As these surgeries are performed more frequently, they may become ambulatory surgery. Yet, new neurosurgeries are likely for conditions not now treatable such as stroke, tremors, and traumatic injuries.

Baylor Medical Center in Irving, Texas recently opened a Neuro-ICU and equipped a $1.2 million neurosurgery operating room targeted to a niche in minimally invasive spine surgery. Baylor is participating in a variety of clinical studies in neurosurgery including minimally invasive spine surgery, inpatient stroke, epilepsy, Parkinson's disease, and tumors.

In July 2003, North Shore-Long Island Jewish Health System in New York opened an institute to treat patients with Chiari malformation, a rare cerebellar structural condition that includes a complex group of disorders characterized by herniation of the cerebellum through the large opening in the base of the skull into the spinal canal. Chiari malformation often presents in children who complain of headaches and pain at the base of their head or upper neck and can progress to scoliosis and cerebellar dysfunction (especially balance, coordination, and disequilibrium). The Chiari Institute at North Shore-Long Island Jewish Health System now handles more than 400 Chiari cases per year from around the world.

Other hospitals have been successful with non-invasive procedures for brain tumors. They have kept physicians up to date about Gamma Knife and CyberKnife and advertised directly to consumers and others (including media) to "ask your doctor" for information about minimally invasive surgical technologies. Georgetown Hospital in Washington, DC acquired a CyberKnife (an advanced stereotactic radiosurgery system for inoperable tumors of the brain, neck, and spine). Georgetown sent more than 50,000 potential referral sources information, including a letter and a CD, about the availability of its new CyberKnife. Stories about the Cyber-Knife at Georgetown appeared on several TV stations and was further elaborated on its own website. Having the high-tech equipment solidified Georgetown's status as a tertiary institution.

Source: Bradley Worrell and Susan J. Alt, "Neurosciences Provide Great Opportunities for Hospitals," *Health Care Strategic Management* (June 2004), pp. 1, 14–19 and Richard L. Cohen, "Neurology: Marketing Non-Invasive Procedures for Brain Tumors," *Healthcare Marketing Report* (September 2003), pp. 1, 8–10.

As illustrated in Perspective 6–9, Carolinas Healthcare System, previously known as Charlotte/Mecklenburg Hospital Authority, demonstrates the successful use of combination strategies. Beginning with a single county hospital as the base, Carolinas Healthcare System used practically every type of adaptive and market entry strategy to achieve its vision of a fully integrated regional health system with Carolinas Medical Center as its foundation.

Exhibit 6–16: Product/Market/Distinctive Competency Choices and Generic Competitive Strategies

	Cost Leadership	Differentiation	Focus
Product Differentiation	By Price	By Uniqueness	Price or Uniqueness
Market Segmentation	Mass Market	Many Market Segments	Only One or a Very Few Segments
Distinctive Competency	Operations and Materials Management	Research and Development/Marketing	Any Kind of Distinctive Competency

Exhibit 6–17: Advantages and Disadvantages of Positioning Strategies

Positioning Strategy	Major Advantages	Major Disadvantages
Cost Leadership	• Provides clear competitive advantage • Provides clear market position • Provides opportunities to spend more than competition	• Must obtain large volume • Product/service must be standardized • Product/service may be viewed as low quality
Differentiation	• Product/service viewed as unique • Often viewed as high quality • Greater control over pricing	• Often difficult to adequately differentiate product or service • Product/service may be higher priced
Focus	• Appeals to specialized market • May develop good relations with market	• Market may be small • Expansion of market may be difficult

In addition to an organization using several different strategies at once, a strategy may have several phases. It may be necessary to "string together" several strategic alternatives as phases or elements to implement a broader strategic shift. In a two-phase strategy, an organization may employ a retrenchment strategy in phase one and an enhancement strategy in phase two. As illustrated in Exhibit 6–19, the strategic manager's vision often extends through several strategic alternatives or phases. Such vision helps provide long-term continuity for the entire management team. However, the strategic manager must be aware that, in a dynamic environment, circumstances may change and later phases may have to be modified or revised to meet the needs of the unique and changing

Perspective 6–9

Integration at
Carolinas Healthcare
System

Carolinas Healthcare System (CHS), once a lone public hospital, is now a regional system overseen by the Charlotte/Mecklenburg Hospital Authority. It is the fourth largest hospital system in America. CHS owns 7 acute care hospitals, a physician network that includes 63 different practices, 6 behavioral health centers, 3 rehab centers, a retirement community, 8 nursing homes, and MedCenter Air, with 2 Bell 230 helicopters and 4 fixed-wing planes (3 Beechcraft Super King Air 200s and one Cessna Citation V Jet). In addition, CHS is the largest not-for-profit hospital management company in America, managing 13 hospitals in 7 counties.

CHS's flagship hospital is the 777-bed Carolinas Medical Center, with eight programs of excellence: Carolinas Heart Institute, Blumenthal Cancer Center, Level I Trauma Center, Carolinas Neuroscience and Spine Institute, the Children's Hospital, Carolinas Orthopedics Institute, the Women's Institute, and Carolinas Transplant Center.

CHS owned an HMO as a way to protect its significant Medicaid business but it proved to be unprofitable and was divested in 2000. CHS has 17,000 employees, serves more than 2 million patients a year, and reported net income of $278.8 million on net patient revenue of $2.4 billion in 2003.

CHS ownership includes:

Carolinas Medical Center
Carolinas Medical Center-Mercy
Carolinas Medical Center-Pineville
Carolinas Medical Center-University
Anson Community Hospital
Avery Health Care System
Charles A. Cannon Jr. Memorial Hospital
Blue Ridge HealthCare System
Grace Hospital
Valdese Hospital
Roper St. Francis Healthcare, Roper Hospital
Roper Berkeley Day Hospital
Bon Secours St. Francis Hospital
Roper Rehabilitation Hospital
Cleveland County HealthCare System
Cleveland Regional Medical Center
Crawley Memorial Hospital
Kings Mountain Hospital
Lincoln Medical Center
Union Regional Medical Center
Amethyst at Scotland Memorial Hospital
Behavioral Health Center at Kings Mountain
   Hospital

CMC-Randolph
First Step at Union Regional Medical Center
Grace Center for Behavioral Health
Horizons at Carolinas Medical Center-Mercy
Carolinas Integrative Health
Carolinas Medical Center-NorthCross
Carolinas Sports Performance Center

Rehabilitation Services
Carolinas Physical Therapy Network
Charlotte Institute of Rehabilitation
CMC-Mercy Rehabilitation Center

Post-Acute Care
Cannon Nursing Center
Cleveland Pines Nursing Center
College Pines Nursing Center
Grace Ridge Retirement Community
Grace Heights Nursing Center
Huntersville Oaks
Lillie Bennett Nursing Center
Sardis Oaks
Smith Nursing Center

Source: Lori Johnston, "Weathering Health Care Turmoil: Carolinas Healthcare CEO Harry Nurkin Thinks Toughest Challenge Lies Ahead," *Charlotte Business Journal* (October 6, 2000), pp. 3, 70; Barbara Kirchheimer, "Back to Basics: Carolinas Healthcare System Is Looking to Divest Its Money-losing HMO Business," *Modern Healthcare* 30, no. 45 (October 30, 2000), pp. 10–12; and CHS website (www.carolinas.org).

Exhibit 6–18: Vertical and Horizontal Integration Combination Strategy

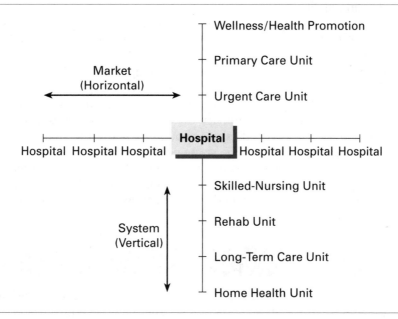

Exhibit 6–19: Vision of Strategy Combinations and Phases

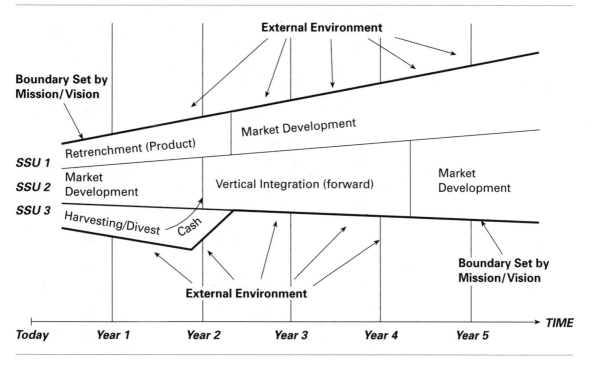

situation. Strategic management is a continuous process of assessment and decision making.

The decision logic for the formulation of the strategic plan was illustrated in Exhibit 6–2. At this point, it would be useful to return to Exhibits 6–2 and 6–4 to review the complete strategy formulation process. After all the strategy formulation alternatives have been selected, creation of a strategy map showing the selected directional, adaptive, market entry, and competitive strategies together will help ensure their consistency and fit. In addition, as a review, Exhibit 6–20 provides summary definitions and examples of all of the strategic alternatives. However, it is not enough to know the strategic logic and range of strategic alternatives. The strategic alternative (or set of alternatives) should be selected that best meets the requirements of the external environment, strengths and weaknesses of the organization, and the directional strategies. Chapter 7 will discuss methods for evaluating the strategic alternatives presented in this chapter.

Summary and Conclusions

This chapter introduces a hierarchy of strategic alternatives as a strategic thinking map for strategic planning. There are several types of strategies, and within each type, several strategic alternatives are available to health care organizations. In addition, there is a general sequential decision logic in the strategy formulation process. First, directional strategies must be articulated through the organization's mission, vision, values, and goals. Second, adaptive strategies are identified, evaluated, and selected. The adaptive strategies are central to strategy formulation and delineate how the organization will expand, contract, or maintain the scope of operations. Expansion strategies include diversification, vertical integration, market development, product development, and penetration. Contraction strategies include divestiture, liquidation, harvesting, and retrenchment. Finally, maintenance of scope strategies include enhancement and status quo.

The third type of strategic decision concerns the market entry strategies. Expansion and maintenance of scope strategies call for a method to carry out the strategy in the marketplace. Therefore, some method for entering or gaining access to that market is required. Market entry strategies include acquisitions and mergers, internal development and internal ventures, alliances and joint ventures, licensing, and venture capital investments. Any of the market entry strategies may be used to carry out an expansion or maintenance of scope adaptive strategy.

The fourth category of strategy includes the competitive strategies. Competitive strategies specify strategic posture of the organization and position the products and services vis-à-vis competitors. The strategic posture should be well thought through by strategic leadership. Strategic posture specifies the organization/market relationship and provides decision and culture guidelines for management. Strategic postures that may be adopted by an organization include

Exhibit 6–20: Definition and Examples of the Strategic Alternatives

Strategy	Definition	Example
Adaptive Strategies		
Related Diversification	Adding new related product or service categories. Often requires the establishment of a new division	Kimberly-Clark designed a Kleenex Anti-Viral tissue that claims to kill 99.9 of cold and flu viruses
Unrelated Diversification	Adding new unrelated product or service categories. Typically requires the establishment of a new division	Sam's Club, a division of Arkansas-based Wal-Mart Stores Inc., will offer group health insurance plans to small businesses beginning in Tennessee and nine other states nationwide
Forward Vertical Integration	Adding new members along the distribution channel (toward an earlier stage) for present products and services or controlling the flow of patients from one institution to another	Community Memorial Hospital (New York) organized 120-bed Crouse Community Center and a 40-bed skilled-nursing facility at Community Memorial to enable the hospital to discharge patients requiring long-term care to facilities offering an appropriate level of care
Backward Vertical Integration	Adding new members along the distribution channel (toward a later stage) for present products and services or controlling the flow of patients from one institution to another	The Children's Hospital of Philadelphia has opened a number of primary care centers (clinics) throughout the city
Market Development	Introducing present products or services into new geographic markets or to new segments within a present geographic market	HEALTHSOUTH Corporation contracted to manage an inpatient rehabilitation hospital and ambulatory surgical center in Saudi Arabia
Product Development	Improving present products or services or extending the present product line	Becton, Dickinson and Company developed safety-engineered syringes, needles, and blood-collection devices designed to prevent accidental needle-sticks
Penetration	Seeking to increase market share for present products or services in present markets through marketing efforts (promotion, channels, or price)	Promotional efforts of New York dermatologist Dr. Zizmor to increase market share have become a well-known cultural phenomenon in New York City
Divestiture	Selling an operating unit or division to another organization. Typically, the unit will continue in operation	Osteopathic Medical Center of Texas in Fort Worth negotiates to sell its clinics while they hope new potential bidders will buy the closed hospital

Exhibit 6–20: (cont'd)

Strategy	Definition	Example
Adaptive Strategies		
Liquidation	Selling all or part of the organization's assets (facilities, inventory, equipment, and so on) in order to obtain cash. The purchaser may use the assets in a variety of ways and businesses	Needing less corporate office space, Unity Health System sold its expansive headquarters in a St. Louis suburb
Harvesting	Products or services typically in late stages of the product life cycle (late maturity and decline) where industry-wide revenues are expected to decline. These products or services will ultimately be discontinued but may generate revenue for some time. Few new resources are allocated to these areas	Glaxo Wellcome continues to sell Imitrex (intended to relieve migraine) while marketing its Amerge (a more potent receptor agonist but designed to do the same thing). Amerge, in time, will end the Imitrex product life cycle
Retrenchment	Reducing the scope of operations, redefining the target market, cutting geographic coverage, reducing the segments served, or reducing the product line	After financial losses, Hillcrest Health Care System in Tulsa sold three of its five health care facilities, but remained in the Tulsa market on a smaller, more focused basis
Enhancement	Seeking to improve operations within present product or service categories through quality programs, increasing flexibility, increasing efficiency, speed of delivery, and so on	1st Medical Network, which covers 650,000 patients, is planning to create a not-for-profit health care quality institute that will use the PPO's database – amounting to 1.7 million claims and growing – as the raw material for utilization review research
Status Quo	Seeking to maintain relative market share within a market	Many public health departments that operate clinics are using a status quo strategy (wait and see what happens) until the impact of managed-care, system integration, and other reforms are clearer
Market Entry Strategies		
Acquisition	Strategy to grow through the purchase of an existing organization, unit of an organization, or a product/service	Kansas-based LabOne Inc. has completed acquisition of the core laboratory run by the Health Alliance of Greater Cincinnati for $38.5 million in cash

Exhibit 6–20: (*cont'd*)

Strategy	Definition	Example
Market Entry Strategies		
Licensing	Acquiring or providing an asset (technology, market, equipment, etc.) through contract	GlaxoSmithKline's Pennsylvania-based North American Consumer Healthcare division has agreed to pay Switzerland's Roche Holdings Inc. $100 million for the rights to sell an obesity drug over the counter in the US
Venture Capital Investment	Financial investment in an organization in order to participate in its growth or receipt of venture capital for startup or expansion	Rightfield Solutions LLC received $4.2 million from private investors to develop an interactive patient education software program called *Emmi*
Merger	Combining two (or more) organizations through mutual agreement to form a single new organization	Sanofi-Synthelabo merges with Aventis to create Sanofi-Aventis, the third largest pharmaceutical company in the world
Alliance	Formation of a formal partnership	The West Central Ohio Regional Healthcare Alliance is a network of allied community hospitals with a shared vision
Joint Venture	Combination of the resources of two or more organizations to accomplish a designated task	The University of Pittsburgh Medical Center Health System and South Hills Health System created a joint venture for providing home health in Western Pennsylvania called UPMC South Hills Health System Home Health
Internal Development	Products or services developed internally using the organization's own resources	Albany Medical Center, a traditional hospital, developed a primary care network using internal resources
Internal Venture	Establishment of an independent entity within an organization to develop products or services	Tenet Healthcare Corporation formed an Internet-based e-learning company to provide educational opportunities for Tenet employees and health care professionals
Competitive Strategies		
Defender	Focus on a narrow market with limited number of products or services and aggressively defend this segment through pricing or differentiation	Suffolk County Department of Health emphasizes differentiating its traditional public health services such as its series of weight management classes for diabetics

Exhibit 6–20: (*cont'd*)

Strategy	Definition	Example
Competitive Strategies		
Prospector	Continuously seek out new products and new markets	St. Jude Children's Research Hospital uses an online auction to raise funds for the not-for-profit hospital
Analyzer	Balance market defense in some markets with selectively entering a limited number of markets or products	Baldwin Area Medical Center (Wisconsin) defends its traditional health services but also has entered selected "complementary medicine" markets such as acupuncture and massage therapy
Cost leadership	Low-cost/price strategy directed toward entire market	Roche pharmaceuticals incorporated the latest technologies and production processes in its Sisseln, Switzerland plant in order to be the global cost leader in the production of vitamin E
Differentiation	Development of unique product/service features directed toward entire market	Phoenix's Good Samaritan Regional Medical Center differentiated its hospital by constructing a 12,500 square foot outdoor "healing garden" to help patients relax as they await treatment or recover from surgery
Focus – Cost Leadership	Low-cost/price strategy directed toward a particular market segment	Metro Med Inc., a physician practice management company, emphasizes cost leadership through group purchasing agreements for a variety of medical devices
Focus – Differentiation	Development of unique product/service features directed toward a particular market segment	Primary stroke centers specializing in the diagnosis, treatment, and prevention of strokes; pain management clinics designed to contain both acute and chronic pain

defender, analyzer, prospector, or reactor (although the latter usually indicates the lack of a strategy). In addition, there are the positioning strategies (often called generic strategies). These include cost leadership and differentiation, both of which can be applied as marketwide strategies or focus strategies (a market segment strategy). Each of the generic strategies places different demands on the organization and requires unique resources, competencies, and capabilities.

The strategy formulation decision logic provides a sequence for making the strategic decisions. However, the selected strategic alternatives must be viewed together to ensure their fit and consistency. In addition, it is unlikely that a single strategy will suffice for an organization. Several strategic alternatives may have to be adopted and used in combination. For instance, one service category may require market development whereas a different service category may require harvesting. One division may be a defender positioned as a cost leader and another may be a prospector pursuing differentiation. Furthermore, several strategic alternatives may be seen as phases or sequences in a broader strategic shift.

Key Terms and Concepts in Strategic Management

Acquisition
Adaptive Strategy
Alliance
Analyzer Strategic Posture
Backward Vertical Integration
Combination Strategy
Competitive Strategy
Concentric Diversification
Conglomerate Diversification
Contraction of Scope Strategy
Cooperation Strategy
Corporate-Level Strategy
Cost Leadership
Defender Strategic Posture
Development Strategy
Differentiation
Diversification
Divestiture

Divisional Strategy
Ends–Means Chain
Enhancement
Expansion of Scope Strategy
Focused Factory
Focus Strategy
Forward Vertical Integration
Feneric Strategy
Harvesting
Horizontal Integration
Implementation Strategy
Internal Development
Internal Venture
Joint Venture
Licensing
Liquidation
Maintenance of Scope Strategy
Market Development

Market Entry Strategy
Marketwide Generic Strategy
Merger
Penetration Strategy
Positioning Strategy
Product Development
Prospector Strategic Posture
Purchase Strategy
Reactor Strategic Posture
Related Diversification
Retrenchment
Status Quo
Strategic Posture
Strategy Formulation
Unrelated Diversification
Venture Capital Investment
Vertical Integration

QUESTIONS FOR CLASS DISCUSSION

1. What four types of strategies make up the strategy formulation process? Describe the role each plays in developing a strategic plan.
2. Why are the directional strategies both a part of situational analysis and a part of strategy formulation?
3. How is strategy formulation related to situational analysis?
4. Name and describe the expansion, contraction, and maintenance of scope strategies. Which of the adaptive strategies are corporate and which are division level? Under what conditions may each be appropriate?
5. Why does the selection of the strategic alternatives create "direction" for the organization?
6. What is the difference between related diversification and product development? Provide examples of each.
7. What is a market-driven or focused factory strategy? Identify some organizations that have employed this type of market development strategy.
8. Many organizations engaged in vertical and horizontal integration in the 1980s and 1990s. At the beginning of the new century the pace of integration slowed. Why have vertical and horizontal integration become less popular for health care organizations?

9. Describe vertical integration in terms of patient flow.
10. Explain the difference between an enhancement strategy and a status quo strategy.
11. How is market development different from product development? Penetration? Provide examples of each.
12. Compare and contrast a divestiture strategy with a liquidation strategy.
13. Which of the market entry strategies provides for the quickest entry into the market? Slowest?
14. What is strategic posture? How does a decision concerning the strategic posture help create decision guidelines for management and affect the organization's culture?
15. Explain Porter's generic strategies. How do they position the organization's products and services in the market?
16. How might a retrenchment strategy and a penetration strategy be linked together? What are some other logical combinations of strategies? How may a combination of strategies be related to vision?
17. Work through Exhibit 6–4, "Strategic Thinking Map – Hierarchy of Strategic Decisions and Alternatives," for several organizations with which you are familiar. Practice selecting different alternatives under each strategy type.

NOTES

1. Warnock Davies, "Understanding Strategy," *Strategy & Leadership* 28, no. 5 (September–October 2000), pp. 25–30.
2. Richard Farson, *Management of the Absurd* (New York: Simon and Schuster, 1996), p. 21.
3. For example, see John C. Peirce, "The Paradox of Physicians and Administrators in Health Care Organizations," *Health Care Management Review* 25, no. 1 (winter 2000), pp. 7–28; John D. Blair and G. Tyge Payne, "The Paradox Prescription: Leading the Medical Group of the Future," *Health Care Management Review* 25, no. 1 (winter 2000), pp. 44–58; and G. Tyge Payne, John D. Blair, and Myron D. Fottler, "The Role of Paradox in Integrated Strategy and Structure Configurations: Exploring Integrated Delivery in Health Care," in John D. Blair, Myron D. Fottler, and Grant T. Savage (eds) *Advances in Health Care Management* (New York: Elsevier Science, 2000), pp. 109–141.
4. Chris Zook and James Allen, "Growth Outside the Core," *Harvard Business Review* 81, no. 12 (2003), pp. 66–73.
5. Jay Greene, "Diversification, Take Two," *Modern Healthcare* 23, no. 28 (1993), pp. 28–32.
6. Leslie E. Palich, Laura B. Cardinal, and C. Chet Miller, "Curvilinearity in the Diversification–Performance Linkage: An Examination of Over

Three Decades of Research," *Strategic Management Journal* 21, no. 2 (February 2000), pp. 155–174.
7. Ibid.
8. Myron D. Fottler, Grant T. Savage, and John D. Blair, "The Future of Integrated Delivery Systems: A Consumer Perspective," in John D. Blair, Myron D. Fottler, and Grant T. Savage (eds) *Advances in Health Care Management* (New York: Elsevier Science, 2000), pp. 15–32.
9. Ibid.
10. Gloria J. Bazzoli, Stephen M. Shortell, Nicole Dubbs, Cheeling Chan, and Peter Kralovec, "A Taxonomy of Health Networks and Systems: Bringing Order Out of Chaos," *Health Services Research* 33, no. 6 (1999), pp. 1683–1717.
11. Gloria J. Bazzoli, Benjamin Chan, Stephen M. Shortell, and Thomas D'Aunno, "The Financial Performance of Hospitals Belonging to Health Networks and Systems," *Inquiry* 37, no. 3 (2000), pp. 234–252.
12. VHA, Inc. and Deloitte & Touche LLP, *Health Care 2000: A Strategic Assessment of the Health Care Environment in the United States* (Irving, TX, and Detroit, MI: VHA, Inc. and Deloitte & Touche, LLP, 2000), p. 65.
13. Stephen S. Mick and Douglas A. Conrad, "The Decision to Integrate Vertically in Health Care

Organizations," *Hospital & Health Services Administration* 33, no. 3 (fall 1988), p. 352.

14. Fottler, Savage, and Blair, "The Future of Integrated Delivery Systems," p. 18.

15. Regina E. Herzlinger, *Market-Driven Health Care: Who Wins, Who Loses in the Transformation of America's Largest Service Industry* (Reading, MA: Addison-Wesley Publishing Company, 1997), p. xxi.

16. E. Gardner, "Baptist Uses Expansion Alliances to Bypass Mayo Jacksonville Beachhead," *Modern Healthcare* 20, no. 32 (August 13, 1990), pp. 34–39.

17. Mick and Conrad, "The Decision to Integrate Vertically," p. 348.

18. Charles L. Breindel, "Nongrowth Strategies and Options in Health Care," *Hospital & Health Services Administration* 33, no. 1 (spring 1988), p. 42.

19. Larry Selden and Geoffrey Colvin, "M&A Needn't Be a Loser's Game," *Harvard Business Review* 81, no. 6 (2003), p. 75.

20. Dennis Carey (Moderator), "A CEO Roundtable on Making Mergers Succeed," *Harvard Business Review* 78, no. 3 (May–June 2000), pp. 145–154.

21. Bazzoli, Chan, Shortell, and D'Aunno, "The Financial Performance of Hospitals Belonging to Health Networks and Systems," pp. 234–252.

22. Joanne Spetz, Shannon Mitchell, and Jean Ann Seago, "The Growth of Multihospital Firms in California," *Health Affairs* 19, no. 6 (2000), pp. 224–230.

23. Jeffrey F. Allen, "Franchise Issues – Exclusivity of Territory," *Inquiry* 39, no. 1 (2000), pp. 8–11.

24. Ibid.

25. Edward B. Roberts and Charles A. Berry, "Entering New Businesses: Selecting Strategies for Success," *Sloan Management Review* 25 (spring 1985), p. 7.

26. Shattuck Hammond Partners/Pricewaterhouse-Coopers Securities, *Healthcare Venture Capital Report: Third Quarter 2000 Results* (PricewaterhouseCoopers, 2001), pp. 1–11 (and http://www.pwchealth.com/venture.html).

27. Sharon Roggy and Ron Gority, "Bridging the Visions of Competing Catholic Health Care Systems," *Health Care Strategic Management* 11, no. 7 (1993), pp. 16–19.

28. Thomas P. Weil, "Management of Integrated Delivery Systems in the Next Decade," *Health Care Management Review* 25, no. 3 (summer 2000), pp. 9–23.

29. Ibid.

30. Howard S. Zuckerman and Arnold D. Kaluzny, "Strategic Alliances in Health Care: The Challenges of Cooperation," *Frontiers of Health Services Management* 7, no. 3 (1991), p. 4.

31. Michael E. Porter, *The Competitive Advantage of Nations* (New York: Free Press, 1990), p. 65.

32. Seungwha (Andy) Chung, Harbir Singh, and Kyungmook Lee, "Complementarity, Status Similarity, and Social Capital as Drivers of Alliance Formation," *Strategic Management Journal* 21, no. 1 (January 2000), pp. 1–22.

33. Toby E. Stuart, "Interorganizational Alliances and the Performance of Firms: A Study of Growth and Innovation Rates in a High-Technology Industry," *Strategic Management Journal* 21, no. 8 (August 2000), pp. 791–811.

34. Joel A. C. Baum, Tony Calabrese, and Brian S. Silverman, "Don't Go It Alone: Network Composition and Startups' Performance in Canadian Biotechnology," *Strategic Management Journal* 21, no. 3 (March 2000), pp. 276–294.

35. Leonard H. Friedman and James B. Goes, "The Timing of Medical Technology Acquisition: Strategic Decision Making in Turbulent Environments," *Journal of Healthcare Management* 45, no. 5 (September–October 2000), pp. 317–330.

36. Sandra Pelfrey and Barbara A. Theisen, "Joint Ventures in Health Care," *Journal of Nursing Administration* 19, no. 4 (April 1989), p. 39.

37. Lawton R. Burns, Gloria J. Bazzoli, Linda Dynan, and Douglas R. Wholey, "Impact of HMO Market Structure on Physician–Hospital Strategic Alliances," *Health Services Research* 35, no. 1 (April 2000), pp. 101–132 and Michael A. Morrisey, Jeffery Alexander, Lawton R. Burns, and Victoria Johnson, "The Effects of Managed Care on Physician and Clinical Integration in Hospitals," *Medical Care* 37, no. 4 (1999), pp. 350–361.

38. Roberts and Berry, "Entering New Businesses," p. 6.

39. Pelfrey and Theisen, "Joint Ventures in Health Care," pp. 39–41.

40. Ibid., p. 42.

41. Donna Malvey, "Hospital–Physician Joint Ventures: Unstable Strategies for a Rapidly Changing Environment," Unpublished Working Paper, School of Health Related Professions, University of Alabama at Birmingham (1994).

42. James Bamford, David Ernst, and David G. Fubini, "Launching a World-Class Joint Venture," *Harvard Business Review* 82, no. 2 (2004), pp. 90–100.

43. Raymond E. Miles, Charles C. Snow, Alan D. Meyer, and Henry J. Coleman, Jr., "Organizational Strategy, Structure, and Process," *Academy of Management Review* 3, no. 3 (1978), pp. 546–562.

44. Monique Forte, James J. Hoffman, Bruce T. Lamont, and Erich N. Brockmann, "Organizational Form

and Environment: An Analysis of Between-Form and Within-Form Responses to Environmental Change," *Strategic Management Journal* 21, no. 7 (July 2000), pp. 753–773.

45. Miles, Snow, Meyer, and Coleman, Jr., "Organizational Strategy, Structure, and Process," pp. 546–562.

46. Forte, Hoffman, Lamont, and Brockmann, "Organizational Form and Environment," pp. 753–773.

47. For a review of research on Porter's generic strategies see Colin Campbell-Hunt, "What Have We Learned About Generic Competitive Strategy? A Meta-Analysis," *Strategic Management Journal* 21, no. 2 (February 2000), pp. 127–154.

48. Michael E. Porter, *Competitive Strategy* (New York: Free Press, 1980), p. 35.

49. Ibid.

ADDITIONAL READINGS

Christensen, Clayton M. and Michael E. Raynor, *The Innovator's Solution: Creating and Sustaining Successful Growth* (Boston, MA: Harvard Business School Press, 2003). It is a paradox of business history that yesterday's story of success is tomorrow's story of failure. Although virtually everyone favors innovation, the truth is that neither business nor health care is very good at it. Most of what is called innovation is really just tinkering with existing products and services. The authors skillfully distinguish between disruptive and sustaining innovations. Instead of tinkering with existing products and services, bold leaps of creativity are needed to create entirely new markets.

Hitt, Michael A., Jeffery S. Harrison, and R. Duane Ireland, *Creating Value through Mergers and Acquisitions* (Oxford: Oxford University Press, 2001). The authors assert that acquisition strategies are among the most important corporate-level strategies in the new millennium. They take the reader step by step through the merger and acquisition (M&A) process, starting with the elements of a successful merger, due diligence to ensure that the target firm is sound and fits well with the acquiring firm, and the financing of mergers and acquisitions. They move on to explore finding partners/targets for acquisitions that have complementary resources and finding partners with which integration and synergy can be achieved. Finally, they discuss the potential hazards found in M&As and how to avoid them, how to conduct successful cross-border acquisitions, and how to ensure that ethical principles are not breached during the process.

Pablo, Amy L. and Mansour Javidan (eds) *Mergers and Acquisitions: Creating Integrative Knowledge* (Malden, MA: Blackwell Publishing Company, 2004). Virtually every industry, including health care, has experienced consolidation over the past several decades. However, much remains to be learned about mergers and acquisitions. The contributors to this book review successful and unsuccessful mergers and acquisitions and draw upon scholarly research to identify lessons that can be learned. Attention is given to the important processes involved in the successful implementation of mergers and acquisitions.

Wilson, Ian, *The Subtle Art of Strategy* (Westport, CT: Praeger Publishing, 2004). The author looks at examples where strategic planning has failed and attempts to understand the reasons for the failures. Using examples and illustrations, Wilson reformulates strategic planning as a long-term, holistic art form. The book provides a different and interesting way of thinking about strategy and strategic management that is both practical and theoretically sound.

Zook, Chris, *Beyond the Core: Expand Your Market Without Abandoning Your Roots* (Boston, MA: Harvard Business School Press, 2004). Growth is an imperative. However, growth involves risks. Only about one quarter of growth initiatives succeed. Most of the business disasters of the past five years were growth initiatives gone awry. Most enduring performers succeeded by focusing on one or two well-defined dominant core abilities. Many organizations fail because they prematurely abandon their core to chase after a hot topic or fad.

Zuckerman, Alan M. and Russell C. Coile, Jr., *Competing on Excellence: Healthcare Strategies for a Consumer Driven Market* (Chicago: Health Administration Press, 2003). Consumer-driven health care organizations gain market share by demonstrating outstanding clinical outcomes and customer service. This book serves as a guide for developing excellence in health care operations. Principles, programs, and strategies for making clinical programs excellent are provided.

7 *CHAPTER*

Evaluation of Alternatives and Strategic Choice

"Getting the facts is the key to good decision making. Every mistake that I made – and we all make mistakes – came because I didn't take the time. I didn't drive hard enough. I wasn't smart enough to get the facts."

Charles F. Knight
Chairman, Emerson Electric

Introductory Incident

Analytical Tools for Strategy Decisions

The yearly Bain survey of companies found that managers are using more tools than ever to cope with difficult economic times. The typical organization in the survey used 16 tools and relied more than ever on tried and true techniques such as strategic planning, benchmarking, and mission and vision statements. Respondents' choice of tools revealed a clear preference for growth over cost cutting. The message is clear – we are moving ahead, not retrenching. Growth is critical to the control of an organization's destiny.

The determination to find opportunities in economic hard times showed up in the types of tools companies adopted in the most recent survey. Overwhelmingly, senior executives employed tools that helped sharpen strategies and prepared managers for the challenges to growth. Proven techniques such as strategic planning and core competencies received rave reviews – again – for helping companies stay on course.

The survey provides these important tips for successful use of the tools of strategic management:

1. *Get the facts*. All tools, even mission and vision statements, have strengths and weaknesses. It is important to understand all the possible effects of a particular tool. Use available research, talk to managers who have experience using the tools, and do not expect a tool to provide a simple, easy solution. A tool is only as good as the way it is used.

2. *Champion enduring and proven strategies, not fads*. Although advocates of particular tools can

▶

provoke stimulating discussion, they rarely know what is best for a given organization. Managers who promote fads undermine the confidence of employees and generate increased skepticism for any of their programs. One Bain survey respondent explained what makes fads attractive: "It's a fear of being left behind." However, executives should choose tools cautiously and put their reputations behind those that can provide realistic goals and strategic direction. Mission, vision, and value statements have shown through their continued inclusion in the survey that they are more than passing fads.

3. *Choose the best tools for the job.* Managers need a system for selecting, implementing, and integrating the tools and techniques appropriate for their organizations. Before adopting a tool, managers should determine that it helps uncover yet unaddressed customer needs, builds distinctive competencies, and exploits competitor vulnerabilities.

4. *Adapt tools to the organization's system (and not vice versa).* Most tools gain exposure because an advocate touts them. They will point the way to reorient management structures and processes. Often this is not practical. Most organizations use multiple tools – 16 on average. Managers cannot keep rebuilding their organizations around each new tool. Tools come and go, but corporate cultures last. Therefore, the organization's structure, culture and management processes should dictate the way a tool is implemented – not vice versa.

Source: Darrell Rigby, "Management Tools Survey 2003: Usage Up as Companies Strive to Make Headway in Tough Times," *Strategy & Leadership* 31, no. 5 (2003), pp. 4–7.

Learning Objectives

After completing this chapter the student should be able to:

1. Understand the rationale underlying the various strategic thinking maps used to evaluate strategic alternatives.

2. Discuss, evaluate, and select appropriate adaptive strategic alternatives for a health care organization.

3. Discuss, evaluate, and select appropriate market entry strategic alternatives.

4. Discuss, evaluate, and select appropriate strategic posture and generic positioning alternatives.

5. Determine whether selected strategies are consistent, coordinated, and fit the situation.

6. Understand the role of the service delivery and support strategies.

Evaluation of the Alternatives

There are several frameworks or maps that may be used to guide strategic thinking about the appropriate strategic alternatives for an organization. These strategic thinking maps incorporate the results of external and internal analyses, as well as the development of directional strategies. As suggested in the Introductory Incident there are many possible tools for strategy analysis. Thoughtful analysis to understand the internal requirements and external conditions of the strategic alternatives is essential to assure a coherent and integrated strategy.

The strategic thinking maps for evaluating and selecting strategic alternatives are actually constructs or frameworks for helping managers strategically think about the organization and its situation (strengths and weaknesses) relative to the general environment, competitors, and consumers. In other words, the maps help strategic managers work through the variables in their strategic decisions, allowing them to consciously balance organizational motives with community health needs. Thus, market share and revenue issues may be seen in a context of providing health and well-being to real people. However, none of the strategic thinking maps provides a definitive answer to the question of appropriate strategy. None of the frameworks actually makes the strategic choice. Rather, the maps aid in organizing and demonstrating relationships inherent in the situation. The various strategic thinking maps help to structure the thought processes of decision makers.

Although the evaluation of strategic thinking maps fine-tunes the manager's perspective and organizes thinking, ultimately, the strategic manager must make the decision. Strategic managers need to understand the risks, make judgments, and commit the organization to some course of action. Therefore, the strategic thinking maps cannot be used to obtain "answers," but they can be used to gain perspective and insight into a complex relationship between organization and environment. There is no right answer. As Peter Drucker has pointed out: "It is a choice between alternatives. It is rarely a choice between right and wrong. It is at best a choice between 'almost right' and 'probably wrong' – but much more often a choice between two courses of action neither of which is probably more nearly right than the other."[1] As suggested in Perspective 7–1, in order to have the proper perspective, it is important that strategic managers be involved with customers, vendors, and the organization and talk to people to get a real feel for the culture, competitive advantage, and organizational opportunities and threats.

Evaluation of the Adaptive Strategies

As discussed throughout Chapter 6, once the directional strategies have been developed, consideration is given to the adaptive strategies. The adaptive strategies are central to strategy formulation and are the broadest interpretation of the directional strategies. This level of strategic decision making specifies whether the organization wants to grow (expansion of scope), become smaller (contraction of scope), or remain about the same (maintenance of scope). Once the decision has been made to grow, contract, or remain the same, the methods to accomplish expansion, contraction, or maintenance of scope (diversification, divestiture, enhancement, and so on) must be formulated.

Several constructs help strategic managers think about adaptive strategic decisions. However, as expressed previously, these constructs help show

Perspective 7–1

Managing By
Wandering Around

Tom Peters and Robert Waterman popularized the term "managing by wandering around" (MBWA) in their book *In Search of Excellence*. They found that excellent companies are a vast network of informal, open communications. Getting managers out of their offices to see things for themselves was cited as a major contributor to informal exchanges. Later, Tom Peters and Nancy Austin devoted an entire chapter to the concept in *A Passion for Excellence*. Peters and Austin posit that a major managerial problem is leaders who are out of touch with their people, customers, and vendors. Simple wandering – listening, empathizing, and staying in touch – leads to better communication and "hands-on" problem solving. Being in touch cannot be achieved without being there.

Recently, numerous hospitals are improving their bottom line by performing a contemporary form of MBWA – "executive rounds." John McWhorter of Baylor University Medical Center in Dallas began making executive rounds to improve patient satisfaction. He believes that two major benefits occur for the organization:

1. Executive rounds demonstrate that leadership is committed to listening to patients' and staffs' concerns (which have been reported more frequently and candidly), and
2. Service improvements accrue that might not otherwise have been addressed.

Crystal Haynes, CEO of St. Louis University Hospital, makes rounds to keep her pulse on the life in the wards, to improve satisfaction among the hospital's physicians, patients, and employees, and to let the nursing staff know that she understands the difficulties they face in delivering outstanding patient care. A result has been a decrease in the nursing turnover rate from 20 percent to 15 percent in less than a year.

Partners HealthCare System in Boston used the concept to improve patient safety. "Patient Safety Leadership WalkRounds" are formal rounds of patients at the system's Brigham & Women's Hospital to ask specific questions about adverse events, near misses, and factors that might have led to the events. The information gathered is used to identify quality improvement initiatives.

In 2003, Abington Memorial Hospital won the American Hospital Association's Quest for Quality prize and the John Eisenberg Award for its safety improvement initiatives that were a result of "rounding." CEO John Kelley is a strong advocate of executive rounds because he believes that detachment from clinical processes has grown as layers of management have increased and managers spend more on time managing.

Source: Thomas J. Peters and Robert H. Waterman, Jr., *In Search of Excellence* (New York: Harper & Row Publishers, 1982); Tom Peters and Nancy Austin, *A Passion for Excellence: The Leadership Difference* (New York: Warner Books, 1985); and Bonnie Darves, "Executive Rounds Improve Performance, Boost Patient Satisfaction," *COR Healthcare Strategist* (December 2003), pp. 1, 17–19.

relationships of the organization to its markets and competitors; they do not make the decision. Methods to evaluate the adaptive strategies include:

- threats, opportunities, weaknesses, and strengths (TOWS) matrix;
- product life cycle (PLC) analysis;
- Boston Consulting Group (BCG) portfolio analysis;
- extended portfolio matrix analysis;
- strategic position and action evaluation (SPACE); and
- program evaluation.

For the most part, any of these methods may be used to evaluate the adaptive strategic alternatives for all types of health care organizations – for-profit as well as not-for-profit. As illustrated in Perspective 7–2, the strategic thinking requirements and resultant strategies are often quite similar for both types of institutions.

Because strategy formulation is a matter of "fitting" the organization to its environment, each of these evaluation methods uses the organization's external opportunities and threats and internal factors as inputs to the strategic thinking. The competitively relevant threats, opportunities, weaknesses, and strengths constitute the *strategic assumptions* on which strategic decision making will be grounded. Although the strategic assumptions are based on extensive information gathering and analysis, managers cannot always be certain that the assumptions are correct. Therefore, it is often useful to have more than one set of likely strategic assumptions, particularly regarding the external environment. This provides several "backdrops" or contexts for the formulation process and facilitates strategic thinking. Depending on the environmental analysis method used, several sets of simple trend, expert opinion, stakeholder, scenario, or competitor analysis (see Chapters 2 and 3) assumptions may be generated to evaluate strategy. For example, in evaluating the adaptive strategic alternatives, several possible scenarios about the external environment (refer to Exhibit 2–9) or service area structure analyses (refer to Exhibit 3–5) may be used as a basis for evaluating alternatives. Different strategic assumptions can provide the basis for contingency plans should the assumptions prove to be wrong or change over time. This strategic thinking process is important because each organization is unique and in a unique situation. As indicated in Perspective 7–3, copy cat strategies or following the crowd may be inappropriate and ineffective.

Perspective 7–2

For-Profits and Not-for-Profits Pursue Similar Strategies

Of particular significance in the development of hospital systems is the blurring of differences between investor-owned systems and not-for-profit systems. With the exception of large public hospital systems (and even here the distinctions are fading), the not-for-profit systems are behaving more like investor-owned systems in terms of increasing attention given to balance sheets, the external environment, and competitive strategies. Not-for-profit systems have adopted corporate models, established for-profit subsidiaries, and narrowed the profitability gap when compared to investor-owned systems. Meanwhile, the role of the large investor-owned system has been diminishing. Recognizing that health care is a local business and that survival depends on dominance in local and regional markets, investor-owned systems are no longer focusing on national competition. Instead, they are pursuing growth strategies similar to not-for-profit systems. Investor-owned systems are concentrating on smaller local and regional markets and are abandoning markets where they are poor competitors. These systems have streamlined, reorganized, and refinanced, plus divested themselves of unprofitable acquisitions.

Source: Donna Malvey, PhD, College of Public Health, University of South Florida.

Perspective 7–3

Academic Health Centers: The Phenomenon of Strategy Similarity

The health care environment poses numerous threats and challenges to academic health centers (AHCs). Whether through market forces or governmental reforms, AHCs face a marketplace in which managed care pressures demand more cost-effective, high-quality care to compete. Yet recent research suggests that many AHCs are implementing strategies that are similar to those used by local, and often competing, community hospitals and regional systems.

AHCs are pursuing expansion strategies that involve building primary care physician practices and adding hospitals through cooperative and collaborative arrangements such as mergers and affiliations. However, such "copy-cat" strategies are counterintuitive to strategic planning because of differences in missions and environmental challenges. AHCs have multiple missions that are very different from other hospitals and systems, including teaching, research, patient care, and providing more than 40 percent of the indigent care in the United States. Because of multiple missions, AHCs produce costly clinical services that are inconsistent with the demand for less expensive services in today's competitive health care environment.

Drastic cuts in government funding have undermined educational and research missions. Furthermore, AHCs have different strengths and weaknesses and confront different threats and opportunities than their nonacademic counterparts. For example, AHCs have enjoyed a privileged place atop the health care pyramid as a niche provider of very expensive tertiary services. However, more recently the majority of services provided by AHCs are available elsewhere, such as local community hospitals and specialty private medical practices. With such dissimilarities, why are AHCs imitating the strategies of their nonacademic counterparts? What is the motivation?

One explanation is that AHCs are copying strategies because others are copying strategies as well. After all, the health care literature repeatedly recommends the same generic strategies such as "build your own system," "find a partner," and "add primary care capabilities." Health care executives are provided with what might be called a "cookbook" method of strategic planning. In addition, it is possible that a "one size fits all" strategic approach results from many of the AHCs using the same consultants. Another possible explanation is that AHCs simply may be following the leader. Because hospitals that are out in front strategically tend to have status, reputation, and influence over other hospitals and systems, these other hospitals and systems mimic the leaders' behavior.

To behave strategically, AHCs must ensure that assumptions about the environment, their missions, and core competencies are integral in the planning process. Recent evidence suggests that some AHCs are forging unique strategic paths that reflect their distinct missions and environments. New Mexico Health Sciences Center, for example, has implemented population-based strategies that are aimed at generating strong and enduring AHC–community alliances while simultaneously enhancing economic viability.

Source: Donna Malvey, PhD, College of Public Health, University of South Florida.

TOWS Matrix

Within a framework provided by the mission, vision, values, and goals, the internal and external factors may be combined to develop and evaluate specific adaptive strategic alternatives using a TOWS (threats, opportunities, weaknesses, strengths)

matrix.[2] As illustrated in Exhibit 7–1, the internal strengths and weaknesses that result in competitive advantages and disadvantages for the organization are summarized on the horizontal axis and the external environmental opportunities and threats are summarized on the vertical axis. The *TOWS matrix* indicates four strategic conditions that the organization may encounter. Adaptive strategic alternatives may be developed by matching the organization's competitively relevant strengths with external opportunities, strengths with threats, competitively relevant weaknesses with opportunities, and weaknesses with threats.

Adaptive strategic alternatives are suggested by the interactions of the four sets of variables. In this example, the primary concern is the adaptive strategic alternatives, but this analysis could also be applied to the development of any type of strategy.[3] In practice, particularly in open discussion sessions, some of the alternatives developed through the TOWS matrix may be adaptive, market entry, competitive, or value adding service delivery and support strategies.

Exhibit 7–1: *TOWS Matrix*

	List Internal Strengths (competitive advantages) 1. 2. 3. 4.	List Internal Weaknesses (competitive disadvantages) 1. 2. 3. 4.
List External Opportunities 1. 2. 3. 4.	**4** ***Future Quadrant*** • Related Diversification • Vertical Integration • Market Development • Product Development • Penetration	**2** ***Internal Fix-It Quadrant*** • Retrenchment • Enhancement • Market Development • Product Development • Vertical Integration • Related Diversification
List External Threats 1. 2. 3. 4.	**3** ***External Fix-It Quadrant*** • Related Diversification • Unrelated Diversification • Market Development • Product Development • Enhancement • Status Quo	**1** ***Survival Quadrant*** • Unrelated Diversification • Divestiture • Liquidation • Harvesting • Retrenchment

Source: Adapted from Heinz Weihrich, "The TOWS Matrix: A Tool for Situational Analysis," *Long Range Planning* 15, no. 2 (1982), p. 60. Reprinted by permission of Elsevier Science Ltd., The Boulevard, Langford Lane, Kidlington OS5 1GB, UK.

The Survival Quadrant

An organization faced with both external threats and significant internal weaknesses that result in competitive disadvantages is in a difficult position. Because the organization must attempt to minimize both weaknesses and threats, this quadrant is often referred to as the *survival quadrant*. Obviously, the organization must respond to this situation with an explicit strategy. Adaptive alternatives that may be pursued by an organization in this situation include unrelated diversification (if financial resources are available), divestiture, liquidation, harvesting, and retrenchment. For instance, a preferred provider organization may have the internal weaknesses of declining enrollments and an image of declining quality (both significant competitive disadvantages) in the face of growing external threats from health maintenance organizations, accountable health plans, and industry-wide consolidation. Such conditions may suggest retrenchment.

The Internal Fix-It Quadrant

The *internal fix-it quadrant* indicates that managers should attempt to minimize competitively relevant internal weaknesses and maximize external opportunities. Typically, an organization will recognize an external opportunity but have a competitive disadvantage that prevents it from taking advantage of the opportunity. Therefore, this quadrant is referred to as the internal fix-it quadrant.

If actions are taken to strengthen the organization (often a value adding action plan), it may be able to pursue the opportunity. Strategies in this quadrant may require two phases (a combination strategy): first, correcting the internal weakness and thus eliminating or reducing the competitive disadvantage; and, second, pursuing the opportunity. Strategic alternatives that are frequently selected in this quadrant include retrenchment, enhancement, market development, product development, vertical integration, and related diversification. For example, a for-profit hospital may have an external opportunity to enter an attractive new market but presently may not have the financial resources to do so (a competitive disadvantage). After addressing this weakness (perhaps by selling additional stock), the opportunity may be pursued (market development).

The External Fix-It Quadrant

In the *external fix-it quadrant*, the organization recognizes that it has significant competitively relevant strengths but that it must deal with external environmental threats. Therefore, managers must attempt to maximize the organization's competitive advantages manifest in its strengths and minimize the external threats. As in the internal fix-it quadrant, strategies in this quadrant may require two phases. Strategies that are often employed in this quadrant include related and unrelated diversification, market development, product development, enhancement, and status quo. For instance, an investor-owned skilled-nursing home with competitive advantages of strong management, financial resources, and customer loyalty may encounter the external threat of a powerful new competitor planning to enter the service area. The nursing home may use a preemptive strategic response by engaging in status quo in the skilled-nursing home segment while using related diversification into domiciliaries and retirement communities to expand its presence in the market.

THE FUTURE QUADRANT

The *future quadrant* represents the best situation for an organization as it attempts to maximize its competitively relative strengths and take advantage of external opportunities. It represents the strategies that the organization will adopt for future growth. Strategies in this quadrant lead from the strengths (competitive advantages) of the organization and use its internal resources to capitalize on the market for its products and services.[4] Typical strategic alternatives that might be selected in this quadrant include related diversification, vertical integration, market development, product development, and penetration. For example, a metropolitan hospital with the competitive advantages of access to technology, economies of scale in purchasing, and capable management may be presented with an external opportunity to initiate affiliations with several rural or specialty hospitals and thus create a more extensive referral system for the hospital (vertical integration).

Product Life Cycle Analysis

Product life cycle (PLC) analysis can be useful in selecting strategic alternatives based on the principle that all products and services go through several distinct phases or stages. These stages relate primarily to the changing nature of the marketplace, the product-development process, and the types of demands made on management. In evaluating product life cycles, the evolution of service category sales and profits (or a surrogate for sales such as the number of subscribers, hospital visits, or competitors) is tracked over time. This evolution will have strategic implications for the organization. A typical PLC and the attributes of each stage are presented in Exhibit 7–2.

Products and services have an introductory stage during which sales are increasing yet profits are negative. In this stage, there are few competitors, prices are usually high, promotion is informative about the product category, and there are limited distribution outlets. In the growth stage, sales and profits are both increasing, and, as a result, competing organizations enter the market to participate in the growth. During this stage, prices are still high but may begin to decline, promotion is directed toward specific brands, and there is rapid growth in the number of outlets.

The maturity stage of the PLC marks the end of rapid growth and the beginning of consolidation. In addition, market segmentation (defining narrower and narrower segments of the market) occurs. In this stage, prices have stabilized or declined, price promotion becomes common, and distribution is widespread.

Exhibit 7–2: The Product Life Cycle

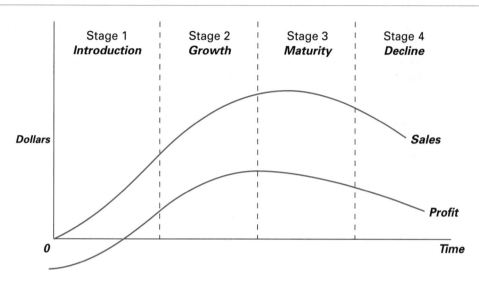

PLC Stage Characteristics

	Introduction	Growth	Maturity	Decline
Sales/Revenue	Low	Rapid growth	Slow growth	Declining
Profits	Negative	Peak levels	High	Low
Competitors	Few	Growing	Many	Declining
Cost/Customer	High	Average	Low	Low
Capital Access	Venture	Equity/debt	Debt/internal	Minimal

Source: Adapted from Philip Kotler and Kevin Lane Keller, *Marketing Management*, 12th edn (2006), p. 332. Reprinted by permission of Simon & Schuster.

In the decline stage, total revenues and profits for the product or service are declining and will likely continue to decline over the long term. Perspective 7–4 describes the PLC for health maintenance organizations.

There are two important questions for strategy formulation when using product life cycles: "In what stage of the life cycle are the organization's products and services?" "How long are the stages (and the life cycle itself) likely to last?"

STAGE OF THE PRODUCT LIFE CYCLE

The stage in the product life cycle for a product or service indicates a likely strategic response and a level of resources that might be committed to a particular product or service. Exhibit 7–3 shows logical strategic alternatives for each stage of the PLC.

LENGTH OF THE PRODUCT LIFE CYCLE

The relevance of the strategies shown in Exhibit 7–3 depends on management's perception of the timing of the cycle. Products and services that management determines have lengthy stages (or a long PLC) will require dramatically different strategies than those that management concludes have short stages or a short PLC. For instance, extensive vertical integration may be justified in the growth stage and even in the mature stage of the PLC if the cycle is judged to be a long one. However, the investment in and commitment to the product required in vertical integration may not be justified when the PLC is viewed as being relatively short.

DETERMINING THE PLC STAGE AND ITS LENGTH

To determine the stage of the PLC, management must use a great deal of judgment. Total service category revenues and profits may be monitored as an initial

---

Perspective 7–4

The Product Life Cycle Concept Applied to Health Maintenance Organizations

The health maintenance organization (HMO) in-dustry is an excellent example of long introductory and growth stages of the product life cycle (PLC). HMOs had an extended introductory period. The first HMO prototype, the Ross-Loos Clinic in Los Angeles, became operational in 1929. Forty years later, in 1970, there were only 33, generally not-for-profit, HMOs in the United States, serving approximately 3 million enrollees.[1]

The boost that pushed HMOs from introduction into growth included the passage of the Health Maintenance Organization and Resources Act of 1974, which provided development funding of over $350 million for ten years.[2] Additionally, the market for HMOs was expanded with the passage of the HMO Act Amendments.

In addition to the federal funding for development and growth, HMOs sought additional capital in the early 1980s. One method to accomplish this was to convert from a not-for-profit to a for-profit HMO. US Healthcare Systems, Inc. (then known as HMO of Pennsylvania), converted to for-profit status in 1981 and obtained a venture capital investment of $3 million from Warburg, Pincus and Co., Inc. Two years later, US Healthcare Systems, Inc., became the first HMO to offer stock to the public and raised $25 million in two public offerings. Others followed suit and for several years HMOs were the darlings of Wall Street as record growth and earnings were reported. Not-for-profit HMOs also sought additional capital to fund growth. Kaiser Permanente Medical Care Program, the country's largest HMO, offered $75 million in tax-exempt bonds. By 1983, there were 280 HMOs serving some 12 million enrollees.

Signs of the shift to maturity were typified by the acquisition of Health-America Corporation by Maxicare Health Plans, Inc., in late 1986. In many parts of the country HMOs were changing hands as the returns began to decrease and the growth phase entrepreneurs and investors pulled out.[3]

By the mid-1990s, many urban markets experienced high managed care penetration signifying local maturity. HMO consolidation in major markets continued and company strategies were typical of market maturity – price competition, extensive channel development, aggressive promotion, and product ▶

differentiation. In addition, few new players were entering the market in these areas. However, as suggested in the bar graph, HMO enrollment in the United States appeared to be in the late growth stage but growth could continue through the end of the decade. Confusing the picture are the rural and nonurban markets that continue to adopt managed care very slowly because of a lack of economies of scale and an insufficient number of providers. In addition, few new players are entering the market in these areas. Overall enrollment shows growth, but hides two separate HMO life cycles that are in different stages – urban maturity, perhaps toward decline, along with rural/nonurban growth.

Americans Move into HMOs

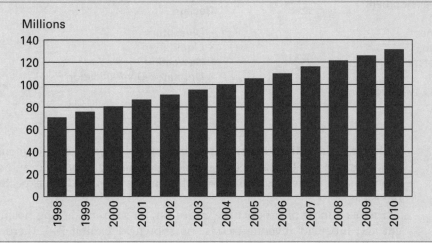

Source: Group Health Administration of America, Interstudy, American Association of Health Plans.

Despite its limitations, PLC analysis is a useful tool for business planning. It provides a framework for assessing existing activities as well as new products/services. The decomposition and critical review of market characteristics in conjunction with the PLC can serve as a guideline for strategy development. A PLC framework is particularly useful for product, marketing, and management strategies. In addition, it can clarify access and types of capital available as well as the intrinsic PLC risk.

In the consideration of new product/service lines, a PLC analysis can help to answer questions about not only whether an activity is attractive for the organization, but also what the best market entry strategy is. Historically, hospitals have developed the businesses or services that they offer. However, development makes sense only if the business is in introductory or growth stages of the life cycle. If the hospital chooses to enter a mature business, it is usually better to joint venture the business with an experienced party or acquire an existing provider. Introducing new products during late maturity or decline carries great risk.

Notes

1. Susanna E. Krentz and Suzanne M. Pilskaln, "Product Life Cycle: Still a Valid Framework for Business Planning," *Topics in Health Care Financing* 15, no. 1 (fall 1988), pp. 47–48.
2. 42 US Code sec. 300e.
3. J. Graham, "Initial Public Offerings Slow as HMOs Fail to Extract Substantial Profits," *Modern Healthcare* 16, no. 13 (1985), p. 62.

Exhibit 7–3: Strategic Choices for Stages of the Product Life Cycle

Stage 1
Introduction

- Market Development
- Product Development

Stage 3
Maturity

- Market Development
- Product Development
- Penetration
- Enhancement
- Status Quo
- Retrenchment
- Divestiture
- Unrelated Diversification

Stage 2
Growth

- Market Development
- Product Development
- Penetration
- Vertical Integration
- Related Diversification

Stage 4
Decline

- Divestiture
- Liquidation
- Harvesting
- Unrelated Diversification

indicator. In addition, information obtained in external environmental analysis concerning technological, social, political, regulatory, economic, and competitive change is valuable in assessing both the current stage and the expected length of the cycle.

The usefulness of product life cycles can be seen in tracking hospital outpatient and inpatient revenue trends. As shown in Exhibit 7–4, there has been a reduction in the percentage of hospital inpatient revenues to total health care revenue since 1993 (and there was an even greater reduction in the 1983 to 1993 period). This decline can be attributed largely to a shift to less costly services, efforts by public and private payors to contain their outlays for health care, and hospital efforts to contain or reduce staff and beds. As a result, outpatient visits, revenues, and the percent of outpatient revenue to total gross revenue have been on the increase. Declines in the percentage share of total revenue coupled with the high level of industry consolidation signals that inpatient services have reached the mature stage of the PLC, whereas outpatient services appear to still be in a growth stage (even though total revenues for both continue to increase). Administrators of a hospital who are considering product/ service mix decisions may initiate a status quo or harvesting strategy for inpatient services and engage in a market development strategy for outpatient services (or related diversification into outpatient services). In addition, hospital administrators should continue to monitor, forecast, and assess these trends because new forces in the environment could change the life cycles or create entirely new life cycles.

PLC may be represented by tracking and forecasting the number of consumers or, in the case of managed care plans, the number of enrollees. For example, as illustrated in Exhibit 7–5, enrollment in indemnity plans, PPOs, and HMOs is a good indicator of the stage of the product life cycle for each. Traditional

Exhibit 7–4: Percent Inpatient and Outpatient Gross Revenue

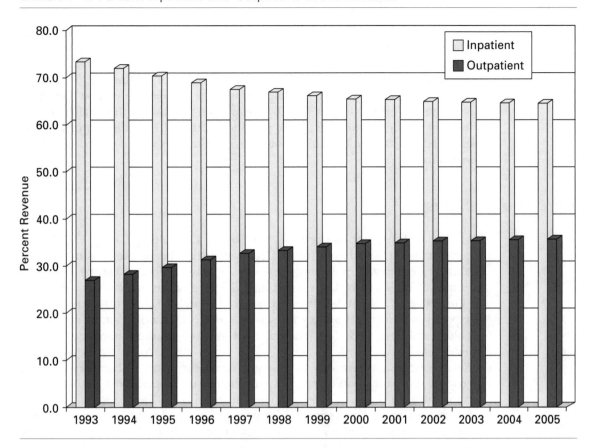

Exhibit 7–5: Indemnity, PPO, and HMO Enrollment

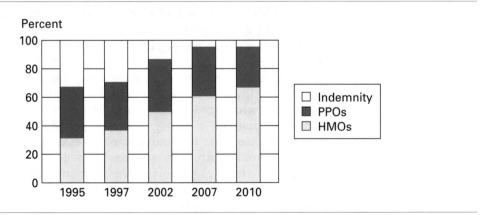

Source: Institute for the future, *Health & Health Care 2010: The Forecast, The Challenge* (San Francisco, Jossey-Bass Publishers, January 2000), p. 43. Reprinted with permission of John Wiley & Sons, Inc.

indemnity health care insurance appears to be in the decline stage of the product life cycle. It is predicted that indemnity plans will increasingly turn into PPOs and continue to decline throughout the period from 2000 to 2010. After a period of fairly stable enrollments (maturity), there are signs of declines in PPO enrollments late in the decade. The principal reason for the decline will be that PPOs have been less effective than HMOs in containing costs and the quality of care often varies widely from provider to provider. After 2010, the distinctions among these products will be difficult to discern, creating a new generation of "HMO descendants."[5]

Portfolio Analysis

Portfolio analysis, popularized by the Boston Consulting Group (BCG), has become a fundamental tool for strategic analysis. The market position of the health care organization as a whole or its separate programs can be examined in terms of its share of the market and the rate of service category growth.[6] As illustrated in Exhibit 7–6, the traditional *BCG portfolio analysis* matrix graphically portrays differences among the various products/services (stars, cash cows, problem children, and dogs) in terms of relative market share and market growth rate.

Relative market share can be thought of as the market share held by the largest rival organization compared with the market share held by others in the service category. Growth rate is usually measured by the changes in level of gross patient service revenues or by population or service utilization growth (admissions or inpatient days).[7] Classification as high, medium, or low may be determined through comparison with national or regional health care growth figures, the prime rate, return on alternative investments, or the stage in the product life cycle.[8]

An example of portfolio analysis for one institution is illustrated in Exhibit 7–7. Cash cow services, such as plastic surgery and substance abuse (lower left quadrant) have achieved high market share but the growth rate has slowed. These services should generate excess cash that may be used to develop stars and problem children services. Service lines in the upper left quadrant such as women's services, geriatrics, cardiology, and so on, have high market growth and a relatively high market share (and most likely high profitability). These services are the most attractive for the institution and should be provided additional resources and encouraged to grow (and become cash cows). Services in the upper right-hand quadrant (neurology/neurosurgery, GI/urology, emergency services, and so on) over time will move into the stars quadrant or the dogs quadrant. It is important to nurture the services that will most likely move to the stars quadrant. Services such as psychiatry, vascular surgery, pediatrics, and so on, have low growth rates as well as a low relative market share (and most likely low profitability) and may be targets for contraction strategies. However, in health care some "dog" quadrant services may be slated for maintenance of scope or even expansion because of community needs.

Exhibit 7–6: BCG Portfolio Analysis

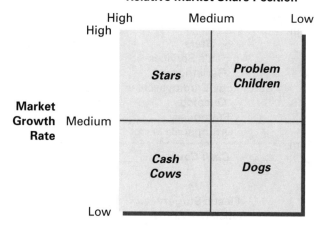

Relative Market Share Position

Stars
Products and services that fall in this quadrant (high market growth and high market share) represent the organization's best long-run opportunity for growth and profitability. These products and
services should be provided resources. Market development, product development, penetration, vertical
integration, and related diversification are appropriate strategies for this quadrant.

Cash Cows
Products and services in this quadrant have low market growth (probably in maturity and decline
stages of the PLC) but the organization has a high relative market share. These products and services
should be maintained but should consume few new resources. For strong cash cows, appropriate
strategies are status quo, enhancement, penetration, and related diversification. For weak cash cows,
strategies may include retrenchment, harvesting, divestiture, and perhaps liquidation.

Problem Children
Problem children have a low relative market share position, yet compete in a high-growth market.
Managers must decide whether to strengthen the products in this quadrant with increased
investment through market development or product development or get out of the product/service
area through harvesting, divestiture, or liquidation. A case may also be made for retrenchment into
specialty niches.

Dogs
These products and services have a low relative market share position and compete in a slow- or no-
growth market. These products and services should consume fewer and fewer of the organization's
resources. Because of their weak position, the products or services in this quadrant are often liquidated
or divested or the organization engages in dramatic retrenchment.

Exhibit 7–7: BCG Portfolio Analysis for a Health Care Institution

Relative Market Share Position

	High	Medium	Low
High **Market Growth Rate** Medium	***Stars*** Women's Services Geriatrics Cardiology/Cardiovascular Oncology Pulmonary Orthopedics		***Problem Children*** Neurology/Neurosurgery GI/Urology Emergency Services Ambulatory Surgery, Adult Ambulatory Surgery
Low	***Cash Cows*** Plastic Surgery Substance Abuse		***Dogs*** Psychiatry Vascular Surgery Pediatrics E.N.T. Ophthalmology General Medicine

Source: Adapted from Doris C. Van Doren, Jane R. Durney, and Colleen M. Darby, "Key Decisions in Marketing Plan Formulation for Geriatric Services," *Health Care Management Review* 18, no. 3, pp. 7–20. Copyright © 1993, Aspen Publishers, Inc. Adapted by permission.

Extended Portfolio Matrix Analysis

Although the BCG matrix may be used by health care organizations, portfolio analysis must be applied with care. For example, health care organizations typically have interdependent programs, such as orthopedics and pediatrics, that make SSU definition difficult. Additionally, underlying the BCG matrix is an assumption that high market share means high profitability and that profits may be "milked" to benefit other programs with growth potential. In health care organizations, however, it is quite possible to have a high market share and no profit. For example, because of reimbursement restrictions, a high number of Medicaid patients may cause a physician practice to be unprofitable. Similarly, programs such as obstetrics, pediatrics, neonatal intensive care, and psychiatry may have high market share but be unprofitable for a hospital.[9]

The profitability issues suggest that portfolio analysis for health care organizations might better utilize an *extended portfolio matrix analysis* that includes a profitability dimension. The profitability dimension is measured by high or low profitability according to positive or negative cash flow or return on invested capital. The expanded matrix is presented in Exhibit 7–8.

Exhibit 7–8: Expanded Product Portfolio Matrix

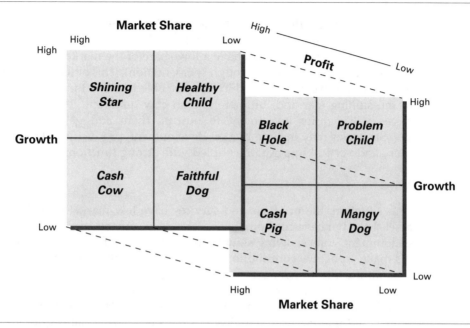

Source: Adapted from Gary McCain, "Black Holes, Cash Pigs, and Other Hospital Portfolio Analysis Problems," *Journal of Health Care Marketing* 7, no. 2 (June 1987), p. 58. Reprinted by permission of the publisher, the American Marketing Association.

SHINING STARS

Shining stars have high market growth (typically in the early stages of the PLC), a high market share, and high profitability. This quadrant represents the best situation for a health care organization. However, it is likely that high profitability will attract competitors. Therefore, aggressive enhancement or product development will be required; market development may be difficult because of the already high market share. In addition, the organization will want to consider vertical integration and related diversification.

CASH COWS

Cash cow products and services have low market growth but a high market share and high profitability. In this situation, the organization has a dominant position in the market (perhaps 100 percent) and further growth is unlikely. Again, the high profitability may attract competition, and the organization may have to defend its market share. Thus, strategies should be directed toward maintaining market dominance through enhancement. If the PLC is viewed to be long, the organization may want to engage in vertical integration or related diversification.

HEALTHY CHILDREN

Healthy children products and services have high market growth, a low market share, and high profitability. This quadrant demonstrates that there are situations in which it is possible to have a low share of the market and be profitable (at least in the short term or through segmentation). This situation is potentially attractive to the organization, which may be able to move the product or service into the shining star and, ultimately, cash cow quadrant. These products and services will require investment to nurture them and gain relative market share. Strategies may include market development, product development, penetration, and vertical integration coupled with strong functional support.

FAITHFUL DOGS

In this situation, the products and services have low market growth and a low market share, but have been profitable. For example, many hospital services involve less-dominant units showing slow growth. However, if they are profitable, such units make a positive contribution to the overall health of the hospital.[10]

For faithful dogs, managers must assess if increased market share will add to profitability. For instance, if profitable segments can be identified, it may be more advantageous to withdraw from broader markets, concentrate on a smaller segment, and maintain profitability. In such situations, a status quo or retrenchment strategy may be appropriate. If profitability is likely to decline over time, a harvesting or divestiture strategy may be employed.

BLACK HOLES

Black hole products and services have high growth and a high market share but low profitability. Not all high-growth, high-share programs are profitable in health care. For instance, costly technological equipment may make an organization the sole provider of a service whose high cost cannot be recovered from individual patients. However, such services may contribute to the overall image of the organization and increase the profitability of other services.

Nevertheless, having a high share for a service that is low or negative in profitability is quite disturbing. There must be a concentrated effort to reduce costs (enhancement strategy) or to add revenue without adding costs to such a program. "When circumstances prevent a service from generating most of its own cash inflow, it becomes a 'black hole' – a collapsed star sucking in light (profit or cash) – rather than shining and generating cash or profits."[11]

If a black hole product or service cannot be made into a shining star, it is likely to become a cash pig. Therefore, enhancement and retrenchment strategies may be most appropriate. In addition, action plan strategies should be employed to reduce costs and increase revenue.

PROBLEM CHILDREN

Problem children are low-share, high-growth, and low-profitability products and services that present both challenges and problems. Some of the products and services represent future shining stars and cash cows, although others represent future black holes and mangy dogs. Management must decide which products and services to support and which to eliminate. For supported products, market development with strong financial commitment is appropriate. For products that management does not feel can become shining stars, divestiture and liquidation are most appropriate.

CASH PIGS

Cash pig products and services have a high or dominant share, are experiencing low growth, and have low profitability. Health care cash pigs are likely to be those well-established SSUs with dominant shares that once were considered to be cash cows. Typically, they have well-entrenched advocates in the organizational hierarchy who support their continuance.[12]

A possible solution to the cash pig problem is to cut costs and raise prices. Therefore, aggressive retrenchment may be required. This strategy may allow the organization to give up the market share to find smaller, more profitable segments and thus create a smaller cash cow.

MANGY DOGS

Products and services with low growth, a low share, and poor profit have a debilitating effect on the organization and should be eliminated as soon as possible. In this situation, it appears that other providers are better serving the market. Probably the best strategy at this point is liquidation, as it will be difficult to find a buyer for products and services in this quadrant.

Strategic Position and Action Evaluation

Strategic position and action evaluation (SPACE), an extension of two-dimensional portfolio analysis (BCG), is used to determine the appropriate strategic posture of the organization. By using SPACE, the manager can incorporate a number of factors into the analysis and examine a particular strategic alternative from several perspectives.[13]

SPACE analysis suggests the appropriateness of strategic alternatives based on factors relating to four dimensions: service category strength, environmental stability, the organization's relative competitive advantage, and the organization's financial strength. The SPACE chart and definitions of the four quadrants are shown in Exhibit 7–9. Listed under each of the four dimensions are factors to which individual numerical values ranging from 0 to 6 can be assigned. The numbers are then added together and divided by the number of factors to yield an average. The averages for environmental stability and competitive advantage each have the number 6 subtracted from them to produce a negative number. The average for each dimension is then plotted on the appropriate axis of the SPACE chart and connected to create a four-sided polygon. Factor scales for each dimension are presented in Exhibit 7–10, which has been filled in for a regional hospital. The

Exhibit 7-9: Strategic Position and Action Evaluation (SPACE) Matrix

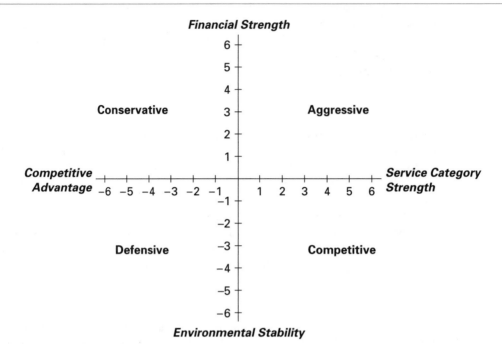

Aggressive Posture
This posture is typical in an attractive service category with little environmental turbulence. The organization enjoys a definite competitive advantage, which it can protect with financial strength. The critical factor is the entry of new competitors. Organizations in this situation should take full advantage of opportunities, look for acquisition candidates in their own or related areas, increase market share, and concentrate resources on products having a definite competitive edge.

Competitive Posture
This posture is typical in an attractive service category. The organization enjoys a competitive advantage in a relatively unstable environment. The critical factor is financial strength. Organizations in this situation should acquire financial resources to increase marketing thrust, add to the sales force, extend or improve the product line, invest in productivity, reduce costs, protect competitive advantage in a declining market, and attempt to merge with a cash-rich organization.

Conservative Posture
This posture is typical in a stable market with low growth. Here, the organization focuses on financial stability. The critical factor is product competitiveness. Organizations in this situation should prune the product line, reduce costs, focus on improving cash flow, protect competitive products, develop new products, and gain entry into more attractive markets.

Defensive Posture
This posture is typical of an unattractive service category in which the organization lacks a competitive product and financial strength. The critical factor is competitiveness. Organizations in this situation should prepare to retreat from the market, discontinue marginally profitable products, aggressively reduce costs, cut capacity, and defer or minimize investments.

Source: Adapted from Alan J. Rowe, Richard O. Mason, Karl E. Dickel, and Neil H. Snyder, *Strategic Management: A Methodological Approach*, 4th edn (Reading, MA: Addison-Wesley Publishing, 1994), pp. 145–150. Reprinted by permission of Pearson Education Inc., Upper Saddle River, NJ.

Exhibit 7–10: Strategic Position and Action Evaluation Factors

Factors Determining Environmental Stability

Factor	Label	0	1	2	3	4	5	6	Label
Technological changes	Many	0	(1)	2	3	4	5	6	Few
Rate of inflation	High	0	(1)	2	3	4	5	6	Low
Demand variability	Large	0	1	2	3	(4)	5	6	Small
Price range of competing products/services	Wide	0	(1)	2	3	4	5	6	Narrow
Barriers to entry into market	Few	0	1	2	(3)	4	5	6	Many
Competitive pressure	High	0	1	(2)	3	4	5	6	Low
Price elasticity of demand	Elastic	0	1	2	3	(4)	5	6	Inelastic
Other: _____	_____	0	1	2	3	4	5	6	_____

Average − 6 = <u>−3.7</u>

Critical factors

Fairly turbulent environment; strong competition; many technological changes.

Comments

Necessary to maintain financial stability because of turbulence in the environment; demand in market segments relatively stable; protect market niche against competition.

Factors Determining Service Category Strength

Factor	Label	0	1	2	3	4	5	6	Label
Growth potential	Low	0	1	2	3	(4)	5	6	High
Profit potential	Low	0	1	2	3	4	(5)	6	High
Financial stability	Low	0	1	(2)	3	4	5	6	High
Technological know-how	Simple	0	1	2	3	4	(5)	6	Complex
Resource utilization	Inefficient	0	1	2	3	(4)	5	6	Efficient
Capital intensity	High	0	1	(2)	3	4	5	6	Low
Ease of entry into market	Easy	0	(1)	2	3	4	5	6	Difficult
Productivity, capacity utilization	Low	0	1	2	3	4	(5)	6	High
Other: <u>Flexibility, adaptability</u>	<u>Low</u>	0	1	2	3	4	(5)	6	<u>High</u>

Average <u>3.7</u>

Critical factors

Good growth and profit potential; strong competition.

Comments

Very attractive service category, but strong competition; degree of capital intensity increasing.

Exhibit 7–10: (cont'd)

Factors Determining Competitive Advantage*

		0	1	2	3	4	5	6	
Market share	Small	0	1	②	3	4	5	6	Large
Product quality	Inferior	0	1	2	3	4	5	⑥	Superior
Product life cycle	Late	0	1	2	③	4	5	6	Early
Product replacement cycle	Variable	0	1	2	3	④	5	6	Fixed
Customer/patient loyalty	Low	0	1	2	3	④	5	6	High
Competition's capacity utilization	Low	0	1	2	3	④	5	6	High
Technological know-how	Low	0	1	2	3	④	5	6	High
Vertical integration	Low	0	1	②	3	4	5	6	High
Other: _____	_____	0	1	2	3	4	5	6	_____

Average – 6 = –2.4

Critical factors

Market share low; product/service quality very good.

Comments

The organization still enjoys slight competitive advantage because of quality and customer loyalty; can be expected to diminish, however, because of improving performance of competitive organizations.

Factors Determining Financial Strength

		0	1	2	3	4	5	6	
Return on investment	Low	0	1	2	3	④	5	6	High
Leverage	Imbalanced	0	①	2	3	4	5	6	Balanced
Liquidity	Imbalanced	⓪	1	2	3	4	5	6	Balanced
Capital required/capital available	High	0	①	2	3	4	5	6	Low
Cash flow	Low	0	①	2	3	4	5	6	High
Ease of exit from market	Difficult	0	1	2	3	④	5	6	Easy
Risk involved in business	Much	0	①	2	3	4	5	6	Little
Other: Inventory turnover	Slow	0	①	2	3	4	5	6	Fast

Average 1.6

Critical factors

Very little liquidity; too much debt.

Comments

Financial position very weak; cash inflow has to be increased in order to improve liquidity; outside financing difficult because of high leverage.

* Represent important competitive advantages.

Source: Adapted from Alan J. Rowe, Richard O. Mason, Karl E. Dickel, and Neil H. Snyder, *Strategic Management: A Methodological Approach*, 4th edn (Reading, MA: Addison-Wesley Publishing, 1994), pp. 148–149. Reprinted by permission of Pearson Education Inc., Upper Saddle River, NJ.

resulting shape of the polygon can be used to identify four strategic postures – aggressive, competitive, conservative, and defensive. The quadrant with the largest area is the most appropriate general strategic position.

The factor scales shown in Exhibit 7–10 are for a California-based regional hospital system specializing in health services for the elderly and chemically dependent. This hospital system is operating in a fairly turbulent environment with many competitive pressures and many technological changes (environmental stability axis). However, the hospital's service category segments show good growth potential that attracts strong competition. Increasing competition requires increased investment in new facilities and technology. The hospital still has a competitive advantage (competitive advantage axis) derived from early entry into the market and it has been able to retain customer loyalty because of high-quality service. However, the hospital's financial position (financial strength axis) is weak because it financed new facilities through a substantial amount of debt. Its liquidity position has eroded and cash flow continues to be a problem.

Which of the adaptive strategic alternatives is most appropriate for this regional system? The dimensions for this organization are plotted on the SPACE matrix shown in Exhibit 7–11, demonstrating that the hospital is competing fairly well in an unstable but attractive service category segment. This organization

Exhibit 7–11: SPACE Profile for a Regional Hospital System

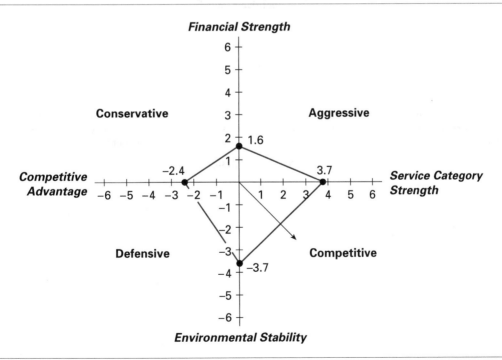

Exhibit 7–12: Space Strategy Profiles

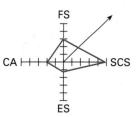 **Aggressive Profiles**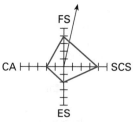

A financially strong organization that has achieved major competitive advantages in a growing and stable service category

An organization whose financial strength is a dominating factor in the service category

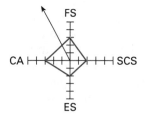 **Conservative Profiles**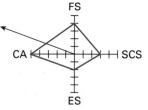

An organization that has achieved financial strength in a stable service category that is not growing; the organization has no major competitive advantages

An organization that suffers from major competitive disadvantages in a service category that is technologically stable but declining in revenue

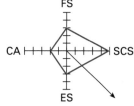 **Competitive Profiles**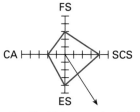

An organization with major competitive advantages but limited financial strength in a high-growth service category

An organization that is competing fairly well in a service category where there is substantial environmental uncertainty

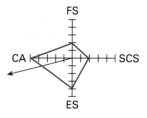 **Defensive Profiles**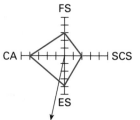

An organization that has a very weak competitive position in a negative-growth, stable but weak service category

A financially troubled organization in a very unstable and weak service category

Source: Adapted from Fred R. David, *Strategic Management,* 2nd edn (Columbus, OH: Merrill Publishing Co., 1989), p. 216.

cannot be too aggressive because it has few financial resources and the environment is a bit unstable. Therefore, it should adopt a competitive posture.

It is important to remember that the SPACE chart is a summary display; each factor should be analyzed individually as well. In particular, factors with very high or very low scores should receive special attention.[14] Exhibit 7–12 examines various possible strategic profiles that may be obtained in a SPACE analysis and Exhibit 7–13 shows the adaptive alternatives for each strategic posture.

The SPACE plot for the regional hospital system examined previously resulted in a competitive profile. Accordingly, the most appropriate strategic alternatives are penetration, market development, product development, status quo, or enhancement, with the most likely being enhancement. The hospital should continue to differentiate itself but must rectify its financial position because an unstable environment may place unanticipated demands on the organization that will require an additional infusion of capital. In light of its financial problems, the hospital may have to pursue its goals (for example, market development) through a cooperation market entry strategy. A cooperation strategy – joining a network – may be important in an environment where health care systems, continuums, and referral networks are the key to market development and penetration. In the end, the adaptive and market entry strategic decisions are inextricably linked.

Exhibit 7–13: Strategic Alternatives for SPACE Quadrants

Conservative
- Status Quo
- Unrelated Diversification
- Harvesting

Aggressive
- Related Diversification
- Market Development
- Product Development
- Vertical Integration

Defensive
- Divestiture
- Liquidation
- Retrenchment

Competitive
- Penetration
- Enhancement
- Product Development
- Market Development
- Status Quo

Program Evaluation

Program evaluation is especially useful in organizations where market share, service category strength, and competitive advantage are not particularly important or are not relevant. Such organizations are typically not-for-profit, state- or federally-funded institutions such as state and county public health departments, state mental health departments, Medicaid agencies, community health centers, and public community hospitals. Despite the fact that these organizations are public and not-for-profit, they should develop explicit strategies and evaluate the adaptive strategic alternatives open to them. Although TOWS and a form of portfolio analysis may be used to evaluate public health programs,[15] evaluation methods that consider increasing revenue and market share may be inappropriate or difficult to use. Perspective 7–5 provides an overview of the public health system and its essential services.

Public and not-for-profit institutions typically maintain any number of programs funded through such sources as state appropriations, federal grants, private donations, fee for service, and so on. In a public health department, such programs might include HIV/AIDS education, disease surveillance, disease control, immunizations, food sanitation inspection, on-site sewage inspection, and many more. Usually, these programs have been initiated to fill a health care need within the community that has not been addressed through the private sector. These "health care gaps" have occurred because of federal or state requirements for coordination and control of community health and because of the large number of individuals without adequate health care insurance or means to pay for services.

Within the context provided by an understanding of the external environment, internal environment, and the directional strategies, these not-for-profit institutions must chart a future through a set of externally and internally funded programs. The set of programs maintained and emphasized by the organization constitutes its adaptive strategy. The degree to which they are changed (expansion of scope, contraction of scope, maintenance of scope) represents a modification of the adaptive strategy. Public health departments (both state and local) often add initially federally funded programs (following grants), become spread too thin, and become less effective as they move more distant from their core competency. This grant-seeking approach can stretch an agency's core capabilities and push it in unintended directions.[16] The fundamental question is, "Does our current set of programs effectively and efficiently fulfill our mission and our vision for the future?" This question may be addressed through a process of program evaluation. Two program evaluation methods that have been used successfully are needs/capacity assessment and program priority setting.

NEEDS/CAPACITY ASSESSMENT

The set of programs in not-for-profit organizations such as public health departments essentially are determined by (1) community need and (2) the organization's capacity to deliver the program to that community. Of course, some

Perspective 7–5

Overview of Public
Health In the
United States

The work of public health developed over time in response to community need and is carried out at federal, state, and local levels. In 1988, after an intense study of public health in six states, the Institute of Medicine defined the basic functions of public health as assessment, policy development, and assurance. The Centers for Disease Control and Prevention (CDC) proposed ten organizational practices to implement the three core functions. In spring 1994, a national working group composed of representatives of the Public Health Services Agencies and the major public health organizations developed a consensus list of the "essential services of public health." The new statement on essential services provided a vision for public health in America – "Healthy People in Healthy Communities" – and stated the mission of public health – "Promote physical and mental health and prevent disease, injury, and disability." The statement included two brief lists that described what public health seeks to accomplish in providing essential services to the public and how it carries out these basic public responsibilities.

The Essential Services

The fundamental obligation or purpose of public health agencies responsible for population-based health is to:

- prevent epidemics and the spread of disease,
- protect against environmental hazards,
- prevent injuries,
- promote and encourage healthy behaviors and mental health,
- respond to disasters and assist communities in recovery, and
- assure the quality and accessibility of health services.

Part of the function of public health is to assure the availability of quality health services. Both distinct from and encompassing clinical services, public health's role is to ensure the conditions necessary for people to live healthy lives, through community-wide prevention and protection programs.

Public health serves communities (and individuals within them) by providing an array of essential services. Many of these services are invisible to the public. Typically, the public only becomes aware of the need for public health services when a problem develops (for instance, when an epidemic occurs). The practice of public health is articulated through the list of "essential services."

Assessment services include:
- Monitoring health status to identify community health problems;
- Diagnosing and investigating health problems and hazards in the community;
- Researching for new insights and innovative solutions to health problems.

Policy development services include:
- Informing, educating, and empowering people about health issues;
- Mobilizing community partnerships and actions to identify and solve health problems;
- Developing policies and plans that support individual and community health efforts.

Assurance services include:
- Enforcing laws and regulations that protect health and ensure safety;
- Linking people to needed personal health services and ensuring the provision of health care when otherwise unavailable;
- Assuring a competent public and personal health care workforce;
- Evaluating effectiveness, accessibility, and quality of personal and population-based health services.

Source: Ray M. Nicola, MD, MHSA, FACPM, Senior CDC Consultant to the Turning Point National Program Office.

programs may be mandated by law, such as disease control, disease surveillance, and the maintenance of vital records (birth and death records). However, the assumption is that the legislation is a result of an important need and, typically, the mandate is supported by nondiscretionary or categorical funding (funding that may be used for only one purpose). Therefore, in developing a strategy for a public health organization or not-for-profit organization serving the community, a *needs/capacity assessment* must be undertaken – community needs must be assessed vis-à-vis the organization's ability (capacity) to address those needs.

Community need is a function of (1) clear community requirements (environmental, sanitation, disease control, and so on) and personal health care (primary care) gaps, (2) the degree to which other institutions (private and public) fill the identified health care gaps, and (3) public/community health objectives. Many not-for-profit institutions enter the health care market to provide services to those who otherwise would be left out of the system. Despite efforts to reform health care, these gaps are likely to remain for some time. Health care gaps are identified through community involvement, political pressure, and community assessments such as those carried out by the Centers for Disease Control and Prevention (CDC). These gaps exist because there are few private or public institutions positioned to fill the need. Where existing institutions are willing and able to fill these gaps, public and not-for-profit organizations should probably resist entering the market. In addition, public and community health objectives must be considered when developing strategy. National, state, and community objectives such as the Healthy People 2010 objectives should be included as a part of a community needs assessment.[17]

Organizational capacity is the organization's ability to initiate, maintain, and enhance its set of adaptive strategy programs. Organizational capacity is composed of (1) funding to support programs, (2) other organizational resources and skills, and (3) the program's fit with the mission and vision of the organization. Availability of funding is an important part of organizational capacity. Many programs are supported with categorical funding and accompanying mandates (program requirements dictated by a higher authority, usually federal or state government). Often, however, local moneys supplement federal- and state-funded programs. For other programs, only community funding is available. Thus, funding availability is a major consideration in developing strategy for public and not-for-profit organizations. In addition, the organization must have the skills, resources, facilities, management, and so on to initiate and effectively administer the program. Finally, program strategy will be dependent upon the program's fit with the organization's mission and vision for the future. Programs outside the mission and vision will be viewed as luxuries, superfluous, or wasteful.

Exhibit 7–14 presents the adaptive strategic alternatives indicated for public organizations as they assess community needs and the organization's capacity to fill the identified needs. Where the community need is assessed as high (significant health care gaps, few or no other institutions addressing the need, and the program is a part of the community's objectives) and the organization's capacity is assessed as high (adequate funding, appropriate skills and resources, and fit with mission/vision), then the organization should adopt one of the expansion

Exhibit 7–14: Public Health and Not-for-profit Adaptive Strategic Decisions

Organizational Capacity

	High	Low
High (Community Need)	**Expansion Strategies** • Vertical Integration • Related Diversification • Product Development • Market Development • Penetration	**Maintenance/Contraction** • Enhancement • Status Quo • Retrenchment • Harvesting
Low (Community Need)	**Contraction/Maintenance** • Related Diversification • Retrenchment • Harvesting • Status Quo	**Contraction** • Liquidation • Harvesting • Divestiture • Retrenchment

of scope adaptive strategies (upper left-hand quadrant). Appropriate strategies might include vertical integration, related diversification, product development, market development, and penetration. When the community need assessment is low (no real need, the need has abated, need is now being addressed by another institution, or the need does not fit with community objectives), but organization capacity is high (adequate funding, appropriate skills and resources, and fit with mission/vision), there should be an orderly redistribution of resources, suggesting contraction and maintenance of scope adaptive strategies (lower left-hand quadrant). Contraction of scope strategies should be given priority as the community need diminishes. However, phasing out a program may take some time or, alternatively, the uncertainty concerning the changing community needs may dictate maintenance in the short term. Appropriate adaptive strategies include related diversification, retrenchment, harvesting, and status quo.

Where community needs have been assessed as low (no real need, the need has abated, need is now being addressed by another institution, or the need does not fit with community objectives) and the organization has few financial or other resources to commit to programs (low organization capacity), one of the contraction of scope adaptive strategies should be adopted (lower right-hand quadrant). These strategies include liquidation, harvesting, divestiture, and retrenchment. When community needs have been assessed as high but organizational capacity is low, maintenance and contraction of scope strategies are appropriate (upper right-hand quadrant). Maintenance of scope strategies should be given priority because of the high community need but, if resources dwindle or funding is reduced, contraction may be required. Appropriate adaptive strategic alternatives include enhancement or status quo (maintenance of scope) and retrenchment or harvesting (contraction of scope). As resources become available, and organization capacity increases, programs in this quadrant will move to the upper left-hand quadrant, enabling more aggressive (expansion) strategies to be selected.

PROGRAM PRIORITY SETTING

The second method of developing adaptive strategies for not-for-profit or public programs involves ranking programs and setting priorities. *Program priority setting* is significant because community needs (both the need itself and the severity of the need) are constantly changing and organizational resources, in terms of funding and organization capacity, are almost always limited. Invariably more programs have high community need than resources are available. Therefore, the most important programs (and perhaps those with categorical funding) may be expanded or maintained. The organization must have an understanding of which programs are the most important, which should be provided incremental funding, and which should be the first to be scaled back if funding is reduced or eliminated.

The nature and emphasis on programs is the central part of strategy formulation in many public and not-for-profit organizations. However, a problem in ranking these programs is that typically all of them are viewed as "very important" or "essential." This is particularly true when using Likert or semantic differential scales to evaluate the programs. Therefore, it is necessary to develop evaluation methods that further differentiate the programs. One method that can be used is to list all the programs of the agency or clinic, each on a separate sheet of paper posted in different areas of the room. Use three different colors or types of stickers, one for each of the adaptive strategies – expand the scope, contract the scope, and maintain the scope. Each member of the management team is asked to sort the organization's programs into categories – those that should be expanded, those that should be reduced, or those to remain the same – based on the perceived importance of each to the organization's mission and vision. The group may agree on several programs. Discussions can then be focused on those programs where there is disagreement. After points have been raised and discussed, the programs can be ranked again, hopefully leading to greater consensus from the group.

The Q-sort method provides a more formal method of differentiating the importance of programs and setting priorities. Q-sort is a ranking procedure that forces choices along a continuum in situations where the difference between the choices may be quite small. The *program Q-sort evaluation* is particularly useful when experts may differ on what makes one choice preferable over another. By ranking the choices using a Q-sort procedure, participants see where there is wide consensus (for whatever reasons used by the experts) and have an opportunity to discuss the choices for which there is disagreement (and, hopefully, reach greater consensus).

The Q-sort is a part of Q-methodology, a set of philosophical, psychological, statistical, and psychometric ideas oriented to research on the individual. Q-sort evaluation helps overcome the problem of all programs being ranked as very important by forcing a ranking based on some set of assumptions. Fred N. Kerlinger, in *Foundations of Behavioral Research*, characterized the Q-sort as "a sophisticated way of rank-ordering objects."[18] Once the Q-sort has rank-ordered a series of objects (programs), then numerals may be assigned to subsets of the objects for statistical purposes.

Q-sort focuses particularly in sorting decks of cards (in this case each card representing a program) and in the correlations among the responses of different individuals to the Q-sorts. Kerlinger reports good results with as few as 40 items (programs) that have been culled from a larger list. However, greater statistical stability and reliability usually results from at least 60 items, but not more than 100.[19]

For ranking an organization's programs, only the first step in using Q-methodology is used – the Q-sort. In the Q-sort procedure, each member of the management team is asked to sort the organization's programs into categories based on their perceived importance to the organization's mission and vision. To facilitate the task, the programs are printed on small cards that may be arranged (sorted) on a table. To force ranking of programs, managers are asked to arrange the programs in piles from most important to least important. The best approach is that the number of categories be limited to nine and that the number of programs to be assigned to each category be determined in such a manner as to ensure a normal distribution.[20] Therefore, if a public health department had 49 separate programs that management wished to rank (culled from a larger list of programs), they may be sorted as shown in Exhibit 7–15. Notice that to create a normal distribution (or quasi-normal), 5 percent of the programs are placed in the first pile or group, 7.5 percent in the second group, 12.5 percent in the third, and so on. In this case, there are two programs in the first group, four programs in the second group, six in the third, and so on.

Depending on in which group it is placed, each program is assigned a score ranging from 1 to 9, where 1 is for the lowest and 9 is for the highest ranked programs. The score indicates an individual's perception of that program's importance to the mission and vision of the organization. A program profile is developed by averaging individual members' scores for each program.

Based on the results of the Q-sort, programs may be designated for expansion, contraction, or maintenance of scope. For the public health programs in Exhibit 7–15, food sanitation and epidemiology, sewage planning and operation, sexually transmitted disease (STD) control, and so on, might be earmarked for expansion. Cancer prevention, lodging/jail inspection, injury prevention, and so on, might be slated for maintenance of scope, whereas plumbing inspection, hearing aid dealer board regulation, and animal control may be marked for contraction.

The Q-sort procedure works well using several different sets of strategic assumptions or scenarios. For example, the programs may be sorted several

Exhibit 7–15: Department of Public Health Q-Sort Results*

Most Important	Next Most Important	Next Most Important	Next Most Important	Next Most Important	Next Most Important	Next Most Important	Next Most Important	Next Most Important
				Cancer Prevention 4.88				
			Seafood Sanitation 6.11	Lodging/Jails Inspection 4.88	Microbiology 4.44			
			Infection Control 5.77	Injury Prevention 4.77	Home Health 4.22			
		Immunization 6.99	Health Education 5.66	Disaster Preparedness 4.77	Quality Assurance 4.11	Administrative Support 3.99		
		Tuberculosis Control 6.88	Family Planning 5.66	Public Health Nursing 4.75	Primary-Care Support 4.11	Vector Control 3.99		
	Sewage Regulation 7.22	Licensure and Certification 6.77	Child Health 5.55	Lead Assessment 4.62	School Health Education 4.0	Dental Health 3.87	Medicaid Waiver 3.33	
	STD Control 7.22	Newborn Screening 6.62	Emergency Medicine 5.50	HMO Regulation 4.55	WIC 4.0	Diabetes 3.77	Swimming Pools 3.11	
Food Sanitation 8.0	Milk Sanitation 7.0	Health Statistics 6.44	Radiation Control 5.44	Hypertension 4.55	Vital Records 4.0	Indoor Air Quality 3.66	Adolescent Health 2.66	Hearing Aid Regulation 1.88
Epidemiology 8.0	HIV/AIDS Planning and Control 7.0	Solid Waste 6.33	Maternity 5.22	Myco-bacteriology 4.55	Serology 4.0	Public Health Social Work 3.44	Plumbing Inspection 2.55	Animal Control 1.44
5%	7.5%	12.5%	15%	20%	15%	12.5%	7.5%	5%

* Program name and mean score in each box.

times, each based on a different scenario. Then the group can determine which of the scenarios is most likely and make decisions accordingly.

Evaluation of the Market Entry Strategies

Once expansion of scope or maintenance of scope through enhancement adaptive strategies are selected, one or more of the market entry strategies must be used to break into or capture more of the market. All of the expansion adaptive strategies require some activity to reach more consumers with the products and services. Similarly, enhancement strategies indicate that the organization must undertake to "do better" what it is already doing, which requires market entry analysis. Contraction of scope strategies are methods to either rapidly or slowly leave markets and therefore do not require a market entry strategic decision.

The market entry strategies include acquisition, licensing, venture capital investment, merger, alliance, joint venture, internal development, and internal venture. Although any one (or several) of these strategies may be used to enter the market, mergers and alliances received most of the media attention throughout the 1990s. Mergers and alliances are the principal cooperation strategies.

The specific market entry strategy considered to be appropriate depends on (1) the external conditions, (2) the pertinent internal strengths and weaknesses based on the organization's resources, competencies, and capabilities, and (3) the goals of the organization. Each of these three areas should be scrupulously evaluated.

External Conditions

The first consideration in the selection of the market entry strategy is the evaluation of the environment. A review of the external environmental opportunities and threats and supporting documentation (see Chapters 2 and 3) should provide information to determine which of the market entry strategies is most appropriate. Exhibit 7–16 provides a list of representative external conditions appropriate for each of the market entry strategies.

Internal Resources, Competencies, and Capabilities

Each market entry strategy requires different resources, competencies, and capabilities (see Exhibit 7–17). Before selecting the appropriate market entry strategy, a review of the internal competitively relevant strengths and weaknesses should be undertaken (see Chapter 4). If the required skills and resources, competencies, and capabilities (strengths) are available, the appropriate market entry strategy may be selected. On the other hand, if they are not present, another alternative should be selected or a combination strategy of two or more phases should be adopted. The first phase would be directed at correcting the weakness prohibiting selection of the desired strategy, and the second phase would be the initiation of the desired market entry strategy. In some cases a total redesign, or *reengineering*, of a process may be required before a strategy may be implemented. Perspective 7–6 provides some insight into the requirements of reengineering.

Organizational Goals

Along with the internal and external factors, organizational goals play an important role in evaluating the appropriate market entry strategies. As shown in Exhibit 7–18, internal development and internal ventures offer the greatest degree of control over the design, production, operations, marketing, and so on of the product or service. On the other hand, licensing, acquisition, mergers, and venture capital investment offer the quickest market entry but control over design, production, marketing, and so on is low in the short term (in the longer term the organization can take complete control). Alliances and joint ventures offer relatively quick entry with some degree of control. The trade-off between speed of

Exhibit 7–16: External Conditions Appropriate for Market Entry Strategies

Market Entry Strategy	Appropriate External Conditions
Acquisition	• Growing market • Early stage of the product life cycle or long maturity stage • Attractive acquisition candidate • High volume economies of scale (horizontal integration) • Distribution economies of scale (vertical integration)
Licensing	• High capital investment to enter market • High immediate demand for product/service • Early stages of the product life cycle
Venture Capital Investment	• Rapidly changing technology • Product/service in the early development stage
Merger	• Attractive merger candidate (synergistic effect) • High level of resource required to compete
Alliance	• Alliance partner has complementary resources, competencies, capabilities • Alliance partner has similar status • Market demands complete line of products/services • Market is weak and continuum of services is desirable • Mature stage of product life cycle
Joint Venture	• High capital requirements to obtain necessary skills/expertise • Long learning curve in obtaining necessary expertise
Internal Development	• High level of product control (quality) required • Early stages of the product life cycle
Internal Venture	• Product/service development stage • Rapid development/market entry required • New technical, marketing, production approach required

entering the market and organizational control over the product or service must be assessed by management in light of organizational goals.

Evaluation of the Competitive Strategies

After the market entry strategies have been selected, the strategic posture must be specified and the products/services must be positioned within the market using the generic strategies of cost leadership, differentiation, or focus. All of the adaptive strategies (expansion, contraction, and maintenance of scope) require explicit strategic posture and positioning strategies.

Exhibit 7–17: Appropriate Internal Resources, Competencies, and Capabilities for the Market Entry Strategies

Market Entry Strategy	Appropriate Resources, Competencies, and Capabilities (Strengths)
Acquisition	• Financial resources • Ability to manage new products and markets • Ability to merge organizational cultures and organizational structures • Rightsizing capability for combined organization
Licensing	• Financial resources (licensing fees) • Support organization to carry out license • Ability to integrate new product/market into present organization
Venture Capital Investment	• Capital to invest in speculative projects • Ability to evaluate and select opportunities with a high degree of success
Merger	• Management willing to relinquish or share control • Rightsizing capacity • Agreement to merge management • Ability to merge organizational cultures and organizational structures
Alliance	• Lack of competitive skills/facilities/expertise • Desire to create vertically integrated system • Need to control patient flow • Coordinate board/skills • Willing to relinquish share control
Joint Venture	• Lack of a distinctive competency • Additional resources/capabilities are required • Not enough time to develop internal resources, capabilities, or competencies • Venture is removed from core competency • Lack required skills and expertise
Internal Development	• Technical expertise • Marketing competency • Operational capacity • Research and development capability • Strong functional organization • Product/service management expertise
Internal Venture	• Entrepreneur • Entrepreneurial organization • Ability to isolate venture from the rest of the organization • Technical expertise • Marketing competency • Operational capacity

Perspective 7–6

Reengineering – Rethinking Health Care Delivery

Reengineering has been used as part of strategic planning to help organizations rethink the way processes are managed in organizations. Many health care organizations are using reengineering to cut across departmental lines to completely redesign a process. Its founders and leading proponents, Michael Hammer and James Champy, define reengineering as "the fundamental rethinking and radical redesign of process to achieve dramatic improvements in critical, contemporary measures of performance, such as cost, quality, service, and speed." Key words in this definition are radical and process.

Reengineering goes beyond quality improvement programs that seek marginal improvements. It asks a team to "start over" and completely and radically redesign a process. It does not mean tinkering with what already exists or making incremental changes that leave basic structures intact. It ignores what is and concentrates on what should be. The clean sheet of paper, the breaking of assumptions, the throw-it-all-out-and-start-again flavor of reengineering has captured and excited the imagination of managers from all industries. Radical redesign requires creativity and a willingness to try new things, questions the legitimacy of all tasks and procedures, questions all assumptions, breaks all the rules possible, and draws upon customer desires and needs.

A process is a complete end-to-end set of activities that together create value for a customer. Many organizations have become so specialized that few people understand the complete process of creating value for the customer. In the past, organizations have focused on improving the performance of individual tasks in separate functional units rather than on complete processes that typically cut across many functions. Everyone was watching out for task performance, but no one was watching to see whether all the tasks together produced the results they were supposed to for the customer. Dramatic improvement can be achieved only by improving the performance of the entire process.

To be successful, management must be willing to destroy old ways of doing things and start anew. Many changes take place in an organization or unit when reengineering is initiated:

- Work units change – from functional departments to process teams.
- Jobs change – from simple tasks to multidimensional work.
- People's roles change – from controlled to empowered.
- Job preparation changes – from training to education.
- The focus of performance measures and compensation change – from activity to results.
- Advancement criteria change – from performance to ability.
- Values change – from protective to productive.
- Managers change – from supervisors to coaches.
- Organizational structure changes – from hierarchical to flat.
- Executives change – from scorekeepers to leaders.

Michael Hammer identified seven principles for organizational reengineering:

1. Organize around outcomes, not tasks. By focusing on the desired outcome, people consider new ways to accomplish the work.
2. People who use the output should perform the process.
3. Include information processing in the "real" work that produces the information.
4. Treat geographically dispersed resources as if they were centralized.
5. Link parallel activities rather than integrate them. By coordinating similar kinds of work while it is in process rather than after completion, better cooperation can be fostered and the process accelerated.
6. Let "doers" be self-managing. By putting decisions where the work is performed and building in controls, organizations can eliminate layers of managers.
7. Capture information once and at its source.

Source: Michael Hammer and James Champy, *Reengineering the Corporation: A Manifesto for Business Revolution* (New York: HarperBusiness, 1994); Michael Hammer, *Beyond Reengineering: How the Process-Centered Organization Is Changing Our Work and Lives* (New York: HarperBusiness, 1996); and Michael Hammer, "Reengineering Work: Don't Automate, Obliterate," *Harvard Business Review* 68, no. 4 (July–August, 1990), pp. 104–112.

Exhibit 7–18: Market Entry Strategies and Organizational Goals

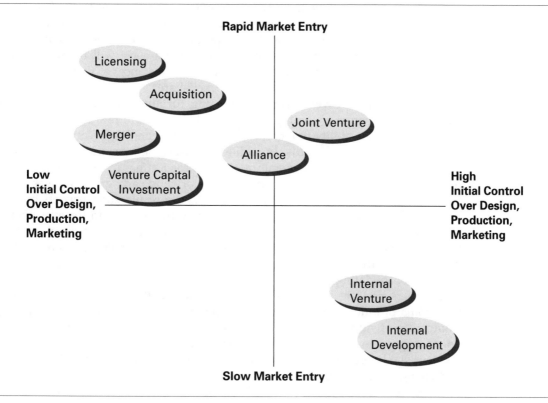

Strategic Posture

Strategic posture concerns the relationship between the organization and the market and describes the pattern of strategic behavior. Appropriate strategic postures include defender, prospector, and analyzer. Any of these may be appropriate, subject to: the external environment; the changing nature of the market; competition; the resources, competencies, and capabilities of the organization; and the vision and values. It is important to make sure the strategic posture is linked to and fits with the adaptive and market entry strategies.

EXTERNAL CONDITIONS

External conditions are very important in the selection of strategic posture. Defender strategies tend to be successful when the external environment is relatively stable (change is slow and reasonably predictable). In such environments competitive rivalry is low and the barriers to entering the market are high. Indeed the cost-efficiency strategy of the defender tends to push entry barriers even higher. Because defender organizations focus on a narrow product line, the strategy works best when relatively long product life cycles are expected. Long product life cycles allow the organization to commit to vertical integration, develop cost efficiency, and create routine processes. Defender strategies are most effective in the mature stage of the product life cycle. The risks associated with the defender posture are that the product life cycle will be dramatically shortened by external change (new technology, for instance) or that a competitor can somehow unexpectedly take away market share.

Prospectors operate well in rapidly changing, turbulent environments. In these environments change is coming so rapidly that there are few rewards for efficiency. Rather, the ability to incorporate the latest technology, feature, or design will reap the greatest rewards. In addition, prospectors are successful by utilizing a technology across several markets (prospecting in new high-growth markets). Products are usually in the introductory and early growth stages of the PLC and the cycle tends to be relatively short. As a result, entry barriers may be low and the intensity of rivalry typically is low (there is room for everybody). As products or services mature, prospector organizations move on to new products and services, typically in introductory stages of the PLC. Prospectors divest their maturing products and services to successful defender organizations that are consolidating.

Analyzers operate well in environments where there is moderate change with some product categories that are quite stable and some that are changing. Competitive rivalry tends to be relatively high and these organizations cannot afford to ignore new product developments, markets, or product categories. PLCs for their stable products are moderately long but there are periodic innovations and changes. Therefore, these organizations must enter new markets and new product areas. Analyzers typically do not enter the market in the introductory stage of the PLC. Instead they carefully watch product and market developments (the prospectors) and enter the most promising ones in the early growth stage of the product life cycle (using one of the market entry strategies). Analyzers attempt to maintain balance with both mature- and growth-stage products or services and markets.

The external conditions appropriate for each of the strategic postures are summarized in Exhibit 7–19.

INTERNAL RESOURCES, COMPETENCIES, CAPABILITIES

As shown in Exhibit 7–20, there are certain strengths associated with each of the strategic postures. For the defender posture the organization must be able to develop a core technology and be very cost efficient. Defender organizations try to drive costs down through vertical integration, specialization of labor, a well-defined organization structure, centralized control and standardization, and cost reduction while maintaining quality. Prospectors, on the other hand, are continuously moving in and out of products and markets looking for high growth. Therefore, they need organization structures, systems, and procedures that are flexible. Prospectors rely on decentralized control. These types of organizations do not concentrate on developing efficiency but, rather, focus on the development and early

Exhibit 7–19: External Conditions Appropriate for Strategic Postures

Posture Strategy	Appropriate External Conditions
Defender	• Stable external environment • Predictable political/regulatory change • Slow technological and competitive change • Products or services in mature stage of PLC • Relatively long PLCs • High barriers to entry
Prospector	• Turbulent environment • Rapid technological, political/regulatory, economic change • Introduction and early growth stages of PLC • Technology may be employed across markets • Low intensity of competitive rivalry • Numerous market and product opportunities • Fairly low barriers to market entry
Analyzer	• Moderately changing environment • Technological, regulatory, economic, social, and competitive change open new opportunities • Some competitive rivalry in old and new markets • Some stable products and markets • Some new market and product opportunities • Growth and mature stage of PLC for existing products • Growth stage of PLC for new products

adoption of new products and services. Analyzers attempt to balance defender strategies in stable markets with some prospecting in selected developing markets. Managing these organizations is often difficult because they must mix high levels of standardization and routinization with flexibility and adaptability.

Positioning Strategies

As discussed in Chapter 6, products/services may be positioned marketwide or for a particular market segment. Cost leadership and differentiation are used as marketwide strategies or they are used to focus on a specific segment of the market.

Presence in a market requires that the products and services be positioned vis-à-vis competing products and services. Similar to the other strategy types, positioning depends upon the strengths and weaknesses of the organization and the opportunities and threats in the external environment. In other words, how a product or service is positioned depends on the organization's competitive situation. Therefore, the positioning strategies must be selected based on resources, competencies, and capabilities (strengths), as well as environmental risks. For

Exhibit 7–20: Appropriate Internal Resources, Competencies, and Capabilities for Strategic Postures

Posture Strategy	Appropriate Internal Conditions (Strengths)
Defender	• Ability to develop a single core technology • Ability to be very cost efficient • Ability to protect market from competitors • Capacity to engage in vertical integration strategy • Management emphasis on centralized control/stability • Structure characterized by division of labor • Well-defined hierarchical communications channels • Cost control expertise • Well-defined procedures and methods • High degree of formalization, centralization
Prospector	• Ability to adjust organization to a variety of external forces • Technological and administrative flexibility • Ability to develop and use new technologies • Ability to deploy and coordinate resources among numerous decentralized units • Decentralized planning and control • Flexible structure • Marketing plus research and development expertise • Low degree of formalization (few well-defined procedures and methods)
Analyzer	• Ability to mix high levels of standardization and routinization of core products and markets with flexibility and adaptation for new products and markets • Structure accommodates both stable and dynamic areas of operation • Effective lateral and vertical communication channels • Many different management skills required • Effective strategy and planning team

example, it would be difficult for an urban public community hospital dependent on limited county funding to be positioned as the high-technology hospital in the region (differentiation strategy). Conversely, a well-funded hospital using the latest technology is unlikely to be positioned as the cost leader.

EXTERNAL CONDITIONS

Each of the generic positioning strategies has its own external risks that must be evaluated by the organization (see Exhibit 7–21). Perhaps the biggest risk for cost leadership is technological change. Technological change in processes may allow competitors to achieve cost advantages. Technological change in products/ services may result in differentiation, making the cost leader's product less desirable. The most significant risks for the organization that chooses a differentiation strategy are that emphasis on differentiation pushes costs too high for the

Exhibit 7–21: External Risks Associated with Positioning Strategies

Generic Strategy	External Risks
Cost Leadership	• Technological change that nullifies past investments or learning • Low-cost learning by industry newcomers or followers, through imitation or through their ability to invest in state-of-the-art facilities • Inability to see required product or marketing change because of the attention placed on cost • Inflation in costs that narrow the organization's ability to maintain sufficient price differential to offset competitors' brand images or other approaches to differentiation
Differentiation	• The cost differential between low-cost competitors and the differentiated firm is too great for differentiation to hold brand loyalty; buyers therefore sacrifice some of the features, services, or image possessed by the differentiated organization for large cost savings • Buyers' need for the differentiating factor diminishes, which can occur as buyers become more sophisticated • Imitation narrows perceived differentiation, a common occurrence as the industry matures
Focus	• Cost differential between broad-range competitors and the focused organization widens to eliminate the cost advantages of serving a narrow target or to offset the differentiation achieved by focus • Differences in desired products or services between the strategic target and the market as a whole narrows • Competitors find submarkets within the strategic target and outfocus the focuser • Focuser grows the market to a sufficient size that it becomes attractive to competitors that previously ignored it

Source: Adapted from Michael E. Porter, *Competitive Strategy: Techniques for Analyzing Industries and Competitors* (1980), pp. 40–41. Copyright © 1980, 1998 by The Free Press. All rights reserved. Adapted by permission of Simon & Schuster Adult Publishing Group.

market or that the market fails to see, understand, or appreciate the differentiation. In addition, there are risks for the organization adopting a focus strategy. Often, the focusing organization is dependent on a small segment that may diminish in size, or purchasers may turn to the broader market for products or services. Movement toward marketwide products and services will occur if the differences in cost or differentiation become blurred.

INTERNAL RESOURCES, COMPETENCIES, AND CAPABILITIES

Exhibit 7–22 presents the appropriate internal strengths for each of the positioning strategies. For an organization to use a cost leadership strategy, it must have or develop the ability to achieve a real cost advantage (not price) through state-of-the-art equipment and facilities and low-cost operations. This competitive advantage must be maintained through tight controls and emphasis on

Exhibit 7–22: Appropriate Internal Resources, Competencies, and Capabilities for the Positioning Strategies

Generic Strategy	Resources and Competencies	Organizational Capabilities
Cost Leadership	• Sustained capital investment and access to capital • Process engineering skills • Intense supervision of labor • Products and services that are simple to produce in volume • Low-cost delivery system	• Tight cost control • Frequent, detailed control reports • Structured organization and responsibilities • Incentives based on meeting strict quantitative targets
Differentiation	• Strong marketing abilities • Product/service engineering • Creative flair • Strong capability in basic research • Reputation for quality or technological leadership • Long tradition in the industry or unique combination of skills • Strong cooperation from channels	• Strong coordination among functions in R&D, product/service development, and marketing • Subjective measurement and incentives instead of quantitative measures • Amenities to attract highly skilled labor, scientists, or creative people
Focus	• Combination of the preceding skills and resources directed at a particular strategic target	• Combination of the preceding organizational requirements directed at a particular strategic target

Source: Michael E. Porter, *Competitive Strategy: Techniques for Analyzing Industries and Competitors* (1980), pp. 40–41. Copyright © 1980, 1998 by The Free Press. All rights reserved. Adapted by permission of Simon & Schuster Adult Publishing Group.

economies of scale. Differentiation requires the ability to distinguish the product or service from other competitors. Typically, this requires technical expertise, strong marketing, a high level of skill, and an emphasis on product development. A focus strategy is directed toward a particular segment of the market. However, either cost leadership or differentiation may be used. Therefore, the appropriate competencies are the same for either market segment or marketwide strategies. It is important that organizations adopting a focus strategy closely monitor their market so that specialized needs may be fully addressed and changes in the segment carefully tracked. Otherwise, changes in the market may negate the differentiation or cost leadership. Often *benchmarking* (see Perspective 7–7) can be used to assess current internal strengths for successfully implementing strategies.

Fit with Situational Analysis and Strategy Mapping

After all of the strategy formulation decisions have been made, they should be evaluated in combination to ensure they are logical and fit together. As suggested at the beginning of Chapter 6 and illustrated in Exhibit 6–1, the strategies selected must address an external opportunity or threat, draw on an internal and

Benchmarking is a management process of comparing one organization with a set of its peers. Benchmarking is generally considered to be part of an organization's "learning" or continuous-improvement efforts. As a concept, benchmarking is akin to "taking a picture" of one's organization and comparing this picture with pictures of other organizations. Some organizations simply identify a peer organization and try to emulate it. However, this Perspective deals with benchmarking in the context of an ongoing, long-lived process for senior management that is designed to gather and disseminate both process and performance information throughout an organization.

The benchmarking process begins with the identification of a set of peers. The peers should be organizations that are similar, but not necessarily identical, to the organization and should operate on a scale that will not distort the understandings. The peers should not be direct competitors because of the collaborative nature of the process that will ensue. For example, a steel fabricator with sales of $200 million may seek a paper converter with $50 million in sales as a benchmarking peer or a large health care system might use a telecommunications company as a benchmarking peer.

Senior management of the peer organizations should be contacted to initiate a dialog. The initiator of the benchmarking process is seeking a group of senior managers with whom every intimate detail concerning the strategies of the organizations may be shared. In other words, the initiator should describe the desire to share strategies, financial data, personnel data, and so on, as though the benchmarking participants are part of the senior management team of each organization. The number of participants in a benchmarking group probably should be limited to seven or fewer in order to allow all participants equal opportunities to participate and gain from the experience.

Once a set of willing participants has been recruited, an initial meeting should be scheduled for the purpose of establishing protocol – a set of ground rules for the operation of the benchmarking group. Although there is no well-established standard for such a protocol, it should focus on creating an atmosphere in which full disclosure and frank discussion is facilitated. The meeting can be held at the location of one of the participants or it can be at a neutral site. Ground rules should deal with frequency of meetings, confidentiality, format of the meetings, processes for establishing the agenda for subsequent meetings, and the process of choosing the locations for meetings.

It may be useful to hire a professional facilitator for the first meeting and to determine whether such a person would be helpful in further meetings of the group. Each participant should leave the first meeting with the agenda for the second meeting and a set of work assignments to be completed by the next meeting. Work assignments might include detailed descriptions of the handling of customer complaints, how orders are processed and filled in a minimum of time, or whatever activities were identified as worthy of discussion by the group. At each meeting, detailed minutes (perhaps a transcript) of the meeting should be taken, produced, and distributed to the participants in a timely manner. The purpose of the minutes is to formalize the process and to minimize misunderstandings that may arise from failed memories.

The formal agenda for subsequent meetings should include reports from each of the participants. The frequency of meetings should be such that they impact the practices and procedures of the participants. For the most positive impact, meetings should occur at least on a quarterly basis.

The benchmarking process is not completed when the meetings end. The lessons learned and the insight gained must be shared with subordinates. Participants in the benchmarking process should schedule regular meetings with subordinates for dissemination of information. In other words the lessons should be shared widely within the organization to gain the greatest impact.

Source: Andrew C. Rucks, PhD, School of Public Health, University of Alabama at Birmingham.

competitively relevant strength or fix a competitively relevant weakness, keep the organization on mission, move the organization toward the vision, and make progress toward achieving one or more of the organization's goals. Each strategy should be checked to determine if it meets these criteria.

The strategies of the organization should be mapped and evaluated. Each strategy ends–means chain should be clearly shown. The interdependence of strategies requires managers to evaluate them in concert for consistency and compatibility. Evaluating all the strategic decisions together provides the "big picture" of where the organization is going and helps determine if the vision is really being achieved. In the process of evaluating the strategic map, adjustments may be made and the strategies (each ends and means) reconsidered. For example, a vertical integration adaptive strategy and a prospector strategic posture may not work together well. Similarly, a product development or diversification adaptive strategy through an internal development market entry strategy may be inconsistent with an analyzer strategic posture. In addition, the map provides useful shorthand for communicating and discussing the strategy of the organization.

Strategic Map: An Example

A strategic map for a long-term care organization is shown in Exhibit 7–23. This long-term care organization has been a free-standing, independent institution for some time. However, because of the growth of managed care and emergence of integrated health systems in the area, the organization's leadership has decided that it needs to be part of a system to provide a steady referral base. Therefore, vertical integration as an adaptive strategy was selected. To accomplish the vertical integration strategy, management decided to develop an alliance with a nearby local hospital. The strategic posture is one of aggressively defending the organization's traditional market (private pay and insurance), but management is willing to enter new products and markets if the viability seems reasonable. In addition, management has selected market development directed toward entering into the Medicare segment of the market and has decided that the organization has the internal resources to accomplish Medicare certification. Furthermore, product development has been selected and management is planning to add an independent living facility on the organization's campus to complement the current assisted living and nursing facilities. The product development strategy will be accomplished through a joint venture with a regional hotel chain. The organization's leadership believes the market and product development strategies are consistent with their analyzer strategic posture. The organization plans on developing an extensive advertising campaign (penetration strategy) aimed at communicating its highly effective differentiation strategy based on quality, high level of service, and caring. The organization has committed to install a sophisticated information system including bedside terminals to further differentiate itself from its competition.

Such a strategy map provides a broad overview of the organization's direction and a basis for the development of effective implementation strategies to

Exhibit 7–23: Map of Selected Strategies for Long-Term Care Organization

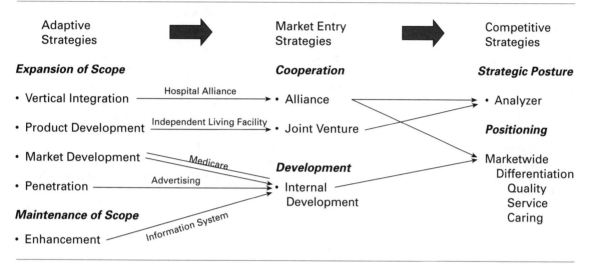

carry out the organization's overall strategy. These maps need not be complicated. Indeed, at this level, simple is better. In stable markets, strategic managers can rely on complicated strategies built on detailed predictions of the future. But in complicated, fast-moving markets where significant growth can occur, unpredictability reigns. When "business" becomes complicated, strategy should be simple.[21]

Managing Strategic Momentum – Adaptive, Market Entry, and Competitive Strategies

Managing strategic momentum at this level is not a matter of keeping the organization on track: rather, it entails deciding if a completely new track or approach is warranted. Managers must decide if conditions require a change in the organization's fundamental strategies. Lorange, Morton, and Ghoshal have called this decision "managing the strategic leap." They suggest:

> Here the challenge is to reset the trajectory of the strategy as well as to decide on the relative levels of thrust and momentum for the new strategic direction. The critical underlying assumptions that underpin the strategy are no longer viable, and the rules that govern the strategy must be redefined. This situation involves a mental leap to define the new rules and to cope with any emerging new environmental factors. Such a recalibrating of strategy requires a personal liberation from traditional thinking, an ability to change one's mindset and confront the challenge of creating advantage out of discontinuity. The question now is how to achieve a quantum leap in one's strategy to capitalize on emerging environmental turbulence. One must proceed by redefining the rules rather than by clinging to the unrealistic hope that the old rules are still valid.[22]

Exhibit 7–24: Managing Strategic Momentum – Adaptive Strategies

1. Are all the important assumptions on which the strategy is based realistic (external environment, competitive environment, internal environment)?
2. Has the strategy been tested with appropriate strategic thinking tools?
3. Have the major stakeholders, inside and outside the organization, that will be most influential in ensuring the success of the strategy been identified and evaluated?
4. If the adaptive strategy is to fill a currently unfilled niche in the market, has the organization investigated whether the niche will remain open long enough to return the capital investment?
5. Has the adaptive strategy been tested with appropriate analysis, such as return on investment and the organization's ability and willingness to bear the risks?
6. Is the payback period acceptable in light of potential environmental change?
7. Does the strategy take the organization too far from its current products and markets?
8. Is the adaptive strategy appropriate for the organization's present and prospective position in the market?

Exhibit 7–25: Managing Strategic Momentum – Market Entry Strategies

1. Is the market entry strategy the most appropriate way to achieve the mission, vision, and goals of the organization?
2. Is the market entry strategy consonant with the values of the organization?
3. Is the market entry strategy the best way to accomplish the adaptive strategy?
4. Is the market entry strategy compatible with the adaptive strategy?
5. Does management understand the unique requirements of the market entry strategy (purchase, cooperation, development)?
6. Does management understand the important market forces?
7. Have adequate financial resources been allocated to enter the market?
8. Does the selection of the market entry strategy affect the ability of the organization to effectively position its products/services in the market?
9. Is the market entry strategy compatible with the competitive strategies?
10. Does the market entry strategy place unusual strains on any of the functional areas?
11. Have new stakeholder relationships developed as a result of the market entry strategy (customers, vendors, channel institutions, and so on)?
12. Has the relationship between the desire and need for rapid market entry been properly analyzed?
13. Has the relationship between the desire and need for control over the products and services been achieved?
14. Have the trade-offs between costs and control been properly analyzed?

Changes in one organization's adaptive strategy create significant changes for other organizations. Such dramatic change is relatively rare in stable environments but somewhat more frequent in dynamic environments. Signals that the basic strategy for the organization needs to be changed must be carefully monitored because the change will have serious long-term consequences. The questions presented in Exhibit 7–24 are helpful in surfacing such signals, and they provide a starting point for discussion of the appropriateness of the organization's adaptive strategy. The assumption underlying Exhibit 7–24 is that the mission, vision, values, and goals are still appropriate but that the organization's adaptive strategy should be questioned.

Changes in market entry strategies represent a "new way of doing business" for an organization. For example, developing alliances as a means of accomplishing market development is quite different than an internal development strategy and changes the whole orientation of the organization. Evaluation of the effectiveness of the market entry strategies provides insight into how well the adaptive strategies are being carried out in the marketplace (see Exhibit 7–25). Similarly, a change in an organization's strategic posture or positioning represents a revolutionary change. For example, moving from a differentiation strategy to cost leadership initiates substantial change throughout the organization. The adaptive strategies and market entry strategies may be appropriate, but if the product or service does not have the appropriate strategic posture or is not positioned effectively the organization may not achieve its goals (see Exhibit 7–26).

Summary and Conclusions

Several strategic alternatives are available to health care organizations. To initiate strategic thinking and planning, it is important that the organization has a process in place for understanding the internal and external environments and methods for evaluating strategic alternatives. This chapter provides a number of frameworks for evaluating adaptive strategies, market entry strategies, and competitive strategies.

There are several methods for deciding which of the adaptive strategic alternatives is most appropriate for an organization. The TOWS (threats, opportunities, weaknesses, and strengths) matrix, product life cycle (PLC) analysis, portfolio analyses (BCG and extended), strategic position and action evaluation (SPACE) analysis, and program evaluation were examined in considerable depth. Using these methods, managers can classify internal and external factors to gain perspective on which adaptive strategic alternative or combination of alternatives is most appropriate.

Once the most appropriate adaptive strategy (or combination of adaptive strategies) has been determined, a market entry strategy must be selected. Expansion and maintenance of scope strategies are initiated through one or more of the market entry strategies. Entry strategies include acquisition, licensing, venture capital investment, merger, alliance, joint venture, internal development, and internal venture. The organization's internal resources, competencies, and capabilities (strengths), the external conditions, and the organization's objectives will determine which of these strategies is most appropriate.

After the market entry strategy has been selected, competitive strategies, which include strategic posture and positioning strategies, should be evaluated and selected. Strategic postures include defender, prospector, and analyzer strategies. Positioning strategies include marketwide or focus strategies of cost leadership or differentiation. The external conditions and internal resources,

Exhibit 7–26: Managing Strategic Momentum – Competitive Strategies

Strategic Posture

1. Is the strategic posture sustainable?
2. Have there been external developments (technological, social, regulatory, economic, or competitive) that have shortened product life cycles?
3. Are there new market opportunities that suggest the organization should move more toward a prospector posture? Analyzer strategy? Defender strategy?
4. Has the organization developed the right mix of centralization and decentralization for the selected strategic posture?
5. Is the level of standardization and administrative flexibility appropriate to the strategic posture?
6. Is the level and type of communication appropriate for the strategic posture?
7. Is the strategic posture appropriate given the barriers to market entry?
8. Has the level of vertical integration been appropriate for the strategic posture?
9. Has the organization been caught by surprise too often?
10. Are the overall strategy, strategic posture, and value adding strategies compatible?
11. Does the organization need to evolve its strategic posture?

Positioning

1. Is the product or service positioned appropriately in the market?
2. Can the organization use one of the other generic positioning strategies?
3. Is the positioning strategy appropriate considering the external opportunities and threats?
4. Will market forces allow the selected positioning?
5. Is the positioning strategy best suited to capitalize on the organization's strengths and minimize its weaknesses?
6. Is the positioning of the organization's products and services unique in the marketplace?
7. Is the positioning strategy defensible against new players trying to position themselves in a similar fashion?
8. Is the positioning strategy compatible with the market entry strategy?
9. Does the positioning strategy provide the appropriate image for the organization?
10. Is the positioning strategy sustainable?
11. Is the appropriate distribution channel being used?
12. Is the current promotional strategy appropriate?
13. Is the pricing strategy appropriate?

capabilities, and competencies influence strategic posture and positioning strategies. Therefore, the most appropriate strategic posture and positioning strategy may be selected through an evaluation of the internal skills and resources of the organization and the external conditions.

Chapters 8 through 10 discuss implementation strategies. Chapter 8 will address strategy implementation through value adding service delivery strategies.

Key Terms and Concepts in Strategic Management

BCG Portfolio Analysis
Benchmarking
Community Need
Extended Portfolio Matrix
  Analysis
External Fix-It Quadrant
Future Quadrant

Internal Fix-It Quadrant
Needs/Capacity Assessment
Organizational Capacity
Product Life Cycle (PLC)
  Analysis
Program Evaluation
Program Priority Setting

Program Q-Sort Evaluation
Reengineering
SPACE Analysis
Strategic Assumptions
Survival Quadrant
TOWS Matrix

QUESTIONS FOR CLASS DISCUSSION

1. Explain how external opportunities and threats are related to internal strengths (competitive advantages) and weaknesses (competitive disadvantages) to develop strategic alternatives.
2. Using the TOWS matrix, what adaptive strategic alternatives might be appropriate for each quadrant?
3. Describe the product life cycle. How is it useful for thinking about the adaptive strategy of a health care organization?
4. Why is the length of the product life cycle important for strategy formulation?
5. What adaptive strategic alternatives are indicated for each stage of the product life cycle?
6. Is BCG portfolio analysis useful for developing adaptive strategic alternatives for health care organizations?
7. Explain the rationale for expanding the traditional BCG portfolio matrix.
8. Identify appropriate adaptive strategic alternatives for each quadrant in the expanded portfolio matrix.
9. Explain the strategic position and action evaluation (SPACE) matrix. How may adaptive strategic alternatives be developed using SPACE?
10. Why should program evaluation be used for public health and not-for-profit institutions in the development of adaptive strategies?
11. What are the critical factors for determining the importance of programs within a not-for-profit organization?
12. Why should public health and not-for-profit organizations set priorities for programs?
13. Describe program Q-sort. Why would an organization use program Q-sort?
14. How are market entry strategies evaluated? What role do speed of market entry and control over the product or service play in the market entry decision?
15. How are the strategic postures and the product life cycle related?
16. How may the positioning strategic alternatives be evaluated?
17. Do health care organizations change directional and adaptive strategies often?
18. How can "doing the strategy" (managing the strategic momentum) provide information about changing the strategy?
19. As managers learn by doing, what strategies are most likely to change: adaptive, market entry or competitive?

NOTES

1. Peter F. Drucker, *Management: Tasks, Responsibilities, Practices* (New York: Harper & Row Publishers, 1974), p. 470.

2. Heinz Weihrich, "The TOWS Matrix: A Tool for Situational Analysis," *Long Range Planning* 15, no. 2 (1982), pp. 54–66.

3. Ibid., p. 61.

4. Ibid.

5. Institute for the Future, *Health & Health Care 2010: The Forecast, The Challenge* (San Francisco: Jossey-Bass Publishers, January 2000), p. 43.

6. Robin E. Scott MacStravic, Edward Mahn, and Deborah C. Reedal, "Portfolio Analysis for Hospitals," *Health Care Management Review* (fall 1983), p. 69.

7. Gary McCain, "Black Holes, Cash Pigs, and Other Hospital Portfolio Analysis Problems," *Journal of Health Care Marketing* 7, no. 2 (June 1987), p. 56.

8. Ibid., pp. 56–57.

9. MacStravic, Mahn, and Reedal, "Portfolio Analysis for Hospitals," p. 70.

10. McCain, "Black Holes, Cash Pigs," p. 60.

11. Ibid., p. 61.

12. Ibid., p. 62.

13. Alan J. Rowe, Richard O. Mason, Karl E. Dickel, and Neil H. Snyder, *Strategic Management: A Methodological Approach*, 3rd edn (Reading, MA: Addison-Wesley, 1989), p. 143.

14. Ibid., p. 145.

15. Peter M. Ginter, W. Jack Duncan, Stuart A. Capper, and Melinda G. Rowe, "Evaluating Public Health Programs Using Portfolio Analysis," *Proceedings of the Southern Management Association*, Atlanta (November 1993), pp. 492–496.

16. Rangan V. Kasturi, "Lofty Missions, Down-to-Earth Plans," *Harvard Business Review* 82, no. 3 (2004), p. 112.

17. US Department of Health and Human Services, *Healthy People 2010* (Washington, DC: US Government Printing Office, 2000). This publication presents the 467 national health objectives that cover 28 priority areas. US Department of Health and Human Services, *Tracking Healthy People 2010* (Washington, DC: US Government Printing Office, November, 2000). This publication is a statistical compendium that provides information on measuring the 2010 objectives, technical notes, and operational definitions.

18. Fred N. Kerlinger, *Foundations of Behavioral Research* (New York: Holt, Rinehart & Winston, 1973), p. 582.

19. Ibid., p. 584.

20. J. Block, *The Q-Sort Method in Personality Assessment and Psychiatric Research* (Palo Alto, CA: Consulting Psychologist Press, 1978), p. 137.

21. Kathleen M. Eisenhardt and Donald N. Sull, "Strategy as Simple Rules," *Harvard Business Review* 79, no. 1 (January 2001), pp. 107–116.

22. Peter Lorange, Michael F. Scott Morton, and Sumantra Ghoshal, *Strategic Control* (St. Paul, MN: West Publishing, 1986), p. 11.

ADDITIONAL READINGS

Barca, **Mehmet,** *Economic Foundations of Strategic Management* (Burlington, VT: Ashgate Publishing, 2003). To what extent can economic theory provide the theoretical foundations of strategic management? This book attempts to address and answer this question. It integrates insights from the philosophy of science, microeconomic theory, and other approaches to strategic management. The author illustrates that many of the propositions of strategic management can be traced to a variety of economic theories.

Forgang, **William G.,** *Strategy-Specific Decision Making: A Guide to Executing Competitive Strategy* (Armonk, NY: M. E. Sharpe, Inc., 2004). This book contains a number of theoretical and practical approaches to the design and implementation of corporate strategies. The author presents a view of strategy from the operations level using a comprehensive case study to illustrate concepts and issues. A variety of tools and techniques are presented that are useful in thinking about strategy in all types of organizations.

Longest, **Beaufort B.,** *Managing Health Programs and Projects* (Indianapolis, IN: Jossey-Bass, 2004). The author develops principles and practices for program and project management in public health, community health, and health services organizations. The book looks at both the technological and soft sides of program and project management. The decision-making process is explored in detail and the importance of communicating the results of decision making are emphasized.

Schwartz, Peter, *Inevitable Surprises: Thinking Ahead in A Time of Turbulence* (New York: Penguin Publishers, 2004). An internationally known author presents ideas on the use of scenario analysis to offer views of how the world of tomorrow might appear. A helpful book for understanding the possible uses of scenario planning, Schwartz presents a convincing argument for the use of strategic thinking in all areas of business.

Surowiecki, James, *The Wisdom of Crowds: Why the Many Are Smarter than the Few and How Collective Wisdom Shapes Business, Economies, Societies, and Nations* (New York: Doubleday, 2004). People seem to naturally distrust decisions made by groups, crowds, and teams. Yet, when properly formulated, collective wisdom can far exceed that of any single individual. This book provides numerous examples of how large groups can make very effective decisions.

White, Colin, *Strategic Management* (London: Palgrave Macmillan Publishing, 2004). Various theories and approaches to strategy are included in this book. The author asserts that the best way to assist managers of the future in problem solving is to illustrate how to conceptualize and generalize their problems. Philosophical topics are discussed without a loss of the practical aims of aiding managers in developing better strategies for success.

8 CHAPTER

Value Adding Service Delivery Strategies

"Discovery consists of seeing what everybody else has seen and thinking what nobody else has thought."

Albert Szent-Gyorgyi Von Nagyrapolt,
Hungarian-born US biologist

Introductory Incident

Eliminate Appointments, Serve Patients Better

It may sound crazy but an increasing number of physicians believe the best and most efficient way to serve patients is to eliminate appointment systems – and some convincing data exist to back this assertion. A system known as open access scheduling developed by Mark Murray, MD and Catherine Tantau (part of a more comprehensive reengineering process called idealized design of clinical office practice – IDCOP) is based on the premise that today's work should be done today.

Years ago people who needed to see a doctor simply went to the office, "took a number," and waited their turn. This wait-your-turn system overwhelmed doctors and patients; appointments were welcomed as bringing order to chaos. However, the increasing demand for patient services resulted in appointment systems that were ever-more complex and frustrating. Despite the fact that appointments were scheduled, they were rarely honored. Double and triple booking to account for no shows resulted in *de facto* wait-your-turn systems. The uncertainty with regard to timely access encouraged patients to seek high-cost emergency room care. Studies have shown, for example, that almost half of some HMO patients who presented for emergency room care would have preferred a

▶

day or two wait for a primary care physician if they could have been assured of seeing a doctor in a day or two rather than "next week."

Open access scheduling means that patients call and are asked whether they would prefer to come in today or tomorrow and given a time to see the doctor. Approximately one-third of the appointment times are reserved for required rechecks, but if they are not filled they are made available. Depending on the practice type, the number of held appointments would vary – pediatricians have more rechecks than many other practice types, for instance. Contrary to popular belief, physicians were not overwhelmed by a guarantee of same-day scheduling. Moreover, the fear of not having full appointment books (with consequent reductions in revenue) appeared to be unfounded. In one study, medical practices' total patient visits actually increased more than 7 percent during the first year of same-day scheduling, 12 percent in the second year, and a little more than 15 percent in the third year.

Medical practices can create considerable value by enabling patients to see the doctor promptly. Adding value in this manner provides an advantage over competitors who require long waits. Since the appointment system is essentially the gatekeeper into the system, any improvement in this area can represent a significant competitive advantage.

The Jefferson County (Alabama) Department of Health provides primary care in health clinics located throughout the county. Before the health department implemented the same-day scheduling system, patients were keeping only about 50 percent of their appointments. The typical patient had to wait from one to three months for an appointment and physicians were routinely overbooked because of the high no-show rate. Countless appointment guidelines, including type of appointment (routine physical versus acute illness and so on) and time slots (must schedule 15 minutes or 30 minutes, and so on for the type of appointment), were possible, transforming the county's appointment system into a clerical nightmare.

A pediatrician in one of the health clinics read reports on reengineering medical practices and was taken by Dr. Murray's advice, "To gain control over your schedule you must do the unthinkable: offer every patient an appointment for today." The pediatrician convinced the Health Officer to pilot test same-day scheduling in one clinic. Prior to initiating the same-day scheduling system, baseline data were collected for six months. The average number of pediatric visits per month was 382; the average number of new patients per month was 78; and the mean waiting time for the next available appointment was 46 days. The average no-show rate was 56 percent and physician productivity averaged 89 percent.

After the six-month period, same-day scheduling was initiated in the clinic. The results were impressive. Average waiting time for the next available appointment was reduced from 46 days to 5 days. The no-show rate was reduced from 56 percent to 19 percent. At the test site new patients per month increased from 78 to 95 and provider productivity increased to 122 percent (a productivity level greater than 100 percent was possible if the provider saw patients at a rate that exceeded the national average). The results of the pilot program were so impressive that all the county health clinics converted to the same-day scheduling system.

Some of the lessons learned from this pilot study include:

1. Simple systems are better than complex systems and doing today's work is preferable to pushing today's work to the next day, week, or month.
2. People have to be willing to think outside the box and be willing to do things differently.
3. Health professionals have to be willing to get rid of systems that no longer work.
4. Open access created considerable value among clinic patients and is instrumental in increasing the desirability of the practice.

Source: Stephen D. Mallard, Terri Leakeas, W. Jack Duncan, Michael E. Fleenor, and Richard J. Sinsky, "Same-Day Scheduling in a Public Health Clinic: A Pilot Study," *Journal of Public Health Management and Practice* 10, no. 2 (2004), pp. 148–155.

Learning Objectives

After completing this chapter the student should be able to:

1. Understand the decision logic for developing implementation strategies.

2. Understand that the service delivery portion of the value chain is key in the implementation of strategy.

3. Link the results of internal analysis and the development of service delivery implementation strategies.

4. Understand how the pre-service, point-of-service, and after-service strategies of an organization are the means to achieve directional, adaptive, market entry, and competitive strategies.

5. Understand that competitive advantage may be created inside the organization through implementation of the service delivery strategies.

6. Understand that through service delivery strategies the organization itself is changed, strengthening competitive advantages and improving competitive disadvantages.

7. Create service delivery strategies that carry out the directional, adaptive, market entry, and competitive strategies.

Implementation Strategies

Once the directional, adaptive, market entry, and competitive strategies have been planned, planning for implementation strategies commences. Further strategic thinking is required to determine how to achieve the decisions previously made in strategy formulation. As introduced in Chapter 1 (refer to Exhibit 1–3), the implementation strategies include two different sets of value adding strategies – value adding service delivery strategies and value adding support strategies. In addition, planning strategy implementation includes the setting of organizational objectives, development of plans, and agreement on budgets that translate the organization's overall strategy into specific action plans.

Strategies Based on the Value Chain

Chapter 4 presented strategic thinking maps for evaluating the strengths and weaknesses of the organization. This approach focused on evaluating those components of the organization that create value and, ultimately, competitive advantage – the value chain (see Exhibit 8–1). Recall that the upper portion of the value chain focuses explicitly on the primary activities of the organization – the delivery of services. The lower portion of the value chain contains the value adding support activities

Exhibit 8-1: The Value Chain

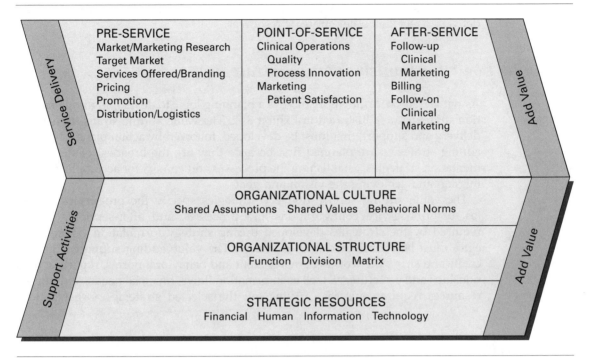

Source: Adapted from Michael E. Porter, *Competitive Advantage: Creating and Sustaining Superior Performance* (New York: Free Press 1985), p. 37.

that include the organization's culture, structure, and strategic resources. The components depicted in the value chain are the principal means of creating value for the organization and developing competitive advantages. These activities are major elements of strategy implementation and are shaped by strategic thinking and strategic planning.

As the activities are completed, strategies are implemented, the goals are achieved, and the organization moves toward the vision. This movement by one organization changes the environment; it creates new issues, trends, events, or forces for the other organizations' environments. In other words, it changes the world – if ever so slightly. At the same time, completion of the activities changes the organization itself. This continuous movement creates "permanent white water for ourselves and others" and, if successful, weaknesses are strengthened and strengths are made more sustainable.[1]

The categories depicted in the value chain have been well documented as key elements that create value in an organization. It is important to remember that service delivery strategies and support strategies are not separate but, rather, inter-act and complement each other. The organization's culture, structure, and strategic resources are in reality an inherent part of the pre-service, point-of-service, and after-service activities. Thus, a change in the culture of the organization

– human competencies – is clearly reflected in service delivery. Further, an enhanced information system – a resource – can benefit all aspects of service delivery as well as other strategic resources.

Planning Logic for Implementation Strategies

As with strategy formulation, there is a planning logic to developing implementation strategies, as illustrated in Exhibit 8–2. The value adding strategies (service delivery and support) first must be developed, followed by action plans. The value adding strategies are planned first because they are the broadest of the implementation strategies, establishing the processes and context for accomplishing the mission and achieving the vision and goals.

The value adding service delivery strategies specify the pre-service activities, point-of-service configurations and processes, and after-service activities required by the strategies developed during strategy formulation. These strategies must be coordinated and consistent. The value adding support strategies create and shape the working environment and behavioral norms, reporting relationships and structure, as well as information flows, financial needs, and human resources requirements for carrying out the selected strategies. Organizations

Exhibit 8–2: Planning Logic for the Value Adding Strategies

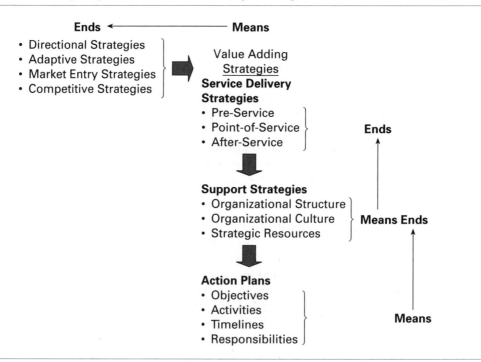

that do not have the appropriate culture, structure, or strategic resources cannot implement effective plans. Finally, for the organizational units, specific objectives may be developed, activities necessary to accomplish the objectives established, and financial resources committed to the activities. Clearly, the culture, structure, and strategic resources must be shaped and provided direction by strategic managers developing the overall strategic plans of the organization.

As with the strategy formulation phase, implementation strategies form an ends–means relationship. The value adding strategies must accomplish the directional, adaptive, market entry, and competitive strategies and the action plans must accomplish the value adding strategies. The action plans link the individual organizational units to the overall strategy. Units are typically functional, such as operations (surgical units, Alzheimer's units, well-baby care, and so on), marketing, finance, human resources, and so on. Operations and marketing are the primary work of the organization – the value adding service delivery activities – because providing a product/service and delivering it to customers are the central activities of organizations.

The major emphasis of human resources, finance, facilities management, and information systems typically will be directed toward achieving the support strategies. These functions support the accomplishment of the primary work of the organization.

Developing Value Adding Strategies

Each area of the value chain was evaluated during internal analysis as part of situational analysis (Chapter 4) and the conclusions used as inputs to strategy formulation. Each of the strategic decisions (directional, adaptive, market entry, and competitive) made to this point move the organization closer to accomplishing its mission and vision and at the same time make special demands on the organization that require explicit action. The requirements of directional, adaptive, market entry, and competitive strategies have been discussed in Chapters 5 through 7. Based on the results of the comparison of the current situation and what strategic managers want the organization to be, value chain components may need to be maintained or changed to carry out the strategy.

The logic of developing specific strategies for each component of the value chain is illustrated in the strategic thinking map in Exhibit 8–3. The resulting decision matrix is shown in Exhibit 8–4. As suggested by the decision matrix, for each component of the value chain, a strategic decision must be made (maintain or change) and general direction provided to the organizational units as to how that decision is to be accomplished. Later more specific organizational unit strategies (action plans) that carry out the value adding strategies will be developed. This chapter discusses the organizational requirements for the value adding service delivery strategies. Value adding support strategies will be discussed in Chapter 9 and the translation of the value adding strategies into specific organizational objectives, action plans, and budgets will be discussed in Chapter 10.

Exhibit 8–3: The Process of Developing Value Adding Strategies

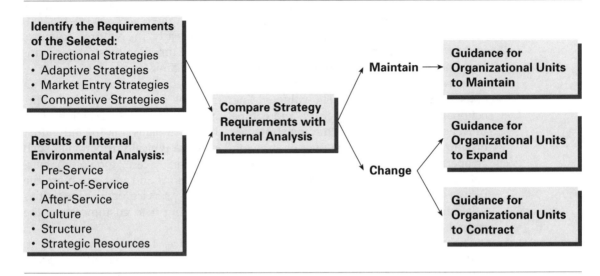

Exhibit 8–4: Strategic Thinking Map for Developing Value Adding Strategies

Value Adding Service Delivery Strategies	Results of Internal Analysis	Requirements of Selected Strategies	Comparison of Strategy Requirements and Internal Analysis	Maintain or Change
Pre-Service				
Market/Marketing Research				
Target Market				
Services Offered/Branding				
Pricing				
Promotion				
Distribution/Logistics				
Point-of-Service				
Clinical Operations				
Marketing				
After-Service				
Follow-up Activities				
Billing				
Follow-on Activities				
Value Adding Support Strategies				

Value Adding Service Delivery Strategies

The *value adding service delivery strategies* include pre-service, point-of-service, and after-service strategies. Value adding service activities are critical to the success of the organization because they are the principal method for creating value. Therefore, explicit strategies must be developed for each. The components must be coordinated and work in concert. It is the role of strategic managers responsible for developing and managing the strategic plan to ensure the compatibility of pre-service, point-of-service, and after-service strategies.

Pre-Service Activities

Pre-service entails the planning and activities that enable the organization to determine its customers and the services that will be offered to them as they enter the system. Marketing is central in developing pre-service strategies. Pre-service marketing entails market and marketing research that enables the organization to determine the appropriate customer (target market), design services that will satisfy that customer, identify the service through branding, price the service at a level that is acceptable to the customer while allowing the organization to survive, and offer the service where the customer wants or is able to obtain it.

Pre-service marketing spills over into pre-service operations. If the organization is already providing a service such as heart catheterizations, pre-service marketing would investigate whether that service should be maintained or changed in some way to meet the needs of customers (both physicians and patients). Pre-service operations – including location, facilities design, medical expertise offered, and so on, in which the operations (or work) of the health care organization will be carried out – has to be thought of in concert with pre-service marketing. For example, during pre-service marketing an organization may determine that becoming a comprehensive long-term facility is not possible given the need in the environment (decreasing population in the area), the number of competitors (strong competition already exists), and the shortage of employees (for minimum wage employees needed as well as RNs). However, further research might suggest a niche market exists for an Alzheimer's unit.

Research by Miles, Snow, Meyer, and Coleman indicates that there is greater performance variation within strategic postures rather than between postures.[2] Their research indicates that prospectors and analyzers place greater emphasis on marketing than do defenders, and prospectors utilize marketing most. Prospectors and analyzers both seek market information in turbulent times to attempt to gain competitive advantage. A strong and enduring relationship with a customer has become the foundation for competitive advantage. "Marketing has much to contribute to the strategy dialogue, including insights on market selection, construction of a consumer value proposition, and business strategy implementation."[3] Once these activities have been completed, the information about the service has to be made available to potential customers.

Market and Marketing Research

Market research is any data gathering about the market itself – potential customers, their wants, needs, and habits in terms of health care, and the services an organization could provide that would satisfy those wants and needs. Market research aids in identifying the target market but must be done in conjunction with identifying the services the organization will deliver.[4] For example, a group of physicians in a medical clinic has internal resources, competencies, and capabilities to provide care. If all the physicians are board certified in plastic surgery, the group could decide to provide comprehensive care including reconstructive and cosmetic surgery or the physicians could decide to focus only on cosmetic surgery "to the stars" with extreme confidentiality in a remote but very comfortable location. The target market has to want or need the services and the organization must have the resources, competencies, and capabilities to provide the services.[5]

Marketing research is data gathering to assist in decision making concerning the components of marketing (the four Ps: product, price, place, and promotion). Because the internal assessment has highlighted the organization's strengths and weaknesses, the external analysis has identified the threats and opportunities in the marketplace, and the organization has identified the strategies it wants to pursue, pre-service strategies attempt to identify the specific target market and the services to be offered.[6]

Service Strategy versus Services Strategies

The marketing of *services*, such as health care services, is not the same as marketing products such as automobiles, beer, or computers. In addition it is important to differentiate between services and service. "Competitors commonly offer the same services and different service."[7] In the early 1980s, when marketers began differentiating between physical goods and services, Len Berry defined a good as an object, a device, or a thing; a *service* was defined as a deed, a performance, or an effort.[8] Because physical goods do contain some elements of service and services contain some physical components, marketers think of products (the inclusive term used to mean goods, services, or ideas) as ranging along a goods–services continuum. As indicated in Exhibit 8–5, most primary health care providers (hospitals, physicians, hospices, and so on) would be located further to the right on the continuum. Secondary providers, such as pharmaceutical manufacturers, would be further to the left on the continuum.

There are several differences that translate into unique marketing problems for health care services:

1. *Intangibility.* Health care is probably the most intangible service because the consumer cannot sample it before the purchase and usually cannot effectively evaluate it after "consumption."
2. *Variability.* The mismatch between consumer expectations and actual delivery may be greater for the health care product because of the uniqueness of individual

Exhibit 8–5: Health Care Goods–Services Continuum

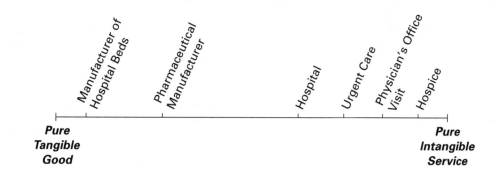

diagnosis and response to medications and treatment. In addition, the multiplicity of health care professionals with whom the patient interacts results in greater variation in the quality of care. Even an individual provider's care will vary based on how he or she feels on a given day.

3. *Perishability.* The demand for a health care product is less predictable, although some possibilities exist to better control usage. For example, incentives can be offered to induce physicians to perform elective surgery in the afternoons and over weekends when the operating room is virtually unused. Emergency rooms need to be staffed, although when emergencies will occur is unknown.

4. *Inseparability.* Distinguishing the decision maker from the consumer may be more involved for the health care product because the physician often recommends specific hospitals, long-term care facilities, home care agencies, therapists, and others to the patient who customarily – but not always – follows that advice. In addition, production and consumption occur simultaneously.

5. Frequently, the patient does not pay directly for the health care service.[9]

Although services, and health care services in particular, have a number of differences in comparison to physical products, they have many more similarities. The basic approach to marketing does not change. Health care organizations, as services providers, need to understand and adopt marketing practices if they are to survive in today's competitive environment. Even so, as pointed out in Perspective 8–1, health care boards of directors and CEOs are calling for hard empirical evidence that proposed marketing expenditures will yield greater profitability.

Identifying the Health Care Customer – Target Market

One of the difficulties with health care marketing is that there are many, very diverse customers to satisfy in the market – physicians, health care consumers (patients) and their friends and families, other health care organizations, third-party payors, and so on. In addition, there are multiple services categories

Perspective 8–1

Return on Marketing
Investment (ROMI)

Increasingly, boards and CEOs are calling for hard empirical evidence that proposed marketing expenditures will yield greater profitability. Organizations are starting to put the foundation for ROMI in place, but even the benchmarking companies have realized that there is a long way to go. Marketers have resisted ROMI because of their belief that marketing is inherently creative and difficult to quantify.

Marketing managers have found that when they cannot show a return on marketing investment, next year's marketing dollars may be diverted or decreased. However, the value of knowing the organization's ROMI is not just about measuring return but more about using the knowledge to better determine how to serve and understand customers, and how existing offers, products, and channels can be matched with the correct customers. According to Drew Eginton of Marketswitch (a software company that enables managers to collect data and determine ROMI), "Marketing is not an expense. It is mission critical if you see consumers as an asset that you cannot afford to lose."

Although ROMI has never been easy to calculate, marketers are investing time and money to improve its measurement. The Advertising Research Foundation's (ARF) ROMI benchmark studies identified three areas that are receiving greater emphasis:

1. *Discipline:* consistent, rigorous follow-through. ROMI-managed companies have a person with sufficient credibility, conviction, and clout to instill a ROMI focus across the organization. The leader in several of the best practice companies has been the CEO, but senior marketing executives have filled the role.
2. *Metrics:* consensus is required on the definitions, measures, and analytic approaches to build ROMI metrics.
3. *Advanced analytics:* in the past three decades marketing measurement has shifted from simple sales tracking to market share tracking to revenue targets with market share as the ROMI metric. Organizations do not want to cede share to the competition, but neither do they want to buy share through lost revenue.

The ARF's ROMI benchmarking studies showed that managers applying ROMI metrics-based decision processes made faster decisions and had fewer criticisms from "Monday morning quarterbacks." Key to their improved decision making was the trust in the system shared by marketers and other managers. They built confidence in a judgment process that was constantly fed new learning through methodical ROMI measurement of marketing activities. Despite the barriers that made capturing ROMI challenging, experts agree that it is just a matter of time before it is required.

Somerset Medical Center in New Jersey decided to change its typical classified newspaper ads for nurses to display ads with a photo of an antacid dissolving in a glass of water. The caption – "Not exactly bubbling over with enthusiasm?" – acknowledged the stresses of nursing but was offset by the hospital's promise to renew enthusiasm through its career environment. The effort resulted in nursing vacancies decreasing from 40 to 13. Return on marketing investment was calculated based on ad cost versus typical recruiting expenses. In addition, costs associated with overtime work and outsourcing to fill vacant shifts was incorporated.

Another ROMI opportunity is to purchase tracking software for the health/medical care organization's website. The number of visitors to a site, the length of time they stay on a page, and whether they take some action can determine the investment's pay-off. Baylor Health Center set up four kiosks in its lobby – for general visitors, patients, recruitment, and donors – and within eight months, 400 individuals had left their email addresses for further contact. Although the number may appear modest, they are qualified names. ROMI can be calculated from the results of each of the kiosks.

Yale-New Haven Hospital in Connecticut was able to reduce its "marketing cost per patient gained" from $1,103 in 2000 to $433 in 2002 by using print banner advertisements. The cost per banner ad ▶

(typically a 2–3″ tall ad that is 5–12″ wide running along the top or bottom of the front page of a newspaper) was less than 3 percent of a display ad because banner ads are generally text only and the cost for placement was about 10 percent of a display ad. During the time the ad ran, consumers associating Yale-New Haven with "advanced medicine" increased from 22 percent to 40 percent and admissions increased from 39,113 to 43,524.

A chest pain center campaign brought in more than $1.25 million in margin contribution while the yearly marketing investment was $250,000. A large group physicians' practice developed a marketing campaign to remind its current patients about recommended screenings and check-ups. Each existing patient received an annual wellness message, based on age and gender, sent within two weeks of the patient's birthday. The practice used a control group (not receiving the messages) to determine that over 20 percent more appointments were made, resulting in ROMI of over $100,000.

Without proven ROMI, marketing budgets may be drastically reduced in this time of declining reimbursements, increasing numbers of uninsured, and falling returns on stocks and bonds.

Source: William A. Cook, "ROMI Outlay Brings High Yields to B-to-B Marketers," *B to B* 89, no. 4 (April 5, 2004), p. 26; William Gombeski, Jr., Jan Taylor, Katie Krauss, and Clayton Medeiros, "Banner Year," *Marketing Health Services* 24, no. 2 (Summer 2004), pp. 32–37; and Arundhati Parmar, "Barriers to Success," *Marketing News* 38, no. 4 (March 1, 2004), pp. 20–22.

– long-term care, emergency medicine, oncology, dermatology, and so on – that determine who the customer will be.[10] Furthermore, within these specializations are customers with varying needs, wants, and desires.

Segmentation is the process of identifying recognizable groups that make up the market and then selecting a group as the *target market*. Several groups may be targeted, but each one requires different marketing activities to achieve customer satisfaction. Exhibit 8–6 illustrates the many customers for a hospital and the segments a physician (one of the hospital's customers) may consider. The process of segmentation for a general medical practice service category would be more challenging than for an oncology (cancer) practice, which is more specialized. However, many segments can be identified among cancer patients – those with leukemia, skin cancer, lung cancer, and so on. Specialization of the hospital, nursing home, or physician's practice would be a first step in the segmentation process, but other demographic, psychographic, geographic, and benefits factors must be considered as well.

PHYSICIANS, PATIENTS, AND THIRD-PARTY PAYORS AS CUSTOMERS

Physicians are a major target for marketing efforts because they recommend other health care providers for their patients. Estimates are that physicians control 80 percent of health care costs, as they prescribe pharmaceuticals and medical equipment, and determine hospitalization and diagnostic and surgical procedures. Doctors are an important customer base for hospitals because almost all patients are admitted by physicians who have staff privileges at the hospital. If physicians choose not to admit patients to a given hospital, the hospital will have no patients.

Exhibit 8-6: Determining the Health Care Customer

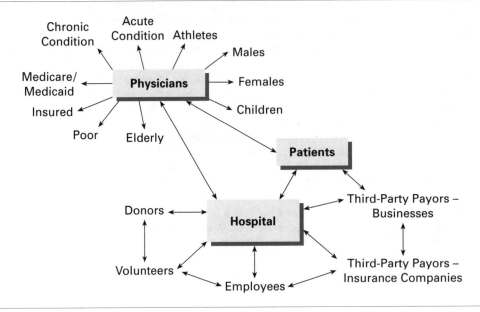

The patients themselves are customers. However, the buyer–seller relationship of traditional exchange processes has to be modified in much of health care because the patient has a professional dependency on the doctor. Most people have no knowledge of medical terminology, or the complexity of medical diagnosis or care, and cannot accurately evaluate the medical care provided.

At one time, patients would never have questioned their doctor's choice of a hospital. Today, a patient whose physician does not have privileges at the hospital of the patient's choice may change physicians. In a national study by Professional Research Consultants and American Hospital Publishing, Inc., more than 42 percent of the participants said they would change physicians to be admitted to the hospital they preferred.[11] When considering maternity care, 58 percent of pregnant women select a hospital before choosing a physician.[12]

Third-party payors (insurance companies and employers) are also customers. These companies must be satisfied that the health care provider is efficiently treating patients or they will use their substantial financial influence to dictate that patients go elsewhere. Considerable insight concerning third-party payors can be gained through quality monitoring organizations.

The National Committee for Quality Assurance (NCQA) is an independent, not-for-profit organization started by a number of large employers in 1991 with a mission to "improve health care quality everywhere." NCQA uses three different methods to assess quality: (1) voluntary accreditation (currently about 50 percent of HMOs are accredited); (2) Healthplan and Employer Data and Information Set (HEDIS), a tool used to measure performance in key areas such as immunizations and mammograms; and (3) a comprehensive member satisfaction survey. NCQA

Perspective 8–2
On the Way to Quality Improvements – Patient Satisfaction and a Malcolm Baldridge Quality Award

SSM Health Care, sponsored by the Franciscan Sisters of Mary in St. Louis, Missouri, is one of the largest Catholic integrated delivery systems, with 4,500 beds. SSM's receipt of the Malcolm Baldrige Quality Award was not the only goal of all its effort to improve patient satisfaction. The desired outcome was a transformation of the organization's culture to one that valued and worked for continuous improvement. In the pursuit of the award, SSM learned four keys to establishing an environment where quality can flourish:

1. *Framework.* The requirements for the award provided a framework for analysis, decision making, and action. It helped the organization focus on the most important things.
2. *Mission.* It took many months and a comprehensive employee survey before SSM was able to consolidate its mission statement into one that every employee agreed with and could recite.
3. *Bias toward Results.* Goals are essential but results are what count. Many health care organizations are confused about accountability. People work hard without achieving the desired results. In SSM's case, if an activity is not getting the results they want, they change the activity. The results are the important thing to SSM.
4. *Dedicated Leadership.* During the process of seeking the award, there was no management restructuring and very few employees left the organization. Leadership became important throughout SSM.

An example of accomplishment will illustrate some of the positive gains made in the process of working toward the award. To improve patient loyalty, SSM considered streamlining measures already in use at some of its hospitals. Among others, these measures include providing immediate results from mammograms, allowing 24-hour family visitation (even in the ICU), and allowing patients to order meals any time of day (similar to room service). The goal is to allow patients more control and to serve them better – not to make the work of the hospital easier.

In the immediate future the organization's leadership is committed to improving two specific measures of patient satisfaction – returning for future care and patients' recommendations of SSM to others. The overall goal is for SSM's 20 acute-care hospitals and three nursing homes to increase their market shares in the communities they serve in Missouri, Illinois, Wisconsin, and Oklahoma.

Each hospital in the SSM system is expected to develop its own market strategy based on the community it serves. On the basis of this strategy some hospitals may decide to eliminate or consolidate product/service lines or make themselves regional centers for specialized treatment.

Building a quality culture is a challenging but satisfying task. Competing for the Malcolm Baldrige Quality Award was one means of focusing on quality. And for SSM it worked.

Source: Anonymous, "SSM Health Care Values Continuous Quality Improvement Results," *Health Care Strategic Management* 22, no. 3 (2004), pp. 11–12.

maintains an up-to-date website available to consumers and employers to determine whether they want to use a specific plan. Because of NCQA's success in the private sector it has expanded to the public sector as well – Medicaid HEDIS is being used in various states.[13] In addition, as described in Perspective 8–2, quality awards, such as the Malcolm Baldrige Quality Award, have been used successfully to assess and improve health care quality.

THE NEW HEALTH CARE CONSUMER

The Institute for the Future has identified a new US customer for the twenty-first century. This new consumer is better educated, has a sizeable income, and is comfortable using information technology. Fifty percent of adults have at least one year of college, tending to make them more analytical and more prone to information processing than those with no college.[14] About 40 percent of US households earn more than $50,000 per year, enabling them to have some discretionary spending. Although 62 percent of US consumers have computers in their households, 83 percent of new consumers own personal home computers.

About half of American households are "new consumers" and share the following characteristics:

- They prefer choice and will seek out information to make a better choice (89 percent will search through at least four different information sources).
- They demand better information and communications.
- They are skeptical of brands based on corporate claims and will investigate to determine value for themselves.
- They are willing to experiment.
- They value convenience (70 percent of US households are dual income and have less time).
- They expect superior service.[15]

To satisfy the new consumers, whether it is with cars or computers or health care, it is important that employees who interact with them have a good attitude, provide solutions rather than sell a particular product, are flexible, listen, show initiative and innovation, possess good interpersonal skills, and have a strong belief in the services they are selling. *Consumerism* (consumers' proactive taking of their rights) is one of the major driving forces in health care today (see Perspective 8–3).

To Brand or Not to Brand Services

A brand is everything the services organization stands for but it does not have any merit if customers do not value it. Every customer evaluates every service experience by dividing quality by price to arrive at a sense of value. It may not be a perfect method, or very accurate, but it is real as far as that consumer is concerned. For services the brand is more important than for tangible products, especially because if performance falls short, the service brand's image and positioning deteriorate more quickly.[16]

Much branding activity in health care has centered on promoting and creating identities for health care systems. However, customers are not interested in abstract systems, but rather the physician and nurses who care for them in a hospital that they have been aware of and perhaps preferred for decades. Although preference for a new brand can be built over time, in most cases it is

Perspective 8–3

Consumerism in Health Care

Gone are the days when physicians told patients what to do, admitted them to the hospital of the physician's choice, and the consumer meekly followed the physician's directives. Consumerism in health care is here – and most agree it will not go away any time soon. There is a fundamental market shift as consumers are becoming better informed, more involved in their own health care, and more demanding.

The following trends are considered to be the most compelling evidence of the consumerism movement in health care:

1. *Success of direct-to-consumer marketing.* For example, drug companies have advertised a variety of prescription drugs directly to consumers and achieved bottom-line success. Consumers visit a physician and ask for the prescription drug by name, armed with information about it.
2. *More demanding patients.* Consumers are using the Internet and other sources to learn more about their health. They are demanding to be involved in health care decision making and challenge physicians over prescriptions, surgery, and so on.
3. *Consumers opt for more choice.* Traditional HMOs have not been growing as they were at the end of the twentieth century; it is the PPO and POS plans that have accounted for the growth in managed care. Consumers favor those plans that offer more choices of physicians and hospitals over a plan that has a slightly lower monthly charge.
4. *Employers are shifting risk by allowing consumers to make more decisions about health care benefits.* Consumer directed health care plans, sometimes referred to as cafeteria plans, allow the employee to choose how a fixed amount of money per month or year is used to receive the benefits the employee determines is best for his or her family. Driven largely by employers to control escalating health care costs, some consumers are expected to resist because the consumer directed health plans have higher deductibles, but the monthly cost is considerably lower and will be attractive to other consumers.
5. *Explosion in alternative medicine.* Complementary and alternative medicine (CAM) is being integrated into many hospitals. A 2003 *Health Forum* study found that half of responding hospitals have or are considering CAM. Currently paid out of pocket, consumers are pressuring employers and managed care plans to cover these benefits. Most commonly paid by insurance are chiropractic, nutritional counseling, and biofeedback.
6. *Demographics favor women.* This is the group most interested in health care, especially the "sandwich generation" (boomers who are responsible for health care of children, themselves, husbands, and parents).
7. *Private-pay health services.* These are sought and paid for by consumers interested in shortening their nose, improving their smile, correcting vision, relieving stress, and so on.
8. *Consumers are accessing health care information online.* Although outdated almost as soon as it is collected, research documenting the number of sites and online use indicates that the number of sites for health care is continuing its explosive growth and the fastest growing segment of users is women who are better educated and older. The most frequently sought online information concerns health care.
9. *Self-care is increasing.* Self-care is being advocated by managed care plans – especially for chronic conditions, such as diabetes and hypertension, where lifestyle has a great deal of impact.

Source: Steve Davis, *Consumer-Directed Health Care: Facts, Trends, and Data 2004–2005* (Washington, DC: AIS Atlantic Information Services, Inc., 2004); Sita Ananthe, *Hospital & Health Networks*, www.hhnmag.com/hhnmag/hospitalconnect/ (January 15, 2004); Elizabeth Fischer and Dean Coddington, *Beyond Managed Care: Consumers and Technology Are Changing the Future of Health Care* (San Francisco, CA: Jossey-Bass, 2000).

less expensive and more effective to leverage and extend the existing brand name. HCA–The Healthcare Company has used this strategy effectively.

A brand represents three things: what an organization offers to the market, what an organization does, and what an organization is.[17] All three are critically important for health care organizations because the brand is intangible – it is simply a set of promises. It implies trust, consistency, and a defined set of expectations. The strongest brands have a unique position in the mind of the buyers and can usually be articulated. Mayo Clinic and Johns Hopkins are examples of brands that have value for customers. Every person who has contact with a patient at these clinics represents that brand. If housekeeping were to be poorly performed, it hurts the brand; if admitting is poorly done, it hurts the brand; if clinical care is done less well than customers expect, it hurts the brand. Thus, it is critical that every member of the organization realizes that the brand is owned and should be managed by every employee. Another way to define brand is that it is every touch point the organization has with its ultimate customer.[18]

To develop a good branding strategy, answers to three questions have to be understood:

1. How do consumers choose one brand over another?
2. How does your brand stack up against competition?
3. What possibilities exist for potential brand growth and expansion?

Perceptual Gaps in Services Delivery

For health care organizations, one way to determine why customers choose one brand (health care organization) over another is to study the *perceptual gaps in service delivery* that exist in patient expectations for health care service quality – especially because quality from the customer perspective is emerging as a critical issue. Exhibit 8–7 illustrates the service quality gap model. Expectations can be shaped by a number of things including the individual consumer's perceptions, direct inspection of a physical product, and traditional organization-dominated sources of information (advertising, news releases, and so on). Regardless of how an individual's expectations are determined, they serve as a means by which quality is evaluated. Gaps exist at a number of points based on the customer's perceptions and the organization's communications and previous contact with the customer. Gap 5, the difference between customer expectations of service and perceived service delivered, is a direct result of any gaps or combination of gaps in 1 to 4. Gap 5 cannot be minimized directly but improvements result from smaller gaps at 1 to 4.[19]

In a number of studies investigating patient expectations of service quality, researchers found that all groups working in a clinic (administrators, physicians, nurses, and other employees) underestimated their patients' expectations for service reliability, assurance, responsiveness, and empathy, but overestimated their customers' expectations for the tangible dimension. The physician group had the poorest understanding of patient expectations and the administrators came the closest to understanding patient expectations, although they underestimated as

Exhibit 8–7: Conceptual Model of Service Quality

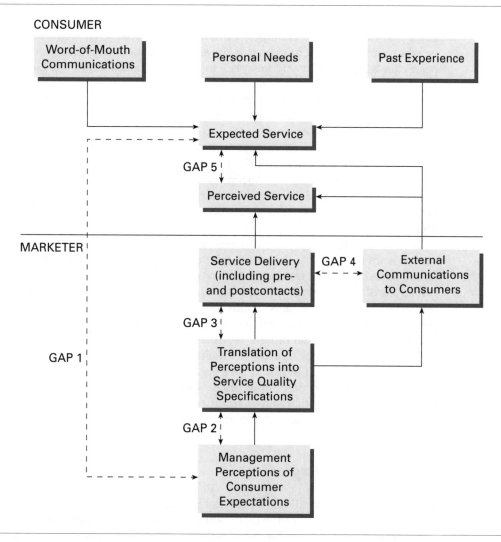

well.[20] A later study of medical and nursing students found that the students came to the health care profession with misunderstandings of patient expectations.[21]

Some physicians believe that patients have unrealistic expectations (often from watching television!). Perhaps it is the role of providers to educate patients to manage those expectations. To ignore the higher expectations of patients is tantamount to sending customers to the competition. Further, "if the organization (administrators, employees, physicians, students) fails to be sufficiently aware as to what patients really expect, any initiatives to bring about improvements in quality will likely fail."[22] To avoid the problem, providers need to determine patient expectations, for example through surveys or focus groups.

Pre-Service Pricing Decisions

Pricing in health care is extremely difficult because it is a service that consumers would rather not have to purchase. In addition, consumer perceptions of "high price equals high quality and low price means low quality" and "you get what you pay for" operate in health care, yet most consumers do not have the ability to judge quality. Further, in many instances third-party payors separate consumers from the actual costs of care. Finally, health care providers often have a great deal of difficulty determining their costs and then deciding on a price. Competitive negotiations with third-party payors that are looking for lower prices have led some health care providers to prices that are too low and threaten the organization's long-term viability. Government reductions for Medicare and Medicaid patients have resulted in reimbursements that are frequently below the cost of providing care. Thus, many providers have opted not to serve Medicare or Medicaid patients.

In health care, low-price strategies must be selected carefully because few people want to think that they are receiving "cheap" (poor quality) care. Although cost leadership strategies are generally associated with having low costs that can be translated into low prices, a high-price strategy can effectively position an organization as a high-quality health care provider. However, the consumer must perceive that the benefits (esthetically pleasing surroundings, attentive care, latest technology, and so on) are worth the high price.

Based on the services offered, the ability of the consumer to pay, and the cost to deliver the service, the health care organization determines a price. There are no magic formulas to determine prices and some government mandates about serving every patient that shows up at the emergency room door, for example, make pricing an even more challenging task.

Pre-Service Distribution/Logistics

The location of the health care provider will impact the number of people who will seek its services. A location that is attractive because of its proximity to patients' homes and work is a valuable asset, especially if other health care providers cannot duplicate the location. Because people do not want to travel great distances for most health care, demographic studies of population are an important part of choosing a location for a facility. Satellite offices and hospital branches have become increasingly important as busy patients value convenience. Although satellite offices/hospitals do not typically cut costs for the organization, they do cut costs for the patient, which can lead to an increased market share and improved efficiency for the health care provider.

Some hospitals are finding it worth while to establish education centers in shopping malls. Other health care organizations have established limited primary care facilities in grocery stores. In Louisville, Kentucky, for example, FastCare began operating medical kiosks in two Kroger grocery stores. The kiosks are staffed by nurse practitioners who offer basic services for ailments such as ear infections, strep throat, and pink eye. Limited lab tests in such areas as cholesterol and drug screenings are offered. According to the vice president for diagnostic services, "The convenience factor is what really drives people in." FastCare leases about 120 square feet near the pharmacy. Each kiosk costs about $150,000 to launch.[23]

Mobile units are another method of achieving the optimum in health care delivery. Long practiced by the Red Cross to gain more blood donations, other institutions are using movable diagnostic equipment to be closer to patients. Approximately 200 mobile mammography units are in operation in the United States to increase women's use of this excellent but expensive tool.[24]

Pre-Service Promotion

Promotion includes: advertising; public relations events (baby birthday parties, health fairs, cancer survivor celebrations, and so on); personal selling; and sales promotion (contests, participation in trade shows, and so on). The promotional elements work in combination to be able to communicate a message to various consumers and stakeholders of health care organizations.

During the 1990s hospitals learned that increased amounts of advertising would not fill more beds and that great advertising might set customer expectations higher than the organization could deliver. Advertising works best when there is an identified product or service that meets consumers' needs. Branding helps consumers know the service to seek and reminds them where they can obtain health care when they have a need for it.

Personal selling has been used more extensively in health care as various organizations compete to be the provider of choice in managed care plans. In addition, personal selling has come into play as health care providers compete for employees that are in short supply. Pharmaceutical companies, long users of personal selling, have realized that their customers are busier than they ever have been and sales reps will probably have less than two minutes to tell a physician about a new drug. Direct-to-consumer advertisements encourage the patient to "ask your doctor" about new drugs.

Matching Pre-Service to the Strategy

It is important that services characteristics and the target market are appropriate for the selected strategy. In addition, the services price, brand, promotional activities, and logistics must contribute to the accomplishment of the directional, adaptive, market entry, and competitive strategies. The services delivery activities were assessed and classified as competitive advantages or competitive disadvantages in the internal analysis phase of situational analysis. As shown earlier in Exhibit 8–3, the attributes of the current pre-service activities must be compared with the service characteristics, target market, price, brand, promotional activities, and services logistics that are required by the strategy. Results of this assessment will determine whether the strategic managers need to create implementation strategies to maintain or change the pre-service activities.

MAINTAINING PRE-SERVICE ACTIVITIES

When the requirements of the strategy match the current pre-service strengths and needs of the customers, then strategic managers should focus on maintaining those strengths, giving particular attention to those areas that have created competitive advantage. For example, if during internal environmental analysis, a brand name was evaluated as a strength having high value (H), was rare (Y), was difficult to imitate (D), and was sustainable (Y), resulting in HYDY, maintaining the effectiveness of the brand name is particularly important. Allowing such a strength to weaken may lead to the loss of an important competitive advantage, particularly when a strong brand name is common (not rare) among competitors (HNDY). Therefore, in maintaining pre-service activities, strategic managers should:

- Engage in periodic customer focus groups and market research to understand the wants, needs, and desires of the organization's target markets and whether they are or are not being satisfied;
- Monitor the demographic, psychographic, and health status characteristics of the service area (with particular attention to trends in the target markets);
- Continually communicate to physicians, patients, third-party payors, and others concerning the type and range of services offered, pricing, and branding;
- Monitor promotional effectiveness; and
- Monitor customer ease of system entry (logistics).

CHANGING THE PRE-SERVICE ACTIVITIES

Pre-service activity changes can be difficult and may require considerable market research as well as promotion. In internal environmental analysis, where the requirements of the strategy call for different services, a different or additional target market, changes in pricing, branding, or promotional activities, change strategies should be initiated. In addition, where significant competitive disadvantages have resulted because of ineffective pre-service activities, it is likely that change strategies will have to be initiated. For example, where the promotional strategy was viewed in internal analysis as a weakness, of high value but common among competitors, difficult to imitate, and sustainable by competitors (HYDY), change strategies should be initiated particularly where competitors may act to develop an effective promotional strategy and achieve a significant competitive advantage. Similarly, where an organization has a weak promotional strategy and other organizations have effective promotions that are difficult to imitate and can be sustained (HNDY), strategic managers will need to initiate change. Strategic managers who want to change pre-service activities should:

- Change the services attributes to better match the expectations of the target market;
- Train employees to better provide the new services;

- Redefine the target market to match the changing demographic, psycho-graphic, and health status characteristics of the service area;
- Provide price discounts or price classes among members of the target market;
- Change the balance among advertising, personal selling, and direct marketing (one-to-one marketing);
- Brand individual products (as opposed to the organization's name as the brand); and
- Redesign parking lots, walkways, signage, and reception.

Point-of-Service Activities

Point-of-service is a transformational process that incorporates an organization's resources – human and nonhuman, competencies, and capabilities: its assets – into value added service delivery. Health care was a cottage industry for centuries. Specialization, cost pressures, and the actual work being done have taken health care from being totally customized for the individual patient in his or her home to an attempt to treat patients more similarly so as to develop economies of scale. Placing people in hospitals, outcomes measures, formularies, and so on, focus on treating patients more alike – the industrialization of health care. Most Americans and their physicians do not like it. The Planetree system was introduced to refocus delivery on patient care (Perspective 8–4). The best services delivery differs for each organization depending on the strategies determined during strategy formulation.

Point-of-Service – Clinical Operations

The appropriate model of health care delivery is based to a great degree on the care required. If health care were divided into three sectors – acute illnesses with quick recovery, significant illnesses (chronic but manageable), and catastrophic illnesses (AIDS, cancer, and so on) – each accounts for approximately one-third of the health care dollar in America. However, the latter two represent 10 percent of the population. In other words, 90 percent of the population represents short-term treatable illnesses where the volume is high, but costs are low per episode and co-payments and deductibles have a measurable impact. Technology can improve efficiencies in this sector. For significant and catastrophic illnesses, health care providers can increase efficiencies through understanding the choice of processes and selecting the one most suitable for patients' care (mass customization).[25]

Mass Customization

Mass customization may be the way to capture the customer-friendly benefits of long-term physician–patient relationships and the cost-careful benefits of capitation for survival in today's health care market. *Mass customization* can be accomplished by a "series of modular approaches to prevention and care, highly

Perspective 8–4

Planetree – Customer Oriented Care

Successful businesses in today's consumer driven environment have identified what is important to consumers – not only the products but also the delivery of the product. For example, a nondescript hotel provides a room that is acceptable to a business traveler; a great hotel knows that particular traveler prefers a non-smoking room on a lower floor farthest from the elevator on the west side. Although most businesses have embraced the consumer revolution and thrived, health care has been slow to change. Health care providers have defined their products too narrowly as a good technical or physical outcome. The "technology may be state-of-the-art, but the delivery has been pathetic." Patients come not only for medical care, nursing care, and health care, they come for caring.

Planetree was founded in 1978 by Angelica Thieriot, an Argentinean married to a prominent San Francisco businessman. She was treated in a US hospital for a rare virus and was appalled by the cold, impersonal, dehumanizing medical care she received. When her son and father-in-law had a similar hospital experience, she began a crusade – leading to the founding of Planetree – dedicated to improving the hospital experience for patients and their families. Named after the tree under which Hippocrates taught the art of healing some 2,500 years ago, Planetree is based on compassion, comfort, dignity, esthetic beauty, shared knowledge, and the freedom of informed choice.

The initial program began in 1981 with the opening of the Planetree Health Resource Center on the 272-bed California Pacific Medical Center campus in San Francisco to provide information that patients and families could easily access to make informed choices. In 1992 the first Planetree units outside California were opened at Beth Israel Medical Center cardiac unit in New York City and a subacute care unit at Delano Regional Medical Center in Delano, California. The first hospital-wide adoption of the concept was at Mid-Columbia Medical Center in The Dalles, Oregon. In 1994 Griffin Hospital in Derby, Connecticut, became the first Planetree affiliate hospital.

Planetree units are designed to soothe and cater to the sick. Families are encouraged to visit at any time and to maintain some semblance of normalcy by eating a home-cooked meal together in a fully equipped kitchen or strolling through a garden. Volunteers bake breads and cookies that make a Planetree hospital smell like no others. Planetree hospital staff – from physicians and nurses to housekeepers – are trained to understand the patient-centered care approach.

Patients are urged to become informed about their illness and participate in the decision making for their care. They are given instructions on how to read their medical record and encouraged to make notes on it. When patients are ready for discharge, they are provided with "take-out" information that documents all medications, the reasons for taking them, the schedule, and so on. The information duplicates what has been discussed in the hospital. Actually the patient begins controlling medications in the hospital as soon as he or she is able (since they will be in charge at home).

The basic Planetree philosophy is comprised of two parts: (1) if patients have access to information regarding their illness and hospitalization they can become active participants in restoring their health, and (2) it is possible to create a healing, caring environment in a hospital setting.

Sixty-two hospitals in 24 different states are members of the Planetree Alliance attempting to improve patient-centered care.

Source: Susan B. Frampton, Laura Gilpin, and Patrick A. Charmel, *Putting Patients First: Designing and Practicing Patient-Centered Care* (San Francisco: Jossey-Bass, a Wiley Imprint Company, 2003).

Exhibit 8–8: Increasing Quality through Mass Customization

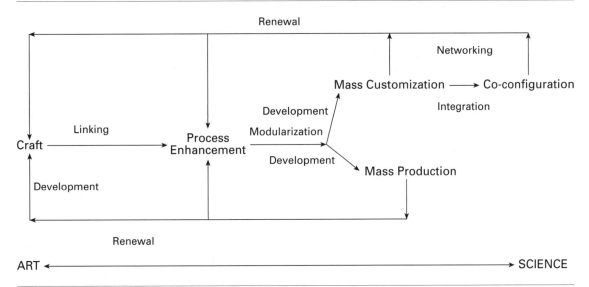

Source: Reprinted from C. P. McLaughlin and A. D. Kaluzny, *Defining Quality Improvement, Continuous Quality Improvement in Health Care*, 2nd edn, p. 15, 1999, Jones and Bartlett Publishers, Sudbury, MA. Reprinted with permission www.jbpu.com.

articulated and well supported by information technology" (Exhibit 8–8). Clinical pathways represent an example of mass customization. Pathways represent the best known way to treat the patient but the path still has to be applied based on the individual patient's background, medical history, health status, and so on. Recognizing that people are different, this "synchronization of the implementation of the modules" or co-configuration, must be determined by the providers.[26]

Mass customization requires that a sufficient number of people have the same disease or diagnosis. For example, with some disease states mass customization lacks the personal appeal needed for involvement. Medco Health Solutions has effectively created mass customization through segmentation. The mass customization "digs down" another level to differentiate clinical needs among people in a single disease category (diabetes) that is large enough to warrant separate contact but not too small to present an administrative burden. In these cases true customization is not cost justified, but "one-size" programs (standardized or mass programs) are not effective either. Mass customization falls somewhere in between and prevents therapy gaps within categories, such as the gap between diabetics who have only a few health problems and diabetics who require frequent medical attention.[27]

QUALITY OF OPERATIONS

The trust in the health care system has diminished because of reports in the media over managed care's failures as well as the Institute of Medicine's study indicating that as many as 98,000 deaths per year are because of medical error. The greatest opportunity a health care organization has is the day-to-day interaction between caregivers and patients.[28] Every person in a health care organization has some responsibility for its image.

Historically hospitals have concentrated on meeting the expectations of physicians, and then more recently physicians and third-party payors. The structure of the health care industry has enabled it to circumvent a customer orientation that most other segments in the services industry have had to adopt.[29] Various environmental changes are creating the need for health care to be more responsive to the wants, needs, expectations, and requirements of patients for information, convenience, and personal control. Recently, there have been attempts to rank health care organizations based on clinical quality. However, as suggested in Perspective 8–5, rankings are difficult because there is a lack of agreement over the assumptions underlying the ranking attributes and some of the implications may be misleading.

The National Committee for Quality Assurance (NCQA) developed by large employers provides the Healthplan Employer Data Information Set (HEDIS) to compare individual managed care health plans. The intent was to create a database that the participants (consumers or employers) could use to compare the performance of their health plans against other health plans on a consistently measured and reported set of criteria.

Neither the Joint Commission (JCAHO) nor the HEDIS data can be correlated with *Consumer Report* satisfaction studies. The fact that mammograms are done (a HEDIS measure) does not mean women are happy with the way they are done (a measure of patient satisfaction). Today, health care providers are more responsive to patients because of excess capacity, the increasing impact of consumerism, deregulation of health care, changes to reimbursement systems, declines in occupancy rates, and corporate restructuring and diversification. Companies are tired of trying to manage the health care of their employees; they are offering programs for employees to choose their own benefits package.

Lakeland Regional Medical Center, an 851-bed facility in Florida, discovered during a planning retreat that the time allocated to coordination and scheduling of procedures was almost the same as the time spent in providing services. Red tape and increasingly specialized jobs made relatively simple procedures seem to be overly complex to the patients. In addition, customers had to repeat the same information to a variety of staff. A patient might come into contact with 60 different employees.[30] The quality of clinical care received by patients was not perceived to be as good as it actually was because of the way care was delivered (see Exhibit 8–9).

Labor-intensive services are difficult to automate, but not impossible. Blood pressure checks have been automated. Additionally, a finger stick for routine blood work could be done by a machine; but would the public accept a machine instead of a nurse? In a different but important service industry, many bankers held on to their belief that consumers would want to talk to a real person when cashing checks or depositing money. Those banks that were the first to automate with teller machines have been very profitable. Similar results may be achieved in health care.

Perspective 8–5
Hospital Rankings – Quality Assessment or a Great Marketing Tool?

Daniel Beckham, a health care consultant, wrote an article about the top ten hospitals based on his assessment of how well the hospital embraced a common set of priorities and, as a result, had succeeded in growing revenues, profits, and market share. Claims of "top ten" status soon appeared in advertising by those hospitals, but there were no questions concerning the actual quality of care delivered. Beckham suggested to HCIA, a Baltimorebased health care information company that was sold in 1998, that it use its database to develop a ranked list of hospitals. The "Top 100" list is now published annually in *Modern Healthcare*. The early rankings relied on utilization and financial data.

A ranking list that is regarded as credible (one done by an organization or group of individuals perceived as having specialized knowledge or expertise) is an excellent means for an organization to position itself in the market. US consumers like lists, believing that the "Top 100" provides assurance and reliability. At most it provides aggregate information that tells consumers how a medical staff or institution performs on average. But no one actually receives care from an organization "on average."

US News & World Report produces the most visible and sought-after rankings in health care. Of the 6,012 US medical centers (military and veterans hospitals are not included), only 2,113 are eligible to be ranked by *US News* based on meeting one of the following three criteria: member of the Council of Teaching Hospitals, affiliation with a medical school, or offering at least nine of 17 technology-related services. Three areas are given approximately equal weight: reputation, mortality, and other factors. *US News* uses surveys of board certified specialists (150 from each ranked specialty for a total of 2,550) surveyed – about one-half of them responded in 2004. Respondents identify five hospitals they consider to be the best in their area of specialization. Mortality ratios are adjusted for severity of condition. "Other factors" are taken from American Hospital Association annual surveys (number of procedures, number of nurses to number of beds, and number of technology services). The model for determining the ranking was created in 1993 by the National Opinion Research Center at the University of Chicago.

In 2004, only 177 medical centers were ranked in at least one specialty and 14 made the "honor roll" that required very high rankings in at least six specialties. For those at the top of the honor roll list, such as Johns Hopkins and Mayo, it provides prestige and increased use of the facility. Specialty category leaders – such as Cleveland Clinic, Mayo Clinic, and Duke University Hospital for heart care; University of Texas M. D. Anderson Cancer Center and Memorial Sloan Kettering for cancer care – allow more facilities to be recognized (and sells more publications).

Rating health care organizations is somewhat different from rating universities or large businesses. Rarely do people seek out number 15 on the list for a life-threatening illness if they can go to number 1.

Clinical quality is still an illusive component in the rankings. Will patient satisfaction studies and actual outcomes data be used in the future?

Source: J. Daniel Beckham, "What the Health Care Ranking Lists Can – and Can't Do," *Health Forum Journal* (January–February 2001), pp. 39–41, 47 and Avery Comarow, "Best Hospitals 2004: Methodology Behind the Rankings," *US News & World Report* 137, no. 1 (July 12, 2004), p. 48.

Exhibit 8–9: Key Questions for Determining Patient- and Family-Oriented Care

Trustees, administrators, and medical and nursing leaders should ask themselves the following key questions to determine whether their organization's environment puts patients and families first:

• Do the hospital's vision, mission, and philosophy of care statements reflect the principles of family-centered care?
• Are the vision, mission, and philosophy communicated clearly throughout the hospital, to patients and families, and others in the community?
• Do patients and families serve as advisors to the hospital? In what ways are the patients and families involved in the orientation and education of employees? In the design planning process?
• Are hospital policies, programs, and staff practices consistent with the view that families are allies and important to patient well-being? Are families considered visitors?
• What systems are in place to ensure that patients and families have access to complete, unbiased, and useful information?
• Does the hospital's human resources system support the practice of family-centered care?
• In academic medical centers, how do the education programs prepare students and professionals in training for family-centered practice?

Source: Institute for Family-Centered Care, Bethesda, Maryland.

CLINICAL PROCESS INNOVATION

Clinical process innovation (or CPI) is defined as "the generation, acceptance, and implementation of new ideas, tools, and/or support systems aimed at improving clinical processes and, ultimately, patient care."[31] It differs from continuous quality improvement (CQI) in that CQI focuses on improving existing clinical processes for performance improvement. CPI is a contextual and critical appraisal of current clinical processes to identify opportunities for more effectively providing care. As Michael Hammer explains, "Operational innovation should not be confused with operational improvement or operational excellence. Those terms refer to achieving high performance via existing modes of operation. . . . Operational innovation means coming up with entirely new ways of filling orders, developing products, providing customer service, or doing any other activity that an enterprise performs."[32]

Through the first decade of the twenty-first century, providers need to realize that consumers who want more control over their health care will have it through consumer advocacy groups, increased competition, and unprecedented access to information. If customers do not receive the care they want, they will change to another provider. Physicians have to be willing to listen to patients talk about other treatments and how alternative therapies might blend with more traditional medicine to improve health. Consumers who use alternative therapies are middle- to upper-class, well-educated people with good jobs and money to spend on whatever they believe to be important for their health care.[33]

Point-of-Service – Marketing

Physicians are an integral part of the health care system. As such, hospitals and health systems have tried a variety of models to incorporate physicians into the new systems. Thus far, none of the models (as depicted in Exhibit 8–10) has really worked. Perhaps that is because none of these models focus on the physician–patient relationship. "A renewed patient focus is not only the best way to serve our customers and patients, it is also a business imperative for any organization that wishes to survive into the next era of health care."[34] Some strategies in which physicians and health systems can work together to achieve patient goals include redesigning services lines around enhancing the patient experience rather than around financial aspects of delivery of care, multispecialty physician care teams based on consumers' needs, physician outreach programs to determine ways that physicians believe patient care can better be delivered, increasing physician–patient communications since physicians are frustrated by the lack of time they can spend with patients, and agreeing on measurements for success.

Health care providers must understand their current situation in the market. How well are they satisfying the various customers they currently serve? Are competitors better meeting customer needs? What new needs will occur in the near future that should be in the planning stages today? Frequently, the necessary information is not available, and marketing research must be conducted to understand patient satisfaction, medical staff satisfaction, competitive offerings, and so on. Often it is important to collect data from patients and staff who do not use (or occasionally use) the facility as well as current users. Another way to collect consistent and reliable data is to use mystery shoppers (see Perspective 8–6).

Matching Point-of-Service to the Strategy

Each strategic alternative selected by an organization may affect the point-of-service delivery strategy. However, as discussed previously, central to point-of-service delivery are issues such as quality, efficiency/speed, innovation, and flexibility (mass customization) of the service. Most organizations are constantly trying to improve point-of-service delivery – employing an adaptive/enhancement strategy.

MAINTAINING POINT-OF-SERVICE ACTIVITIES

When the requirements of the selected strategy match the characteristics of the current point-of-service delivery, the strategic managers should develop strategies to maintain the current strengths of the organization's resources, competencies, and capabilities. As with the pre-service activities, particular attention should be given to those point-of-service delivery areas that have created competitive advantage. In maintaining point-of-service delivery activities strategic managers should:

Exhibit 8–10: A Partnership Model Scorecard

Model	Financial Performance	Strategic/Market Performance	Physician Satisfaction
Employed medical group	• Health system suffers huge operating losses • Physician income is greater than production	Market share does not increase substantially	Health system control mentality is contrary to physician mindset
Managed care organization/ Physician-hospital organization	• Added market leverage is questionable • Capitation has proven difficult to manage	Number of covered/served lives can increase	Physicians often have multiple contracting vehicles and may question the value of this model
Management services organization	• Infrastructure can be expensive • Organization will break even at best	Model typically has no impact	Physicians are typically unhappy with level of service
Shared ownership	• Physicians are reluctant to provide capital • Good investments can result in attractive returns	Model has potential to increase market share	Physician satisfaction is enhanced as physicians feel ownership in the organization
Physician incentives to manage components of care delivery	Health system must be willing to share dollars	Model is primarily a cost reduction strategy	Physicians receive financial rewards for improving quality and reducing cost
Link with major health plan	Organizations must carefully develop appropriate financial incentives	Model can secure a market leader position	Physicians must take on the additional responsibility of controlling the delivery process

Source: "The New Playbook: Transforming Health System-Physician Relationships," © 1999 VHA/Tiber Group.

Perspective 8–6

Mystery Shoppers Aid Health Care Organizations in Developing and Maintaining Business

Standard patient satisfaction surveys do not always reveal to a health care organization the aggregate of things that drive consumers away. Mystery shoppers (often they are actors) are usually hired by an independent agency to check out a health care facility's customer service. They call and report such things as how many rings before the phone was answered, how long and how many times they were put on hold, friendliness and willingness to help, flow and signage, and so on. These things generally will not be identified on a patient satisfaction survey, often because the dissatisfied consumer is no longer a patient – he or she will go elsewhere for health care.

Mystery shopping has not been widely used in health care because of the complexity of carrying it out in such a challenging setting, but it is often the little things that irritate consumers – and they can be improved. Smiling, making eye contact, any staff member stopping to help give directions to someone who ponders a directional sign for an overly long time, making sure a caller is transferred to the correct department, giving correct information on services the health care organization offers and does not offer (but where it can be obtained), and referral to a website (for someone with a computer) or referring to the website themselves and sharing the information with someone who does not have online access – all these actions can be performed by any employee and it says "we care."

Parkview Health System, a four-hospital system in northeast Indiana, credits mystery shoppers along with other internal efforts for the system's increase in patient satisfaction. Before using mystery shoppers, one of its ERs scored 20 percentile in the national Press Ganey study of patient satisfaction in third quarter 1998. After using mystery shoppers and identifying and resolving problem areas, that same ER's score improved to 91 percentile in fourth quarter 1999, positioning it in the top 10 percent nationally.

Source: Karen Southwick, "Mystery Shopping Captures Missed Opportunities," in *Healthcare Growth Strategies 2001* (Santa Barbara, CA: COR Health, LLC, 2000), pp. 43–46.

- Monitor service quality through asking customers (physician, patient, payor, other) if there is a way the experience could be improved – as they are the ones receiving the service;
- Monitor clinical (patient) and organizational (financial) outcomes;
- Institute quality programs in key service areas;
- Benchmark other organizations' processes;
- Measure the organization's efficiency (personnel, assets, costs) against peer organizations and industry standards;
- Revise rules and regulations that limit process innovation; and
- Continue to communicate and emphasize the individuality of customers.

CHANGING POINT-OF-SERVICE ACTIVITIES

If the requirements of the strategy indicate that the present point-of-service delivery processes should be changed, then explicit strategies must be implemented. In addition, where internal environmental analysis indicates that the point-of-service delivery process is a weakness (resulting in competitive disadvantages) or the requirements of the strategy call for new standards of quality, efficiency, or innovation, change strategies should be initiated. Strategic managers who want to change clinical point-of-service activities should consider involving a team of appropriate leadership across disciplines to:

- institute a CPI program for service delivery,
- reengineer critical service delivery activities,
- provide quality enhancement training for service delivery personnel,
- institute a cost-cutting program,
- provide incentives for efficiency suggestions,
- reduce dramatically rules and regulations that limit innovation, and
- provide savings or revenue sharing with employees to encourage innovations.

To change marketing point-of-service activities, strategic managers should:

- target unserved consumers,
- increase market penetration activities,
- serve new markets with existing products,
- offer new products for current consumers, and
- improve differentiation among services offered.

After-Service Activities

After-service includes follow-up (both clinical and marketing), billing, and follow-on activities. They are sometimes referred to as "back office strategies" and are often the final impression (contact) that a customer has with the health care organization.

Follow-Up Activities

Follow-up calling to inquire after the health of a child who was seen in the ER would spotlight a pediatrician as "caring and concerned" and endear him or her to any mother. Calling after outpatient surgery to ask if everything is going as expected or whether additional prescriptions are needed is simply good clinical follow-up (and can save pain, complications, and an office's schedule). Rather than having the consumer feel that he or she is intruding and interrupting the doctor, follow-up calls say "we care" and avoid negative reactions.

Marketing follow-up activities include patient satisfaction studies to determine from a patient's perspective how he or she was treated. All health care providers should be doing follow-up studies with their customers. The studies offer greater insight if they are conducted several days after the health care encounter as bias can be incorporated in on-site collection of data.

With the assistance of Press Ganey, a health care consulting firm, *Hospitals & Health Networks* conducted a survey to determine the use of patient satisfaction studies. Of the 783 respondents, 95 percent said their organization measured patient satisfaction and over 99 percent said there were many opportunities to improve patient satisfaction. However, less than 40 percent said they were doing a better job of it than ten years ago.[35]

Health care purchasing decisions are often made through a third-party payor with little or no consumer involvement. That eventually distances the relationship between the provider and the consumer of health care. Consumers are now spending more out of pocket for co-pays and percentage of the cost yet are not aware of how their money is being used. Pressed for time, they become frustrated if they feel their time is being wasted, as when they have an appointment and sit for an hour waiting for an X-ray or to see a physician. Today, consumers have the knowledge to take their business elsewhere.

Studies of patient satisfaction cannot be merely looked at, plotted as to movement up or down, and put on a shelf. They need to be analyzed to learn what customers expect, what the organization is able or willing to do to meet the expectations (its capabilities), and manage those that they are not willing or able to meet.[36] For example, it may not be possible to shorten the time for test results because of the time it takes to do the test properly. However, patient expectations can be managed by explaining the length of time it takes to do the test and making the information available as soon as possible on a secure Internet website – if the patient wants the information this way – or an immediate call from the physician's office, or at least providing a consumer hot line to call.

Although many health care organizations are undertaking customer satisfaction surveys, they may not be performing them in a rigorous enough manner. Despite all the studies that have been done, quality improvement has not lived up to expectations. To develop satisfaction, customers must be satisfied throughout the value chain from pre-service activities to after-service activities. The problem has been that the studies were not designed with minimal standards of conceptual or methodological rigor; nor were they designed to facilitate quality improvement.[37] Regional coalitions are being used to more rigorously collect data. In Massachusetts, a partnership of health care, business, and government leaders recognized the need for better information and collected data from 24,200 patients discharged from over 50 hospitals. The participants agreed not to use the data for "best" and "worst" lists but to educate and inform hospitals and consumers and to focus and facilitate quality improvement efforts.

Billing Activities

There is more to the patient's determination of the value and quality of the total health care experience than the success or failure of the medical procedure or clinical service itself. Richard L. Clarke, HFMA (Health Financial Management Association) CEO and president has stated: "The best care, and great customer service provided during the patient's hospital encounter can be destroyed quickly by confusing, complicated, and incorrect billing afterwards."[38] Hospital bill features that irritate customers most include:

1. Confusion about what the patient's insurance company has paid;
2. Confusion about the balance the patient owes the hospital once the insurance company pays its share;
3. Use of medical terminology that the patient doesn't understand;
4. Sending a bill to the patient before the insurance company had processed the patient's claims; and
5. Inability to determine exactly what services the hospital has provided and what the patient is being charged for a service.[39]

Greenwich Hospital's convoluted billing statement was reported in the *New York Times* when a freelance writer tried to figure out what he owed the hospital. His very public discussion of the problems with billing began a major change for the hospital. Having undergone the process, Greenwich recommends that when a health care organization realizes that its billing statement needs revision, the task should not be delegated to staff. Rather, a task force of actual customers, physicians, information systems personnel, clinical employees, and billing personnel should be charged with making the bill understandable. Greenwich followed this format and the redesigned billing process dropped consumer complaints from about 30 per week to 5 per week and, interestingly, there was a reduction in accounts receivable and bad debt because people understood their bill and paid it.[40]

When customers call in with questions about their bills, how are the calls handled? More than likely someone has to stop with data entry or analysis of data input to answer a patient's question. Answering customers' questions is not a priority and customers will know it. However, costs are associated with doing things incorrectly. Consider a hospital or nursing home billing statement that contains errors. Not only is there the cost of finding the error and redoing the statement, there is also the cost of losing a positive consumer attitude – and, perhaps, a patient who decides to go elsewhere.

Follow-on Activities

It is almost always preferable to have services recovery occur during services delivery rather than waiting to institute services recovery at a later time. However, health care managers are not always aware of the failure until *follow-on* activities are undertaken (see Perspective 8–7).

After a patient has been seen by a physician or is leaving the hospital after surgery, there is a likely need for further services: a child with an ear infection has to return in ten days for another check-up to make sure the infection is no longer present; after hip surgery a patient may need to be relocated to a rehabilitation facility to learn to walk again. These additional services are called follow-on value adding service activities. A new mom with a child's first ear infection has no idea about returning. An unexpected broken hip, surgery, and then the need for additional care is not something most families research until it happens. If the health care provider has thought through the follow-on care and provides

Perspective 8-7
Win Back Dissatisfied Customers: Focus on Service Recovery

A service organization's best asset is its customers' confidence in the services it provides. Health care customers need to feel confidence in their providers and they need the assurance that they are being cared for by the right people and the right organization. Any service failure damages that confidence and today's consumers have choices for their health care providers.

A fundamental aim of service recovery is to restore confidence that has been shaken. A single service failure is unlikely to destroy confidence in a provider or organization unless the failure is so egregious (such as operating on the wrong knee) that recovery of any type is all but impossible, or the failure is in a pattern rather than being an isolated incident, or the service recovery is weak and compounds the original failure rather than countering it.

Inadequate recovery can demonstrate a pattern of poor service and signals a "We don't care" attitude that is dangerous for a health care organization. In one study of positive and negative service experiences, 43 percent of the negative experiences were actually related to poor service recovery whereas another study demonstrated that satisfactory service recovery sharply increased customers' willingness to recommend an organization and improved overall perception of service quality. Most service recovery activities in health care involve experience quality (what the patient perceives) versus technical quality (what is done medically or surgically by the provider).

Effective recovery enables the organization to resolve the problem and restore confidence. In addition, in the process of service recovery, information can be gleaned to address the cause of the problems within the system and improve overall quality. Five guidelines offered for effective service recovery include:

1. *Embrace recovery* – service recovery is an attitude to be shared. Authorize contact personnel to make amends for service failure. Make service recovery an expectation for everyone's job performance and include it in the employee performance measurement and reward system.
2. *Recover through feedback* – convince patients and employees that the organization really wants to know how to improve. Use proactive methods to gather service problem feedback (1–800 numbers, websites, asking patients, exit interviews, and so on) as well as reactive methods (sending a survey after the hospital stay that the organization reacts to). All feedback needs to be captured and analyzed to change processes and improve.
3. *Recover quickly and simply* – quickest and simplest is to fix a problem before it occurs (use feedback, analysis, and awareness to avoid problems). When a service failure does occur, address it promptly and as effectively as possible.
4. *Recover personally* – a personal and sincere apology signals respect and concern and should never be underestimated (especially because of the litigious health care climate in the United States).
5. *Recover fairly* – reactions to unfairness are pronounced. Although challenging in health care, consider a service guarantee (for things over which the organization has control, such as wait times, returning phone calls, and so on).

Source: Leonard L. Berry and Jonathan A. Leighton, "Restoring Customer Confidence," *Marketing Health Services* 24, no. 1 (Spring 2004), pp. 14–19.

literature, assistance with placement in another facility, and so on, consumers will leave with a more favorable experience.

After a doctor visit, can the patient easily find the appointment desk? Is the employee that handles next appointments knowledgeable concerning the length of time it will take for routine visits? Do these employees know that they represent the entire organization to the patient? Customer capital is the value of customer relationships and the contribution this value makes to future growth prospects. Customer capital includes an organization's customer base, customer relationships, customer potential, and brand recognition. Although the specifics vary by industry, it has been long understood by marketers that it costs more to gain a new customer than it takes to retain a customer. Given that this is true, then it is logical to assume that the customer franchise is an asset of real worth. Establishing lifetime relationships with customers is the focus of the smart twenty-first century organization because it leads to competitive advantage.[41] Follow-on activities can cement or destroy a good customer relationship.

To achieve high levels of patient satisfaction, Baptist Hospital in Pensacola, Florida, felt that it needed to become the employer of choice.[42] It monitors employee satisfaction as well as customer satisfaction. Managers' performance is measured in five areas – customer service, quality (length of stay), expense management, employee turnover, and growth – and compensation is linked to accomplishing objectives.

Matching After-Service to the Strategy

As with pre-service and point-of-service activities, after-service activities must contribute to the accomplishment of the selected strategy. These operations and marketing activities may be quite important in an effective strategy. Follow-up, billing, and follow-on activities humanize the services, reduce hassles and frustration, and provide for continued care. Such activities often make the difference between a positive and negative health care experience and can differentiate the service and create competitive advantage. Effective after-service activities are typically of high value, often rare, fairly easy to develop, and are sustainable. These activities can be the source of at least short-term competitive advantage. However, these areas are often ignored by many health care organizations and thus those organizations that do them well may create a long-term advantage. Therefore, careful attention should be given to understanding the after-service requirements of the selected strategy. Strategic managers must decide if the activities should be maintained or changed.

MAINTAINING AFTER-SERVICE ACTIVITIES

When the requirements of the selected strategy match the characteristics of the current after-service activities, the manager should develop strategies to maintain the current after-service strengths of the organization through its resources, competencies, and capabilities. Likewise, those after-service activities that have resulted in a competitive advantage should be protected and maintained. In maintaining after-service activities, strategic managers should continue to:

- Emphasize and train employees on telephone and email communication and etiquette;
- Emphasize patient satisfaction;
- Improve the "readability" of billing statements;

- Stress the importance of correct billing statements and ensure their accuracy; and
- Develop relationships in the referral network to facilitate follow-on activities.

CHANGING AFTER-SERVICE ACTIVITIES

If the requirements of the strategy indicate that the present after-service activities should be changed, then explicit strategies must be implemented. In addition, where internal environmental analysis has indicated that follow-up, billing, or follow-on is a weakness resulting in competitive disadvantage, change strategies should be developed. Strategic managers who want to change after-service activities should:

- Make follow-up an explicit part of patient (customer) care;
- Keep a log of patient follow-up as a part of the patient/customer record;
- Train employees on telephone and email communication and etiquette;
- Emphasize customer satisfaction at staff meetings;
- Redesign the billing statement with the assistance of a variety of stakeholders, including patients;
- Inform customers about billing procedures;
- Clear confusion about billing charges and which charges are to be paid by insurance;
- Create a clear, easy-to-read billing statement, including definitions of complicated medical terms;
- Continue to improve relationships with payors;
- Develop more and better relationships with referral organizations; and
- Develop a list of options for referral patients, explaining the characteristics and pricing of each.

Extending the Strategic Thinking Map

The value adding service delivery strategies translate the directional, adaptive, market entry, and competitive strategies into action. As a critical component of the value chain, value adding service delivery strategies coupled with the value adding support strategies set the stage for maintaining strategic momentum through the action plans and control of the strategies.

No position of leadership lasts forever. Every health care organization that succeeds at differentiation serves as a model for new competitors.[43] The dynamic health care market and ever-changing technology mean that no competitive advantage can be sustained in the long run without a great deal of thought and effort. To further complicate the strategic process, the long run itself is becoming shorter as the rate of change becomes increasingly rapid.

In conjunction with external environmental analysis, service area competitor analysis, and internal analysis, the value adding service delivery strategies attempt to keep repositioning the health care organization in its environment to create new competitive advantages. Although there are maps for developing value adding service delivery strategies (see Exhibit 8–11 for an example), using a compass to creatively develop new strategies for pre-service, point-of-service, and after-service delivery can rejuvenate competitive advantage.

Exhibit 8–11: Strategic Thinking Map for Value Adding Support Strategies for a Long-term Care Organization

Adaptive Strategy: Vertical integration – enter into a system of care.
Market Entry Strategy: Enter into an alliance with a hospital to assure referral network.
Strategic Posture: Move from defender posture to analyzer posture.
Positioning Strategy: Differentiation based on quality, upscale image.

Value Adding Service Delivery Strategies	Characteristics/Attributes		Evaluation			Support Strategy
	Results of Internal Analysis	Requirements of Selected Strategies	Comparison: Strategy Requirements – Internal Analysis Results	Maintain	Change	Guidance for Organizational Units (Basis for Unit Action Plan Development)
Pre-Service • Market/Marketing Research • Target Market • Services Offered/Branding • Pricing • Promotion • Distribution/ Logistics	Target market: upscale families, private pay. Prestige pricing in this step-down facility that offers long-term care and skilled nursing. Word-of-mouth is relied on as well as the publicity about the CEO's mother residing there. Excellent location – upscale neighborhood with excellent shopping and recreation nearby.	Become Medicare and Medicaid qualified to meet hospital's needs. Intensify branding efforts to combat new competition. Maintain upscale appearance, caring staff. Add new services to be "full-service."	Fairly good match. Expansion of the target market may impact upscale image. Word-of-mouth promotion not sufficient to develop brand awareness. Maintaining the current competitive advantage will be challenging with an expanded target market.	X		**Marketing** – enhancement: Develop a promotional campaign to enhance brand awareness, redesign of the logo and new signage, consider comparative advertising with other local upscale facilities. **Operations** – enhancement: modify procedures to be consistent with Medicare and Medicaid regulations, ensure facilities are clean/neat to reflect upscale image, make facilities modifications to meet Medicare and Medicaid requirements, ensure recruitment of caring professionals.
Point-of-Service • Service Delivery	Patients/families indicate care delivery is outstanding. Facility is clean, does not smell like a nursing home. Food is tasty and nutritious – like home cooked. Families do not want to move the loved one if other problems associated with aging occur.	Expand services: Alzheimer's care, senior day care, rehabilitation.	Fairly good match. Services differentiation strategy requires improved information system to track care. Enhancement strategy requires process innovation while maintaining caring environment, cleanliness, great food. Product development offers opportunities.	X		**Clinical** – status quo: maintain service delivery at its current high level of quality and caring, continue quality food service/dining. **Marketing** – product development analysis: Alzheimer's care and senior day care units. **Operations** – enhancement: work with IS to enhance tracking of care, improve activities and social opportunities for residents, develop procedures for operating Alzheimer's and day care units. Work with Facilities Management on the facilities requirement for Alzheimer's and day care units.
After-Service • Follow-up Activities • Billing • Follow-on Activities	"No need" for patient/family satisfaction studies. Billing process: give an accumulated bill to a family member when they stopped in for a visit. If the patient needs care from a specialist, referrals are prompt, transportation arranged.	Satisfaction studies to track improvements. Billing procedure to provide consistent revenue stream.	Not a good match. IS upgrade needed to match the hospital's system for timely, accurate billing to increase customer satisfaction. Expanded target market requires careful tracking to maintain image.		X	**Marketing** – initiate patient/family satisfaction studies, make recommendations to leadership based on results of the study, track brand awareness and image in an expanded target market. **Operations** – work with IS to change billing system, coordinate with alliance hospital for consistency in billing procedures.

Managing Strategic Momentum – Service Delivery Strategies

Just as the success of the directional, adaptive, market entry, and competitive strategies of the organization must be evaluated as an ongoing part of managing the strategy, the service delivery strategies often must be adjusted as managers learn by doing. This type of change represents an evolutionary alteration or a strategic adjustment. Lorange, Morton, and Ghoshal referred to this as managing the strategic momentum and explained, "The basic continuity of the business is still credible, and one can hence speak of an extrapolation of the given strategy, even though a lot of operational changes may be taking place. The challenge here is to manage the buffeting of the given strategy and to maintain the strategy on course."[44]

In the end it is implementation that has to be effective and efficient. Changes in the "way we do things" represent evolutionary change. Each of the value adding strategies – service delivery and support – should be examined separately to determine whether management has correctly defined the role of these strategies in supporting the organization's overall strategy. Strategic managers must determine whether the service delivery, the support strategies, and action plans are well integrated and support one another. The questions presented in Exhibit 8–12 provide an evaluation of the effectiveness of the service delivery strategies. The logic underlying these questions is that the organization's strategy is fundamentally sound but the organization's performance in carrying out service delivery may not be as effective or efficient as it could be. Adding value is an ongoing process and requires the value adding support strategies to be in concert with the value adding service delivery strategies. The value adding support strategies are discussed in Chapter 9.

Exhibit 8–12: Strategic Thinking Map for Evaluating Service Delivery Strategies

1. Have the pre-service activities provided customers with need satisfying services?
2. Have the pre-service activities provided the right price, level of information to current and potential customers, and locations?
3. Are the pre-service logistics appropriate to the service?
4. Are the point-of-service activities sensitive to changing customer needs?
5. Are the point-of-service activities efficient? Effective?
6. Has the quality of the services changed?
7. Has the organization innovated in the delivery of its services?
8. Is the delivery of services flexible (can accommodate special customer needs)?
9. Is there proper follow-up with customers?
10. Is the billing system timely, accurate, and user friendly?
11. Are the follow-on strategies appropriate?

Summary and Conclusions

Because of the competition and complexity in the market, health care providers must add value to survive. The value chain consists of value adding service delivery strategies that are primarily operations (clinical) and marketing oriented as well as value adding support strategies that include organizational culture, organizational structure, and strategic resources.

The chapter illustrates how the directional, adaptive, market entry, and positioning strategies are implemented through value adding service delivery, including pre-service, point-of-service, and after-service strategies. Pre-service activities include market research to understand the customer and marketing research to understand the customer's reactions to the organization's marketing efforts. A variety of health care customers – including physicians, patients, third-party payors, volunteers, employees, and so on – are discussed and their interdependence illustrated. Patients have to be admitted to a hospital by a physician; third-party payors influence physician choice, length of stay, and so on; volunteers and employees may also be patients; government entities interpret the need for additional health care subsidies from the public. In addition, pre-service includes segmentation to select the target market and determination of the services that will satisfy the target market. Further, decisions have to be made concerning branding as well as pricing, promotion, and distribution/logistics.

Point-of-service delivery is oriented around patient care and delivery – clinical and marketing activities. Marketers study the customer and market to suggest the manner of care delivery, while clinical personnel deliver care. Mass customization is proposed as a way to deliver efficient and effective care. Product development, market development, penetration, enhancement, and differentiation are examples of strategies that marketing implements.

After-service activities include both clinical (next appointments, further services) and marketing (determining how to satisfy customers through new products/services that are needed) follow-up activities. Staff could make clinical calls to inquire how the patient is doing and whether additional medication is needed. Marketing follow-up is generally in the form of patient satisfaction studies. Billing is another important after-service activity, as it is the time when the consumer decides if value has been received. Follow-on activities include nursing home care arrangements after hospitalization, arranging home care, and other similar activities.

Key Terms and Concepts in Strategic Management

After-Service Strategy
Consumerism
Follow-On
Follow-Up
Marketing Research
Market Research

Mass Customization
Perceptual Gaps in Service
 Delivery
Point-of-Service Strategy
Pre-Service Strategy

Service
Services
Target Market
Value Adding Service Delivery
 Strategies

QUESTIONS FOR CLASS DISCUSSION

1. Explain the linkage between internal environmental analysis and the value adding service delivery and support strategies. How are the value adding strategies linked with action plans?
2. Explain the difference between pre-service, point-of-service, and after-service. What elements are central to each? Provide an example of how an organization might create a competitive advantage in each of these areas.
3. Explain why pre-service, point-of-service, and after-service activities are fundamentally marketing and clinical in nature.
4. How does the marketing of a service differ from the marketing of a physical product (good)?
5. Discuss the various ways that health care providers can define the market that they want to serve.
6. What role does marketing play in the implementation of adaptive strategies for expansion? Is marketing ever involved in contraction?
7. Does marketing have a role to play in the market entry strategies? Explain your answer.
8. What is mass customization? Under what circumstance does mass customization become useful?
9. What is "evolutionary" strategic change?

NOTES

1. Peter B. Vaill, *Learning as a Way of Being: Strategies for Survival in a World of Permanent White Water* (San Francisco: Jossey-Bass Publishers, 1996), p. 17. See also Michele Murphy-Smith, Barbara Meyer, Jeffrey Hitt, Margaret A. Taylor-Sheehafer, and Diane O. Tyler, "Put Prevention into Practice Implementation Model: Translating Practice to Theory," *Journal of Public Health Management and Practice* 10, no. 2 (2004), pp. 109–115.
2. Raymond E. Miles, Charles C. Snow, Alan D. Meyer, and Henry J. Coleman, "Organizational Strategy, Structure, and Process," *Academy of Management Review* 3, no. 3 (1978), pp. 546–562.
3. Stanley F. Slater and Eric M. Olson, "Strategy Type and Performance: The Influence of Sales Force Management," *Strategic Management Journal* 21, no. 5 (May 2000), p. 826.
4. Sharon Ponsonby and Emily Boyle, "The 'Value of Marketing' and 'The Marketing of Value' in Contemporary Times – A Literature Review and Research Agenda," *Journal of Marketing Management* 20, no. 3/4 (2004), pp. 342–356.
5. John Callahan and Eylan Lasry, "The Importance of Customer Input in the Development of Very New Products," *R & D Management* 34, no. 2 (2004), pp. 107–121.
6. Jacquelyn S. Thomas, Robert C. Blattberg, and Edward J. Fox, "Recapturing Lost Customers," *Journal of Marketing Research* 41, no. 1 (2004), pp. 31–40 and Cheryl L. Stavins, "Developing Employee Participation in the Patient-Satisfaction Process," *Journal of Healthcare Management* 49, no. 2 (2004), pp. 135–140.
7. Valarie A. Zeithaml, A. Parasuraman, and Leonard L. Berry, *Delivering Quality Service* (New York: Free Press, 1990), p. 11.
8. Leonard L. Berry, "Services Marketing Is Different," *Business* (May–June 1980), pp. 24–30.
9. Karen Russo France and Rajiv Grover, "What Is the Health Care Product?" *Journal of Health Care Marketing* 12, no. 2 (June 1992), p. 32.
10. Ed Finkel, "A Well-Oiled ER: Streamlined Emergency Room Procedures Improve Everyone's Satisfaction," *Modern Healthcare* 33, no. 50 (December 15, 2003), pp. 26–27 and Koichiro Otani and Richard S. Kurz, "The Impact of Nursing Care and Other Healthcare Attributes on Hospitalized Patient Satisfaction and Behavioral Intentions," *Journal of*

Healthcare Management 49, no. 3 (2004), pp. 181–198.

11. "Smart Consumers Present a Marketing Challenge," *Hospitals* (August 20, 1990), pp. 42–47. See also Sunil Gupta, Donald R. Lehmann, and Jennifer Ames Stuart, "Valuing Customers," *Journal of Marketing Research* 41, no. 1 (2004), pp. 7–14.

12. "It's a Woman's Market . . . ," *Hospitals and Health Networks* 67, no. 18 (September 20, 1993), p. 30.

13. http://www.ncqa.org/Pages/about/overview3.htm

14. Katherine Kress, Nancy Ozawa, and Gregory Schmid, "The New Consumer Emerges," *Strategy & Leadership* 28, no. 5 (2000), pp. 4–9.

15. Ibid., p. 5.

16. Kevin Clark and Mary McNeilly, "Case Study: IBM's Think Strategy – Melding Strategy and Branding," *Strategy & Leadership* 32, no. 2 (2004), pp. 44–49 and J. Daniel Beckham, "Marketing vs. Branding," *Health Forum Journal* 43, no. 2 (March–April 2000), pp. 64–68.

17. Scott M. Davis, "The Power of the Brand," *Strategy & Leadership* 28, no. 4 (2000), pp. 4–9 and M. Tolga Akcura, Fusun F. Gonul, and Elina Petrove, "Consumer Learning and Brand Evaluation: An Application on Over-the-Counter Drugs," *Marketing Science* 23, no. 1 (2004), pp. 156–170.

18. Davis, "The Power of the Brand," ibid.

19. A. Parasuraman, Valarie A. Zeithaml, and Leonard L. Berry, "A Conceptual Model of Service Quality and Its Implications for Future Research," *Journal of Marketing* 49, no. 2 (1985), pp. 41–50.

20. Stephen J. O'Connor, Richard M. Shewchuk, and L. W. Carney, "The Great Gap: Physicians' Perceptions of Patient Service Quality Expectations Fall Short of Reality," *Journal of Health Care Marketing* 14, no. 2 (1994), pp. 32–38.

21. Stephen J. O'Connor, Hanh Q. Trinh, and Richard M. Shewchuk, "Perceptual Gaps in Understanding Patient Expectations for Health Care Service Quality," *Health Care Management Review* 25, no. 2 (2000), p. 19.

22. Ibid.

23. Jennifer Gordon, "Medical Kiosks at Kroger Stores Add Laboratory Services," *Business First* 20, no. 29 (February 20, 2004), pp. 6–7.

24. Mary Wagner, "Mobile Mammography Tries to Enhance Its Image; Revenue Through Strategic Ties," *Modern Healthcare* (January 8, 1990), pp. 78, 286.

25. Curtis P. McLaughlin and Arnold D. Kaluzny, "Building Client Centered Systems of Care: Choosing a Process Direction for the Next Century," *Health Care Management Review* 25, no. 1 (Winter 2000), pp. 73–82.

26. Ibid.

27. Julie Miller, "Mass Customization Suits Varied Needs of Large Employers: Not Too Big and Not Too Small, Disease Subcategories Reduce Administrative Burdens of Disease Management," *Managed Healthcare Executive* 13, no. 9 (September, 2003), pp. 46–48.

28. Julie T. Chyna, "Enhancing Your Public Image," *Healthcare Executive* 16, no. 1 (January–February 2001), pp. 7–11.

29. Robert C. Ford and Myron D. Fottler, "Creating Customer-Focused Health Care Organizations," *Health Care Management Review* 25, no. 4 (fall 2000), pp. 18–33.

30. Ellen G. Lanser, "Ensuring a Customer-Focused Experience: Two Success Stories," *Healthcare Executive* 15, no. 1 (January–February 2000), pp. 8–23.

31. Lucy A. Savitz, Arnold D. Kaluzny, and Diane L. Kelly, "A Life Cycle Model of Continuous Clinical Process Innovation," *Journal of Healthcare Management* 45, no. 5 (September–October 2000), p. 308.

32. Michael Hammer, "Deep Change: How Operational Innovation Can Transform Your Company," *Harvard Business Review* 82, no. 4 (2004), p. 86.

33. Jill L. Sharer, "The New Medical Team: Clinicians, Technicians, and Patients?" *Healthcare Executive* 15, no. 1 (January–February 2000), pp. 12–17.

34. Julie T. Chyna, "Physician–Health System Partnerships: Strategies for Finding Common Ground," *Healthcare Executive* 15, no. 2 (March–April 2000), pp. 12–17.

35. "Patient Satisfaction Survey," *Trustee* 53, no. 9 (October 2000), p. 24.

36. Julie T. Chyna, "The Consumer Revolution: An Age of Changing Expectations," *Healthcare Executive* 15, no. 1 (January–February 2000), pp. 7–10.

37. Paul D. Cleary, "The Increasing Importance of Patient Surveys: Now that Sound Methods Exist, Patient Surveys Can Facilitate Improvement," *British Medical Journal* 319 (September 18, 1999), pp. 720–721.

38. "Anxious to Please Patients, Hospitals Should Remember that Bills Anger Customers Most," *Health Care Strategic Management* 18, no. 11 (November 2000), p. 12.

39. Ibid., p. 14.

40. Ibid.

41. Jan Duffy, "Measuring Customer Capital," *Strategy & Leadership* 28, no. 5 (2000), p. 11.

42. Ed Egger, "Inspiring Patient, Employee Satisfaction Turns Florida Hospital into Top Performer," *Health Care Strategic Management* 17, no. 6 (June 1999), p. 13.

43. George S. Day, *Market Driven Strategy, Process for Creating Value* (New York: Free Press, 1990), p. 163.

44. Peter Lorange, Michael F. Scott Morton, and Sumantra Ghoshal, *Strategic Control* (St. Paul, MN: West Publishing, 1986), p. 11.

ADDITIONAL READINGS

Entoven, Alain and Laura A. Tollen (eds) *Toward A 21st Century Health System: The Contributions and Promise of Prepaid Group Practice* (Indianapolis, IN: Jossey-Bass, 2004). This series of essays discusses a wide range of topics dealing with American health care. The papers present a variety of examples of effective systems that already exist and are capable of meeting the challenges of twenty-first century health care. Some arguments are presented as to why the American health care system continues to be such an underachiever in light of the resources it consumes.

Hartman, Amir, *Ruthless Execution* (New York: Prentice Hall Financial Times Publishing, 2004). Strategies for dealing with business slumps are discussed and numerous case studies are provided to illustrate how ruthless execution has led to business success. To help stalled companies on the road to renewal, Hartman presents strategies for renewal and a plan that rebalances performance and growth. The goal is to promote accountability, define the right metrics, and promote discipline in the absence of bureaucracy.

Herzlinger, Regina E., *Consumer-Driven Health Care: Implications for Providers, Payers, and Policy-Makers* (Indianapolis, IN: Jossey-Bass, 2004). Consumer-driven health care is rapidly becoming the topic of an important debate in health care strategy. The author argues that the future of our health care system depends to a great extent on people becoming empowered as active consumers and purchasers of health benefits and services. The book offers an intriguing vision of a health care system built to satisfy the needs of the people it serves.

Keagy, Blair and Marci Thomas (eds) *Essentials of Physician Practice Management* (Indianapolis, IN: Jossey-Bass, 2004). A readable book with case examples, it is a comprehensive reference on a number of areas of physician practice management. Information on operations, financial management, strategic planning, human resources, and community relations is provided.

Nalbantian, Haig R., Richard A. Guzzo, Dave Kieffer, and Jay Doherty, *Play to Your Strengths: Managing Your Internal Labor Markets for Lasting Competitive Advantage* (New York: McGraw-Hill, 2004). The largest asset of many organizations is its human capital combined with the system that manages it. However, many managers treat employees as if they were costs to be minimized rather than investments that could be encouraged to add value to the products or services of the organization. It is important to align an organization's human capital strategy with its business strategy to develop a true competitive advantage.

Thomas, Richard K., *Marketing Health Services* (Arlington, VA and Chicago: AUPHA/HAP, 2005). *Marketing Health Services* is a comprehensive guide. Its contents run the gamut from understanding health care markets to applying marketing techniques to evaluating the marketing effort. The latest thinking on health care marketing, including factors that drive marketing approaches and consumer behavior in health care, practical tips on devising a marketing strategy and managing its progress, critical analysis of the marketing techniques currently used in health care, strategies to consider when initiating market research, and case studies illustrating various marketing techniques are included.

Zuckerman, Alan M. and Russell C. Coile, Jr., *Competing On Excellence: Healthcare Strategies for a Consumer Driven Market* (Chicago: Health Administration Press, 2003). Consumer-driven health care organizations gain market share by demonstrating outstanding clinical outcomes and customer service. This book serves as a guide to develop excellence in health care operations. Principles, programs, and strategies for making clinical programs excellent are provided.

CHAPTER **9**

Value Adding Support Strategies

"Never tell people how to do things. Tell them what to do and they will surprise you with their ingenuity."

George Patton

Introductory Incident

Safer. Smarter. Digital.

Mercy Hospital of Port Huron, Michigan is the guinea pig for a $200 million investment in computerized order entry and electronic medical records systems that eventually are to be installed in 16 more member organizations of the Trinity Health System. Computer screens literally line the hallways at Mercy, with one outside each patient room plus several at each nursing station. In addition, there are computers on rolling carts and wireless laptops that can be checked out by clinicians who prefer to carry their order entry device with them.

Project Genesis, as the effort is known, will take until 2008 to fully implement and will eventually alter the work habits of every physician and nurse in the Trinity System. Trinity's CEO regards Project Genesis as an opportunity to help health care information technology overall and in the process transform the organization. The CEO provided the staff with the freedom to do what was necessary to make Project Genesis acceptable to the institution's

almost 200 physicians. The CEO knew that as private practitioners the physicians were under no obligation to implement the system, yet without their acceptance it could not be successful. Most of the physicians came on board even though they were busy and learning a new system was an additional demand on their time.

One example of improvement is the adverse-drug-event alerting system. An interface connects the pharmacy to the lab information systems and whenever a medication order conflicts with a lab result an alert is printed. Systemwide, 15,000 alerts were printed every month; the alerts resulted in about 1,300 changes in care. A pilot study estimated that the alerts provided potential savings of $27,000 to $160,000 per month from averted errors. Of course, error reporting is a touchy subject. To overcome some of the reluctance to report errors, Trinity developed the potential event/error reporting system (PEERS) modeled after the airline

▶

industry. The system is anonymous, voluntary, and nonpunitive. Through a simple Internet interface employees or physicians who want to alert management to a problem can do so without the risk of exposing themselves to retaliation.

In 2003, PEERS reporting led to 72 facility improvements, 29 new policies or procedures, 36 revisions of existing procedures, and 179 revisions in existing processes. For example, PEERS reporting highlighted a cluster of complaints in one hospital about physicians not responding to their pagers. Investigation showed that all the "guilty" doctors were in one area of the hospital that turned out to be a "dead zone" for pagers. The installation of an extra antenna solved the problem immediately.

The day the computer system made its debut at Mercy, physicians entered 23 percent of their orders themselves. A year later almost half of the physicians' inpatient orders were placed online – excellent progress in a community hospital setting where most clinical order-entry systems average about 30 percent. Not all the doctors are enthusiastic about the system – especially internists and family physicians whose orders tend to be more intricate and varied than those of surgeons and specialists. However, as the chief of the medical staff states, "The hospital administration has been great – absolute superstars. Their support, energy, and effort have been outstanding, and they've done a great thing."

Source: Elizabeth Gardner, "Pulling It Together," *Modern Healthcare* 34, no. 25 (June 14, 2004), pp. 8–9.

Learning Objectives

After completing this chapter the student should be able to:

1. Understand that the value adding support strategies are important elements in the implementation of strategy.

2. Appreciate the importance of aligning the value adding support strategies to ensure they point the organization toward achieving its vision and goals.

3. Link the results of internal environmental analysis of the support activities to the implementation of value adding support strategies.

4. Understand how the culture, structure, and strategic resources of an organization must be explicitly linked to directional, adaptive, market entry, and competitive strategies, as well as the value adding service delivery strategies.

5. Understand that through the value adding support strategies the organization itself is changed, creating or solidifying competitive advantages and strengthening weaknesses to overcome competitive disadvantages.

6. Understand that the value adding support strategies provide guidance for the development of organizational objectives and action plans.

7. Create value adding support strategies that help accomplish directional, adaptive, market entry and competitive strategies, as well as value adding service delivery strategies.

Implementing Support Strategies

As indicated in Chapter 8, implementation strategies take a decidedly internal focus. Effective and efficient operations make strategies work. Along with the pre-service, point-of-service, and after-service strategies, the value adding support strategies should be developed and specified. Similar to the service delivery strategies, the value adding support strategies are implementation strategies directed toward accomplishment of all the other strategies including the directional, adaptive, market entry, competitive, and service delivery strategies. As introduced in the strategic thinking map of the value chain shown in Exhibit 8–1, the value adding support strategies are based on the elements of the lower portion of the value chain and are the means for accomplishing the decisions made in strategy formulation. Once the support strategies are determined, more specific action plans may be developed (see Chapter 10).

Value Adding Support Strategies

The lower portion of the value chain contains the *value adding support activities* and includes the organization's culture, structure, and strategic resources. More specifically, the support strategies concern areas such as the behavioral norms, structural standardization and flexibility, human resources, finance, information systems, and technology, and will play a major role in the implementation of the organization's overall strategy. Each of these areas adds to value creation in the organization. Thus, strategies are required to maintain or enhance the organization's competitive advantages or strengthen areas where the organization has identified competitive disadvantages.

As with the service delivery strategies, value adding support strategies must be consciously aligned to accomplish the strategy. Strategic managers should take care to ensure that the support strategies are consistent and compatible with each other as well as inclined to contribute to the accomplishment of the organization's overall strategy. Therefore, the support strategies for each area cannot be evaluated or developed in isolation. It is the strategic manager's responsibility not only to make decisions concerning each support strategy but also to ensure that these elements are aligned and coordinated to help achieve the overall strategy of the organization. Strategic thinking, strategic planning, and managing strategic momentum are central to this process.

Decision Logic for the Value Adding Support Strategies

Once the service delivery strategies (the primary value adding activities) are formulated, support strategies that provide the appropriate organizational context and resources to carry out the organization's strategy may be developed. As with the value adding service delivery strategies, the results of the internal environmental analysis identify the strengths and weaknesses related to the current resources, competencies, and capabilities for the support activities. Each of these value chain support areas was evaluated in situational analysis (Chapter 4) and the conclusions used in strategy formulation. Similarly, the appropriate directional, adaptive, market entry, and competitive strategies have been discussed in Chapters 5 through 7. Depending on the results of this comparison, the support areas may need to be maintained or changed to carry out the selected strategy. A strategic thinking map depicting this rationale in the form of a table is in Exhibit 9–1. In this chapter each of the value adding support strategies will be examined and key decision areas identified to suggest support strategies.

Organizational Culture as a Value Adding Support Strategy

Culture permeates the organization and successful strategic managers understand its importance. Studies have demonstrated that in addition to strategy, execution, and structure, the proper culture was imperative for organizations that outperformed their industry peers.[1] To successfully implement strategy, strategic managers must know how to maintain as well as change organizational culture. Organizational culture may be supportive of strategic efforts and, therefore, there is no requirement to change the culture. In this case, a policy of maintaining the culture is necessary. On the other hand, the current culture may inhibit changes that alter the accepted ways of doing things. If this situation occurs, the implementation process will require modification of the culture as its first effort. Although culture change is difficult, it is often an important factor in moving the organization toward realizing its vision.

Understanding Organizational Culture

Most managers agree that there is something that characterizes a health care organization's customary way of doing things, the values that most members

Exhibit 9–1: Strategic Thinking Map for Developing Value Adding Support Strategies

Value Adding Support Strategies	Results of Internal Analysis	Requirements of Selected Strategies	Comparison of Strategy Requirements and Internal Analysis	Maintain or Change
Organizational Culture				
Organizational Structure				
Strategic Resources				

of the organization share, and the things that must be learned and subscribed to by new members if they are to be satisfied and productive in their jobs. This customary way of doing things, referred to collectively as the culture of an organization, is important in assessing competitively relevant strengths and weaknesses, and ultimately in building sustained competitive advantage, because it can either aid or hinder an organization's response to external opportunities and threats.

A Definition of Organizational Culture

Organizational *culture* is defined as the "implicit, invisible, intrinsic, and informal consciousness of the organization that guides the behavior of individuals and shapes itself out of their behavior."[2] Therefore, organizational culture may be thought of as:

- shared assumptions,
- shared values, and
- behavioral norms.

Assumptions and values are the basis for an informal consciousness and persist over time even when the membership of the organization changes. *Shared assumptions* include a common understanding of "who we are" (mission) and "what we are trying to accomplish" (vision and goals) and the belief in the values of the organization. *Shared values* represent the understanding of "the way we do things" and may or may not reflect the organization's "stated" values – it is the actual members' values that create the organization's culture. The behavioral expectations or *behavioral norms* that are common among the members of a group are the visible consequence resulting from the informal consciousness. Organizational culture possesses three important characteristics – culture is learned, culture is shared, and culture is both subjective and objective.

ORGANIZATIONAL CULTURE IS LEARNED

The culture of a health care organization is made meaningful by experience. Those who work in an organization gradually accept its expectations. Culture influences all aspects of what goes on in the organization, including what employees think is important or unimportant.[3] For example, consider an organization such as the Mayo Clinic that has a strong culture. Mayo is built on three primary values that permeate its culture and can be traced directly to the founders: (1) pursuit of service rather than profit; (2) concern for the care and welfare of individual patients; and (3) interest by every member of the staff in the progress of every other member.[4] Anyone working at the Mayo Clinic will soon be confronted with these three core values and that person's success will depend to a great extent on how well these values are learned, accepted, and reflected in his or her behavior.

Organizational Culture Is Shared

Shared understandings and meanings are important because they help employees know how things are to be done. If an employee knows that the culture of the hospital dictates that the patient is all-important, decisions can be made according to this understood value system, even when a policy, procedure, or rule is not available in a particular situation.[5]

People who "fit in" at the Mayo Clinic soon find themselves sharing the culture with others. When the Mayo Clinic made a strategic decision to geographically expand by aggressively establishing a presence in Florida and Arizona, one of the greatest concerns was whether the "Rochester ethic" (culture) could be transferred to the Sun Belt.[6]

Culture Is Subjective and Objective

Shared assumptions, meanings, and values are subjective. The objective aspect of organizational culture can be heard and witnessed. Health care organizations are often quite rich in objective culture, which includes the heroes of the organization, the stories that are told from one generation of employees to another, the ceremonies and rituals of the organization, and so on.

Culture and the Bottom Line

Some organizational cultures have the potential to inspire aggressive and calculated managerial action, whereas other cultures do little more than encourage managers to be mere caretakers. Cultures build group cohesiveness and when members of the group insist on high levels of performance, each individual is encouraged to do his or her best.[7] A surgical team performing complex operations is a good example of how the culture of the group demands that each individual perform at the highest possible level if membership is to be maintained.

Unfortunately, very cohesive cultures can discourage change. When organizations become too committed to "how we do things around here" and "what we believe in," it may be difficult, at least in the short run, to change the culture. Opportunities can be missed and competitive advantages can be lost simply because the culture is so strong that it will not tolerate new ideas and directions. However, organizational cultures, when they encourage mission-critical factors such as patient-centered care, can be positive contributors to the overall success of an organization. Even emphasis on intangible concepts such as ethical behavior and values can have a positive effect on the bottom line, as demonstrated by Memorial Hermann Healthcare System in Perspective 9–1.

Developing Cultures that Are Adaptive

Kotter and Heskett reviewed much of the literature on organizational culture and studied numerous organizations in an attempt to understand the relationship

Perspective 9–1
A New Model of Strategic Leadership

Recent unethical practices in business and health care have resulted in a loss of confidence in corporate leadership. The cry for greater accountability has given rise to a new leadership model – one that focuses on spirituality. Spiritual leadership emphasizes ethical behavior, values, relationship skills, and a healthy balance between work and self.

During his years as CEO of Memorial Hermann Healthcare System in Houston, Dan Wilford looked for ways to nurture spirituality within his organizational initiatives. In 1996 Wilford recognized that modern leadership models were exhausted and conceptualized the Spiritual Leadership Institute. He sought out the ideas and commitment of a small group of people – a healthcare futurist, a strategic planning consultant, an organizational psychologist, a managing partner of a prominent law firm, president of a Baptist University, and two Methodist ministers. The present CEO of Memorial Hermann has continued to emphasize spirituality in the workplace and created programs for clinical personnel and other employees.

According to the Dean of the Spiritual Leadership Institute, other forms of leadership are geared toward meeting economic benchmarks. Spiritual leadership emphasizes a high interest in ethics, relationship skills, and a balance between work and self. Spiritual leadership occurs when the following behaviors are practiced.

- *Focus on values.* Embracing values such as ethics, quality, diversity, and spirituality will influence the way executives lead, the programs they develop and support, and the standards they set for the organization. In addition, the executives need to focus on aligning the values of employees, managers, executives, clinicians, and board members.
- *Provide employees with an opportunity to explore and express their spirituality.* People enter health care because they consider it a calling and want to help people. Through the Institute, Memorial Hermann introduced more than 1,000 executives and 1,500 employees to the concept of spiritual leadership. The intent is to have participants come away from the program with more positive feelings about the organization, a stronger sense of its values, a deeper commitment to the employer, and a better understanding of themselves.
- *Plan for and encourage community involvement.* An organization that values caring for others will reach beyond its walls and care for those in need. The leaders at Memorial Hermann, for example, established a tithing program whereby they give 10 percent of the health system's netrevenue to community organizations of the employees' choice. As one executive pointed out, from the time the tithing program began, Memorial Hermann has improved its bottom line every year.

Although spiritual leadership focuses on intangible concepts, it can have very tangible outcomes. Since the leadership model was implemented at Memorial Hermann, patient satisfaction, employee evaluations, and employee recruitment and retention have all improved. Spiritual leaders should be an inspiration to the people they serve. People in health care are already motivated and the Institute helps organizations capitalize on that motivation and inspiration.

Source: Emily J. Wolf, "Spiritual Leadership: A New Model," *Healthcare Executive* 19, no. 2 (2004), pp. 22–26.

between an organization's culture and its long-term performance.[8] They found that the strength of an organization's culture and its "fit" with the demands of the external environment only partially explained the culture–performance relationship. Instead, adaptive cultures or those cultures that assisted in anticipating and adapting to environmental changes were associated with superior performance over the long run.[9]

An adaptive culture is one that allows for reasonable risk taking, builds on trust and a willingness to allow people to fail, and exhibits leadership at all levels. In organizations with adaptive cultures everyone, regardless of position, is encouraged to initiate changes that are in the best interests of patients, employees, and managers. The fear of failure is reduced by tolerating creative, and sometimes risky, efforts to make the organization a better place to work and more responsive to all stakeholders. In other words, adaptive cultures are necessary for organizational excellence.

Matching Culture and Strategy

Mission, vision, values, and strategic goals (discussed in Chapter 5) provide the linkage between strategy and culture. Just as these directional strategies were a major input to the selection of the adaptive, market entry, and competitive strategies, they play a major role in shaping the appropriate organizational culture. How the organization defines itself, what it wants to be, how it accomplishes its tasks, and what it wants to achieve, shape the culture of the organization. The directional strategies can be powerful forces in maintaining or changing the culture.

Strategic mangers must decide if the organizational culture can help achieve the strategy. Therefore, they must assess what assumptions, values, and behavioral norms are necessary to most effectively carry out the strategy. Attributes of the current assumptions, values, and behavioral norms must be compared with the assumptions, values, and behavioral norms required by the strategy. For example, if a market development strategy is being pursued, strategic managers may have to maintain the current culture; for new entrepreneurial ventures or product development, however, the culture may have to change. As discussed in Chapter 6, strategies that involve acquisitions, mergers, and alliances usually have organizational culture implications. Incompatible cultures can contribute to failure of the strategy.

During the situational analysis of the strategic management process, the mission, vision, values, and goals (the directional strategies) were evaluated. The leader must assess whether these directional strategies are still appropriate and are actually reflected in the culture of the organization. Results of this assessment will determine whether the leader needs to create implementation strategies to maintain or change organizational culture.

In addition to the comparison of the requirements of the overall strategy to current culture, results of the internal analysis itself may suggest action. The internal analysis specifies whether the organization's culture is a strength or weakness and whether it might create a competitive advantage or disadvantage. Therefore, the results of the internal analysis must also be incorporated into the decision to maintain or change the culture.

Maintaining Organizational Culture

Despite a good match between the attributes of the current culture and requirements of the strategy, the work of management is not complete. Maintaining culture often requires a great deal of hard work. In internal environmental analysis, if aspects of culture are evaluated as a strength having high value (H), are not rare (N), are easy or difficult to develop (E or D), and are sustainable (Y) – resulting in HNEY or HNDY – maintaining culture is particularly important because culture can be a source of short-term or long-term competitive advantage. Culture can be a powerful weapon in recruiting, efficiency, and innovation. Allowing this strength to deteriorate will lead to competitive disadvantage, particularly when it is common (not rare) among competitors.

Therefore, in maintaining culture, managers should:

- Communicate often the mission, vision, values, and goals – verbally and in writing;
- Behave in ways that are consistent with the values and vision – first through their personal behavior, and then through who they hire, who they promote, and what they reward; and
- Review and discuss the values and behavioral norms periodically.

Changing Organizational Culture

Changing organizational culture can be difficult and requires a great deal of planning, time, and energy. Michael Beer and Russell Eisenstat pointed out, "We've become convinced that the most powerful way for leaders to realign their organization is to publicly confront the unvarnished truth about the barriers blocking strategy implementation. Typically this involves looking closely at the roles and decision rights of various parts of the business, as well as changing the behavior of people at all levels."[10]

When culture is viewed as a weakness (from internal environmental analysis) or the requirements of the strategy call for a different culture, culture change strategies should be initiated. In cases where ineffective culture is assessed as a common weakness but as easy to correct (HYEY or HYEN), competitors may be moving to build their own organizational culture to create competitive advantage; therefore, culture change actions are warranted. Even when effective culture is a weakness, but among competitors the weakness is not common and is difficult to develop (HNDY and HNDN), change strategies should be initiated, particularly where competitors may act and achieve a significant competitive advantage. The most serious situation, of course, is where an organization has a weak culture and other organizations have effective cultures (weak culture is not common), and it is difficult to develop a new culture (HNDY and HNDN). Effective culture most often is difficult to develop and a significant competitive disadvantage when competitors have effective cultures. Strategic managers who want to create culture change should focus their energies on a few critical activities:

- Clarify the mission and vision and discuss the types of values and behaviors that would best achieve the vision.
- Discuss and codify the values and behavioral norms.
- Live by the values from the very beginning.
- Review and discuss the values and behavioral norms periodically.
- Create an atmosphere of perceived "crisis" in the organization. Without dissatisfaction with the current state, there is little incentive for managers to change familiar patterns of behavior.
- Clarify the vision and indicate what changes are necessary to achieve the vision. People need a clear sense of where the organization is going and where they should be headed.
- Communicate the mission, vision, values, and goals widely and repeatedly. Strategic managers should use simple, powerful, and consistent language.
- Model the kinds of behaviors and practices they want infused into the organization through their own actions. "Walking the talk" gives credibility to the words and provides examples to others in the organization of what behavior is expected.
- Empower other people to start acting in ways that are consistent with the desired values, and to implement new behaviors and practices. Part of empowering others is removing barriers within the organization that are in the way of the desired behavior.
- Look for some quick but sustainable successes. Short-term successes are critical to provide the change effort with some credibility, keep people motivated, and demonstrate positive results to the organization.
- Demonstrate patience and persistence. Major culture change takes a long time – years not months – and the willingness to persist in the face of obstacles and setbacks is critical.[11]

Organizational Structure as a Value Adding Support Strategy

Similar to culture, the organizational structure must facilitate rather than impede the implementation of the overall strategy. As Alfred Chandler observed, "Matching organization structure to the strategy is a fundamental task of the strategist."[12] Once the directional, market entry, competitive, and service delivery strategies have been developed, management must determine what organizational structure will best facilitate the strategy. This strategic thinking activity matches the requirements of strategy with the advantages and disadvantages of various organizational structural options. In addition, it should be acknowledged that an organization's current organizational structure might limit the strategic options or at least their initiation in the short run. Over time, the structure can be changed to meet the needs of the proposed strategy. At some point, the strategist must decide if the present structure should be maintained or changed.

Organizational Structure Building Blocks

Organizational hierarchy remains the basic structure of most, if not all, large organizations. As Harold Leavitt has written, ". . . just about every large organization remains hierarchical."[13] Organizations, whether loosely coupled, networked, or divisionalized, seem to be no more than modifications of the same basic design. Leavitt concludes that, ". . . hierarchies remain the best available mechanism for doing complex work."[14] There are three fundamental organizational hierarchical designs that form the basic building blocks for organizations:

- functional structure,
- divisional structure (strategic business or service units), and
- matrix structure.

FUNCTIONAL STRUCTURE

Functional structures organize activities around the mission-critical activities or processes of the organization and are the most prevalent structures for single product/service and narrowly focused organizations. A functional structure might include departments such as clinical operations, marketing, finance, information systems, and so on. However, activities will vary from one organization to another. Often parts of an organization are structured around processes. For example, in health care organizations, clinical operations are mission critical and the clinical function may be at the center of a functional structure. The clinic may then be organized around separate clinical processes such as registration, testing, examination, lab, and so on.

A functional structure builds a high degree of specialization and expertise within the functions or processes and can foster efficiency, particularly when tasks are routine and repetitive (such as in clinics). Moreover, in this type of organizational structure, control of strategic decisions is highly centralized. However, functional structures sometimes foster "silo thinking," slowing down decision making and inhibiting horizontal communication. As a result, it becomes a major task of strategic management to keep functional managers focused on the broader mission and the organization's vision (beyond their own functions) and to ensure coordination and communication across the functions. Exhibit 9–2 illustrates a functional organizational structure for clinical operations (organized around processes) and summarizes the advantages and disadvantages of functional structures.

DIVISIONAL STRUCTURE

Divisional structures are common in organizations that have grown through diversification, vertical integration, and aggressive market or product development. As organizations grow and become more diverse, divisional organizational structures are used to break the organization down into more manageable and focused parts. Therefore, a divisional structure creates several smaller, more focused,

Exhibit 9–2: Functional Structure Combined with Process Structure

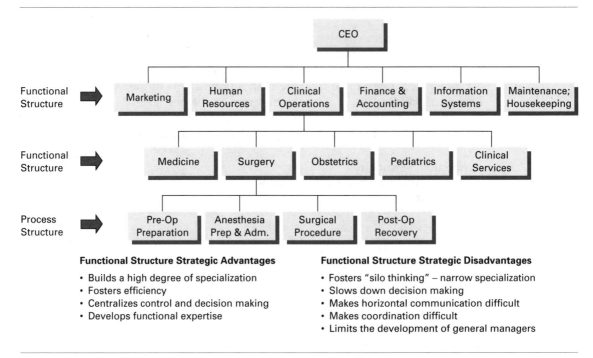

Functional Structure Strategic Advantages

- Builds a high degree of specialization
- Fosters efficiency
- Centralizes control and decision making
- Develops functional expertise

Functional Structure Strategic Disadvantages

- Fosters "silo thinking" – narrow specialization
- Slows down decision making
- Makes horizontal communication difficult
- Makes coordination difficult
- Limits the development of general managers

semi-autonomous strategic business/service units (SBUs/SSUs). Typical divisions might be based on geography (markets) or products/services or customers.

Structures with geographic divisions allow each division to tailor strategy and differentiate products/services based on the unique needs or characteristics of the geographic area or market. Local responsiveness will usually result in enhanced performance because communication and coordination within a target market will be improved. When organizations have unique multiple products/services, a divisional structure that places organizational emphasis on these products/services may be most appropriate. This structure gives the product division managers authority and responsibility to formulate and implement a product/service strategy. In addition, the structure allows functional areas to specialize around each product/service, thus increasing the coordination and communication. Divisions based on products/services increase the focus on products, markets, and quick response to change.

Divisional structures are not without problems. Divisional structures make it difficult to maintain a consistent image or reputation, add layers of management because of duplicate services and functions, and require carefully developed policy guidelines for the SBU/SSU. In addition, divisional structures may create competition for resources among the divisions. Exhibit 9–3 illustrates an organizational structure with product divisions (organized geographically) and summarizes the advantages and disadvantages of divisional structures.

Exhibit 9–3: Divisional Structure – Product with Geographic Divisions

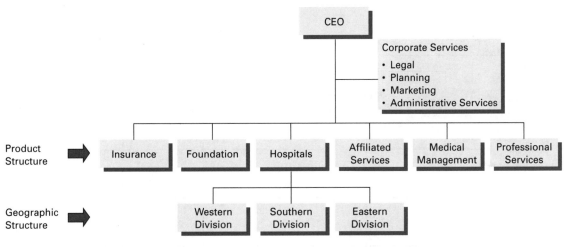

Divisional Structure Strategic Advantages

- Forces decision making down the organization
- Allows different strategies among divisions
- Fosters improved local responsiveness
- Places emphasis on the geographic region or product/service
- Improves functional coordination within the division
- Identifies responsibility and accountability
- Develops general managers

Divisional Structure Strategic Disadvantages

- Makes it difficult to maintain a consistent image/reputation
- Adds layers of management
- Duplicates services and functions
- Requires carefully developed policies and decision-making guidelines
- Creates competition for resources

MATRIX STRUCTURES

A *matrix structure* may be most appropriate when organizations have numerous products or projects that draw on common functional expertise. The fundamental rationale underlying a matrix structure is to organize around problems to be solved rather than functions or products or geography. Matrix organizations develop expertise and allow product areas or projects to use that expertise as needed. Therefore, in this structure, functional specialists may work on a number of different projects and with a number of project managers over time. Matrix structures foster creativity and innovation in the organization and, therefore, the structure is particularly effective for rapid product development and can accommodate a wide variety of product or project activities.

Matrix structures are difficult to manage – no one disputes that fact. The structure violates the "unity of command" (people report to only one boss) principle and, as a result, employees are often confused on priorities and "who is the boss." Therefore, this type of structure requires a great deal of coordination and communication and some degree of negotiation and shared responsibility between

Exhibit 9–4: Matrix Structure

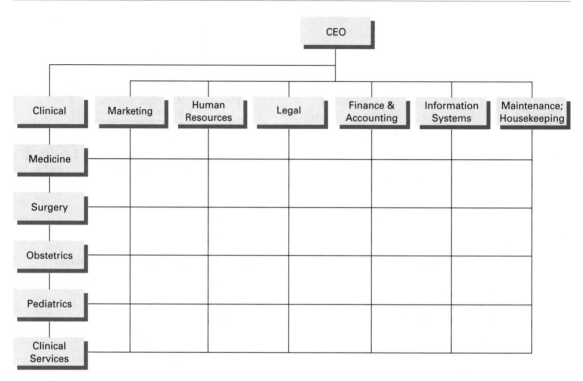

Matrix Structure Strategic Advantages

- Develops functional expertise
- Allows for a variety of product/project developments
- Allows for the efficient use of functional expertise
- Encourages rapid product development
- Fosters creativity and innovation

Matrix Structure Strategic Disadvantages

- Causes difficulties in management
- Violates the unity of command principle
- Creates coordination and communications problems
- Requires negotiation and shared responsibility
- Allows for confusion on priorities

project managers and functional managers. Exhibit 9–4 illustrates a matrix structure and summarizes the advantages and disadvantages.

COMBINATION STRUCTURES

Determining the most effective basic structure that will carry out the strategy is critical for all organizations. However, most health care organizations are rarely organized using just a single structural building block. Rather, health care organizations find it necessary to mix and often supplement the basic design. These designs are *combination structures*. For example, functional organizations often are supplemented with cross-functional teams to improve coordination and communication. Geographic divisions may be organized around functions or products. Product divisions may have geographic divisions as well as functional components. Organizational structure should enable the strategy and managers should select the most appropriate set of organizational structure building blocks.

Although the organizational structure building blocks set the basic design of the organization, seldom is it adequate alone for carrying out the strategy and work of the organization. Therefore, most organizations modify their basic structure with some type of coordinating structures. These coordinating structures are sometimes referred to as the *collateral organization* – a system of task forces, committees, and ad hoc groups used to bring different perspectives on issues to the table for discussion and resolution. No organization can function for long without an effective collateral organization.[15] Collateral structures include:

- *Project and product teams* – created to undertake well-focused projects (typically short term) or to develop new products.
- *Cross-functional task forces* – created to bring together specialists from several functional areas and address threats or opportunities. Typically, task forces take on a major project such as reorganization or the building of new facilities.
- *Venture teams* – created outside the normal organizational structure, they are not bound by the normal "rules" of the organization. Because they develop new products or processes, the creation of venture teams is sometimes called "intrapreneuring."
- *Reengineering teams* – created to evaluate and reconfigure an organizational process (such as service delivery). Such teams are asked to disregard the current way of doing things and to redesign a process from scratch.
- *Executive and standing committees* – created to make organization-wide decisions. Executive and standing committees provide wide representation for key decisions and facilitate communication of the organization's direction and strategy implementation.

Matching Structure and Strategy

Strategic managers should strive to keep their structures (and processes) as simple as possible and trim every vestige of unnecessary bureaucracy – for example, extra layers of management.[16] Fundamentally, the structural decision is one of prioritizing standardization versus flexibility and selecting the basic structure that best achieves the required priority. Therefore, strategic managers must evaluate the advantages and disadvantages of each of the structural building blocks and match them with the requirements of the strategy. For example, a different structure may be required to carry out a defender/cost leadership competitive strategy than that for a prospector/differentiation strategy. Defender strategies require a high degree of structural standardization to create cost efficiencies while prospector strategies require a great deal of structural flexibility to develop new technologies and innovative products and services. The strategic thinking map shown in Exhibit 9–5 provides guidance concerning the most appropriate basic organizational structure based on the strategy requirements of standardization or flexibility.

Exhibit 9–5: Strategy Requirements and Organizational Structure

Strategy Requirements	High Standardization ← → High Flexibility		
	Functional	**Divisional**	**Matrix**
High level of coordination	X		
High level of standardization	X		
Area/Functional expertise	X		
Main goal of efficiency	X		
High level of control	X		
Develop general managers		X	X
High degree of operating autonomy	X		
Decentralized decision making geared to market		X	
High need to customize product or services to market		X	
Consistent image	X		
Need local coordination		X	
Many projects using similar technologies			X
Need high level of creativity and innovation		X	X
Need high level of stability	X		
Need to develop new technologies			X
Need to be a cost leader	X		
Need to have service diversity		X	
Large organization		X	

MAINTAINING THE STRUCTURE

If there is a good match between the characteristics of the current organizational structure and the requirements of the strategy, then the present basic structure should be maintained. However, additional coordinating mechanisms may be required. It is not often that organizational structure alone will create long-term competitive advantage. However, structure is a key implementation area (especially when coupled with an effective culture). When it is viewed as an organizational strength, efforts should be made to keep it effective – whether it is or is not rare among competitors. In maintaining the present structure management should:

- Evaluate the present level of communication and coordination and discuss needed additional communication channels and coordinating mechanisms;
- Evaluate the present structure to ensure there are opportunities for innovation where appropriate;
- Evaluate the management team to ensure that the leadership skills match their positions; and
- Inventory the present skills to ensure that they are matched to the structure and strategy.

CHANGING THE STRUCTURE

If the comparison of the present structure and requirements of the strategy suggest a need to change the basic organizational structure, then management must develop a plan and move very carefully. Ineffective or inappropriate organizational structure can debilitate the organization's strategy – such as might be the case with too many organizational layers, thus delaying decision making – but by itself structure is not generally seen as a significant long-term competitive disadvantage. However, where the organizational structure is viewed as a weakness, action must be taken. Reorganization represents a significant change for employees and is often viewed as threatening. To help managers think though reorganization, a reengineering approach may be taken. Reengineering reconsiders and changes how tasks connect to each other to produce more efficient overall systems of work.[17] Therefore, when changing the structure, management should:

- Develop a flow chart of the total process, including its interfaces with other value chain activities;
- Simplify first, eliminating tasks and steps where possible and analyzing how to streamline the performance of what remains;
- Determine which parts can be automated (usually those that are repetitive, time consuming, and require little thought or decision);
- Consider introducing advanced technologies that can be upgraded to achieve next-generation capability and provide a basis for further productivity gains in the future;
- Evaluate each activity to determine whether it is strategy critical (strategy-critical activities are candidates for benchmarking to achieve best-in-industry performance status);
- Weigh the pros and cons of outsourcing activities that are noncritical or that contribute little to the organizational capabilities and core competencies;
- Compare the advantages and disadvantages of the organizational building blocks regarding standardization and flexibility; and
- Design a structure for performing the activities that remain, then reorganize the personnel and groups who perform these activities into the new structure.[18]

Changing the organizational structure can be a difficult task and may require some new thinking and new approaches to old problems. Reengineering efforts that have been undertaken by health care organizations indicate that the use of integrating mechanisms, such as codifying the process, and the use of internal teams and committees during implementation appear to be most effective.[19] In addition, as they undertake restructuring, strategic managers need to evaluate what competitive benefits are actually accruing to ensure that managers are not just reorganizing to be like everyone else, but for improved outcomes – they must understand how reengineering affects their competitive position.[20]

Strategic Resources as Value Adding Support Strategies

Effective development and use of key organizational resources are critical in carrying out the selected strategies. Key *strategic resources* include financial, human, information systems, and technology.

Financial Resources

The financial resources of the organization are evaluated during internal environmental analysis and are an input to strategy formulation. Therefore, to this point the financial resources have provided a framework for developing a realistic strategy. Once the strategy has been selected, finance becomes a way to implement the strategy. All organizational strategies have financial implications and most likely will require an assessment of needed capital and a method to access capital (see Perspective 9–2). Expansion, contraction, or maintenance of scope adaptive strategies will require a financial implementation strategy.

Expansion and maintenance of scope strategies frequently make it necessary for health care organizations to enter the capital market or make arrangements to borrow money from one or more financial institutions. Expansion of scope, such as market development, may be realized through acquisition of a competitor (horizontal integration) and involve hundreds of millions of dollars. Expansion carried out through cooperation strategies similarly may require additional financial resources. For example, joint ventures are often financed by attracting other individuals, such as physicians, to invest in promising ideas or equipment along with the hospital. Organizations with sufficient financial resources may even act as venture capitalists for new ideas (see Perspective 9–3). Similarly, maintenance of scope strategies directed toward enhancement of facilities, equipment, quality of services, and so on will often require new capital and operating funds. For example, an organization may have to acquire new property and relocate in its efforts to change the image held by physicians who might join its staff and the patients who might use its facilities. New technology may be demanded as well for this change in image or for significant improvement of services.

Contraction of scope strategies require equally challenging financial decision making. Divestiture, liquidation, harvesting, and, in some cases, retrenchment all convert financial resources, at least temporarily, into cash or near cash assets. This forces strategic managers to consider alternatives for the funds to ensure that they are appropriately invested until they are needed for other uses. Contraction requires careful reevaluation and possible redirection of the use of financial resources. For example, a hospital experiencing financial distress, after careful analysis, might decide that its emergency room is too expensive to continue to operate in view of limited demand by the community. The high level of specialized staffing for around-the-clock operations is a financial burden that cannot be justified economically. The decision to close the emergency room would temporarily

Perspective 9–2

Accessing Needed Capital

In 2002 the total amount of capital available to not-for-profit hospitals and health systems from traditional sources – tax-exempt bonds, equity issues, bank loans, philanthropy, and equipment leases – declined by 29 percent. However, the proportion of funding raised by alternative financial vehicles, such as joint ventures, has risen steadily since 1997.

For health care organizations, seeking new techniques to access needed capital is like a baseball pitcher learning new trick pitches. Forkballs and knucklers may be fine but it is important to master the basic fastball and curveball first. The same is true for hospitals. Before pursuing fancy financing options, the health care organization needs to make sure its profit margins are solid. Having said this, it is important to keep an open mind about alternative sources of capital. Obviously an organization has a limit to the amount of debt that is available, requiring that future projects be funded by a variety of techniques such as philanthropy, joint ventures, and so on. The stronger the organization is financially, the more options it has at its disposal. If a hospital has an AA credit rating, it has many opportunities. If its rating is BBB, it has fewer options.

After falling on hard times, Catholic Health Initiatives in Denver used a variety of approaches to improve its standing in the capital market. In 1999 three credit rating agencies downgraded it to AA–. By improving operations, Catholic Health was able to eliminate the minus sign in 2002. Catholic's CFO said they did not do anything fancy. They just made the improvements the old fashioned way – through hard work. The CFO concentrated on operating performance and a strong balance sheet to improve the organization's access to capital.

As a general rule, health care organizations look to five basic sources when they attempt to obtain more capital. These are:

1. *Operations.* Improving cash flow from operations is an industry mantra. Many health care organizations have focused on revenues. By collecting money owed to them, organizations can improve their operations and strengthen their balance sheet as they improve their cash position.
2. *Debt.* Private sector debt models have become very complex and risky. Some health care organizations have developed complicated debt structures as well. Risk is increased but the innovative financing often pays off.
3. *Investments.* An increasing number of health care systems are using derivative products to lower the cost of capital and make capital projects more affordable. Hospitals, according to industry experts, need to stay current on investment techniques because at some point it becomes a competitive issue if an organization is not investing enough. Most importantly, the organization has to be sure to invest in core assets and attempt to rid itself of noncore assets.
4. *Partnerships.* Joint ventures have become a popular way to share risk and expertise as well as to accommodate physicians who want some ownership in various ventures. Some possible advantages of joint ventures include better management expertise, higher quality products, broader coverage of regional markets, and risk sharing.
5. *Philanthropy.* Contributions to health systems have been difficult to obtain in recent years. Health care organizations may need to become more aggressive in seeking support to pay for mission-related activities.

Source: Dave Carpenter, "Better Access to Capital," *Hospital & Health Networks* 78, no. 5 (2004), pp. C10–C13.

What will happen next? A Virginia hospital system has joined forces with East Coast investors to launch one of the nation's few hospital-backed venture capital funds. Carillon Health System, a nine hospital system, joined Virginia Polytechnic Institute (VPI) and Third Security, LLC to create the New River Valley Investment Fund. Carillon and VPI contributed $5 million each and Third Security supplied $2 million. With this money as backing, the group launched the fund and attracted five existing venture capital funds to join the Consortium, bringing its total to around $43 million.

Because Carillon was already investing a portion of its reserves in out-of-state venture capital funds, joining with VPI and Third Security seemed a logical move and had the effect of improving the local economy. As a not-for-profit health system, Carillon's fortunes rise and fall with the health of the local community; investing in this way seemed in the best interest of all concerned.

The goal of the venture capital fund is to provide funding for start-up companies founded by entrepreneurial graduates of Virginia colleges as well as to attract promising out-of-state start-ups to Virginia. Fund partners are particularly interested in companies in the medical instrumentation and medical information fields.

Already the fund has invested in a small generics research firm and is actively pursuing firms to move to the area. Carillon believes that a flourishing group of start-up firms in the region will not only be good for the local community but for the health system as well. Carillon's CEO Edward Murphy, MD, stated, "Our first responsibility is to provide a broad range of high-quality health care services to the community. But economic development and growth is good for us as an organization, too."

As with any venture capital investor, the goal of the Consortium will be to assist entrepreneurial firms by providing start-up capital. In doing so, the investors hope to invest in some stars that will provide handsome returns in the future.

Source: Richard Haugh, "Investing in Growth," *Hospital & Health Networks* 78, no. 6 (2004), pp. 20–21.

free financial resources that could be allocated to more profitable areas and relieve some of the cost pressure on the hospital.

In developing financial strategies to carry out the organization's overall strategy, two issues typically predominate – increasing financial resources and better management of the organization's current financial resources. Important options for increasing financial resources to carry out the strategy include:

- capital acquisition (equity and debt),
- other forms of debt acquisition, and
- fund raising and philanthropy.

CAPITAL ACQUISITION – EQUITY AND DEBT

Capital investments are significant financial challenges because they involve large sums of money and they cover long time periods. The larger sums cause greater exposure to financial risks, and the longer time periods commit management to actions that are not easily altered.[21]

Capital investments are extremely important to health care organizations because the industry is very capital intensive. State-of-the-art medical equipment is essential to the delivery of quality medical care, but this type of equipment is very expensive. The inability or unwillingness of a hospital to obtain the most advanced technology can result in a loss of medical staff, patients, reputation, and, ultimately, market share.[22] The ability of a health care organization to effectively manage its capital investments is an important strategic strength. Management of capital investments requires an understanding of such specific techniques as the time value of money and the benefits of collecting income streams as soon as possible to take advantage of reinvestment opportunities. In addition, it requires the ability to use suitable financial management concepts necessary to evaluate long-term capital projects.

ACQUIRING EQUITY FUNDS

In the health care industry, equity funding comes from several sources. Financing mergers, acquisitions, and other market entry strategies may require that private health care organizations issue new stock or pursue increased investment from existing owners. If a health care organization is closely held, it may be built with personal investments from physicians and other interested investors who see an opportunity for a good return on their money. If it is a larger facility, it may have the ability to raise funds by going public and offering equity (shares of stock) to investors throughout the region or nation. In many cases, joint ventures between a health care organization and physicians or other firms represent equity investments. Equity funding may be obtained through the reinvestment of profits as well.

Recently, health care organizations have been successful at raising capital through initial public offerings (IPOs). This approach has been particularly common in the high-technology health care segments such as biotechnology, medical devices, and other proprietary and patented specialty medical products. However, as suggested in Perspective 9–4, the performance of IPOs in health care has been quite variable so far.

ACQUIRING DEBT

Long-term debt in the form of tax-exempt bonds has been one of the largest single sources of capital funds for hospitals over the past two decades. However, demands to increase public services and the reluctance of elected officials to enact more taxes cause many citizens to question whether or not governments at all levels will continue to allow tax exemptions for not-for-profit health care organizations. To qualify for the federal tax exemption, bonds are issued by a state or local authority and the health care facility leases the financed assets from the authority that holds the title until the indebtedness is repaid.[23]

Risk is an important consideration. To a great extent, the coupon or interest rate that must be paid for a bond reflects the perceived risk by the investors. However, the organization that issues long-term debt must consider the risks as

Perspective 9–4

Equity Alternative – Available but Beware

A renewed interest in initial public offerings (IPOs) by health care firms emerged early in 2004. During the first four months of the year, 17 health care companies – biotechnology, surgical centers, and medical equipment firms – had gone public, representing an astounding 38 percent of all IPOs for the time period. These 17 IPOs surpassed the number of health care firms going public in 2003 and 2002 combined. At the present pace, 2003 was projected to be even bigger for health care IPOs than 2001, when 23 companies went public.

In fairness it should be noted, however, that the total value of all 17 of the health care IPOs in the first four months of 2004 (about $1 billion) was $1 billion less than the total value of the Google deal. Only three of the 17 health care IPOs raised more than $100 million. Despite the smaller value, 2004 health care deals by May ranked third behind financial services and technology. In addition, of the 17 IPOs, nine were officially priced below the lowest figure in their original price range and two were priced above the highest price in the original range. The others were located in the original range.

By eight months into the year, the number of health care IPOs had almost doubled the number of the entire year of 2001. Thirty-nine biotech, pharmaceuticals, medical devices, medical equipment, and health services firms had successfully gone public. Only 44 firms in this category had gone public in the previous three years combined. Clearly, the equity market was looking more attractive for health care executives and investors. Equity money appeared to be available once again for new ideas and new technology.

Unfortunately, the after-market performance was not impressive. By the end of August 2004, the majority of these IPOs had presented investors with discounted prices and many were even trading below the discounted prices. According to Renaissance Capital, almost 60 percent of the 2004 health care IPOs had offering prices below their original ranges; for IPOs in all other industries, the average was about 38 percent below the original ranges. Although this statistic does not speak well for 2004 IPOs in general, health care discounts were even greater than the total sample.

All the news was not bad. When the current price (as of the end of August 2003) was compared with offering price, health care companies represented four of the ten best performing IPOs in the previous 12 months. Pharmion had an astounding 229 percent return, NitroMed posted a 68 percent return, and Eyetech Pharmaceuticals and Kinetic Concepts were providing investors a 60 percent return.

At the same time, health care IPOs accounted for seven of the 25 worst performing offerings of the previous 12 months. Myogen, for example, was the fourth worst performer, with a share price that dipped 57 percent below its offering price. The story remains the same. Do not be overly impressed by the prospects of the equity market. Very often in health care, as in other businesses, simply going to the market is not always the best way to raise needed capital.

Source: Robert Steyer, "Mixed Prognosis for Health Care IPOs," *TheStreet.com* (May 13, 2004); Robert Steyer, "Health Care Crowds IPO Sick List," *TheStreet.com* (August 25, 2004); www.IPOhome.com/marketwatch/review/2004review.asp.

well. If debt is issued at a time when interest rates are very high, it may be desirable to build in a "call feature" whereby the debt can be refinanced when interest rates are lower. Despite a prepayment fee being charged, it may be beneficial to call in the debt if interest rates drop significantly.

Another aspect of risk is the ability of the organization to service the debt. If revenues are not available to pay the interest in a timely manner and retire the debt, closure is possible. Therefore, margin is an important indicator of a health care organization's ability to effectively service its debt payments (interest and contribution to loan reduction). In recent years, hospitals in particular have recorded lower margins. This results from accelerating expenses and shorter lengths of stay. At the same time, margins have been reinforced by increases in admissions and outpatient visits.[24]

In deciding whether to use long-term debt, strategic managers are favorably influenced by the fact that control over operations and decision making can be maintained more easily than with equity financing. Although it is true that creditors can require restrictive covenants that reduce flexibility and control, the organization's ability to obtain financing for a promised return, without having to broaden participation in decision making, is attractive.

Other Forms of Debt Acquisition

Health care organizations may prefer to deal with a single financial institution rather than numerous individuals and underwriters in the capital market. In such a case, funds can be borrowed from banks or other financial institutions. The risks of bank financing, however, are the same as with other forms of debt. Of course, the attractiveness of debt financing is influenced primarily by interest rates. Because rates were at all-time lows during most of the 1990s and the first five years of the twenty-first century, debt financing has been particularly appealing. In 2005 the economy was improving yet there was uncertainty with interest rate fluctuations as the Fed attempted to stimulate the economy but avoid inflation.

FUND RAISING AND PHILANTHROPY

During a time when capital markets are uncertain, when there is public resistance to tax increases (some of which might eventually assist health care organizations), and when a host of other problems complicate long-term financing, philanthropy is being "rediscovered" and pursued seriously by many health care organizations. Because of the need for earnings, the cost of public offerings, and the desire of many health care organizations to retain their tax-exempt status, private philanthropy has become more important as a source of funds in health care. Giving to health-related causes ranks high in overall terms (almost 10 percent of total gifts). However, it is about the same amount that is given to human services and falls far behind religious and educational causes.

Private individual, corporate, and foundation gifts will remain an important source of funds for health care organizations. However, as with many other areas of activity, fund raising is more competitive than ever. Educational, religious, and environmental organizations are actively seeking and acquiring funds. In the future, hospitals and other health care organizations will be pressured to become even more aggressive and innovative just to maintain their historical share of available gifts.

Effective Management of Financial Resources and Investment

Prior to pursuing the acquisition of new capital and operating funds, a careful examination of the utilization of existing financial resources should be conducted. Moreover, some strategic alternatives might actually be able to be funded through the better utilization of existing financial resources. For example, if the leadership of a long-term care facility determines that enhancing quality demands significant increases in training expenditures, the funds for training might be acquired by reducing the amount in the cash account, more carefully managing and reducing inventories, or similar actions.

Important issues in effective management of financial resources to carry out the strategy include:

- managing existing financial resources,
- managing cash flow, and
- budgeting and financial planning.

Human Resources

It is clear that a successfully implemented strategy is inextricably connected to having committed, high-performance employees.[25] As pointed out in Perspective 9–5, it takes strong leadership and a positive organizational culture to keep employees motivated and productive. Motivated employees are the key to any strategy. However, human resources requirements of the selected strategies will vary considerably depending on whether the organization is expanding, contracting, or maintaining scope. For example, expansion strategies, such as related diversification, will make it necessary to recruit new personnel with skills and talents similar to those already in the organization. On the other hand, unrelated diversification and backward and forward vertical integration will create the need for human resources with skills and talents quite different from those presently employed. The necessity of recruiting, hiring, and leading individuals with different skills and talents is a major reason that these strategies are "riskier" than related diversification. Any one of these strategies requires the merger of similar or dissimilar organizational cultures, presenting yet another human resources challenge.

Diversification and integration are two very different strategic choices, but they require similar types of organizational and human resources management responses. When diversification or integration is selected as a strategic alternative, the potential exists that organizational size and diversity will increase, as will the demand for more specialized human resources management services.

Although the problems are difficult and demanding, expansion is always more fun to manage than maturity and decline. During maturity, the emphasis is on efficiency. Human resources management practices must be constantly refined and improved to ensure that things are done in the best way at the least cost.

Perspective 9–5

Strong Health
Care Leaders
Build Employee
Commitment

More than 11 million people are employed in the health services industry. Keeping employees motivated and inspired is a daunting task for any
manager. Leaders face many challenges – finding the right people for the
job, equipping them with the skills they need to do their jobs (as well as
personal and professional growth), and retaining good employees once
they are hired.

Studies show that at any given time as much as 40 percent of the health
care workforce plans to leave the field in the next few months. Replacing
a trained employee can cost more than two times their annual salary in recruitment time, fees, and retraining. In many cases, disillusion with managers is a primary reason for discontentment. Of the employees
asked to rank their bosses in key skill areas:

- 34 percent thought their supervisor's ability to achieve results through his or her management style
  was not meeting expectations;
- 37 percent indicated that their supervisor's ability to create an environment of mutual trust, respect,
  and open communication was not meeting expectations; and
- 36 percent were not confident that their supervisor had the ability to foster the growth and development of the work team.

Traditional supervisors are often seen as babysitters, primarily ensuring that the work is done. They
accomplish the task by enforcing rules and requiring people to follow standard operating procedures.
Traditional supervisors cannot build effective teams because they take away the thinking work from team
members. Traditional supervisors believe that it is their job to think for their employees. A more effective approach is to coach employees. Coaches are supervisors that develop the abilities of employees to
independently solve problems and implement improvements. Coaches focus on the development of self-
directed individuals and then lead these individuals to solve more complex problems and implement
more complex problems through self-directed teams.

Leaders need to stay on top of the perceptions of employees. They should take the results of employee
surveys seriously and use the data in the strategic planning process. Leaders should be held accountable
for changing negative perceptions. Health care organizations are offering innovative opportunities for
leaders to develop the tools they need to become more effective. Each organization's management team
has the responsibility to look at its current culture and face the reality that em-ployees may not think the
leaders are as effective as the leaders think they are. Steps should be taken to correct inadequacies and
initiate development and team building programs that foster commitment from employees and build healthy
relationships over the long term.

Source: Erin Wilkins, "Healthcare Employee Commitment Rises among Strong Leaders," *Managed Healthcare Executive* 14,
no. 6 (2004), pp. 44–46.

However, organizations do not always successfully manage maturity, and markets erode and even disappear. Therefore, it is important for the strategic health
care manager to understand how to manage the organizational and human
resources aspects during market contraction.

Contraction involves different human resources management skills. Incentives
must be devised to encourage employees to find other jobs or to retire earlier
than anticipated. For some, layoffs may be necessary, and the organization will
be forced to determine its responsibility in assisting displaced employees to find

alternative employment opportunities. At times, health care organizations may assist employees by retraining them for different tasks that will be needed as contraction takes place.

In Chapter 6, several contraction strategies, such as divestiture and liquidation, were discussed. Although terms such as "divestiture" and "liquidation" imply financial actions, they have important human resources implications in the form of restructuring and reorganizing, early retirements, layoffs, and so on.

The benefits of systematically managing the human resources dimension under expansion and contraction strategies are somewhat obvious. The need for carefully managing maintenance of scope strategies is equally important, if not as obvious. Maintenance strategies almost always require training and development activities. Enhancement strategies through total quality management programs involve significant commitments to continuous learning on the part of the individual and the organization. Status quo requires the challenging task of keeping people motivated in the face of career plateaus.

When an organization reaches a point in its life cycle where it is no longer growing, it must work extremely hard to keep from contracting. Strategic decision makers may adopt a conservative strategy, such as managing the steady state or status quo. As was noted in Chapter 6, the assumption underlying this strategy is that the expansion phase of the organization's evolution is over, maturity has been achieved, and acceptable market shares have been attained. The organization attempts to replace personnel with employees of similar skills and training, and works to keep existing personnel up to date and technologically prepared to perform their jobs at high levels of effectiveness.

Maintaining scope can present an opportunity to enhance current levels of operation. This stage of organizational development can be looked on as a temporary "breather," and preparation can commence for the next period of growth. Or, decision makers can simply think of maintaining scope in a dynamic sense and recognize that they must work hard just to hold their current position. In this case, they may choose to enhance their facilities, improve the quality of their services, increase the speed with which they respond to patients and make decisions, and create new and better ways of doing things. Human resources strategies are important to support any attempt at enhancement because ultimately it is the employees that must improve quality, innovate, and work faster if things are to improve.[26]

Information Resources

Information systems (ISs) are an essential competitive resource for health care organizations and are critical in supporting strategic decision making, administrative operations, and patient care in an increasingly information intensive industry. Information systems in health care may be divided into four general categories: clinical, management, strategic decision support, and electronic networking and e-health applications.[27] Competitive advantage may be created in each of these areas, and strategic managers should therefore play a key decision-making role in defining and shaping these systems, as illustrated in the Introductory Incident. Such systems draw on both internal data from clinical and administrative systems in the organization as well as external data on community health, market demography, and activities of competitors.[28] To meet strategic objectives and develop high-priority applications, the health care organization must make decisions about hardware configurations (architecture), network communications, degree of centralization or decentralization of computing facilities, and types of computer software required to support the network.[29] The strategic information system may be effectively used to consider and help implement adaptive, market entry, and competitive strategies.

A *strategic information system* (SIS), sometimes referred to as a *decision support system*, attempts to take vast quantities of unorganized data and turn them into useful information to enable managers to make better decisions. Such information systems involve organizing the data, selecting the models that will analyze the data, and interpreting the output. However, it is not sufficient simply to provide the reports to the strategist. Sometimes there is a need to interpret and clarify the data relative to the assumptions that were used. Because decision support systems attempt to investigate future activities, the assumptions are critical. The organization that can design a strategic IS that is pertinent, relatively accurate, and timely will have developed a competitive advantage. "Inappropriate use and interpretation of decision support models can be dangerous, but appropriate use of these models can be a powerful tool in the hands of an informed decision maker."[30] For example, as explained in Perspective 9–6, geographic information systems (GIS) are increasingly being used in health care to provide decision support.

Administrative information systems support areas other than direct patient care and include financial information systems, human resources systems, payroll, billing, purchasing, materials and facilities management, outpatient clinic scheduling, office automation, and so on. Clinical information systems support patient care and include computerized patient records systems, automated medical instrumentation, patient monitoring systems, nursing information systems, laboratory information systems, pharmacy information systems, clinical decision support systems, and information systems that support clinical research and education. Most information systems in the health care industry focus on the financial and administrative aspects of the practice of medicine and much less on the clinical decision making.[31] However, clinical information systems are growing in importance, creating significant competitive advantage through increased efficiency and effectiveness of patient care. Basic clinical information systems provide a "dictionary" of health problems for clinicians or display background information on specific patients. More sophisticated systems, often referred to as expert or knowledge-based systems, can actively assist clinicians in the decision-making process.[32] Such functions include:

- assistance with diagnosing a patient's condition;
- assistance in determining proper drug dosage;
- reminders to administer preventive services to patients at specific times; and

- assistance in carrying out diagnostic or therapeutic procedures, such as recommending specific treatments, reminders to perform procedures, alerts regarding potential adverse events, feedback based on previous orders, and prompts for testing or treatment options.[33]

In today's information-intense environment, seamless integration and information sharing are becoming increasingly important. Most health care organizations

Perspective 9–6

Strategic Decision Making Using a Geographic Information System (GIS)

Despite a vast network of public and private health services staffed by a large number of health professionals, "health for all" still remains a distant reality, partly because of limited access to health services and the explosive cost of utilization. Poor geographical distribution of health services is an important reason for inadequate access to care and disparities in health outcomes. Using geographical information system technology, spatial analysis can be used to improve access, minimize cost, and improve quality of health service delivery. In addition, a GIS functions as a strategic tool for planning, implementing, and evaluating market availability, viability, and penetration.

GIS is an automated system for the capture, storage, retrieval, analysis, and display of spatial data. IT requires data to be captured and stored via spatial information, such as zip codes, addresses, or census tract. GIS can integrate attribute data with spatial information to allow for more complex data processing, analysis, and modeling. Layered information, displayed as maps, can assist in the understanding of complicated strategic, spatial, and informational relationships. For example, GIS can be used to:

- determine geographic distribution of diseases,
- analyze spatial and temporal demographic trends,
- map populations at risk,
- stratify risk factors,
- assess resource allocation,
- plan and target interventions,
- analyze referral patterns,
- monitor diseases and interventions over time, and
- evaluate marketing campaigns.

A geographical information system was used to analyze the spatial distribution of orthopedic patients around local orthopedic centers in Birmingham, Alabama (see the map). Patients were evenly distributed in the identified catchment areas according to GIS analysis; there were no clusters around any particular center. However, certain clinics did not attract patients from surrounding zip codes. Based on the GIS analysis, the centers that were not attracting patients planned to implement a marketing campaign to raise awareness of their centers in those particular zip code areas.

Historically, GISs have been used in the health care arena for epidemiological research, such as determining cancer mortality or food illness outbreaks by zip code, county, or census tract. However, given the power of GISs and the massive amounts of collected data in health care organizations, GIS analysis can provide valuable insight for decision makers. A GIS is an effective and necessary tool for strategic leaders. The challenges of planning, implementing, and evaluating strategies can be greatly enhanced by applying GIS technology to improve health care access and quality as well as enhancing the strategic management process.

Source: Maziar Abdolrasulnia, PhD student, Administration-Health Services, University of Alabama at Birmingham.   ▶

Patient Distribution Around Two Orthopedic Centers

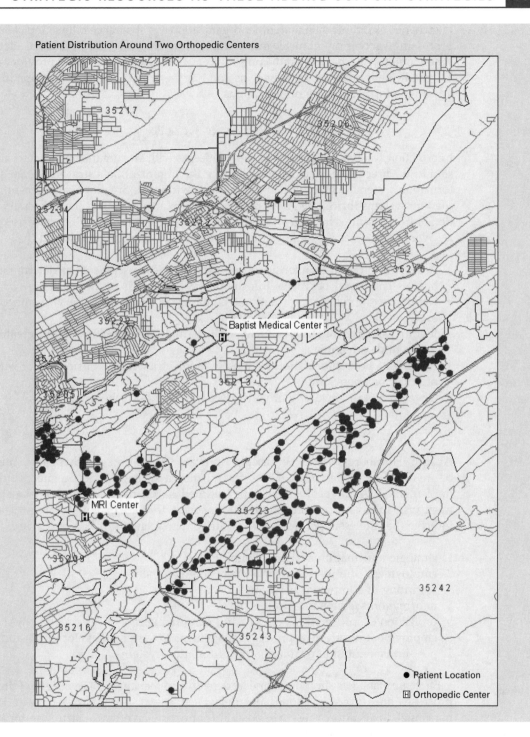

interchange electronic data with other organizations for insurance billing and claims processing, accessing clinical information from regional and national databases, online purchasing, and communications between affiliated providers.[34] Telemedicine is a part of such systems and has the potential to create competitive advantage for health care organizations.

LINKAGE OF IS STRATEGY TO THE ORGANIZATIONAL STRATEGY

Information systems initiatives and capabilities, as with any organizational resource, should be directed to support and advance the organization's strategic goals. Information systems achieve strategic alignment within the organization by ensuring that the systems formulate goals, activities, and plans that effect the implementation of IS capabilities in a way that leverages the organization's ability to carry out its overall strategies.[35] In taking full advantage of ISs, managers should:

- Assess the information intensity of service categories or segments by determining how essential and pervasive information processing is in the segment;
- Determine the role of information technology in defining the service category or segment;
- Identify and rank the ways in which information technology might create a competitive advantage;
- Investigate how information technology might spawn new businesses or ways of doing business; and
- Develop a plan for taking advantage of information technology.[36]

THE STRATEGIST ROLE IN IS

Austin, Hornberger, and Shmerling indicate that strategic managers must be involved in IS decisions if the organization's strategy is to be successfully implemented. As a result, they have outlined seven major executive management principles and responsibilities for ensuring that ISs fit with strategy. They indicate that the essential tasks for executive management in IS strategy are:

1. strategic information systems planning,
2. employment of a user focus in systems development,
3. recruiting of competent personnel,
4. information systems integration,
5. protection of information security and confidentiality,
6. employment of effective project management in systems development, and
7. post-implementation evaluation of information systems.[37]

Strategic managers should assume leadership and management oversight of these processes and typically should not delegate these responsibilities to technical personnel. In addition, these responsibilities provide an efficient structure for the performance of a systematic audit to determine how well information systems are planned, integrated, and managed in furtherance of organizational priorities.[38]

DEVELOPING COMPETITIVE ADVANTAGE

In today's fast-paced environment, health care professionals are searching for any competitive advantage that might be available. Important contributions of IS are to develop competitive advantage by lowering costs, enhancing differentiation, changing competitive scope, and improving customer service levels. Examples of information systems that increase market share, raise profitability, add value to products, and change the competitive position of an organization have many CEOs reexamining the role of information resources in their corporate strategy.[39]

More specifically, IS may be utilized to provide a competitive advantage in four general ways:

1. Leverage organizational processes – improve organizational processes by making them faster, less expensive, less error prone, more convenient, and more available.
2. Enable rapid and accurate provision of critical data – improve strategic, administrative, and clinical information.
3. Enable product and service differentiation, and, occasionally, creation – add value though product enhancements and customizations or new products themselves, such as web-based information services.
4. Support the alteration of overall organizational form or characteristics – improve service quality orientation, communication, decision making, and collaboration.[40]

Information systems assist in improving quality, as pointed out in Perspective 9–7. Medical errors have become a significant health care quality problem.

Strategic Technologies

The technologies selected by the organization are dictated by the chosen strategies. Broadly, *strategic technologies* concern the type of facilities, type and sophistication of equipment, and management of technology employed within the organization. Each of these activities is critical to the successful implementation of the organization's strategy.

FACILITIES

Strategic facilities is the broad term used to delineate the physical environment of the health care organization. It is the "shell" in which health care is delivered. It generally includes such diverse areas as design and construction of new facilities and renovation of older facilities, key equipment, clinical engineering, environmental services, safety and security, materials management, and food service. Each component affects the health care organization's ability to implement its strategy.

Facilities management is an area of increasing concern to strategic managers of health care organizations for a variety of reasons. One of the most important

Perspective 9–7

A Prescription for
Medical Errors

"First, do no harm" is a phrase recited by every physician taking the Hippocratic oath. However, based on the human predisposition for making errors, this can be a lofty goal. In fact, a recent Institute of Medicine (IOM) report suggests that as many as 100,000 Americans die annually because of medical errors.

Medical errors happen when the intended patient intervention is improperly executed or when the wrong course of action was pursued in the first place. When caring doctors and nurses make mistakes it is often no different from the simple mistakes people make every day, but theirs can have devastating consequences on patients.

Errors can happen during even the most routine tasks, such as when a hospital patient on a salt-free diet is given a high-salt meal. More serious errors can occur when a pharmacist misinterprets an illegible prescription and dispenses a potentially fatal drug to a patient. Research indicates that the most preventable errors occur during the entire process of administering drugs.

Experts believe information systems can greatly reduce the number of medical errors. Computerized physician order entry systems have thus far proven the most effective. By computerizing the prescription order process, structure and control are introduced. The system forces the indication of a precise dose, route, and frequency. In addition the system can eliminate the problem of illegible handwriting, incomplete or lost information, and make every prescription traceable to the provider. These systems can provide the latest information about a drug and cross-reference allergies, interactions, and other problems of a patient with the chemical entity being prescribed.

Furthermore, when computerized physician order entry systems are implemented in combination with other information technologies (such as computer-based patient records, decision support systems, and so on) an even greater reduction in medical errors can be realized.

If the IOM report is correct, more people die from medical errors than from motor vehicle accidents, breast cancer, or AIDS. Information systems can prevent these needless deaths. Noted Harvard physician, Lucian Leape, stated it best when he said, "Although human errors are excusable, ignoring them is not."

Source: Nir Menachemi, PhD, School of Medicine, Florida State University.

is the changing technology that has fostered tremendous growth in the number and kind of alternative delivery systems requiring different strategies for success. Free-standing outpatient clinics, ambulatory (same day) surgery centers, diagnostic and imaging centers, and others, are challenging traditional inpatient health care delivery. To survive, hospitals have altered their strategies to expand vertically and horizontally or to diversify into these new delivery systems. However, each type is subject to entirely different design needs for buildings as well as different regulatory guidelines – a challenge for the facilities manager.

A variety of components should be considered in the design of a health care facility: medical technology, the full range of medical procedures from routine exams to complicated life-saving activities, medical staff, sanitation, prevention of injury, economics, patients, and visitors. From the patients' perspective, the facility includes "curb appeal," ease of access to the main entrance, ease of parking, ease of wayfinding (finding the department, room, diagnostic area, or other area where the patient is expected), comfort, and convenience. Designing the facility with the human experience in mind recognizes that people's perceptions of health care are multidimensional; the facility helps them define the care they receive. Sending a "we care" message cannot stop with the staff but must be designed into the facility itself.[41]

When the health care organization decides on a high-tech, a high-touch, or some other strategy, the facility provides the first impression. The design, layout, color scheme, and so on, should reflect the desired image to improve the implementation of the strategy. "Unlike the quality of medical care, health facility design is something that can readily be understood and judged, for better or worse, by the public."[42]

Equipment

Closely associated with strategic facilities is the choice of equipment and technology management. The choice of the type and sophistication of equipment and effective technology management is an integral part of strategic management and should be approached in a systematic way. Because health care technology changes rapidly, is costly, and often requires changes in the facility, it must be assessed and planned for carefully to operate the facility to its greatest potential. Physicians generally want the latest technology – using the "latest" equipment or newest procedure provides prestige with colleagues and patients and may save more lives or provide less discomfort to patients. The decision concerning the use of the latest technology must fit with the strategy (differentiation based on high-technology image).

Technology decisions involve technology assessment, planning, acquisition, and management.[43] They advocate that a committee assess requests for new and emerging technology alongside the capital budget requests for new and replacement technology. The committee should report to senior management and should set mission-based, strategic priorities for new, emerging, and replacement technologies. Many hospitals do not incorporate into the budget the costs of redesign and "space" for new technology; nor do they investigate ways to reduce maintenance, insurance, and outside service contract costs. The planning process has to take into account what the competition is planning to acquire in terms of new and emerging technology as well as assessing the services offered by competitors.

Clinical engineering (sometimes called biomedical engineering) is a relatively new area in most health care organizations. Its responsibilities include: applying engineering technology to diagnostic and treatment devices used by health care facilities through testing, maintaining, and repairing equipment; training; consultation with clinical staff concerning the capabilities, efficiencies, and accuracy of the equipment; environmental testing; and incident and recall investigations that involve diagnostic or treatment equipment. The number and sophistication of technologies within health care institutions has increased significantly in the past decade. Because of the expertise required for such a large variety of equipment, some health care organizations use outside service contracts for some or all of their technological equipment.

Maintaining Strategic Resources

If there is a match between the present level of strategic resources and the requirements of the strategy, then efforts should be made to maintain the financial, human, information, and technology resources. These areas may represent key competitive advantages or disadvantages for an organization. Care should be taken to maintain those areas that are valued by customers and are a strength of the organization. In maintaining strategic resources the leader should do the following:

FINANCIAL

- Evaluate whether current financial resources are being used efficiently.
- Determine whether the liquidity is appropriate for meeting ongoing expenses.
- Seek ways to increase profitability without sacrificing other mission-critical factors.
- Assess the current level of leverage to determine if there is an appropriate level of risk.
- Determine whether asset activity can be improved.
- Assess cash-flow management.
- Consider investment opportunities for idle cash.

HUMAN RESOURCES

- Develop training programs to maintain the current human expertise and capabilities.
- Develop a management succession plan.
- Develop a job market network.

INFORMATION SYSTEMS

- Assess information systems growth needs.
- Develop information systems plans for operations and upgrades.

TECHNOLOGIES

- Make sure there is a plan for facilities and equipment maintenance.
- Develop a facilities and equipment replacement schedule.
- Periodically review the operating procedures, policies, and rules in order to keep them "lean."
- Review environmental services activities and procedures.
- Evaluate current security procedures.
- Evaluate food service activities.
- Evaluate operation and maintenance procedures.

Changing Strategic Resources

If there is a poor match between the present level of strategic resources and the requirements of the strategy, the process should be to change the financial and human resources, information systems, and strategic technologies to meet the needs of the strategy. As with the service delivery strategies and other support strategies, the organization must be particularly sensitive to situations where it is easy to build a strength (ours or the competition's) because the competition may create a long-term competitive advantage. For example, there is evidence that the early adoption of technology is often driven by technological competition where competitive rivalry is high (thus the need to eliminate competitive disadvantage). On the other hand, late adoption of technology may be more a result of revenue considerations (the threat of losing revenue).[44]

Changing the type or nature of the financial and human resources, information systems, or facilities and equipment can be a difficult and long-term project. To change these strategic resources, the leader should do the following:

FINANCIAL

- Assess whether the current revenue can finance the change.
- Investigate the opportunities to finance the change through the issuance of stock and the infusion of additional equity.
- Investigate the opportunities to finance the change through bonds, mortgages, bank loans, fund raising, or philanthropy.

HUMAN RESOURCES

- Assess job markets to determine the availability of individuals possessing the new required skills.
- Begin recruiting for new skills.
- Develop training programs to retrain individuals with skills no longer needed.

INFORMATION SYSTEMS

- Consider outsourcing information systems change needs.
- Assess the impact of change needs on ISs.
- Assess needs of information systems in pre-service, point-of-service, and after-service activities.

TECHNOLOGIES

- Identify the exact specifications of the need for facilities, equipment, or processes.
- Perform cost analysis on the required changes.
- Develop timelines for changing the technologies.
- Investigate the financing alternatives for the required changes.
- Investigate any new required skills or experience to operate or maintain the new facilities or equipment.

- Specify any new required processes or ways of doing things.
- Initiate the facilities, equipment, and technology management renewal.

Extending the Strategic Thinking Map

There are many ways to add value in organizations. The value adding support strategies provide a powerful means to change the organization and create competitive advantage, especially because some of the value adding support activities are less visible to those outside the organization, making the competitive advantage much more difficult to imitate or duplicate. Decisions concerning the organization's culture, structure, and resources are strategic in nature and should be made by strategic thinkers. The effectiveness of the organization's overall strategy may be influenced or even determined by the effectiveness of these implementation strategies. Exhibit 9–6 shows a completed strategic thinking map that compares the results of an internal environmental analysis and the selected strategy requirements and proposed value adding support strategies for a long-term care organization. This map extends and further articulates the strategic thinking maps developed in strategy formulation and the development of the value adding service delivery strategy. In addition, as with the service delivery strategies, guidance for managing the strategic momentum is provided so that unit managers may develop effective action plans that are tied directly to the organization's strategy.

Managing Strategic Momentum – Support Strategies

The actual management of the support strategies includes the managerial processes, procedures, style, and technologies of the organization and is an inherent part of the organization and the way it operates. Strategic thinking and strategy evaluation should be regarded as a normal and necessary part of what the organization and its managers do. Through the setting of objectives, the performance appraisal process, the compensation program, and so on, managers' actions are coordinated toward agreed-upon organizational objectives. Strategic thinking and strategic evaluation become part of the operating procedures and culture (shared values) of the organization. Additional questions to aid strategic managers in managing the support strategies and evaluating their progress and appropriateness are presented in Exhibit 9–7.

Summary and Conclusions

The value chain activities provide the basis for strategy implementation. After the value adding service delivery strategies have been developed, the value adding support strategies should be formulated. The value adding support strategies are key in implementing the overall strategy and include organizational culture,

Exhibit 9–6: Strategic Thinking Map for Value Adding Support Strategies for a Long-term Care Organization: An Example

Adaptive Strategy: Vertical integration – enter into a system of care.
Market Entry Strategy: Enter into an alliance with hospital to assure referral network.
Strategic Posture: Move from defender posture to analyzer posture.
Positioning Strategy: Differentiation based on quality, upscale image.

	Characteristics/Attributes		**Evaluation**			**Support Strategy**
Value Adding Support Strategies	**Results of Internal Analysis**	**Requirements of Selected Strategies**	**Comparison of Strategy Requirements and Results of the Internal Analysis**	**Maintain**	**Change**	**Guidance for Organizational Units (Basis for Unit Action Plan Development)**
Organizational Culture • Assumptions • Values • Behavior Norms	Strong, positive culture based on religious affiliation, caring environment with appropriate behavioral norms, (seen as competitive advantage: valuable, rare, difficult to imitate, and sustainable)	Culture reflects upscale differentiation positioning strategy	Good match. However, culture (values and behavior norms) will need to be transferred to alliance partner (requires major organization effort to maintain competitive advantage)	X		**HR** – Emphasize importance of the organization's culture and image, review and discuss the values/behavior norms, discuss mission, vision, values and strategic goals with new alliance partner
Organizational Structure • Function • Division • Matrix	Strong functional structure (some communication problems across functions, seen as short-term competitive disadvantage: valuable but fairly easy to fix)	Strategy requires specialization, vertical integration through alliance moves organization toward more decentralization	Fairly good match. However, need to increase coordination and communication, improve communications and coordination through executive and standing committees. Cross-functional task force needed to plan and facilitate alliance	X		**All units** – more discussion at executive and departmental meetings, create cross-functional task force to plan and implement alliance with appropriate hospital, initiate training program on communication and coordination

Exhibit 9–6: (cont'd)

Adaptive Strategy: Vertical integration – enter into a system of care.
Market Entry Strategy: Enter into an alliance with hospital to assure referral network.
Strategic Posture: Move from defender posture to analyzer posture.
Positioning Strategy: Differentiation based on quality, upscale image.

	Characteristics/Attributes		Evaluation			Support Strategy
Value Adding Support Strategies	Results of Internal Analysis	Requirements of Selected Strategies	Comparison of Strategy Requirements and Results of the Internal Analysis	Maintain	Change	Guidance for Organizational Units (Basis for Action Plan Development)
Strategic Resources • Human Resources • Information Systems • Strategic Technologies • Financial	Shortages of clinical personnel, reward system not tied to performance (not seen as competitive disadvantage because the problems are common in the industry). Little management depth, information system weak, many billing problems (competitive disadvantages) Excellent facilities, recently remodeled, equipment is state-of-the-art, effective management facilities and technology (competitive advantage: valuable, rare, difficult to imitate, and sustainable) Strong financially	Strong staff to provide long-term continuity of care and maintain image Superior IS to support differentiation strategy Positioning strategies (upscale differentiation) requires quality facilities and technology	Poor match in the areas of HR and IS. Need to be improved to implement strategy. Most problems in HR concern personnel shortages, lack of management depth, and the reward system. Need major emphasis on recruitment of management and technical staff Information system outdated Need development of patient record and billing system. IS critical to the selected positioning strategy Good match: facilities and technology, continual upgrade and maintenance needed Finances available to support the strategy		X	**HR** – create recruitment package to attract and retain key management personnel and technical personnel, develop performance/reward proposal tied to behavior norms identified in internal analysis
					X	**IS** – purchase new billing system, create overall information systems strategy
					X	**Technologies** – install maintenance and upgrade schedule, ensure state-of-the-art facilities and equipment, ensure housekeeping keeps appearances up to high standards, state-of-the-art facilities and equipment in promotional materials, continue image promotions that emphasize differentiation strategy
				X		**Finance** – budget for facilities and equipment upgrades utilizing current revenues

Exhibit 9–7: Strategic Thinking Map for Evaluation – Support Strategies

1. Is the organization's culture appropriate for the overall strategy?
2. Are the organization's values reflected in the service delivery?
3. Are the behavioral norms appropriate for the strategy?
4. Are the management processes (the way we do things) appropriate for the strategy?
5. Does the organizational structure help facilitate the overall strategy?
6. Is there a balance between standardization and flexibility?
7. Are additional coordinating or collateral structures required?
8. Does the organization have the financial resources to carry out the strategy?
9. Does the organization have the appropriate human resources, skills, policies, and procedures for the strategy?
10. Is the management talent appropriate?
11. Do the information systems help facilitate the strategy?
12. Are the facilities and equipment up to date and appropriate to carry out the overall strategy?

organizational structure, and strategic resources. It is important that these strategies work together with the service delivery strategies to effectively implement the organization's strategy.

As with the service delivery strategies, the results of the internal environmental analysis for each of the support activities in the value chain must be compared with the requirements of the strategies selected in the strategy formulation stage of the strategic management process. Results of that comparison indicate whether there needs to be a strategy that maintains the current status of the support activity or a strategy that changes the support area. Value adding support strategies typically maintain current strengths or build new ones, or correct weaknesses in the support activities. For each of the value adding support areas, actions for maintaining or changing the area are recommended as a way to initiate strategic thinking.

The organizational culture permeates the organization and is defined in terms of the shared assumptions, shared values, and accepted behavioral norms. Culture is learned. It is based on shared understandings and meanings within the organization. Culture is subjective in its interpretation but can be objectively observed through its heroes, stories, and ceremonies and rituals. It is important that culture be linked to the proposed strategy.

The organizational structure should help implement the strategy. The fundamental building blocks of organizational structure are functional, divisional, and matrix designs. Each structure has its advantages and disadvantages, and the decision concerning which structure is best to carry out the strategy is based on the need for standardization versus flexibility. Where a high degree of standardization is required, functional structures are desirable. Where a high level of flexibility is required because of diversity of product or markets, or where markets are rapidly changing, divisional or matrix structures may work best. Most organizations use a combination of designs supplemented with coordinating structures such as project teams and cross-functional task forces.

An organization's strategic resources are critical for most strategies – directional, adaptive, market entry, and competitive. Adequate resources allow for a number of strategic alternatives, whereas having few strategic resources inhibits strategy implementation. Strategic resources include financial, human, information, and technological resources. Organizations may finance strategy through equity, debt, fund raising or philanthropy, and efficiently managing existing capital. People are always key and different strategies require different human talents. Responsibility for recruiting and developing the right human resources for the strategy falls to leadership. Strategic information systems and decision support systems can create competitive advantage for organizations through improved customer service and more efficient and effective service delivery. The selection of the strategic technologies is a decision of the strategic leader and is central to strategy implementation. Strategic technologies include the type of facilities and the type and sophistication of equipment. The strategic technologies decisions set physical context and level of sophistication for service delivery and affect everything from the organization's image to patient satisfaction.

An example of value adding support strategies developed through a comparison of the results of an internal analysis and the requirements of the selected strategies for each are presented to extend strategic thinking. Chapter 10 demonstrates how individual organizational units must set objectives and develop action plans based on the value adding service delivery strategies and support strategies selected to achieve directional and adaptive strategies.

Key Terms and Concepts in Strategic Management

Behavioral Norms	Divisional Structure	Strategic Information System
Collateral Organization	Functional Structure	(SIS)
Combination Structure	Matrix Structure	Strategic Resources
Culture	Shared Assumptions	Value Adding Support
Decision Support System	Shared Values	Strategies
(DSS)	Strategic Technologies	

QUESTIONS FOR CLASS DISCUSSION

1. What part does internal environmental analysis play in the development of value adding support strategies? What part does strategy formulation play?
2. How do the value adding support strategies create the "context" for strategy implementation?
3. What is organizational culture? How does it implement strategy?
4. Why is culture change so difficult in health care organizations? What are some ways strategic managers could make culture change easier?
5. What are the basic building blocks of structure? What are the advantages and disadvantages of each?
6. In what circumstances might a high level of standardization be required? A high level of flexibility?

7. Which do you think changes first, strategy or structure? After formulating your answer and making your case, argue the opposite position.

8. What are the primary differences in the financial strategies needed for expansion, contraction, and maintenance of scope?

9. How may a growth strategy be financed? What are the advantages and disadvantages of each option?

10. Why is cash flow important in implementing strategy?

11. What are the primary differences in the human resources strategies needed for expansion, contraction, and maintenance of scope? Which type of adaptive strategy is most difficult to implement from a human resources perspective? Why?

12. What are the general categories of information systems? What are the attributes of each?

13. How can information systems be used to develop competitive advantage?

14. What changes are information systems bringing to health care?

15. Why is facilities management an increasing concern for strategic management?

16. How do facilities affect a health care organization's strategy?

17. How can the equipment–technology decision create competitive advantage?

18. How might future internal analyses be affected by the value adding support strategies?

NOTES

1. Nitin Nohria, William Joyce, and Bruce Roberson, "What Really Works," *Harvard Business Review* 81, no. 7 (2003), p. 47.

2. Ralph Stacey, "Strategy as Order Emerging from Chaos," *Long Range Planning* 26, no. 1 (1993), pp. 10–17. See also Harry C. Triandis, "The Many Dimensions of Culture," *Academy of Management Executive* 18, no. 1 (2004), pp. 88–93.

3. R. H. Kilmann, M. J. Saxton, and R. Serpa, "Issues in Understanding and Changing Culture," *California Management Review* 28, no. 2 (1986), pp. 87–94.

4. Robert W. Fleming, "Understanding the Mayo Culture," *Medical Group Management* (May–June 1989), pp. 46–49 and Charles S. Lauer, "Culture Matters," *Modern Healthcare* 34, no. 27 (July 5, 2004), pp. 27–29.

5. B. Z. Posner, J. M. Kouzes, and W. H. Schmidt, "Shared Values Make a Difference: An Empirical Test of Corporate Culture," *Human Resource Management* 24, no. 3 (1985), pp. 293–309.

6. J. E. Sheridan, "Organizational Culture and Employee Retention," *Academy of Management Journal* 35, no. 4 (December 1992), pp. 1036–1056.

7. D. R. Denison, "Bringing Corporate Culture to the Bottom Line," *Organizational Dynamics* 12, no. 12 (Autumn 1984), pp. 5–22.

8. John P. Kotter and James L. Heskett, *Corporate Culture and Performance* (New York: Free Press, 1992).

9. Ibid., p. 44.

10. Michael Beer and Russell A. Eisenstat, "How to Have an Honest Conversation About Your Business Strategy," *Harvard Business Review* 82, no. 2 (2004), p. 83.

11. James M. Higgins and Craig McAllister, "If You Want Strategic Change, Don't Forget to Change Your Culture," *Journal of Change Management* 4, no. 1 (2004), pp. 63–74.

12. Alfred C. Chandler, *Strategy and Structure* (Cambridge, MA: MIT Press, 1962).

13. Harold J. Leavitt, "Why Hierarchies Thrive," *Harvard Business Review* 81, no. 3 (2003), p. 98.

14. Ibid., p. 102.

15. John R. Griffith and Kenneth R. White, *The Well-Managed Healthcare Organization*, 5th edn (Chicago: Health Administration Press, 2002), p. 163 and M. C. Moldeveanu and Robert M. Bauer, "On the Relationship between Organizational Complexity and Organizational Structuration," *Organization Science* 15, no. 1 (2004), pp. 98–119.

16. Nohria, Joyce, and Roberson, "What Really Works," p. 49 and Bruce A. Waters and Shahid N. Bhuian, "Complexity Absorption and Performance: A Structural Analysis of Acute-Care Hospitals," *Journal of Management* 30, no. 1 (2004), pp. 97–122.

17. Stephen L. Walston and Richard J. Bogue, "The Effects of Reengineering: Fad or Competitive

Factor?" *Journal of Healthcare Management* 44, no. 6 (November–December 1999), pp. 456–474.

18. Judy Wade, "How to Make Reengineering Really Work," *Harvard Business Review* 71, no. 6 (November–December 1993), pp. 119–131.

19. Stephen Lee Walston, Lawton Robert Burns, and John R. Kimberly, "Does Reengineering Really Work? An Examination of the Context and Outcomes of Hospital Reengineering Initiatives," *Health Services Research* 34, no. 6 (February 2000), pp. 1363–1388.

20. Ibid.

21. J. H. Arnold, "Assessing Capital Risks: You Can't Be Too Conservative," *Harvard Business Review* 64, no. 5 (September–October 1986), pp. 113–121.

22. William O. Cleverley, "Assessing Present and Future Capital Expense Levels Under PPS," *Healthcare Financial Management* 40, no. 9 (September 1986), pp. 62–72.

23. Frank Cerne, "Street Wise," *Hospitals and Health Networks* 69, no. 6 (March 20, 1995), p. 42.

24. David Burda, "AHA Paints Gloomier Portrait of 1995's Hospital Performance," *Modern Healthcare* 26, no. 10 (May 20, 1996), p. 3.

25. Joseph F. Michlitsch, "High-performing, Loyal Employees: The Real Way to Implement Strategy," *Strategy & Leadership* 28, no. 6 (November–December 2000), pp. 28–33 and Barry A. Colbert, "The Complex Resource-Based View: Implications for Theory and Practice in Strategic Human Resource Management," *Academy of Management Review* 29, no. 3 (2004), pp. 341–358.

26. Bryan Dieter and Doug Gentile, "Improving Clinical Practices Can Boost the Bottom Line," *Healthcare Financial Management* 47, no. 9 (September 1993), pp. 38–40 and Lynda Gratton and Catherine Truss, "The Three-Dimensional People Strategy: Putting Human Resources Policies into Action," *Academy of Management Executive* 17, no. 3 (2003), pp. 74–86.

27. Charles J. Austin and Stuart B. Boxerman *Information Systems for Health Services Administration*, 6th edn (Chicago: Health Administration Press, 2003), p. 11.

28. Ibid.

29. Ibid.

30. Homer H. Schmitz, "Decision Support: A Strategic Weapon," in Marion J. Ball, Judith V. Douglas, Robert I. O'Desky, and James W. Albright (eds) *Health Information Management Systems* (New York: Springer-Verlag, 1991), p. 47.

31. Holly J. Wong, "The Diffusion of Decision Support Systems in Healthcare: Are We There Yet?" *Journal of Healthcare Management* 45, no. 4 (July–August 2000), pp. 240–249.

32. Ibid.

33. Office of Technology Assessment, *Bringing Health Care Online: The Role of Information Technologies* (Washington, DC: US Government Printing Office, 1995).

34. Austin and Boxerman, *Information Systems*, p. 6.

35. John P. Glaser and Leslie Hsu, *The Strategic Application of Information Technology in Healthcare Organizations: A Guide to Implementing Integrated Systems* (New York: McGraw-Hill, 1999), p. 8.

36. Michael Porter and V. Millar, "How Information Gives You a Competitive Advantage," *Harvard Business Review* 63, no. 4 (July–August 1985), pp. 149–160.

37. Charles J. Austin, Keith D. Hornberger, and James E. Shmerling, "Managing Information Resources: A Study of Ten Healthcare Organizations," *Journal of Healthcare Management* 45, no. 4 (July–August 2000), pp. 229–238.

38. Ibid.

39. David D. Moriarty, "Strategic Information Systems Planning for Health Service Providers," *Health Care Management Review* 17, no. 1 (Winter 1992), p. 85.

40. Glaser and Hsu, *The Strategic Application*, p. 40.

41. Janet R. Carpman and Myron A. Grant, *Design That Cares: Planning Health Facilities for Patients and Visitors*, 2nd edn (Chicago: American Hospital Publishing, 1993).

42. Ibid., p. 19.

43. David A. Berkowitz and Melanie M. Swan, "Technology Decision Making," *Health Progress* 74, no. 1 (January–February 1993), pp. 42–47.

44. Leonard H. Friedman and James B. Goes, "The Timing of Medical Technology Acquisition: Strategic Decision Making in Turbulent Environments," *Journal of Healthcare Management* 45, no. 5 (September–October 2000), pp. 317–330.

ADDITIONAL READINGS Berg, Marc, *Health Information Management* (New York: Routledge Publishing, 2004). An introduction to the challenges of health information management. Particular attention is given to the nature of information demands in the twenty-first century health care organization. The book illustrates how many technological decisions influence the day-to-day practice of clinicians and eventually impact patients.

Carr, Nicholas G., *Does It Matter? Information Technology and the Corrosion of Competitive Advantage* (Boston, MA: Harvard Business School Press, 2004). Has information technology become so pervasive that it no longer provides any opportunity for competitive advantage? The author suggests that organizations might save money and reduce risks by allowing competitors to take the lead in new technologies. This strategy, of course, creates risks of its own.

Orna, Elizabeth, *Information Strategy in Practice* (Burlington, VT: Ashgate Publishing, 2004). An extensive analysis of the theory and practice of information policy and strategy formation. Examples are provided of information strategy in practice. Advice is provided concerning the development of information strategies. The book is written in an informal style and is easy reading on a topic that is often complicated and abstract.

Prahalad, C. K. and Venkat Ramaswamy, *The Future of Competition* (Boston, MA: Harvard Business School Publishing, 2004). Why are companies unable to satisfy customer needs and sustain growth and profitability in an environment of seemingly unlimited business opportunities? One reason is that customers have evolved from passive recipients to active co-creators in the value creation process. To effectively compete in this new marketplace, organizations must fundamentally alter their value creation infrastructures. Information and operations have to become transparent and accessible to all collaborators and interactions with customers must be transformed from transactions to dialogues.

Roberts, John, *The Modern Firm: Organizational Design for Performance and Growth* (New York: Oxford University Press, 2004). This book develops a number of approaches for analyzing organizational design features, competitive strategies, and environmental forces. Historical as well as contemporary examples are used to develop and illustrate concepts. Roberts provides interesting insights into changes taking place in modern organizations.

Torbert, William R., *Action Inquiry: The Secret of Timely and Transforming Leadership* (Williston, VT: BK Publishers, 2004). Organizations and managers are so occupied with the frantic pace of day-to-day operations that they rarely take time to learn from experience. Action inquiry is a process that helps managers go beyond the daily hassle and demonstrate transforming power and timely action. Action inquiry allows managers to correct mistakes before they have negative consequences and create a climate for ongoing individual and organizational learning.

10 *CHAPTER*

Communicating the Strategy and Developing Action Plans

"There is nothing so useless as doing efficiently that which should not be done at all."

Peter F. Drucker

Introductory Incident

Partners HealthCare System – Action Planning for Service Lines

As costs rise and competition increases, health care organizations are forced to look for new ways to increase market share. Some have chosen to approach this problem by deliberately developing and positioning the services they offer through service line planning. That is, the development of a business plan (action plan) for a specific service, such as cardiac care, orthopedics, and so on within the broader portfolio of services offered by the organization. Generally, service lines that are thought to have the most strategic value for health care organizations include cardiology, cancer, neurosciences, orthopedics, pediatrics, and women's services. Defining the service line using a patient-flow/ consumer-driven perspective is recommended over a physician specialty-driven perspective.

Service line planning is an important tool for understanding the competitive nature of an organization's service lines. When service lines are carefully and strategically selected, the organization has a better rationale for resource allocation decisions. To be successful, the planning process must make it clear who is responsible for managing and implementing service line strategies and how accountability will be established and enforced.

Partners HealthCare System, an integrated delivery system in eastern Massachusetts, includes Massachusetts General Hospital, Brigham and Women's

Hospital, Dana-Farber Partners Cancer Care, McLean Hospital, and four community hospitals. Partners Community HealthCare Network comprises more than 7,900 primary care and specialty physicians. The total operating revenue of Partners is more than $3.4 billion and the system employs 33,000 people.

In preparation for its budget cycle, the financial leadership of Partners analyzed the value of four of its specialty areas (cardiac services, orthopedic services, cancer services, and psychiatry/mental health) relative to the overall organization. On the basis of this analysis, the System Integration Committee, a group of Partners' senior administrative and medical leadership charged with developing programs that promoted system integration, adopted a goal to establish business plans for two system-wide services that would focus on growing top line revenue through competitive market share growth and system-wide collaboration. New market share was expected when service line planning:

- focused on growth within an overall system-wide business plan,
- leveraged system-wide strengths,
- reduced the potential for internal competition through collaboration,
- built on clinical expertise to improve quality throughout the system,
- identified areas where operating efficiencies could be improved, and
- improved financial performance.

The cardiology program was selected to be the first to tackle the planning initiative. Cardiology began by delineating the service line – 19 cardiac diagnosis related groups (DRGs) – and organizing them into three clinical areas – cardiac surgery, interventional cardiology, and clinical cardiology. The planning group, including cardiac physician leaders from each of the Partners hospitals, evaluated the competitive environment and identified several areas of vulnerability. Primary research was conducted among referring physicians and customers. Finally, the regulatory environment was assessed.

The information developed was used to construct and select several scenarios for growth. The physician planning team recommended three actions: (1) physician network development, (2) branding, and (3) communication. Because the Massachusetts legislature enabled more community hospitals to offer cardiac services as the planning

committee was working, the team emphasized the necessity of developing and maintaining a loyal physician network and identified actions to support and expand the network.

Marketing research suggested that Massachusetts General Hospital and Brigham and Women's Hospital were recognized and trusted brand names among customers and physicians. A series of actions was designed to leverage these brand names outside the downtown Boston area. Finally, innovation, invention, and new technologies were identified as the attributes that differentiated the cardiac programs at Massachusetts General Hospital and Brigham and Women's Hospital. An ongoing communication program was developed to inform customers and physicians about these advantages.

A number of important lessons have been learned by Partners in the development of a business plan for a service line:

1. Physicians must have an opportunity to work together as a group before meaningful progress can be made.
2. Service line planning can serve as a catalyst for enhanced clinical and operational integration.
3. Because the initiative was led by a senior administrator from Massachusetts General Hospital and a senior physician from Brigham and Women's and supported by a director of business development (a new position created for the service line), organizational acceptance of the planning team's analyses, assumptions, and recommendations was easier to gain.
4. Financial considerations should be included during plan development, with leadership from the finance area engaged during the planning process.
5. The funding mechanism for the plan must be identified before recommendations are presented.
6. In large complex organizations with multiple stakeholders, communication is critical.
7. When moving from planning to implementation, service line leadership needs to balance communication and collaboration with action.

Source: Elizabeth Greenspan, Susanna E. Krentz, and Molly K. O'Neill, "Strategic Service Line Planning Builds Competitive Advantage: Senior Financial Executives Play a Critical Role in Developing an Organization's Service Line Plans," *Healthcare Financial Management* 57, no. 13 (2003), pp. 72–78.

Learning Objectives

After completing this chapter the student should be able to:

1. Describe the interrelationship among situation analysis, strategy formulation, value adding service delivery and support strategies, and action plans.

2. Understand the manner in which strategies are translated into action plans.

3. List the components of an action plan and explain the function of each component.

4. Cite some reasons that cause strategies to be difficult to implement in health care organizations.

5. Suggest some effective ways to overcome barriers to the implementation of strategies.

6. Understand the need for contingency planning and know when contingency plans should be undertaken.

7. Relate the map and the compass metaphor to strategic thinking, strategic planning, and managing the strategic momentum.

Implementation Through Action Plans

The situational analysis discussed in Chapters 2 through 5 culminates with a series of strategic goals that, along with the mission, vision, and values, are directional strategies that provide focus for the organization. Adaptive, market entry, and competitive strategies are designed to accomplish the strategic goals and move the organization in the desired direction. Value adding service delivery and support strategies further shape the strategy and provide guidance and direction to managers who are responsible for implementing action plans.

The desired direction and organizational momentum have been discussed and consensus reached during the strategic planning process, yet no movement has taken place. For real movement to take place, action plans will have to be developed throughout the organization. As Peter Drucker stated, "[strategic] insights are 'bled off' and converted into tasks and work assignments."[1]

Implementation strategies have been referred to by various terms. Some organizations refer to implementation strategies as "tactical plans," while others may use "business plans," and still others, many in health care, have adopted the term "action plans." Action plans is the most descriptive term as it connotes the actions required to carry out strategies and meet objectives. The term action plans may also be applied to the several different levels within organizations that must develop implementation strategies and thus lessens confusion.

The Level and Orientation of the Strategy

This chapter concerns communicating the overall strategy to those who must develop specific action plans to accomplish the strategy and providing them with a consistent format for implementation. However, it is important to note that strategy may be carried out at several different levels. A large integrated health care system may develop strategy at a number of levels – a corporate level, divisional level, organizational level, and a functional level. If the strategy has been developed at the corporate level, action plans will be for entire divisions. If the strategy has been developed at the divisional level, action plans will be for individual institutions or organizations comprising the division, such as a hospital (within the hospital division) or a long-term care facility (within the long-term care division). If strategy has been developed for an individual organization, such as a hospital, the action plans will be developed by functional units within the hospital (such as surgery or pharmacy). Thus, strategies may be developed for large, complex organizations or small, well-focused units; therefore, action plans to implement the strategies will be developed at different levels as well. Trinity Health, introduced in Chapter 1 and illustrated in Exhibit 1–7, portrays the organizational levels and the different orientations.

An effective *action plan*, regardless of level, consists of objectives that specify how the unit (division, hospital, pharmacy) is going to contribute to the strategy, what actions will be required to achieve the objectives and within what time period, who is responsible for the actions, the resources required to achieve the objectives, and how results will be measured. These elements are required whether the action plan is for entire divisions as part of a complex corporate-level strategic plan or for functional units contributing to the strategic plan of a small organization. Identifying objectives, determining who is responsible to accomplish them, the resources required, and how results will be measured is an approach that keeps the strategic plan straightforward and comprehensible. A simple understandable plan is always preferable to a complex incomprehensible plan (see Perspective 10–1).

Action Plan Development Responsibilities

Not everyone can realistically be involved in the strategic planning process. Rather, it involves a number of key participants working together to develop a strategy. A few key players – senior staff, top management, or a leadership team – are needed to provide balanced and informed points of view. Therefore, the development of the initial plan is usually the product of a relatively small number of strategic thinkers. Margaret Meade challenged us to "never doubt that a small group of thoughtful, committed people can change the world; indeed, it's the only thing that ever has!"[2] A small group of thoughtful, committed people can reshape even the most rigid organization. Even so, as pointed out in Perspective 10–2, engaging in strategic change may foment resistance from some within the organization.

Perspective 10–1

Manage Simply

Einstein is credited with the statement "Everything should be made as simple as it possibly can and no simpler." Managers and those seeking to become managers should keep Einstein's idea in mind. Think of it as a manager's vision – seek simplicity, if one confronts complexity; work to simplify; lead to simplify; organize to simplify. Keep simplicity a primary focus of management style. What follows are a few ideas to assist in developing "manage simply" techniques.

- Less management is better than more management. Managing is controlling, but controlling may not be managing. When overdone, control is the dark side of management. It is the nature of management to focus and control behavior, but a light touch is needed rather than a firm grip.
- Create teams and promote teamwork by teaching the team how to manage itself. Minimize rules, policies, and procedures. Resist the temptation to fix everything with a new rule or policy; to the contrary, eliminate as many restrictions on innovation as possible.
- Broad strokes are better than narrow strokes. Vision and future orientation are essential. Constantly keep "what's ahead" in front of the team by communicating a vision in terms that they understand. Avoid micromanagement. Know which details are important, but leave the attention to these details to the authority of another responsible person.
- Processes are not ends in themselves but are viewed that way over time. Goals and objectives are the ends, focus on the ends. Reward innovation and change. Never permit "It's always been done this way" to remain an acceptable process.
- Managers will never get it quite right. Objectives, needs, influences, solutions, and systems constantly evolve. Interpret striving for perfection as continuous improvement. Never make perfection a prerequisite for progress.
- One size does not fit all. Although some order is necessary, blind application of one solution or pattern leads to a dysfunctional workforce. When choosing between centralization and decentralization, customize the solution to fit the circumstances. When in doubt about what to do, decentralize. Be aware that there are many problems with common systems such as personnel evaluations, salary ranges, and so on. To identify which common systems are problems, simply ask around; they will be widely known.
- All solutions are temporary. Remember that "necessity is the mother of invention" and because needs change, the requirement for innovation is constant. Thus, no solution will last very long. Don't work so hard for closure to a problem; be open to and encourage change and innovation.
- Do what is best for each individual and the organization will prosper. Usually what is best for the organization is the sum of what is best for the individuals in the organization. Pay employees as much as possible. Encourage and allow people to do what is best for themselves and this will make the work and the organization hard to leave; in other words, create the greener pasture. Encourage learning and fun.
- Practice "one-level" management. Although someone must be the boss, don't make the organizational hierarchy seem important. Everyone in the organization should be treated as a peer – this is equality. Peers can and will share ideas, opinions, and solutions. The team deserves respect. Simple courtesies are important – be polite, acknowledge their presence, say "hello," and know everyone's name. Casual is better than formal because casual is easier for everyone to achieve and does not have as many rules.
- Make the manager's job harder and others easier. Identify and satisfy internal customers. Remember that subordinates are customers, too. Constantly seek to identify barriers. View the job as that of removing barriers, whatever they may be.

Source: Andrew C. Rucks and Peter M. Ginter, School of Public Health, University of Alabama at Birmingham.

Perspective 10–2

Stages of Resistance to Change

Often people do not like change, and their first reaction may be to resist any changes management may wish to make. When instituting changes in an organization, whether it is initiating the strategic planning process, changing the strategy, or attempting to change the culture, managers find people in various stages of resistance. It is often necessary to "pull" people through these stages if the change is to be successful.

Stage One: Resistance

Often the first reaction to something new is to resist the change. Because organizations have frequent changes and in many instances management has tried several techniques before, employees may see a new program or management effort as another fad that will soon go away (as have the others). Therefore they openly resist (or even sabotage) the proposed change. In this stage managers often hear such comments as, "Here we go again, new manager, new program, new technique" or "This will never work" and "We tried this ten years ago."

Stage Two: Passiveness

In stage two, employees are not resistant; they simply do not want to get involved. These people do not like change and believe that if they bury their heads in the sand (go about their usual work), the change will just go away. In many cases these people do not understand the vision for the future, or they have never been told about it or how they fit in it. In this stage, managers often hear such comments as, "This is just a job" or "I put in my eight hours" or "I'll be here when they're gone."

Stage Three: Convince Me

Some people in organizations are ready to change and will work hard if they believe it will really improve the organization. However, they have been "let down" by the organization before. Perhaps programs were started or promises were made but management neither completed the programs nor fulfilled the promises. These people will give it their best if management can show them that the result will be worth their effort. In this stage, managers often hear such comments as, "Show me that we can improve the way we work and I'll be your biggest supporter" or "Give me some indication that this can be an interesting and challenging place to work, and I'll give it a shot."

Stage Four: Hope

Many people, especially when they start their careers, want to be a part of something important – to make a difference. They have hope that they can make the organization better and be a part of something significant. These people are usually willing to try anything and want to be a part of meaningful change. However, the managers should follow through because if previously proposed changes have not occurred, these people will be difficult to convince the next time management wants to change something. In this stage, managers often hear such comments as, "I don't know if we can succeed but look at the possibilities if we do" or "Wouldn't it be great if we actually pulled it off?"

Stage Five: Involvement

In this stage, people typically understand that the organization must change and continually renew itself if it is to succeed. They are willing to get involved and be a part of any change that will keep the organization viable. They understand that some new things do not work very well and therefore other change agents must be tried. In this stage, managers often hear such comments as, "I don't know if this will work, but we have to try something" or "The world is changing and we have to change with it."

Stage Six: Advocacy

People in this stage believe not only that change is important in a changing world but that this program can really make an important difference. They are ready for a long-term commitment to the program or process and will lead and be responsible for its implementation and progress. These people will convince others to be a part of the change and will keep the process on track. In this stage, managers often hear such comments as, "This is our chance for real long-term success" or "I'm a believer; this can work if we stay committed over the long term."

Because of its involvement in developing strategy, the strategic planning team determines the "broad strokes" of strategy. The team should shape the organization through: a review or revision of the organization's mission, vision, values, and goals; development of strategy through service delivery and support strategies; and providing guidance for what needs to be accomplished. However, action plans should be left to the organizational units. Senior managers shape strategic direction less by deciding the specific strategic content than by framing the context – creating "a sense of purpose that not only provides an integrating framework for bottom-up strategic initiatives but also injects meaning into individual effort."[3] Others in the organization should use their ingenuity to develop action plans and carry out the strategy. As George Patton once said, "Never tell people how to do things. Tell them what to do and they will surprise you with their ingenuity."

Communicating Strategy to Initiate Action Planning

Because everyone cannot be directly involved, many employees within the organization do not know the underlying issues and assumptions that were used to develop the strategy; nor do they know the goals for which they will develop objectives. Therefore, successive layers of management must communicate the overall strategy and provide "maintain or change" *guidance* for the various units that will need to be engaged if the strategy is to be achieved. For example, if management has determined that an expansion strategy is required, guidance is needed as to which parts of the organization have been identified for the expansion. Managers in the identified part or parts then determine the objectives to accomplish the expansion in that area. When different units have overlapping or integrated activities, multiple groups have to coordinate planning. Communication from the top down and the bottom up – as well as across – is required to engage everyone to do his or her part.

Specific milestones in the strategic planning process should include updates for all employees, telling them that the process is ongoing and explaining expected timelines for the strategy to be handed over to those who will be responsible for carrying it out. In addition, successes can be shared and celebrated, and challenges can be identified and monitored. For example, Sharp Healthcare holds quarterly "All Staff Assemblies" to provide open communications with all employees and maintain their engagement in carrying out the organization's strategy. Other organizations have team meetings. It is typically challenging in health care to have a meeting of all employees because a certain number of them always have to be taking care of patients. However, it is also challenging to implement strategy if the employees are not engaged. If top management determines that it is impossible to hold a meeting for all employees, the question should be asked: "Why isn't it possible?" Then, much thought should be given to the question of how management expects to accomplish any strategy if the first decision is "We can't do that."

Developing Action Plans

Although implementation strategies may be carried out at various organizational levels, implementation plans should have common characteristics. These plans concern translating directional, adaptive, market entry, and competitive strategies into tasks and work assignments (specific actions that accomplish the mission, vision, values, goals, strategies, and value adding service delivery and support strategies). In addition, these actions must be the responsibility of individuals within the organization and made an integral part of their job. As pointed out in Perspective 10–3, each job should be structured to show how it contributes to the strategic plan. In general, action plans address the following questions:

- What objectives should units establish?
- What actions are required to accomplish unit objectives? In what sequence should the actions be accomplished?

Perspective 10–3

Performance Appraisal and Compensation

People in organizations do what they get rewarded for doing and ignore most other organizational dictates. As Steve Kerr stated in a classic management article, often management expects "A," but rewards "B," and then cannot understand why "A" never occurs. If strategic management is to become a philosophy or way of managing an organization, people must see a connection between what they do and strategic management. Therefore, unless strategic management is translated into individual efforts and acknowledged through the performance appraisal and reward systems, it is unlikely that everyone will work for the strategic plan. Just as organizational divisions and units must be linked to the strategic plan, so should the work of the individuals involved.

After initiating a strategic planning effort, it is necessary to rewrite job descriptions and performance appraisal standards. Every position, from secretary to CEO, should be linked back to the strategic plan. An effective way to accomplish this linkage is to create duties within the job description related specifically to strategic management processes. Thus, each job description should have sections entitled "Contribution to Vision," "Contribution to Mission," "Contribution to Values," "Contribution to Strategic Goals," "Contribution to Strategy," and "Contribution to Strategy Implementation." Each job should be structured to show explicitly how it contributes to one or more of these processes. There is no justification for any activity that does not specifically contribute to the organization's strategy.

An effective way to redesign job descriptions is to ask three strategic questions for each position:

1. To make the maximum contribution, what is this person not doing now that he or she should be doing?
2. To make the maximum contribution, what is this person doing now that he or she should not be doing?
3. To make the maximum contribution, what is this person doing now that he or she should continue to do but in a different way?

Similarly, performance appraisal forms should be structured around the strategic management processes. Then compensation may be tied directly to the employee's contribution to the strategy.

- Who will be responsible for accomplishing each action by the designated time?
- What organizational resources will be required to accomplish each action in a timely manner?
- How will results be measured?

The answers to these questions form the basis for action plans. Action plans initiate the strategy – start the work – and serve as a blueprint for managing the strategy. As indicated in previous chapters, managers must be ready to think strategically and learn as they carry out their implementation plans. Learning by doing may modify the implementation, the strategy itself, or assumptions underlying the strategy.

Action Planning

As Peter Drucker indicated, "The statement, 'This is what we are here for,' must eventually become the statement, 'This is how we do it. This is the time span in which we do it. This is who is accountable. This is, in other words, the work for which we are responsible.' "[4] A critically important responsibility of the health care organization's leadership is to carefully articulate its strategy to the unit managers. Unit managers should be provided guidance or strategy statements regarding their responsibility to change or maintain the scope of their respective areas. These managers, in turn, are obligated to continue the communication by articulating the manner in which each unit is expected to contribute to service delivery or support services as well as adaptive, market entry, and competitive strategies. Unit manager action plans in aggregate represent the implementation plan for the organization.

Action Planning Example – Community Hospital Pharmacy

The middle section of the strategic management model (see Exhibit 1–3) provides a step-by-step strategic thinking map to illustrate that strategic planning links situational analysis through strategy formulation and planning the implementation. Action plans provide unit managers with a more detailed blueprint that links unit planning activities to the strategy.

To illustrate, consider the implementation responsibility of the head of pharmacy in a community hospital. Strategic leaders determined through a comprehensive strategic thinking effort that the hospital should become more of a health resource to the community at large – enhancement strategy. Leaders provided value chain guidance statements regarding the hospital's commitment to become more community focused to all managers of service delivery and support activities. These managers, in turn, discussed the community focus with the members of the functional units under their respective area or areas of responsibility. The head of clinical operations, for example, held discussions with pharmacy, laboratories, and other ancillary service areas and challenged them to develop plans for expanding the role of the hospital as a community health resource.

The pharmacy might propose that one way the hospital could increase its positive impact on the community would be in the area of outpatient pharmacy services. Community access to health services could be enhanced and hospital revenues could be increased if outpatient pharmacy operations were expanded – the value adding service delivery strategy of point-of-service clinical operations needed to change (expand its services) to better serve the community.

Setting Objectives

The first task of the pharmacy unit is to establish objectives that would accomplish the enhancement strategy. More specific than strategic goals, unit *objectives* should possess the following characteristics.

- Objectives should reinforce organizational strategic goals. Strategic goals relate to mission-critical activities. Reinforcing objectives ensures that the various units contribute to the accomplishment of the organization's mission.
- Objectives should be measurable. The objectives of the individual units are tools for the determination of unit effectiveness, and ultimately resource allocation, so the ability to measure and evaluate unit performance is essential.
- Objectives should identify the time frame for accomplishment.
- Objectives should be challenging but attainable. Objectives that are easy to accomplish do not require stretch. Objectives that are impossible to attain are not motivational.
- Objectives should be easy to understand. Individual group members must accomplish the tasks that result in objective attainment. People work harder to achieve objectives they understand and believe are important.
- Objectives should be formulated with the assistance of the individuals who will be responsible for accomplishing the work. Just as strategic leaders should allow managers discretion in determining how strategies will be achieved, unit managers should allow employee input into the development of unit objectives.

In the action planning process, the head of pharmacy scheduled a meeting of pharmacy employees and encouraged them to suggest ways the pharmacy could aid the hospital in becoming a more valuable community health resource. Although several objectives were actually developed by the pharmacy group, only one objective and its associated action plans are illustrated here. A pharmacy objective that fulfills the criteria for a good objective and contributes to the organization's goal is:

Pharmacy Objective – Revenue Increase. To increase the number of patients served such that the volume of outpatient pharmacy revenues increases by 25 percent by the end of the first year of expanded outpatient operations.

A 25 percent increase in revenue from outpatients in the first year was attainable. This increase in service would contribute significantly to the value adding point-of-service strategy of clinical operations. In addition, accomplishing the objective would be a challenge for the pharmacy. The objective's outcome is measurable and easy to understand by those who will be responsible for making things happen in the unit.

Action Plans and Budget Requests

When unit objectives have been formulated and agreed on, the next step is to identify the actions or activities necessary to accomplish each objective. The expected revenues as well as costs and other resources associated with achieving each activity must be determined to estimate any additional resources needed so they can be incorporated into the unit's budget request.[5] In addition, a timeline should be established for achieving each action to ensure activities remain on schedule. Finally, a specific individual or group of individuals should be assigned the responsibility for ensuring each activity is accomplished.

Beginning and ending dates should be established for each action. This process forces participants to first think sequentially regarding the ordering of actions or activities and, secondly, forces a commitment for completion of the individual activities as well as the overall goal. Thinking sequentially about the required activities essentially develops a process for achieving the goal, as often some activities must be completed before others can begin. Process is defined as, "... a collection of activities that takes one or more kinds of inputs and creates an output that is of value...."[6] Therefore, it is often useful to ask participants to develop a flow chart or to diagram the required activities. A process orientation helps participants sequence activities and establish timing. In addition, through this process, reasonable timelines can be established. Further, setting beginning and completion dates provides personal, unit, and organizational commitment.

In the pharmacy example, an action plan for accomplishing the increase in outpatient pharmacy revenue is presented in Exhibit 10–1. Note that the plan begins with an estimate of the revenue that will be generated from the increase in outpatient pharmacy services. Then, the activities required to accomplish the objective are listed along with the timelines and responsibility assignments. The cost associated with accomplishing each activity is identified. A final column is provided for comments, should clarification be needed regarding an activity, timeline, or responsibility assignment.

This action plan projects a net operating loss of over $43,650 for the outpatient pharmacy during the first year. However, after the first year, additional staff will have been hired and no further hiring is planned, the facilities already will be remodeled, and the introductory promotion expenditures will be reduced significantly to a maintenance level. Therefore, in year two, revenues are expected to exceed costs. The positive impact on the community, however, will begin immediately as access to pharmacy services is expanded. Moreover, as the community discovers that the hospital is providing greater pharmacy service, revenues

Exhibit 10–1: Example of Pharmacy Action Plan

Value Adding Strategy – Clinical Services. Change. Increase role of hospital as community health resource.
Pharmacy Objective – Revenue Increase. To increase the volume of outpatient pharmacy revenues by 25 percent by the end of the first year of expanded outpatient operations.

Activity	Jul	Aug	Sep	Oct	Nov	Dec	Jan	Feb	Mar	Apr	May	Jun	Revenues	Costs	Responsible Person/Group	Comments
New Revenues													$114,750			
Costs																
1. Remodel storage space for waiting area		▮												$12,750	Hospital Facilities Management	Waiting area is the only additional space needed in first year of expanded operations
2. Expand curbside parking near hospital entrance			▮											$4,500	Hospital Grounds and Landscaping	Additional parking spaces will be necessary for customer drop-off and pick-up
3. Add additional telephone line and expand hospital website		▮												$3,150	Telecommunication Services	Additional telephone line required for anticipated increase in volume. Website needed for outpatient pharmacy
4. Contract with marketing firm to promote outpatient pharmacy initiative												▮		$36,000	Head of Pharmacy	Assistance of marketing firm needed to inform physicians and potential customers of new outpatient initiative
5. Recruit and hire up to two additional FTE pharmacy technicians		▮ 1st										▮ 2nd		$49,500	Hospital Human Resources	Increase in volume initially handled by technician. Second may be needed in June depending on volume
6. Recruit and hire one additional 0.5 FTE pharmacist					▮									$52,500	Head of Pharmacy	Anticipated volume will require new pharmacist by end of December
Total Revenue/Cost													$114,750	$153,400		
Net Revenue/Cost														($43,650)		

are expected to increase significantly. This action plan provides the head of pharmacy with the information necessary to develop the budget request and communicate to the manager of clinical services how the pharmacy intends to use the extra resources needed to launch the outpatient pharmacy.

Focusing on Strategy Through Strategy Implementation – Another Approach

The action plan is one of several widely used approaches to assist in the implementation of strategies. Another tool for focusing on implementation as strategy is the *Balanced Scorecard* developed by Robert S. Kaplan of the Harvard Business School and David P. Norton, president of Balanced Scorecard Collaborative, Inc. (see Perspective 10–4). As suggested in the Perspective and illustrated in Exhibit 10–2, the Balanced Scorecard is compatible with, and complementary to, the value chain approach discussed in this text.

The primary value of the Balanced Scorecard approach is to focus the health care organization on those aspects of its operations that most directly impact the accomplishment of its strategies. By identifying those factors that most directly influence successful outcomes and concentrating on accomplishing and improving them, the human and nonhuman resources of the organization can be used most effectively and efficiently.

The Mayo Clinic used a modified version of the Balanced Scorecard to strategically think about implementation. The leadership of outpatient operations at the Mayo Clinic in Rochester, Minnesota, recognized that the competitive environment was changing. Even for the Mayo Clinic it was important to operate in an economically efficient manner while maintaining world-class medical services. Leadership believed that those things that are measured are the things that are managed. Therefore, an effort was made to discover an appropriate measurement system that would contribute to strategy implementation.

Since various perspectives were important, the Balanced Scorecard immediately came to the mind of leaders. This system along with others was analyzed, modified, and ultimately a customized system was developed that was considered to be consistent with Mayo Clinic's mission, vision, and core values. The leadership of outpatient operations believed that to be competitive several competencies were essential. These were (1) clinical quality to maintain and enhance market share; (2) organizational agility in creating and responding to market forces; (3) organizational focus on critical performance metrics; and (4) timely, accurate management information to improve and predict performance.

In the process of customizing the system, managers at the Mayo Clinic learned that performance measurement takes time and continuous commitment; new measurements require new information systems; multiple audiences must understand the performance measures; and performance measurement is an evolving process. In addition, it was noted that strategy implementation cannot be separated altogether from strategy control. People manage what is measured. The

Perspective 10–4	Robert S. Kaplan of the Harvard Business School and David P. Norton, pres-
The Balanced Scorecard	ident of Balanced Scorecard Collaborative, Inc. observed that the traditional

Perspective 10–4

The Balanced Scorecard

Robert S. Kaplan of the Harvard Business School and David P. Norton, president of Balanced Scorecard Collaborative, Inc. observed that the traditional view of corporate performance was developed by, and for, industrial-age companies – a view that is no longer appropriate in an age of information and service. Manufacturers create value by managing tangible assets whereas modern knowledge-based organizations create value by deploying intangible assets such as customer relations, innovative services, high-quality and responsive operations, information technology, databases, and employee competencies. Originally the Balanced Scorecard was about measurement and control. Kaplan and Norton now believe it is a tool for implementing strategy – for dealing with the numerous cases where strategies fail because they are not implemented.

The Balanced Scorecard approach links the organization's strategy to short-term actions. As the concept evolved, four processes were identified for transforming the Balanced Scorecard into a strategic management implementation system: the financial perspective, the customer perspective, the internal perspective, and the learning/growth perspective.

First, if the Balanced Scorecard is to be an effective strategic management system it should be useful in translating the vision into an integrated set of objectives that, when accomplished, contribute to long-term success. Second, successful implementation relies on effective communication with, and linking to, the units that comprise the larger organization. Third, action plans allow the integration of strategic and financial plans. And finally, feedback and learning are developed and nurtured such that consistent decisions are made throughout the organization and resources are allocated in a logical and comprehensible manner.

For example, consider Taiwan, where there has been increased competition in health care markets and the National Health Insurance plan initiated cost controls. Hospitals are experiencing difficulty maintaining their operations and struggling to find ways to achieve their mission and improve financial accountability. Emergency departments are a special problem because the operational processes are very complex and the patients are often critical. Between 40 and 70 percent of the hospitalized cases in Taiwan are admitted from the emergency department, making it the primary revenue generator. Unfortunately, long waiting times to see the physician, time required to obtain necessary laboratory tests, and ever-increasing crowded conditions cause emergency departments to receive more complaints than any other hospital unit.

In a 600-bed church affiliated, not-for-profit hospital located in the Chia Yi City area, the quality improvement team decided to implement a Balanced Scorecard approach in the emergency department on a pilot basis. Four additional hospitals were within a 30-minute drive and competition was intense. The Scorecard used two indicators for three of the four Scorecard areas (only one financial indicator was used). Learning/growth focused on hours of continuing education attended by the staff and staff satisfaction; the internal business process indicators included rate of incomplete laboratory tests within 30 minutes and the average monthly inappropriate return rates; the financial indicator focused on profit (actually measured by percentage increase in revenue); and customer measures included patient satisfaction and the rate of complaints.

Before implementing the Balanced Scorecard, continuing education for all emergency department staff was 4.3 hours per month. After a three-month test period using the Balanced Scorecard, the monthly average increased to 9.7 hours. The mean score for staff satisfaction on a 4.0 scale had been 2.83; however, after implementation of the Balanced Scorecard the satisfaction score increased to 3.29. Relative to the internal business processes perspective, the rate of incomplete tests within 30 minutes reduced from 12.8 percent to 8.3 percent and the average monthly inappropriate return rate decreased from 3.5 percent to 2.1 percent. From the financial perspective, revenues in the emergency room increased from 1.44 percent to 3.27 percent.

The patient satisfaction mean score before implementing the Balanced Scorecard was 3.05 on a 4.0 scale and in three months this average had increased to 3.47. Finally, the rate of patient complaints decreased from 0.28 percent before implementation to 0.1 percent after implementation. Managers concluded that using the Balanced Scorecard approach improved the performance of the hospital both in financial and nonfinancial areas. The results were expected to assist hospital administrators in planning for the future.

Source: Robert S. Kaplan and David P. Norton, "The Balanced Scorecard – Measures that Drive Performance," *Harvard Business Review* 72, no. 1 (1993), pp. 71–79 and Shu-Hsin Huang, Ping-Ling Chen, Ming-Chin Yang, Wen-Yin Chang, and Haw-Jenn Lee, "Using a Balanced Scorecard to Improve the Performance of an Emergency Department," *Nursing Economics* 22, no. 3 (2004), pp. 140–147.

Exhibit 10-2: Health Care Provider Balanced Scorecard Strategy Map

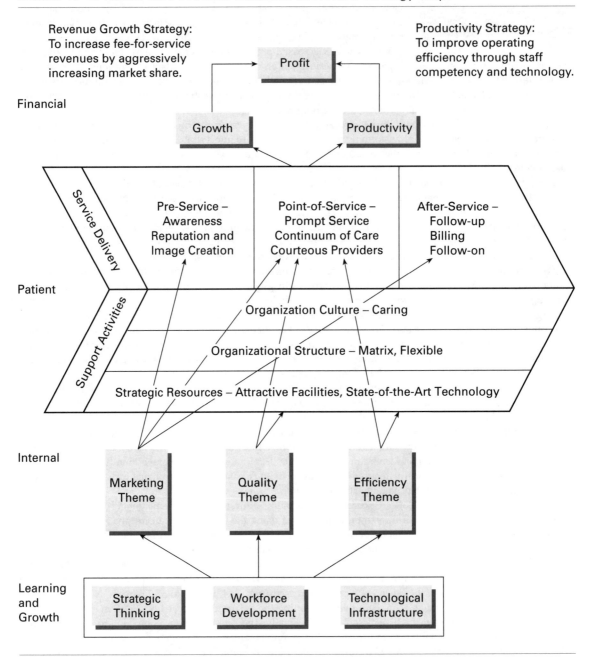

Source: Adapted from Robert S. Kaplan and David P. Norton, "Having Trouble with Your Strategy? Then Map It," *Harvard Business Review* 78, no. 5 (2000), pp. 168–169.

leadership of the Mayo Clinic focused on the Balanced Scorecard, as its developers did early in its evolution, as a performance measurement tool. However, its value as a linkage between strategy implementation and control has become more evident as it has been more widely used.[7]

Managing Strategic Momentum – Evaluating Action Plans

Generally, managing action plans involves agreeing upon objectives, measuring performance, evaluating performance against the objectives, and taking corrective action, if necessary. All of the units act in concert to ensure that the level of actual performance comes as close as possible to a set of desired performance specifications. Managing the strategy provides strategic managers a means of determining whether the organization is performing satisfactorily; it is an explicit process for refining or completely altering the strategy. Therefore, strategic managers must monitor, evaluate, and adjust the action plans. Exhibit 10–3 provides some questions to initiate strategic thinking for assessing the appropriateness and effectiveness of the action plans. These questions may generate information for changing the strategies or action plans. As discussed in Perspective 10–5, planning and replanning are a part of the strategic thinking, strategic planning, and managing the strategic momentum processes.

Implementation Challenges

Although many organizational resources are devoted to strategy formulation, research indicates that many times strategies are not implemented. Furthermore, one study found that more than 40 percent of senior executives and 90 percent of employees did not think they had a clear understanding of their organization's strategy. Ninety percent of these individuals believed that a better understanding of the strategy would improve the likelihood of successful implementation.[8] Understanding the many *paradoxes of strategic management* is a good start in better

Exhibit 10–3: Strategic Thinking Map for Evaluating the Action Plans

1. Has the organization's overall strategy been well communicated to all members of the organizational units?
2. Do the organizational units have the resources required for successful implementation of the strategy?
3. Is there a high level of commitment to the strategy within the organizational unit?
4. Has the organizational unit developed action plans, including realistic objectives, timelines, responsibilities, and budgets?
5. Are the unit objectives consistent and compatible with the strategy?
6. Do the organizational units have the managerial and employee capabilities required for successfully implementing the organization's strategy?
7. Do all the action plans together accomplish the overall strategies of the organization?

Perspective 10–5

Plan and
Replan

The plan is complete and the board has approved it. It has been communicated throughout the hospital through carefully orchestrated "town meetings." The key around which the entire plan revolves is a new multi-million dollar cardiac wing. Two weeks later, the primary cardiology group in town announces they are entering into a joint venture with a private company to open a specialty heart hospital. So much for the strategic plan!

Strategic planning and forecasting are timehonored rituals in hospitals. Yet, many skeptics say that a five-year plan is one part research and forecasting and five parts gazing into a murky crystal ball. So, why bother? It is true that the plan will soon be outdated and the further into the future planners go, the more likely the plan will prove to be inaccurate. In light of the radical changes in health care, can it be that strategic planning is just a waste of time? The Financial Executives Research Foundation discovered that only about one-fourth of their respondents thought the annual planning process was time well spent.

Strategic planning is important precisely because things change so rapidly. A decade ago a developing trend in the Northeast might take a decade to be adopted in the South or Midwest. Today, it may happen in months and managers do not have much time to prepare. Strategic planning should be a dynamic process – not a once a year activity. Although the plan may look ahead for three to five years, it has to be updated periodically and reviewed constantly. The plan must provide for flexibility to cope with rapid, unexpected changes.

Several years ago, for example, St. David's Healthcare Partnership in Austin, Texas spent time and resources formulating a joint venture with Seton Medical Center, an Ascension Health facility. The two organizations' representatives hammered out a plan to increase psychiatric care in the area and were ready to launch the effort when the state's attorney general unexpectedly disallowed the joint venture. When this type of unexpected event occurs, there needs to be a strategy in place for "plan B." Otherwise the organization can be sidetracked, employees can be demoralized, and the leaders move blindly to respond to the unexpected change.

Planning requires management to think about issues that could derail the organization and it is important because those who hold the purse strings expect it, plus financial institutions will demand a plan before investing in a facility. According to Bruce Gordon, senior vice president of health care for Moody's Investors Service, the most important reason for strategic planning is, "If you're planning for growth, you can bet the other guy down the street that you're competing with is doing the exact same thing." If you are not thinking and planning, you are likely to be left behind.

Source: Richard Haugh, "Plan, Replan, Plan Again," *Hospitals & Health Networks* 78, no. 2 (2004), pp. 24–27.

understanding strategy and implementation difficulties. These paradoxes are discussed in Perspective 10–6.

Typically more attention has been given to strategy formulation and its link to organizational performance than to the intervening process of strategy implementation. In addition, the organization's culture and hierarchical structure may have been ignored such that those responsible for implementation may know little about the thinking that provided the basis for the strategy. Research in hospitals has confirmed that consensus around strategic decisions builds commitment to the strategy and commitment leads to successful implementation, although it sometimes progresses at a slow pace.[9]

Perspective 10–6

Strategic Management Paradoxes

- The more chaotic (unpredictable) the external environment, the more strategic planning is needed. Placid environments do not require a great deal of planning. However, where there is a great deal of change, anticipating, recognizing the signals of change, and repositioning the organization are important.
- Strategic management is a top-down, bottom-up process. Top management must initiate and support strategic management – however, organizations must learn by doing. Strategic planning staffs generally are less effective because they do not involve the line managers who must implement the strategy.
- Strategic management is a democratic process where the boss (CEO) is in control. Although everyone has something to offer and should be involved in the process, final responsibility for the viability of the organization rests with the CEO.
- Strategic management is an organized/messy process. There are clear steps in the process of strategic management, but each step raises many questions, controversies, and disagreements. Often, it is an inefficient process of consensus building and decision making.
- Strategic management is about defining the "big picture" and emphasizing the details. The strategic management process defines the organization's relationship with its environment and sets direction. However, implementation involves coordinating numerous details.
- Strategic management concerns destruction and renewal. Sometimes in the process of reinventing an organization, parts of the old organization must first be dismantled to put new processes in place.
- The rules for success are written outside the organization (in the environment), but competitive advantage is created inside the organization. Opportunities and threats are external to the organization. However, management must find the appropriate internal resources, capabilities, and competencies to build sustainable competitive advantage.
- People cannot perform strategic management until they "get it" (understand the process and its implications); and people cannot "get it" until they perform strategic management. Sometimes the full implications of strategic management as a way (philosophy) of managing cannot be fully appreciated until people have experienced it. (You cannot really learn to swim until you have been in the pool.)
- Everybody wants a strategic plan but it is the process that is important. Often managers think the plan (the document) is the objective of strategic management. However, the real objective is to set direction through the processes of communicating, reaching consensus, and decision making.
- Strategic management is easy but difficult. The processes are not complicated but it is often difficult to get people to overcome their fear of change.
- Strategic management is a philosophy composed of techniques. It is management by the compass, but there are many maps to use as a start.
- Strategic management concerns effectiveness and efficiency. Strategic management concerns doing the right thing as well as doing things right.
- Managers seek quantifiable data, but strategic management is fundamentally a qualitative art. Strategic management uses quantifiable data, but basically involves judgment. There are no such things as cold, hard, objective facts – only opinions about those facts. Strategic management is a matter of interpretation and opinion.
- Strategic management controls and empowers. Strategic management focuses organizational efforts toward a vision and well-defined goals; however, the process allows for individual decision making, innovation, and self-expression. If organizations are to successfully renew themselves, there must be enough freedom for employees to question assumptions, strategic decisions, and the way things are done.

Seven deadly sins have been identified that doom effective strategy implementation:

1. The strategy is lacking in terms of rigor, insight, vision, ambition, or practicality. If the strategy is simply more of the same, comfortable, and incremental, it will not create the excitement needed for successful implementation.
2. People are not sure how the strategy is to be implemented. Leaders are too impatient to make the strategy happen so that communicating details about how implementation is to proceed is thought of as time-consuming indecisiveness.
3. The strategy is communicated on a "need to know" basis rather than freely throughout the organization.
4. No one is responsible for every aspect of strategy implementation. Failure to carefully see to all aspects of implementation results in oversights and confusion.
5. Leaders send mixed signals by dropping out of sight when implementation begins. The absence of leadership implies that implementation is not worthy of their attention and, therefore, unimportant.
6. Unforeseen obstacles to implementation will inevitably occur. The responsible people should therefore be prepared for these barriers and be encouraged to overcome them in creative and innovative ways.
7. Strategy becomes all-consuming and details of day-to-day operations are lost or neglected. Strategy is important but so are operations.[10]

Barriers to Implementation

Effective strategy implementation requires the same determination and effort that is devoted to situational analysis and strategy formulation. If the barriers to effective implementation are to be eliminated or overcome, a number of actions will be required.[11] Everyone in the organization has to be a partner in implementation. Strategies are organization-wide and require inter-unit and cross-functional cooperation. It is critically important that everyone understands and supports the strategy. Successful strategies require a willingness to seek the good of the entire organization over any single part. Unit managers have to broaden their view and the organization's leadership has to evaluate success based on contribution to the whole rather than to a single unit.

Strategic managers are responsible for turning vision into a compelling strategy for the future. This compelling vision elevates unclear strategies and conflicting priorities into a consistent pathway to success and makes it "something worth doing." The message from visible and engaged leadership is clear – strategy implementation is important.

If strategy is important, it should be a part of the budgeting, performance evaluation, and reward system of the health care organization. A primary reason why strategies are not implemented is because, in many health care organizations, effective or ineffective implementation makes little or no difference in resource allocation and reward distribution. People, therefore, concentrate on what they perceive as the important things – those things that actually affect their budgets and their paychecks.[12]

Contingency Planning

Contingency planning may be incorporated into the normal strategic management process at any level and is a part of managing the strategic momentum. Contingency plans are alternative plans that are put into effect if the strategic assumptions change quickly or dramatically, or if organizational performance is lagging. Thus, alternative plans are the result of strategic thinking and provide leadership with a different course of action until further analysis can be undertaken and a different strategy – more appropriate for the changed environment – adopted. The more turbulent, discontinuous, and unpredictable the external environment, the more likely it is that unexpected or dramatic shifts will occur and the greater the need for contingency planning. To incorporate contingency planning requires top management to have some very specific triggers that are understood by everyone and significant enough to require a change.

Strategic plans are based on the events and trends that management views to be the most likely (the strategic assumptions). However, these events may not occur, or trends may weaken or they may accelerate far faster than strategic managers anticipated. Therefore, contingency plans are normally tied to key issues or events occurring or not occurring. For instance, if strategic thinkers have based the strategy on an expanding economy but are presented with clear evidence that the economy is slipping into a recession, contingency plans may be activated. Similarly, the announcement that a major competitor is leaving the market may present an opportunity that initiates contingency plans for market development. Such contingency planning forces strategic managers to think in terms of possible outcomes of the strategy.

Specialty hospitals are a good example where the strategic assumptions changed dramatically and contingency plans became important. Cardiac and orthopedic hospitals were aggressively pursuing market development expansion strategies – building free-standing new specialty hospitals in different markets, especially in those states without certificate of need requirements. Congress placed a moratorium (extended to January 1, 2007) that prohibited the construction of any additional specialty hospitals until it was determined whether the impact was too great on traditional community hospitals. New plans were required immediately. What strategies could be pursued to maintain profitability and growth? What should the organization do if the moratorium changed into law prohibiting the construction of specialty hospitals? Contingency plans might be for the organization to change its strategy to one of service improvement (quality) of current operations or cost reduction and efficiency of current operations. If the expansion strategy of market development is no longer an option for increasing profitability, the organization may change to an enhancement strategy or product development (new services such as outsourcing for cardiac or orthopedic units).

To provide strategic control for organizations, effective contingency planning involves a seven-step process:

1. Identify both favorable and unfavorable events that could possibly derail the strategy or strategies.

2. Specify trigger points. Calculate a likely timetable for contingent events to occur.
3. Assess the impact of each contingent event by estimating the potential benefit or harm for each.
4. Develop contingency plans. Be sure that contingency plans are compatible with current strategy and are economically feasible.
5. Assess the counter-impact of each contingency plan. That is, estimate how much each contingency plan will capitalize on or cancel out its associated contingent event. Doing so will quantify the potential value of each contingency plan.
6. Determine early warning signals for key contingent events. Monitor the early warning signals.
7. For contingent events with reliable early warning signals, develop advance-action plans to take advantage of the available lead time.[13]

Strategic Momentum – A New Beginning

The model of strategic management introduced in Chapter 1 presented strategic momentum as the last stage of the model. However, managing the strategic momentum is an inherent part of all the strategic management processes. Strategic managers are managing the strategic momentum as they consider the reasons for strategic change.

Managing the strategic momentum addresses making changes in what the organization is currently doing. Perhaps the best explanation is that strategic management is logically a circular process, and all of its processes are continuous. For instance, strategic thinking and situational analysis are not halted so that strategy formulation may begin. All are continuous and affect one another.

Nevertheless, the act of managing provides the momentum for change, and change is a fundamental part of survival. As health care leaders manage momentum and change their organizations, they chart new courses into the future. In effect, they create new beginnings, new chances for success, new challenges for employees, and new hopes for patients. Therefore, it is imperative that health care managers understand the changes taking place in their environment; they should not simply be responsive to them, but strive to create the future. Health care leaders must see into the future and create new visions for success.

The Map and Compass

Chapter 1 introduced the concept of the map and the compass. Recall that maps provide explicit directions and start the organization on its journey. Sometimes as organizations progress, however, the landscape or landmarks have changed, or in other cases the organization is not really sure exactly where it should be headed. In these instances the compass is more valuable to chart the course. Through strategic planning, organizations create plans (maps) for the future but must be willing to abandon the plan as the situation changes, new opportunities emerge, or managers find out what really works. This requires strategic thinking and leadership – leaders who recognize discontinuities and the need for change before others and commit to managing for the new realities.

Each chapter in this text has presented a strategic thinking map (rational model) for accomplishing strategic management. These maps provide guidelines for strategic management, including general environmental analysis, service area competitor analysis, internal analysis, and so on. The maps keep leaders from being overwhelmed and provide some perspective to chart where they are going and what they want to accomplish. In addition, the maps initiate action toward renewing the organization. Without a map it is difficult to start the journey. However, similar to an organization's plans, these rational models cannot anticipate everything; nor can they be universally applied. They will not be a perfect fit for every organization, yet they can provide the initial logical direction for exploring and learning. They may be used to initiate thinking. Therefore, the organization must reinvent the processes and learn as it goes. True creativity, the kind that is responsible for breakthrough innovations in our society, always changes the rules.

Do not work for the map; allow the map to work for you. When the strategic thinking map no longer provides direction and insight, management must dare to innovate and re-create the process – use a compass. The vision for the organization and its future should be used to determine what to do today to make it happen. To summarize, Perspective 10–7 presents some general dos and don'ts for successful strategic management.

Finally, strategic management requires concentrated effort and takes practice. Lasting change will be made only through a lifelong commitment to a continuing discipline. Lasting organizational change (renewal) comes from thinking strategically and adopting sound management principles that are practiced on a continuing basis. There are no quick fixes. Using strategic thinking, strategic planning, and managing the strategic momentum to go forward enables the organization to change itself, and the world.

Summary and Conclusions

This chapter deals with communicating the strategic plan and developing action plans – the translation of organizational strategies into action plans. Successful implementation relies on this translation. Otherwise, strategy remains little more than wishful thinking. Action plans make strategy happen, yet strategy cannot happen if people do not understand their roles in accomplishing the strategies of the organization.

It is important that the interrelationships among situational analysis, strategy formulation, and action plans are understood by managers and employees. Such understanding is critical because, unless it is achieved, action plans are unlikely to reflect organizational priorities.

Action plans should contain clear objectives that, when accomplished, will achieve the strategies of the organization. These objectives should be measurable, easy to understand, contain timeframes, and involve the individuals responsible for

Perspective 10–7

The Dos and Don'ts of Strategic Management

Do

- Understand that strategic management is a philosophy or way of managing, not simply a technique. Strategic management transcends techniques.
- Remember that in strategic management, the process (strategic thinking) is more important than the product (a plan).
- Involve everyone possible in the process. Those who participate will better understand the benefits and will be more willing to buy into the process.
- Ensure that people within the organization take ownership of the process and its results.
- Realize that because the "rules for success" are written outside the organization, understanding the external environment is an essential task of strategic management.
- Expect that strategic management is really hard work and that it may take years before people really manage (and think) strategically.
- Remember that strategic management is about organizational renewal. Be ready to learn and reinvent the process (and the organization).
- Expect things to get worse before they get better (people are typically confused at first and resistant to change).
- Remember that you will never get it quite right. Strategic management is about constant organizational rethinking, reinvention, re-creation, and renewal.
- Expect the process to be exciting and challenging.

Don't

- Expect strategic management to be the "magic bullet" that will fix everything.
- Start strategic management without full commitment from top management – its support, time, and resources.
- Expect perfection. Strategic management is a "messy" and sometimes inefficient process.
- Rely too much on consultants, outsiders, or a small staff group. It should not be "their" plan, but rather "our" plan.
- Follow the process (map) of strategic management blindly. A compass is necessary to go where the organization has not gone before.
- Expect someone to provide a strategic management "template" that will overlay perfectly with your organization.
- Expect strategic management to be easy or take only a few months or a year.
- Expect that everyone will understand the full implications of strategic management ("get it") at first. People learn by doing.
- Expect immediate results. Strategic management may be a fundamental change in doing business.
- Expect the future to be an extension of the past. The only thing we know for certain is that the future will be different.
- Expect that your organization will survive without change. Organizations that fail to change, fail.

accomplishing them in their formulation. If they are to be effective guides to behavior, unit objectives – whether the unit is a division, a single entity, or a department – must be understood and agreed on by the members of that unit who are responsible for accomplishing the tasks necessary to achieve the objectives.

Action plans are important aids to accomplish the strategies of health care organizations. They outline the activities required for the accomplishment of each unit objective along with an estimate of resources generated and expended in the accomplishment of each unit objective. In addition, action plans specify the time requirements for the accomplishment of each action and the individual or group responsible for ensuring the action is accomplished. Action planning is an effective aid in the formulation of unit budget requests and when rewards are based on action plan accomplishments, everyone recognizes their importance.

The Balanced Scorecard is discussed as a tool for effectively managing strategy implementation as it has evolved from a comprehensive performance measurement tool to a strategy implementation tool.

The strategic management planning process often "falls apart" at implementation. Less attention is given to implementation in most strategic management texts because it is so difficult to provide the specifics (there is no generic implementation strategy but, rather, a series of requirements: objectives, timelines, responsibilities, and measures of success). Implementation is specific to an organization, a strategy, a service area, and a culture. Because strategic assumptions may change, contingency planning is essential to enable an organization to quickly change direction in a fast-paced environment. The map is a useful guide for known destinations whereas the compass aids in times of greater uncertainty.

Key Terms and Concepts in Strategic Management

Action Plan
Balanced Scorecard
Contingency Planning

Guidance
Objectives

Paradoxes of Strategic
Management

QUESTIONS FOR CLASS DISCUSSION

1. Explain the relationship between situational analysis and action plans.
2. List the important components of action plans. Which component do you think is the most important? The least important? Explain your response.
3. How are the action plans for a division (for example, the hospital division) similar to action plans for a department (such as housekeeping)? How are they different?
4. How do action plans assist in the allocation of organizational resources in line with strategies?
5. Are the costs associated with accomplishing the unit objectives the only ones that should be included in budget requests? Why or why not?
6. What are some of the primary barriers to the effective implementation of strategies in health care organizations? How can each be overcome or removed?
7. What are the primary characteristics of unit objectives? Are these characteristics descriptive of good organizational strategic goals? Why or why not?
8. What is a Balanced Scorecard? In what ways is it a means of focusing attention on strategy implementation?
9. Should every organization formulate contingency plans? Why or why not?
10. Explain why strategic momentum may be a new beginning.
11. Explain whether a map or a compass is better for your career path in health care.

NOTES

1. Peter F. Drucker, *Managing for Results* (New York: Harper & Row Publishers, 1964), p. 95.

2. Quoted in Katie Sosnowchik, "A Fierce Momentum," *green@work* (March/April, 2002), p. 6.

3. Christopher A. Bartlett and Sumantra Ghoshal, "Building Competitive Advantage Through People," *MIT Sloan Management Review* 42, no. 1 (Winter 2002), p. 36.

4. Peter F. Drucker, *Managing the Nonprofit Organization: Principles and Practices* (New York: Harper-Collins Publishers, 1990), p. 142.

5. Xiang Li, Cheng-Leong Ang, and Robert Gray, "An Intelligent Business Forecaster for Strategic Business Planning," *Journal of Forecasting* 18, no. 3 (1999), pp. 181–204. See also Alan M. Zuckerman, "Growing Pains: The Difference Between Strategic and Nonstrategic Growth," *Healthcare Financial Management* 58, no. 4 (2004), pp. 102–104.

6. Michael Hammer and James Champy, *Reengineering the Corporation: A Manifesto for Business Revolution* (New York: HarperCollins Publishers, 1993), p. 35.

7. Jonathan W. Cartright, Stephen C. Stolp-Smith, and Eric S. Edell, "Strategic Performance Management: Development of a Performance Measurement System at Mayo Clinic," *Journal of Healthcare Management* 45, no. 1 (2000), pp. 58–68.

8. Yvon Rousseau and Paul Rousseau, "Turning Strategy into Action in Financial Services," *CMA Management* 73, no. 10 (1999), pp. 25–29. Also see Gary P. Latham, "Goal Setting: A Five Step Approach to Behavioral Change," *Organizational Dynamics* 32, no. 2 (2003), pp. 309–317.

9. Robert S. Dooley, Gerald E. Fryxell, and William Q. Judge, "Belaboring the Not-So-Obvious: Consensus, Commitment, and Strategy Implementation Speed and Success," *Journal of Management* 26, no. 6 (2000), pp. 1237–1258 and David Lei and Charles R. Greer, "The Emphatic Organization," *Organizational Dynamics* 32, no. 2 (2003), pp. 142–164.

10. Martin Corboy and Diarmurd O'Corribui, "The Seven Deadly Sins of Strategy," *Management Accounting* 77, no. 10 (1999), pp. 29–30. See also Benson Honig and Thomas Karlsson, "Institutional Forces and the Written Business Plan," *Journal of Management* 30, no. 1 (2004), pp. 29–48.

11. Michael Beer and Russell Eisenstat, "The Silent Killers of Strategy Implementation and Learning," *Sloan Management Review* 41, no. 4 (2000), pp. 29–40. Much of this section was adapted from this source. See also JoAnn Neely, "New Reality: Make the Move to Pragmatic," *Getting Paid in Behavioral Healthcare* 8, no. 5 (2003), pp. 1–5.

12. William S. Birnbaum, *If Your Strategy Is So Terrific, How Come It Doesn't Work?* (New York: AMACOM, 1990), p. 72.

13. Robert Linneman and Rajan Chandran, "Contingency Planning: A Key to Swift Managerial Action in the Uncertain Tomorrow," *Managerial Planning* 29, no. 4 (January–February 1981), pp. 23–27.

ADDITIONAL READINGS

Christensen, Clayton M. and Michael E. Raynor, *The Innovator's Solution: Creating and Sustaining Successful Growth* (Boston, MA: Harvard Business School Press, 2003). It is a paradox of business history that yesterday's story of success is tomorrow's story of failure. Although virtually everyone favors innovation, the truth is that business and health care are not very good at it. Most of what is called innovation is really just tinkering with existing products and services. The authors skillfully distinguish between disruptive and sustaining innovations. Instead of tinkering with existing products and services, bold leaps of creativity are needed to take advantage of emerging new markets.

Forgang, William G., *Strategy-Specific Decision Making: A Guide for Executing Competitive Strategy* (Armonk, NY: M. E. Sharpe Publishing, 2004). A unique approach is presented that emphasizes the implementation of the organization's competitive advantage throughout all levels of the enterprise. A comprehensive case is used to highlight key concepts presented throughout the book. Tools are provided to assess the choices that result in the implementation of the organization's strategy.

Joyce, William, Nitin Nohria, and Bruce Roberson, *What Really Works: The 4+2 Formula for Sustained Business Success* (New York: HarperCollins, 2004). What really works is a great mystery of business life. Everyone has an answer to what works but on investigation it works only for them in many cases. This book reports the results of a ten-year study suggesting that there are four primary practices (strategy, execution, culture, and structure) and two secondary practices (talent and leadership) that lead to sustained double-digit growth.

Kaplan, Robert S. and David P. Norton, *Strategy Maps: Converting Intangible Assets Into Tangible Outcomes* (Boston, MA: Harvard Business School Press, 2004). More than 75 percent of the market value of many companies is from intangible assets. Often traditional metrics simply do not measure this value accurately or completely. The strategy map is a tool for aligning investments in people, technology, and management capital to obtain the greatest outcome. When managers can describe the links between intangible assets and value creation, greater success can be achieved.

Mintzberg, Henry, *Managers Not MBAs: A Hard Look at the Soft Practice of Managing and Management Development* (Williston, VT: BK Publishers, 2004). Reviewers have contended that this book offers the most extensive critique of how managers today are educated and how they manage. The results are not encouraging. It is argued that management education programs often train the wrong people in the wrong ways with the expectation of the wrong outcomes. Suggestions are offered for improving the process.

Peters, Tom, *Re-Imagine* (New York: Dorling Kindersley Publishing, 2003). Organizations are at their best when they are passionate about delivering exciting services to customers and exciting opportunities to employees. However, often all that customers and employees see are barriers, egos, and petty tyrants discouraging the good intentions of enterprising people. Cunning, speed, and surprise are the routes to competitive advantage today and hypercompetition has become the norm. According to Peters, it is time to destroy the myths of business and get to the act of reinvention.

PART 2

Appendices

Analyzing Strategic Health Care Cases A

How do students of management gain experience in strategic thinking and making strategic decisions in health care organizations? One way is to work their way up the organization, holding a variety of positions, experimenting as they develop their decision-making skills, and observing other leaders as they deal with issues and develop strategies. Then, when the opportunity presents itself, they combine what they have learned from others and their own management philosophy, and do the best they can. Unfortunately, learning by experimenting and observing others may be risky in rapidly changing environments and in the often unique situations that health care managers and leaders face.

Hospitals, HMOs, long-term care facilities, public health organizations, and other health services prefer to trust important decision making to experienced managers and leaders. Case studies have been successfully used as a surrogate method to provide aspiring managers and leaders with experience in strategic thinking, strategic planning, and making decisions without undue risk. The best case studies, such as those in this text, contain real situations actually faced by managers and leaders in health care organizations and are documented in a way that makes them useful in providing experience for future strategic decision makers. Because many future health care decision makers are not familiar with how to analyze cases, this Appendix has been included, not to prescribe how cases should always be solved, but to offer some initial direction on how to surface and address the real issues presented in the cases.

An Overview of Case Analysis

Case analysis provides the student of health care an exciting opportunity to act in the role of a key decision maker. From hospitals to community blood centers to physicians' offices, students have the chance to learn about a variety of health and medical organizations and to practice decision-making skills through analyzing cases.

The decisions required to "solve" cases represent a wide range of complexity, so that no two cases are addressed in exactly the same manner. However, the strategic thinking maps presented in this text provide frameworks to aid in strategically thinking about case issues. The fundamental task of the case analyst is to make decisions that will serve as a map to guide the organization into the future. Therefore, most case instructors will expect a comprehensive plan for the organization that addresses relevant current issues and provides a viable and reasonably complete strategy for the future. In order to achieve this goal, the case analyst typically should:

- surface and summarize the key issues,
- analyze the situation,
- develop an organizational strategy,
- develop an implementation plan, and
- set some benchmarks to measure success.

These categories represent the major elements of strategy development and make appropriate section headings for a case analysis written report or presentation. First, using the strategic thinking map presented in Chapter 1 (Exhibit 1–3), it is important to do some serious strategic thinking about the external environment of the organization – the political/legal, economic, social/cultural, technological, and competitive situations faced by the case characters. After gaining knowledge of the issues in the general and industry environments, the service area competitors should be assessed. At this point it is important to relate the resources, competencies, and capabilities of the organization to the external environment, which will require a thorough and objective analysis of the competitively relevant strengths and weaknesses. The value chain provides a useful tool for uncovering these strengths and weaknesses. These strengths and weakness must be evaluated as to their potential to create competitive advantages or disadvantages for the organization. External issues and the organization's competitive advantages and disadvantages provide the basis for strategy formulation. To create the strategy for a health care organization it is necessary to understand its unique mission, vision, values, and goals (directional strategies).

Once the situational analysis is complete, strategic alternatives can be generated as possible solutions to the issues identified in the case. Consideration must be given to the possible adaptive strategies, market entry strategies, and competitive strategies that provide the means for achieving the organization's mission and goals and lead to the accomplishment of its vision. The effectiveness of the chosen alternative for each type of strategy must be evaluated. In addition, at least some thought must be given to the likely outcomes resulting from the different choices. Then a recommendation needs to be made from among the alternatives generated.

Nothing will happen, of course, unless the strategy can be implemented. Therefore, the case analyst must address how the strategy will be carried out. The development of a feasible implementation plan should include specific service delivery and support strategies and, where possible, action plans. These areas are important because they create value for the organization and translate strategy into organizational and individual actions – the work to be done.

Finally, the case analyst should consider how the success of the proposed strategy should be measured. Returning to the mission, vision, values, and goals will provide an initial measure of success. Other measures will include fit with the changing environment, internal changes (development of competitive advantages and lessening of competitive disadvantages), and other more specific measures such as financial measures, market share, growth, and so on.

Although the approach outlined here is logical, it is important to remember that a case should be approached and appreciated as a unique opportunity for problem solving. Cases that everyone agrees have only one solution are not good decision-making aids. Moreover, managers in health care organizations rarely face problems where the solution is obvious to everyone. This does not mean that there are no good and bad answers or solutions in case analysis; some are better than others based on the logic presented. Sometimes the issues presented in a case are not even problems (defined as a negative occurrence that needs to be addressed). Often the greatest challenge facing an organization is recognizing and acting on an opportunity rather than solving a problem. The evaluation of a case analysis is often based more on the approach and logic employed than the precise recommendation offered.

Cases, Strategic Management, and Health Care Organizations

Cases add realism that is impossible to achieve in traditional lecture classes. Realism results from the essential nature of cases, although students may complain that cases fail to provide all the information necessary for decision making. The complaint is valid because cases rarely provide everything that is needed. However, decision makers in health care organizations rarely have all the information they want or need when they face decisions. Risks must be taken in case analysis just as in actual decision making.

Risk Taking in Case Analysis

Any decision about the future involves uncertainty. Decision making under conditions of uncertainty requires that means be devised for dealing with the risks faced by leaders. Cases are valuable aids in this area because they allow the analysts to practice making decisions in low-risk environments. Decisions in a poor case analysis may be embarrassing, but at least they will not result in the closure of a hospital or medical practice. At the same time, the lessons learned by solving cases and participating in discussions will begin to build problem-solving skills.

Solving Case Problems

Solving a case is much like solving any problem. First, information is gathered and issues are defined; the competitive situation is analyzed; alternatives are generated, evaluated, selected, and implemented. Although the person solving the case seldom has the chance to implement a decision, he or she should always keep in mind that recommendations must be tempered by the limitations imposed on the organization in terms of its resources, competencies, and capabilities (although strategies to improve these areas may be required). As the success or failure of the recommendation is analyzed, lessons are learned that can be applied to future decision making.

Alternative Perspectives: Passion or Objectivity

Different hypothetical roles can be assumed when analyzing cases. Some prefer to think of themselves as the chief executive officer or leader to impose a perspective on the problems presented in the case, providing the case analyst with the liberty to become a passionate advocate for a particular course of action. Others prefer to observe the case from the detached objectivity of a consultant who has been employed by the organization to solve a problem.

Either the leader or the consultant perspective may be assumed, but the first offers some unique advantages. To answer the questions from the leader's perspective, it is important to get inside the decision maker's head – to feel the excitement and fear of doing new and innovative things in the dynamic and complex health care environment. However, the passion and frustration of the leader suggest why some case analysts prefer to assume the objective posture of a consultant. Not being in the front line can sometimes suggest alternatives that cannot be seen by those directly involved in making the payroll and paying the bills. The consultant can more easily play the devil's advocate and point out how actions are at odds with current theory. Although the fun and excitement of case analysis is enhanced by assuming the decision maker's role, the options might be expanded through a more objective and detached outlook of an outsider. There are no absolutely correct or incorrect answers to complex cases. The most important lesson is to learn problem solving and strategic management skills.

Reading the Case

Effective case analysis begins with data collection. This means carefully reading the case, rereading it, and sometimes reading it yet again. Rarely can anyone absorb enough information from the initial reading of a comprehensive case to adequately solve it. From the very first reading of the case, the analyst should start to list the external threats and opportunities facing the organization and internal strengths and weaknesses. For example, when a threat is discovered it should be marked for more detailed examination. "Are the threats financial? Do the primary issues appear to be those of human resources, capital investment, or marketing?" Perhaps there are few, if any, apparent threats. The strategic issue facing the organization may be an opportunity to be exploited or it may be both an opportunity and threat. For example, managed care has created some interesting threats and opportunities for many health care organizations.

Listing the possible strengths and weakness in the initial reading provides some perspective concerning the organization's resources, competencies, and capabilities. This list will provide a basis for further investigation and provide a guide for additional information gathering. Once the situation has been reviewed, a better evaluation of the opportunities and threats facing the organization can be made. An effective way of summarizing the results is through the use of a simple two-by-two chart listing the threats, opportunities, weaknesses, and strengths (refer to Exhibit 7–1).

Gathering Information

The information required to successfully analyze a case comes in two forms. The first type of information is given as part of the case and customarily includes history of the hospital, long-term care facility, or home-health care agency; its organizational structure; its management; and its financial condition. Gathering this information is relatively easy because the author of the case has typically done the work.

A second type of information is "obtainable." This information is not provided in the case or by the instructor but is available from secondary sources in the library, familiar magazines and related publications, or over the Internet. Obtainable secondary information helps with understanding the nature of the service category, the competition, and even some managers, past and present, who have made an impact on the service category.

If the case does not include service category information or competitor information, the instructor may expect the class to do some detective work before proceeding. Students should investigate to find out what is happening in the service category and learn enough about trends to position the problems discussed in the case in a broader health care context. The culture of the organization or the style of the chief executive officer may constitute relevant information. Some instructors do not want students to investigate beyond the date of the case or to gather additional service category data. Therefore, students must ask the instructor's preference.

Case Analysis Using the Strategic Thinking Maps

The strategic thinking maps presented in this text provide a means of thinking through strategic management issues and serve as road maps to case analysis. They are useful for analyzing cases and succinctly presenting strategic management decisions in written reports and presentations. The following discussion provides some tips for using the strategic thinking maps in each of the major elements of case analysis – surfacing the issues, situational analysis, development of the strategy, and development of the implementation plan.

Tips on Surfacing the Issues

The discussion and questions in the "Managing the Strategic Momentum" section of each chapter are designed to surface present and potential issues. In case analysis, issues include not only problems but also situations where things may be working well but improvements are possible. The problem may actually be an opportunity that can be capitalized on by the organization if it acts consciously and decisively. With careful analysis, patterns can be detected and discrepancies between what actually is and what ought to be become more apparent. In other words, fundamental issues, not mere symptoms, begin to emerge.

PROBLEMS VS. SYMPTOMS

It is important to realize that the things observed in an organization and reported in a case may not be the real or essential threats and opportunities. Often what analysts observe are the symptoms of more serious core problems. For example, increasing interest rates and cash-flow discrepancies appear to be problems in many case analyses. In reality, the issue is the fundamental absence of adequate financial planning. The lack of planning is simply manifested as a cash-flow problem, and rising interest rates certainly complicate cash flow.

Frequently, hospitals conclude that they have operational problems in the area of marketing when bed occupancy rates decline. Someone may suggest that the marketing department is not doing a good job of convincing physicians to use the hospital. Sometimes people will complain that the hospital is not spending enough on advertising. The real issue, however, might be fundamental changes in the demographics of the market area or an outdated services mix that no amount of advertising will overcome. In organizations as complex as health care, problems may have more than a single cause, so the analyst must not be overly confident when a single, simple reason is isolated. In fact, the suggestion of a simple solution should increase rather than decrease skepticism.

USING TOOLS

Identifying key issues requires that information be carefully examined and analyzed. Often, quantitative tools are helpful. Financial ratio analysis of the exhibits included in the case will sometimes be helpful in the identification of the real problems. In arriving at the ultimate determination of core problems, the analyst should try not to slip into "paralysis by analysis" and waste more time than is necessary on identifying problems. At the same time, premature judgments must be avoided because then real issues may be missed. One general guideline is that when research and analysis cease to generate surprises, the analyst can feel relatively, though not absolutely, sure that adequate research has been conducted and the key issues have been identified.

CHECK FACTS

The issue discovery process should not become myopic. There may be a tendency on the part of individuals interested and experienced in accounting and finance to see all problems in terms of accounting and finance. A physician approaching the same case will likely focus on the medical implications. This is too limited a view for effective strategic decision makers. Strategic analysis effectively transcends a single function. Insistence on approaching case analysis exclusively from the viewpoint of the analyst's expertise and training is not likely to produce an accurate overall picture of the situation facing the organization; nor is this approach likely to improve the organization's performance.

Information, either given or obtained, must never be accepted at face value. If a CEO states that the hospital delivers outstanding quality care, it should not be accepted as a statement of fact without some thought. For example, a character in the case may voice an opinion that is not grounded in fact. The ratios on a long-term care facility's financial statements may look strange, but are they? Before jumping to such a conclusion, analysts should look at the financial ratios in a historical perspective. Even better, they should look at the history (as well as similar ratios) of other long-term care facilities of the same size during the same time period.

RELEVANT ISSUES

Once the issues are identified, they must be precisely stated and their selection defended. The best defense for the selection of the key issues is the data set used to guide the issue discovery process. The reasons for selection of the issues should be briefly and specifically summarized along with the supportive information on which judgments have been based. The issue statement stage is not the time for solutions. Focusing on solutions at this point will reduce the impact of the issue statement. If the role of consultant has been assumed, the issue statement must be convincing, precise, and logical to the client organization, or credibility will be reduced. If the role of the strategic decision maker has been selected, the student must be equally convincing and precise. The strategic decision maker should be as certain as possible that the correct issues have been identified to pursue the appropriate alternatives.

The statement of the issues should relate only to those areas of strategy and operations where actions have a chance of producing results. The results may be either increasing gains or cutting potential losses. Long- and short-range aspects of issues should be identified and stated. In strategic analysis the emphasis is on long-range issues rather than merely handling emergencies and holding things together. However, in some situations, immediate problems have to be solved and then a strategy developed to avoid similar situations in the future (combination strategy).

It is important for students to keep in mind that most strategic decision makers can deal with only a limited number of issues at a single time. Therefore, identify key result areas that will have the greatest positive impact on organizational performance.

Tips on Analyzing the Situation

Situational analysis is one of the most important steps in analyzing a case. In most instances instructors will expect comprehensive external and internal environmental analyses. For external environmental analysis, the case analyst may want to use and present a variety of tools including a trend analysis, stakeholder analysis, the development of a scenario, or service area competitive analysis. Whatever method is used, a clear picture and assessment of the external environment should be presented. Chapters 2 and 3 provide strategic thinking maps for assessing the external environment.

For the internal environment, it is important that the case analyst understand the strengths and weaknesses of the organization in terms of its resources, competencies, and capabilities. Therefore, the case analyst may want to use the value chain, as discussed in Chapter 4, to map resources, competencies, and capabilities and assess their strategic relevance using the criteria of value, rareness, imitability, and sustainability.

Understanding the mission is a good starting point to assess the directional strategies. If a mission statement is included in the case, the analyst should ask "Does it serve the purpose of communicating to the public why the organization exists? Does it provide employees with a genuine statement of what the organization is all about?" In addition, the other directional strategies (vision, values, and goals) should be evaluated as to their appropriateness to the organization and its environment. The vision and goals provide a profile of the future and targets to focus organizational actions. Sometimes the case will indicate what the health care organization plans to achieve in the next year and where it hopes to be in three years, or even in five years. As with mission statements, if the vision and goals are not explicitly stated, there is a need to speculate about them because they will be the standards against which the success or failure of a particular strategy will be evaluated. Moreover because strategic planning is futuristic and no one can predict the future with complete accuracy, vision and goals should always be adaptable to the changing conditions taking place in the organization and in the service category. Sometimes an organization will have to face a major strategic problem simply because it was unwilling to alter its vision and goals in light of changing conditions.

Tips on Formulating the Strategy

After the situational analysis, a recommended course of action – the strategy – must be developed. Thus, adaptive, market entry, and competitive strategies for the organization must be recommended and defended. Exhibit 6–4 provides a strategic thinking map depicting the various alternatives for each of the types of strategy in the strategy formulation process.

EFFECTIVE ALTERNATIVES

If obtaining and organizing information have been done well, the generation of strategic alternatives will be a challenging yet attainable task. Good alternatives possess specific characteristics:

1. They should be practical or no one will seriously consider them. Alternative courses of action that are too theoretical or abstract to be understood by those who have to accomplish them are not useful.
2. Alternatives should be specific.
3. Alternatives should be related to the key issue they are intended to address. If the strategic alternatives generated do not directly address key issues, the analyst should ask how important the issues are to the case analysis; rethinking the issues may be required. Exhibit 6–1 is helpful in demonstrating how the strategic alternatives relate to external and internal issues.
4. Alternatives should be usable. A usable alternative is one that can be reasonably accomplished within the constraints of the financial and human resources available to the organization.
5. Alternatives should be ones that can be placed into action in a relatively short period of time. If it takes too long to implement a proposed solution, it is likely that the momentum of the recommended action will be lost.

ALTERNATIVE EVALUATION

Alternatives should be evaluated according to both quantitative and qualitative criteria. Financial analysis provides one basis for examining the impact of different courses of action. However, a good alternative course of action is more than merely the one with the highest payoff. It may be that the culture of the organization cannot accommodate some of the more financially promising alternative courses of action. For the adaptive strategies, one or more of the decision-making tools discussed in Chapter 7 should be used – TOWS matrix, PLC analysis, BCG portfolio analysis, extended portfolio matrix analysis, SPACE analysis, or program evaluation. For the market entry and competitive strategies, matching the external conditions appropriate for the strategies with the internal requirements of the strategies as discussed in the text with internal strengths and weaknesses and external conditions described in the case provide a basis for selecting and defending these strategies.

The case analyst should be able to map the strategies selected in the strategy formulation process. Strategy maps similar to the one presented in Exhibit 7–23 show the ends–means decision logic for each strategic initiative and provide an excellent overview of the strategy of the organization.

Tips on Developing Implementation Strategies

Once a strategic alternative has been selected, an action plan is required. Action planning moves the decision maker from the realm of strategy to operations. Now the question becomes, "How does the group accomplish the work in the most effective and efficient way possible?"

The task of case analysis does not require that the analyst actually implement a decision; however, because the strategies must be implementable, it is necessary that thought be given to how each strategy would be put into action. Therefore, value adding service delivery and support strategies must be developed as well as action plans. This process is a continuation of the ends–means linkage started in strategy formulation – the implementation strategies are the means to achieve the overall organizational strategies.

Each element of the value chain should be addressed comparing the results of the internal analysis with the requirements of the selected strategy. Matching the present situation with the requirements of the strategy provides a basis to maintain the value chain element or change it to meet the needs of the strategy. Exhibits 8–12 and 9–7 provide examples of what instructors might expect for presenting the value adding strategies.

Next, action plans for the major organizational units affected by the strategy should be developed. Objectives, action plans, and budgets should be addressed if enough detail is provided in the case. Finally, the responsibility for accomplishing the different groups of tasks must be clearly assigned to the appropriate individuals in the organization. Although this is not always possible in case analysis, it is important that consideration be given to how, in a real organization, the recommendations would be accomplished. If, in the process of thinking about getting the different activities completed, it becomes apparent that the organization lacks the resources or the structure to accomplish a recommendation, another approach should be proposed.

The process of developing action plans for important organizational units – whether a highly focused unit, such as a pharmacy, or a broadly focused unit, such as a hospital division for a health system – should not be neglected. Organizations sometimes spend large amounts of money and resources developing strategic plans only to discover that they are not prepared to implement them in an effective manner.

Making Recommendations

Making good recommendations is a critical aspect of successful case analysis. If recommendations are theoretically sound and justifiable, people will pay attention to them. If they are not, little is likely to result from all the work done to this point.

One effective method for presenting recommendations is to relate each one to organizational strengths. Or, if necessary, a recommendation may be related to addressing a weakness. If the organization has sufficient financial strength, the recommendations should highlight how each alternative will capitalize on the strong financial condition. If, on the other hand, the resources are limited, it will be important to avoid recommendations that rely on resources that are not available or to plan a combination strategy to gain new resources.

It will be particularly useful to ask the following questions when making recommendations:

- Does the health care organization have the financial resources needed to make the recommendation work?
- Does the organization have the personnel with the right skills to accomplish what will be required by each recommendation?
- Does the organization have the controls needed to monitor whether or not the recommendations are being accomplished?
- Is the timing right to implement each recommendation? If not, when will the timing be right? Can the organization afford to wait?

Finalizing the Report

Preparation and presentation is the final activity in most case analyses. The report can be either written or oral depending on the preference of the instructor. Although the form is slightly different, the goal is the same – to summarize and communicate in an effective manner what the analysis has uncovered and what the organization should do.

Decision making is the intended result of the report. The analysis must be complete; but the emphasis should be on making the entire report brief enough to encourage people to read it and comprehensive enough to ensure that no major factors are overlooked – especially those that might adversely affect the decision. Therefore, charts and flow diagrams can be effective. In brief outline, the important sections of a case analysis report include:

- Executive summary – usually one page, and rarely more than two pages, it functions as an abstract. Its purpose is to force the writer to carefully evaluate what is really important in all the accumulated facts and data. It is not an introduction.
- Body of the case report
  - *Key Issues*: with the rationale for focusing on them.
  - *Situational Analysis*: results of the external environmental analysis, service area competitor analysis, and internal environmental analysis, as well as analysis of the directional strategies.
  - *Strategy Formulation*: feasible alternatives for directional, adaptive, market entry, and competitive strategies.
  - *Recommendation*: the feasible alternatives, and which one or ones is/are recommended.
  - *Implementation Strategies*: service delivery and support strategies with linkage to the directional, adaptive, market entry, and competitive strategies.

– *Benchmarks for success and contingency plans*: measures of success for the strategy and alternative plans if a major opportunity or threat is subject to change in the short run (contingency plan).

Conclusions

Case analysis is an art. There is no one precise way to accomplish the task, and the analysis has to be adapted to the case problem under review. The analyst must keep in mind that case analysis is a logical process that involves: (1) clearly defining strategic issues; (2) understanding the situation – the organization, service area/service category, and environment; (3) developing a strategy to enable the organization to accomplish its mission and vision; and (4) formulating an implementation plan.

The work of case analysis is not over until all these stages are completed. Often a formal written report or oral presentation of the recommendations is required. Case problems provide a unique opportunity to integrate all that students have learned about decision making and direct it toward specific problems and opportunities faced by real organizations. It is an exciting way to gain experience with decision making. Students should take it seriously and develop their own, systematic, and defensible ways of solving management problems.

Oral Presentations for Health Care Professionals

by Gary F. Kohut and Carol M. Baxter

Health care professionals are required to speak to many different audiences on diverse topics. For example, they may need to persuade supervisors to adopt a new policy, to present a grant proposal to the board of a philanthropic organization, or to discuss a status report with their employees. Whether presenting information to peers, supervisors, community leaders, or members of the health care profession, speakers must use effective oral communication, which involves three major steps: planning, organizing, and delivering the subject matter.

Plan Your Presentation

Planning your presentation effectively is an important step to speaking success. However, before you plan a speech, you must determine the type of presentation you will make, analyze your audience, conduct research, and consider the logistics of the speaking site.

Determine the Type of Presentation You Will Make

The first step in planning is to examine what your goals are for the presentation, since these goals will determine the type of presentation you will make.

Generally, oral presentations are of two types: informative and persuasive. Informative presentations convey information or ideas, whereas persuasive presentations sell an idea or a product to an audience. Informative presentations include progress reports, instructions, explanations, and training programs. For example, you may give a progress report to your supervisor detailing your efforts on a fund-raising project, or you may give similar information to a small group if it is a team-related task. On the other hand, you may be training a group of volunteers, and as coordinator you may inform them about their responsibilities.

Informative presentations can also be instructional. For instance, you might teach individuals how to obtain services for a special group of clients, how to administer a new drug, or how to complete a new form required by a governmental agency. Another variation of the informative presentation is the explanatory presentation, which is very common in the health care industry. An example of this type of presentation is to explain to the media the features of a plan to cut the teen birth rate among Hispanic women. Other examples of explanatory presentations include informing high school students about the health effects of risky sexual behavior and orienting new employees to the policies of an agency.

Persuasive presentations, the second type, include proposals and requests. In some cases, you may have to make a persuasive presentation to obtain authorization for your agency to participate in an experimental drug study. Or, you may present a proposal to your supervisor to conduct research about ways to reach a resistant group of clients. Similarly, in the classroom, when you analyze a case, you are attempting to persuade your audience to understand the logic of your arguments and accept your recommendations. Once you have decided on the type of presentation needed to accomplish your goals, you are ready to consider the audience who will hear your presentation.

Analyze Your Audience

Audience analysis means consciously examining the knowledge, interests, and attitudes of the people who will hear your presentation. Your analysis will help you determine how best to appeal to their concerns, needs, and values; how to organize your material; how to select supporting information; how to choose the appropriate wording; and how to select or prepare appropriate visual aids.

Many presentations may be well delivered, but they fail because speakers do not anticipate audience reaction. You need to consider such characteristics as the size of the group, their level of knowledge about your subject, their interest in the material, their attitude and predispositions toward the subject, and their organizational relationship, if any, to you. For example, if your audience consists of five people, select a site that is small and personal when you present the information. If your audience is large, make sure all members can both hear and see the information you are presenting.

Although individuals within the health care industry tend to be well educated, their technical expertise is usually very specific. Therefore, when planning a presentation, you must ask, "What does this audience already know about this subject?" Never assume that your audience is as knowledgeable about the topic as you are. When analyzing the prospective audience, ask such questions as "What information will I use to get my audience to listen?" and "Will I employ technical data, demonstrations, or statistical comparisons?" Whatever information you use, care should be taken to reach your intended audience. This is particularly true when presenting ideas to laypeople, who generally know much less about the topic than health care professionals. Choose your wording and your examples to match the audience's experience. Within health care, people tend to have high interest in their respective areas but may have less interest in subjects that affect them less directly. Similarly, lay people are often especially interested in their own health but may be easily confused by the technical details about it.

Because all audience members have different perceptions based on personal experiences that have influenced their attitudes about any subject, every audience is unique. Understanding these perceptions will prevent your making bold assumptions that may offend the audience. For example, if your audience consists of people 60–75 years of age, avoid any current slang lest you appear flippant and uncaring. Similarly, if your audience consists of young adults, avoid examples or references to events that they cannot understand because they have not experienced them. Because experience is such an important factor in understanding perceptions, you may not use the same explanations and examples with an audience of parents as you would with a childless audience. Good questions to ask when analyzing an audience are, "What does this group want/need/expect from me?" and "How can I give that to them?"

Once you have answered some of the questions about who your audience is, next ask yourself what type or types of appeal will reach them. When making presentations, you can use the ethical, the emotional, or the logical appeal or any combination of them.

The *ethical appeal* refers to the speaker's or the organization's credibility. It is impossible to separate the speaker's effect on an audience from the content of a message. If listeners regard the speaker highly, they will adopt a more favorable attitude toward the service or idea being presented than if they have a negative impression of the person. Consequently, a speaker must bring to the occasion a strong, positive, personal style. Credibility means believability; you may have a high ethical appeal with members of an audience if they perceive that you have acted with integrity in the past. If, in previous dealings with this audience, you have acted rudely, unethically, or unprofessionally toward them or others, your ethical appeal will be relatively low. Many characteristics such as honesty, dependability, and expertise help to develop credibility. Although it takes some time to establish credibility, it takes only an instant to lose it by saying or doing something unexpected or inappropriate.

The *emotional appeal* uses the audience's motivations to change their thinking or behavior. Because emotion provokes action, speakers often seek to arouse the feelings of their listeners. The emotional appeal is characterized by the use of fear, anger, sympathy, love, jealousy, sex, the desire for attention, the desire for security, or a host of other emotions to persuade the audience. To use the emotional appeal, first analyze the specific emotions to which the audience will respond. Then determine which words, pictures, or actions you can use to best evoke the desired emotion. Once members of the audience are drawn into the persuasion by the emotional "hook," it is easy to ask them to take action to meet the need or to satisfy the emotion that was touched. For example, most people are touched by the vulnerability of children. Therefore, when you show them a touching photograph of a child, you may be able to capitalize on the audience's emotions to get them to do whatever you suggest, such as financially supporting research on childhood diseases. Speakers should be aware, however, that attempts to arouse emotions excessively could lead to a rejection of their arguments by an audience. Thus, the emotional appeal should be used with restraint.

The *logical appeal* draws on an audience's ability to think and reason. This appeal uses sound reasons to show members of an audience why they should change their opinions or actions. The persuasive reasons and the support for those reasons comprise the elements of the logical appeal. For example, if you needed to persuade an audience to follow proper work-related hygiene at a day care facility, you might stress the health and legal ramifications of such behavior. Often, the use of facts and figures is the most effective way to reach audiences that are accustomed to the logical approach in their own work environments.

Conduct Research

Your effectiveness as a speaker depends on what you say about the topic you have selected. Health care research means more than just reading medical journals. Knowing where to look is a starting point for finding the best possible information on your topic, whether it is a classroom case or a work setting. Sometimes the information will come from your personal knowledge, experience, or research. At other times, you may use information collected by others, such as immunization records, census data, admissions/discharge records, inventory records, or pricing information. Furthermore, information from electronic databases or from the Internet can provide current data that may enhance the quality of your presentation.

Your credibility as a speaker – your ethical appeal – will be largely determined by the quality of the information you present. For example, if you are talking about recent trends, data from the 1990 census would damage your credibility unless you want to compare it to 2000 census data. Conversely, up-to-date health care reform legislation passed by various states would be beneficial to an audience that needs to plan strategy in an unstable legislative environment. As you can see, effective speakers always ask what kind of material will meet the needs of the audience.

Consider the Logistics of the Speaking Site

Before you can finalize the organization of your presentation, you must consider some logistical concerns such as the time available for the presentation, the location of the speaking site, and the resources available to deliver the presentation. The first question to ask is, "How much time will I need to give the presentation?" Sometimes you have no control over how long you will speak: you are told the specific amount of time available to you. In such cases, it is imperative that you stay within your time limit. When the time is exceeded, the audience becomes less receptive to your ideas. When given some choice over the length of a presentation, most speakers take too much time. Remember that it is difficult to hold people's attention beyond 20–30 minutes. To improve effectiveness, speakers also need to watch the audience for verbal and nonverbal feedback to evaluate whether their message is being comprehended and accepted.

Second, you need to know where you will make the presentation. You may ask, "Will it be made in a conference room, a traditional classroom, a large auditorium, an office, or a dining hall?" The location of your presentation will determine the kind of delivery and the types of visual aids that you will use as well as how you set up the room. Some guidelines for setting up the speaking site are:

- Arrange seating so that every member of the audience can see and hear you. A semicircular arrangement is preferred if the room and the size of the audience will allow for it.
- Check the lighting, temperature, and noise level of the site to ensure that your audience will be comfortable. Avoid high-traffic areas, such as a room next to a kitchen or one off a busy hallway, which may distract your audience.
- Check any equipment you intend to use to be sure that it can be easily viewed or heard by your audience.
- Remember, if anything can go wrong, it generally will. Therefore, try to anticipate any problems before they occur. For example, when using any kind of projected visual aids, you should carry an extra bulb or have alternate visual aids in case the equipment breaks down. If you are speaking at a site that you have not visited previously, you may even want to bring an extension cord and an adapter plug, tape, push pins, or other supplies that may not be available at the site.

Once you have spent some time planning your presentation, the organization of the information should take much less time.

Organize Your Presentation

In an oral presentation, your audience probably will not have the opportunity to refer to written material; therefore, you must structure the information so that it is very easy to understand the first time it is heard. There is no question that organized or patterned material is easier for an audience to comprehend and retain. Even when you present a lot of detailed information, it will be easier to follow if the overall pattern of organization is simple and clear.

Every effective presentation has an introduction, body, and conclusion. If these are well planned, the audience will be able to follow your ideas easily. We suggest that you prepare a written outline of the information you want to include in these three parts.

Despite the temptation to start with the introduction, we recommend that you start with the core of the presentation, the body. After you have the body developed, then you can attend to the introduction and the conclusion.

Body

When you arrange the body of a presentation, you must remember one thing: a listener's attention span is very limited. Honestly analyze your own attention span – be aware of your own tendency to let your mind wander. You listen to the speaker for a moment, and then perhaps you think of something else, of some problem, or an approaching appointment. Then you return to the speaker. When you become the speaker, remember that people do not hang on your every word.

Various methods are available to develop the body of the presentation. Below are some common ones:

1. Use statistics or other facts.
2. Cite quotations or expert testimony.
3. Employ examples, real or hypothetical.
4. Refer to personal experiences.
5. Use comparisons, contrasts, or analogies to the audience's experiences.

It helps to plan your presentation around intelligent and interesting repetition. Begin by cutting the number of points you intend to cover to a minimum. Build a 5-minute presentation around one point, a 15-minute presentation around two. Even an hour-long talk probably should not cover more than three or four points.

Next, creating suspense as you talk is another way to generate interest from your audience. Try organizing your presentation around the inductive method. That is, give your facts first and gradually build up to the generalizations that they support. If you do this skillfully, using good material, your audience hangs on, wondering what your point will be. If you do not do it skillfully or use dull material, your audience will tune you out and tune into their private thoughts.

Another interest-getting technique is to relate the subject matter to some vital interest of the audience. For example, if you were presenting material to recent heart attack victims on how to live healthier lifestyles, you might begin with a reference to their recent illness. Such an approach, however, might not work with a group of physical therapists who are rehabilitating such individuals.

Introduction

Once the body of the presentation has been prepared, the introduction and the conclusion should be added. After all, you don't know all of what you are introducing until you have prepared the body of the presentation. Good introductions fulfill three purposes: (1) they gain the attention of the audience; (2) they show how the topic is relevant to the audience; and (3) they preview the main points to be covered.

GAIN THE ATTENTION OF THE AUDIENCE

Your first obligation as a speaker is to get the audience interested in your subject with an attention-getting device. Attention-grabbers may include the following:

1. A reference to the event or the occasion. "On Wednesday, April 12, Health Care United treated our 10,000th patient. Although this is only year two of our operation, we cannot rest on our laurels. We need to build a strategic plan for the next decade. That is what I'd like to talk about today."
2. A brief story that allows them to visualize some of the main ideas that you will be discussing. "On June 18, Paul Shivrasta survived complications from an automobile accident the night before. Medical personnel at Our Lady of Mercy Hospital diagnosed his condition and the potential for complications with an RPI404 scanner. This presentation will review the life-saving qualities of this miracle of modern science and its sales potential for the coming year."
3. A quotation by a recognized authority on the subject. "The Surgeon General of the United States has recommended that we reduce our fat intake by 40 percent. Three out of four Americans have too much fat in their diets. This serious problem is one of many reasons why we need to begin our health awareness program."
4. A thought-provoking question that requires the audience members to participate by answering the question or to get involved by raising their hands. "How many of you have been hospitalized in the past year? (Pause for an audience response.) If you have, you know the importance of having a family physician. Today, I'm going to talk about what qualities consumers are looking for in a family physician."
5. A startling statement; it may or may not be a statistic. "If our costs continue to increase over the next three years at the rate they have been over the past decade, we will have to increase our initial office consultation charge to $200. Today, I will present five strategies for reducing costs in . . ."
6. A personal story or reference about the topic. "Seven years ago I suffered from a serious disease. Decatril was prescribed to treat my illness. I'm happy to say that I am fully recovered and owe much of my recovery to this miracle drug. Decatril was just one of the drugs we developed in the past decade. We continue to add new products. This presentation will preview two of them: Daconaise and Zacarin."
7. A joke. This can be particularly tricky in health care as most people feel poor health is not a joking matter. The key is to know your audience and when in doubt . . . don't.

Audiences also respond readily to things that are familiar to them. Events in their hometown, individuals they know, and problems faced by their organizations attract their attention. From your audience analysis, you may be able to make a specific reference to an event or person familiar to this particular group of individuals.

Also, audiences react to the new, the unusual, or the exotic. A promise of new information or knowledge or the description of something beyond their experience will sometimes hold their attention. In other words, show them how they will learn something new as a result of your presentation.

Furthermore, audiences are attracted by competition between principles, organizations, and individuals. The rivalry between two health care organizations can be as dramatic as the competition between baseball teams such as the Boston Red Sox and the New York Yankees.

SHOW HOW THE TOPIC IS RELEVANT TO THE AUDIENCE

Audiences will listen more attentively if you explain "what's in it for them." The relationship of your purpose to your audience and their interests is an important consideration. They will listen more attentively if the topic is vital to them and if it is near in time and place.

PREVIEW THE MAIN POINTS TO BE COVERED

Audiences will listen more attentively if they know where you are going. Previewing the main points of your presentation keeps your audience attuned to what you are saying. Since the attention span of an audience varies from one occasion to the next, clear organization helps increase your credibility and the likelihood that your main points will be remembered.

Conclusion

A presentation can have an excellent introduction and body but still not be effective. Good speakers must leave a favorable impression in the minds of the audience. A good conclusion should accomplish two purposes: (1) the audience should know what is expected of them; (2) they should be in a proper frame of mind to carry it out. To accomplish these goals, the conclusion should consist of two parts: a brief summary of the main points and a final appeal that creates an appropriate ending point. Do not introduce any new information in your conclusion lest you appear unfinished. If some action is expected from the audience, the speaker's expectations should be made clear and easy to follow.

You have probably heard presentations that lacked a real conclusion. The speaker may have looked at his or her watch and announced, "Well, I guess my time is up – that's about all." Since you want your audience to understand something or to take some action, use your conclusion to make a final effort at pushing your main point. Leave the audience with a sense of closure, or completion, that lets them see what you have covered and what you would like to happen next. Conclusions can be developed in a number of ways:

- Summarize your main points.
- Ask the audience to take some action such as buying your product or service or contributing to a particular cause.
- Recall the story, joke, or anecdote in the introduction and elaborate on it or draw a "lesson" from it.

Now that you have structured your presentation, you must find ways to enhance it further. Visual aids are the tools to accentuate the information you want to share.

In summary, introductions and conclusions should be developed after the body of the presentation has been developed. A good introduction gains audience attention, relates the topic to their needs, and previews the organization of the body of the presentation. The conclusion summarizes the main points in the body and provides closure. A good conclusion should leave the audience well disposed to the speaker's purpose.

Internal Transitions and Summaries

Because the audience is listening rather than reading what you are saying, you need to provide ample transitions and internal summaries. Smooth transitions are the key aspect of organization. Transitions serve an important function by linking main points and supporting material. For instance, if your presentation covers three points, one way to transition from point to point is to say "first . . ." (or hold up your index finger), "second . . ." and so on. Other examples include:

- "The first way Daconaise differs from our earlier products is . . ."
- "Now for the second difference . . ."
- "Also . . ."
- "To begin . . ."
- "Finally . . ."

Keep your audience attuned to where you are in the presentation. Listeners do not have the luxury of glancing ahead on a page to see what is coming next; they have to wait for you to say something. Therefore, it is necessary to provide previews to reinforce what is coming next.

Internal summaries are another type of internal organization. Stop at the end of major sections of your presentation to review the main points in that section. This should help the audience retain the main points. No one has ever disputed the old truism (1) tell the audience what you are going to tell them; (2) tell them; and (3) tell them what you just told them. In some situations, speakers provide their audiences with a printed outline of their talk to help them follow the speaker's reasoning.

Prepare Your Visual Aids

Because we live in a visually oriented society, we expect to see as well as hear information. The first purpose of any visual material is to support your message – to enlarge on the main ideas and give substance and credibility to what you are saying. Obviously, the material must be relevant to the idea being supported. Too often a speaker gives in to the urge to show a visually attractive or technically interesting piece of information that has little or no bearing on the subject. Your second reason for using visual aids is to focus attention. A good visual can arrest the wandering thoughts of your audience and bring their attention right down to the specific detail of the message. It forces their mental participation in the subject. When you are dealing with very complex material, as you often will be, you can use a simple illustration to show your audience a single, critical concept within your topic.

Visual material enhances an audience's attention, understanding, and retention. Attention is enhanced when visual material is colorful and attractive. We are more likely to remember material that we both see and hear. In fact, the more senses involved in communicating a message, the more reinforcement there is.

Also, visual material is important for dealing with two potential problems of presentations: length of time and complexity of material. During a long presentation, listeners' minds can wander. Short multimedia segments in the presentation can reawaken or refocus listening. Also, complex material is more easily understood when it can be seen. As a general rule, dollar amounts, percentages, or other numbers as well as unfamiliar material should be seen as well as heard. That means that unfamiliar words, terms, concepts, products, or the like, should be presented visually as well as orally.

Two broad categories of visual aids are available to enhance presentations. One category, *direct viewing visuals*, includes such things as real objects, models, flip charts, handouts, and chalkboards or whiteboards. Real objects are often the best visuals when the audience is small and when seeing "the real thing" will be more convincing than a drawing, diagram, or photograph. For example, if you are touting the quality of a medical device, it might be good to show how a particular component is manufactured – what it looks like, feels like, sounds like, and so forth. Using real items can best do this. To illustrate a key point such as ease of assembly, the object could also be shown both assembled and disassembled.

If the object itself is small enough to handle, it can be an effective visual aid. The use of objects is subject to certain constraints. First, the object and any important components must be clearly visible at about 30 to 35 feet. Ideally, the main parts of the object should be visible from the worst seat in the room. Highlighting certain parts with bright colors can enhance the object's visibility.

Models are very effective for showing how a dialysis unit, operating room, or visitor waiting room will look. This type of visual can be very persuasive if the audience is small enough that everyone can see the model as it is being discussed.

Flip charts are excellent for use with audiences that are small enough to see the information on the chart. Most speakers "write as they talk" when using flip charts. This flexibility gives an informal, conversational tone to a presentation. However, some information, such as key words, may be put on the chart ahead of time and elaborated on during the speech. If this method is used, the words should be covered by leaving the top page blank and lifting it when ready to show the key words. You may prefer to use a flip chart and include only one idea on a page. When you have finished one idea, simply flip the page to the next idea. The final page should include all your key ideas to refresh the listeners' memories during the summary. A word chart or flip chart can also call attention to single words or phrases, technical words, new or seldom-used words, foreign words or phrases, or a list of items. Of course, it does not matter what you put on a word chart or flip chart if the text is too small for easy viewing. Using hard-to-read visuals is one of the most consistent and damaging mistakes made by speakers.

Handouts allow you to fit more information on a printed page than with other visuals, but avoid doing so. Keep handouts simple. Summarize major points, but do not provide the audience with your entire presentation. If possible, distribute the handout when it is needed rather than at the beginning of the presentation. Otherwise, the audience may read the handout while you are explaining background information needed to understand the ideas presented in the handout.

Chalkboards or whiteboards are useful for presenting informal visuals to small groups. Some major problems presented by chalkboards and whiteboards are the time necessary to write the information, lack of cleanliness of some boards, poor penmanship of the user, and failure of the user to erase items once they have been considered. If you plan to use a board, practice and make certain you have all the necessary equipment (appropriate markers, eraser, and so on). If your visual is complex, you may find it helpful to place it on the board before your presentation. Many portable chalkboards or whiteboards have two sides, thus permitting you to keep your material from view until you need it.

The second category of visual aids, *projected visuals*, includes slides, videotapes, overhead transparencies, and computer presentations. Slides can be effective when showing how something looks at particular phases, such as the stages in the progress of a disease. Of course, slides should be organized before they are loaded into the projector. The speaker should practice using them so none are in upside down or backward or out of sequence. Remember to allow enough time to develop the slides if you are producing them yourself.

Videotapes are effective if you need to show a process. Few other types of visuals can capture the drama of a videotape. For example, if you were demonstrating a surgical procedure, a videotape could be excellent. It could show exactly how to perform the surgery and could even be done in slow motion or freeze-frame to allow surgeons to see particularly delicate processes. Or, it could be used to demonstrate the ease of a minor surgical procedure to a patient to dispel anxiety.

Overhead transparencies work best when a large amount of material must be presented and there is little time or money for a more sophisticated type of presentation. Overheads give you a great deal of flexibility. For example, you can circle an important point or change a number or label. In addition, you can place one transparency over another to create a multilayered look. Prepared overheads, such as charts or diagrams, can offer a neat appearance and a more polished presentation. The use of overheads allows you to vary the size of the image through adjusting the distance from the projector to the screen. Finally, even if a transparency is created "on the spot," it still has the advantage of giving you the opportunity to face the audience. In this way you can maintain eye contact and observe audience feedback while you talk about your material.

Computer presentations are being prepared by increasing numbers of speakers. When using presentation software such as Microsoft PowerPoint, Lotus Freelance, and Corel Presentation, speakers should consider the following points:

- Input your ideas into the built-in outliner that will help you organize your thoughts. On-screen assistance is generally available to those needing help with various organizational plans.
- Select features for displaying your text (font, type size, color, texture, border, and so on).
- Edit each visual, indicating the exact sequence of each visual and special effects (graphics, transitions, sounds, and motion).
- Generate printed handouts, slides, transparencies, or a slide show for an on-screen presentation.

Many programs provide templates (prepared designs) that suggest features and colors that work well together. You simply select the template, and your information (text or graphics) is formatted automatically. After viewing the results, you can revise the format if you wish. These templates help the novice presenter resist the temptation to create overwhelmingly complex visuals simply because the technology is available.

Presentation software offers so many choices of typeface, so many sizes of print, and so many choices of color that the temptation is to use some or all of them in your slides or handouts. However, the best slides or handouts are simple ones that follow the guidelines presented below:

- Use no more than three to six lines of text.
- Use phrases rather than sentences.
- Use uppercase and lowercase type (all caps are difficult to read).
- Use a simple typeface.
- Use only one or two fonts to generate text.
- Use bullets or numbering for listing.
- Allow the same amount of space at the top of each visual.
- Use color, boldface, or large-sized type for emphasis.

Running an on-screen presentation takes some practice. Depending on the length of your presentation it may be difficult to remember what information is on each slide. Experience teaches us to rehearse the material to help develop our verbal introduction, develop effective transitions from one slide to another, and conclude effectively. Although they are very effective for large audiences, on-screen presentations may overwhelm a smaller audience. Rather than focusing on the material, the audience may be distracted by the special effects used to move from one idea to another. In addition, on-screen presentations limit audience interaction, which may be an important part of your presentation.

Guidelines for Selecting Visual Aids

Although visual material is almost always a benefit for presentations, its effectiveness depends upon several factors. Certain kinds of topics lend themselves better to visual presentation than others. The speaker and the audience can make a difference as well. The following factors should be taken into consideration when deciding what kind of visual materials to prepare:

1. *The constraints of the topic.* Some topics will limit your choice of visual aids. For example, if you were explaining to a group of laypeople how microsurgery is performed on a hand, you would not use a flip chart because it would be ineffective. Also, you would probably not show a videotape of the surgery being performed because the sight of blood may upset some individuals. Instead, you might use a model of the hand. However, a videotape might be very effective in teaching surgeons how to perform the procedure.

2. *The availability of the equipment.* If the speaking site does not have an overhead projector, you could not use transparencies. Similarly, if the site does not have an electrical outlet near the podium, you would not be able to use a projected visual. Always check to see what equipment is available or bring your own. Also, verify that your computer presentation will run on the version of software installed on the available equipment.

3. *The cost of the visual.* If your budget is very small, a transparency, flip chart, or a handout may be preferable to the more elaborate types of visual aids such as slides or videotapes. A limited budget may have a serious effect on what you produce and how you show it; that is, your budget may affect your effectiveness. A poorly done visual presentation may be more harmful than a presentation without visual material.

4. *The difficulty of producing the visual.* If you have only two days to prepare for your presentation, it may be impossible to assemble a scale model of a labor/delivery room interior or process slides of a sequence of cancer growth.

5. *The appropriateness of the visual to the audience.* The type of audience and the nature of the presentation affect the choice of visual aids. Most people now are accustomed to extremely professional presentations. When you try to use similar techniques, remember that you should use visual aids and techniques that are comfortable for you. Also, bear in mind that your audience may be expecting entertainment along with a substantive presentation. Their expectations may be that speakers always use visual aids. Some charts, graphs, and diagrams may be too technical for anyone but specialists to grasp. Detailed and complicated tables and charts that require considerable time to digest should be avoided. When in doubt, keep your visuals short and simple.

6. *The appropriateness of the visual to the speaker.* Visual aids require skill in order to be effectively presented. A speaker must be able to write large and legibly and draw well-proportioned diagrams to use a flip chart. Projected visuals require skill in handling slides, videotape, or film. Unless you feel comfortable with a particular visual medium, avoid using it. A dynamic speaker who understands the material well probably has less need for visual aids than another speaker, who may be less experienced or dynamic. The use of visual material and multimedia techniques, however, can help an ordinary speaker seem more exciting and can boost the speaker's confidence.

7. *The size of the audience.* The smaller the audience, the easier it is to adapt your information to individuals and to respond to individuals' questions. You cannot respond to larger audiences in such individualized ways, however, and the use of visual materials can help clarify information for larger groups. Of course, the smaller group can more easily see some kinds of visual aids than can larger ones. Larger audiences require larger and bolder visual aids.

8. *The appropriateness of the visual to the time limit.* The speaker should carefully check the time required to display and explain a visual aid to make sure the main ideas of the presentation would not be neglected. Any visual aid that needs too much explanation should be avoided. An appropriate visual aid should be simple, clear, and brief.

Visual aids often increase audience interest. Remember to keep your graphics big and simple. Do not display a visual aid until you want the audience to see it. While the aid is up, call your listeners' attention to everything you want them to see. Take the aid away as soon as you are through with it. If you are using a projection unit, turn it off whenever it is not in use. Be sure to cue every visual aid in your speaker's script. Otherwise you may forget it.

Once you have planned and organized the content of your presentation and prepared your visual aids, you are ready to deliver your presentation.

Deliver Your Presentation

During the first few minutes of a presentation, the audience "sizes up" the speaker and draws conclusions about his or her credibility. Since credibility is essential to achieving their goals, speakers should understand how to gain it.

Establish Credibility

The factors that determine credibility include the speaker's enthusiasm, expertise, and trustworthiness. Enthusiasm is conveyed through tone of voice, eye contact, and energy. Clearly, speakers can display these characteristics by believing in the subject and acting as if they enjoy conveying the information. For example, at the beginning of the presentation, look directly at the audience, give a sincere smile, and say the first few words with energy and excitement. Your credibility will be off to a great start.

Expertise is conveyed through the accuracy of your information, the amount of experience you have had with the subject, and the confidence with which you speak. To guarantee this aspect of your credibility, check your facts, refer to your personal experiences with the topic, and talk about them with confidence.

Trustworthiness refers to the audience's perception that the speaker is unbiased. Consistency in dealing with people over a period of time is important to establish trust. If the audience has had positive dealings with or has heard good things about the speaker, they are likely to perceive him or her as trustworthy.

Reduce Speech Anxiety

Speaking in front of groups has long been recognized as a significant fear. This fear, called speech anxiety, detracts from your credibility. Several techniques can relieve this problem if you are willing to invest a small amount of time in the endeavor. The first technique is borrowed from athletes. Before major events they mentally see themselves doing all the correct things to ensure a win; then they picture themselves winning the event. Speakers should do the same thing. For several nights before the presentation, just before falling asleep, you should close your eyes and picture yourself making a great speech. This positive mental preparation actually works!

Another characteristic of speech anxiety is a lack of control over one's breathing. Again, this can be corrected by practicing an exercise several days before the speech. Select a quiet place where you can sit. Place both feet on the floor and put one hand on your stomach. Now take a deep breath; then exhale deeply (you have done this correctly if you can feel your hand rise and fall on your stomach). Clear your mind of other thoughts and start to focus on the breathing. Continue the deep breathing. Think about how it feels to have the air pass through your nostrils. Think about the pressure on your eyes, the sound of your breathing, and so on. If other thoughts intervene, banish them and return to focus on your breathing. Perform this exercise a minimum of five minutes before you quit. Do this as many times a day as you can to gain control of your breathing. On the day of the presentation, you can do the same exercise for a few seconds just before you speak.

If you suffer from severe speech anxiety and these exercises do not help you, perhaps some work with a therapist will help you uncover the root of your severe anxiety.

Use Your Visual Aids

As we mentioned before, the use of effective visual aids can enhance your presentation and improve your credibility. Conversely, poor use of visual aids can detract from your presentation. Some guidelines for using visual aids are as follows:

1. Avoid turning your back on the audience while you look at or point to a visual aid. Talk to the audience, not to your visuals.

2. Show the visual aid only when you are talking about it; otherwise the audience may be distracted from what you are saying. For example, if you are using transparencies, cover everything except what you are talking about at the moment.
3. Refrain from removing the visual before the audience has had an opportunity to look at the information for themselves. To guarantee that you do not speed past the visuals, make it a point to go over orally everything that is on your visuals.
4. Organize the visuals in the order in which you will use them so you will appear prepared and confident.

Manage Your Nonverbal Communication

Several dimensions of nonverbal communication related to speaking include (1) kinesics, the way people use their bodies to communicate; (2) proxemics, the way people use space to communicate; and (3) paralanguage, the way people use their voices to enhance the verbal message.

When making presentations, two of the most important types of kinetic behavior are gestures and eye contact. Speakers are rarely credible when they stand rigidly behind a podium, grasp it as if it were a crutch, and seldom glance up from their notes to look at the audience. Similarly, poor posture, hands in pockets, and playing with objects, such as chalk or pointers, lessen a speaker's credibility.

Speakers who recognize that "space communicates" will use it wisely. For example, if the audience is small, it may be better to sit at the head of the group than to "stand over them" to deliver the information. Also, if you must deliver unfavorable information, stand close to the audience to appear more sincere and understanding.

Aspects of the voice that affect credibility include volume, rate, pitch, tone, and voice quality. The "sound" of the voice (voice quality) such as raspiness or a nasal sound evokes images in the minds of the listeners; however, it is very difficult to change the voice quality you have. On the other hand, tone, pitch, rate, and volume are easily changed. For example, the person who has a monotone can make the voice seem less monotonous by saying some words softly and others loudly. Even though the tone hasn't changed, the audience perceives that the tone is varied. A low pitch is viewed as more credible in our culture, and a high pitch is often associated with nervousness. Speakers should start talking at the lowest pitch they can achieve. Then if their voice rises a little during the speech, it will seem less offensive than if the speaker begins with a high pitch.

Prepare to Deliver Your Presentation

The situation, the audience, and the speaker determine the type of delivery a speaker will use. The formality or informality of the situation greatly affects delivery. The more formal it is and the larger the audience, the fewer gestures and movements speakers make. They limit themselves more to their position behind the lectern and use a more emphatic speaking voice to compensate for fewer gestures. In very informal situations, speakers are free to move away from the podium and interact with the audience, even strolling between tables or down aisles.

The available equipment will also determine delivery. For instance, if the size of the audience necessitates a microphone, speakers should not move away from the microphone. They may also need to adapt themselves to various tables or other unusual speaking platforms that will hold their notes, visuals, or other forms of support.

The larger the audience, the louder speakers must talk unless there is a microphone. Likewise, eye contact is more challenging with large groups. Therefore, delivery to small groups can be more informal and conversational than with large groups. However, speakers should always look at the audience even if it is impossible to make direct eye contact with members.

Determine the Type of Delivery You Will Use

Several methods for delivering material can be employed, and each has its unique advantages. The four methods of delivery are (1) impromptu, (2) manuscript, (3) memorized, and (4) extemporaneous.

Impromptu delivery requires speaking spontaneously on a topic. This type of delivery is generally inappropriate for technical or complex material because you may forget crucial information if the presentation has not been carefully planned. Impromptu delivery is often used at social occasions such as introductions at an after-dinner speaking engagement or at a professional meeting where you are asked to "sit in" for someone who was going to introduce a speaker but was called out because of an emergency.

Manuscript delivery requires that the speaker read from a prepared text. This type of delivery is ineffective in most presentations because audiences generally prefer more eye contact (they also dislike having material read to them). However, manuscript delivery is a must in one particular situation: when a crisis has occurred. For example, if a client receives the wrong medication and dies as a result, the media is quick to "look for the story." The spokesperson for the organization should never deliver the information in an impromptu manner. Rather, the response should be carefully prepared and read to the media because any misstatement in such a situation could result in litigation against the organization or, at the least, a change in the public's perception of the agency or organization.

Memorized delivery is self-explanatory. In most cases it should be discouraged because memorized presentations usually sound "canned" rather than natural. Worse yet, the speaker may forget part of what was memorized and may lose confidence in himself or herself to remember the rest of the presentation. However, this type of delivery might be appropriate in situations where the presentation will be only a few minutes long, such as introducing a speaker or "saying a few words" about someone at a retirement party.

Extemporaneous delivery is the preferred approach for most presentations. This type of delivery allows the use of notes or an outline to deliver the information.

The speaker should talk in a conversational tone but refer periodically to notes to be sure that all the information is covered. Some people prefer following a precise outline, whereas others prefer using note cards to deliver a presentation. With the use of presentation software such as Microsoft PowerPoint, speakers can even show the audience their "notes" by making them part of certain slides. Each person must find what works best for him or her. Although notes can be a valuable resource for a speaker, they can easily become a psychological crutch. To make sure that they do not become a crutch, remember to use notes only when absolutely necessary. Extemporaneous delivery helps build the speaker's credibility in the eyes of an audience.

Rehearse Your Delivery

Preparation influences a speaker's delivery. A speaker who is well prepared and has something valuable to communicate will be more comfortable physically and vocally. If speakers are unsure of themselves and the material, they may be tempted to read word for word from their outlines. Being too self-conscious or nervous can create physical and vocal qualities and mannerisms that detract from the message. Too much concern with oneself or the ideas and too little concern for the audience will also hinder a speaker's delivery. Always practice aloud what you want to say. You don't need an audience; you can talk aloud to yourself, to your dog or cat, or to the trees. Rehearsing will not only give you confidence but will also help you to hear any awkward phrasing or words that are hard to pronounce. If possible, practice with your visuals so you will know when to use them and how much time it takes to discuss them.

Delivery is not something added to a speech but is an integral part of it. Consider the following when rehearsing your presentation:

1. Practice how you will stand to open the presentation. Will you use a podium or hold your notes?
2. Practice what to do with your hands, but keep them at or above the waist. Gestures give credibility unless they are erratic or overly large and dramatic. Notice if you do anything distracting such as repeatedly scratching your nose or fiddling with your hair.
3. Rehearse projecting your voice; if you will be using a microphone, practice positioning it correctly and holding it to avoid feedback. Practice articulating your words and pronouncing them correctly. A speaker who puts the "-ing" endings on words will seem more educated than one who leaves off the "g".
4. Practice sounding positive and enthusiastic. In a sense, a speaker is a momentary actor and sometimes has to "act" more enthusiastic than his or her normal speech patterns.
5. Rehearse ways to differentiate the main points in some way. Perhaps you will hold up your fingers as you say point 1, point 2, and so on. Or perhaps you will say the points louder or softer or more slowly than the rest of the speech. Or maybe you will pause in some places for emphasis or effect.

6. Involve the audience by practicing eye contact with imaginary audience members in all parts of the room.

After you have rehearsed your speech, you will be prepared for making a dynamic presentation. Before we leave the subject of delivery, we should discuss how to prepare for questions that may arise from your presentation.

Manage Questions from the Audience

Some speaking situations require that the speaker give the audience an opportunity to ask questions. At other times, the speaker may simply want to involve the audience by following a presentation with a question-and-answer session. Whether or not you use this procedure depends on the occasion, the audience, and the amount of time available. You can use this procedure to reinforce key points and gain acceptance of your ideas. Any question-and-answer period should be well organized and brief. To make the most of the available time, follow these guidelines:

- Ask for questions in a positive way. For instance, you could say, "Who has the first question?" If no one asks a question, you may say, "You may be wondering . . ." or "I am often asked . . ." After supplying an answer to the question you have asked, you may ask, "Are there any other questions?"
- Look at the entire audience when answering a question. You are addressing everyone, not just the person asking the question.
- If the question being asked cannot be heard by the entire audience, repeat it for the rest of the group.
- Keep your answers concise and to the point; do not give another speech. You risk losing the audience's attention as well as discouraging further questions.
- Cut off a rambling questioner politely. If the person starts to make a speech without getting to the question, wait until he or she takes a breath and then interrupt with, "Thanks for your comment. Next question." Then look to the other side of the room.
- Remain in control of the situation. Establish a time limit for questions and answers and announce it to the audience before the questions begin. Anticipate the types of questions your audience may ask and think how you will answer. Never lose your temper as you respond to someone who is trying to make you look bad. You may respond with something like, "I respect your opinion even though I don't agree with it." Then restate your response to the issue.
- Watch your nonverbal communication when answering questions. For example, pointing a finger at the audience, putting your hands on your hips, or raising your voice above the pitch of the presentation may give the appearance of authoritarianism and rudeness.
- Look for the unexpected and plan ahead as much as possible. Anticipate questions from your audience and formulate answers.

The question-and-answer session is important to your overall presentation success. Since your credibility can be enhanced or lost in the question-and-answer period, you should prepare intelligently for the session and consider appropriate strategies for handling difficult situations.

Some Final Thoughts

To ensure an effective presentation, you should make sure that everyone involved has the same goal or purpose for the presentation. Once the goal has been established, you must conduct an audience analysis, develop the body of your presentation, organize your visual aid(s), select an introduction, and create a strong conclusion. If appropriate, you should also schedule and practice for a question-and-answer session.

With the growing importance of health care in our society, having the skills and the ability to present your point of view in a convincing manner is essential to reaching your personal and career goals. Presenting information orally is a challenging task. However, if you follow the guidelines for planning, organizing, and delivering that we have suggested, your presentation will be rewarding to both you and your audience.

Cases in the Health Care Sector

The US Health Care System – Participants, Financing, and Trends: An Industry Note

An understanding of the health services environment is provided as a background for the organizationally specific strategic
management cases presented in this book. This Industry Note
describes pivotal historical events, major characteristics, and key
factors for success in the industry as well as the most significant
organizational and professional participants. Part of the students'
job in analyzing the cases will be to evaluate the uncertainties,
determine their importance for the specific issues to be resolved
in the case, and then propose – and be prepared to defend – the
actions that they think are strategically justified.

History of the Health Services Environment

Over the past 50 years, the history of the health services environment was characterized by three basic trends:

1. Growth in the scientific knowledge that underpinned professional practice in health care;

This case was written by Stuart A. Capper, Tulane University. It is intended as a
basis for classroom discussion rather than to illustrate either effective or ineffective handling of an administrative situation. Used with permission from Stuart
Capper.

2. Growth in the percentage of US financial resources allocated to the provision of health services; and

3. Change in the relationships among health care professionals, health service organizations, payors for health services, and health care clients.

These trends did not proceed consistently. Rather, growth in scientific knowledge accelerated over time. Growth in financial resources allocated to health care was rapid between 1950 and 1990, leveled off during the nineties, and accelerated again during the early years of the twenty-first century. The change in organizational relationships was a more recent trend and these relationships continue to evolve. Each trend significantly impacted the health care environment that emerged in the beginning of the twenty-first century.

Growth in Scientific Knowledge

Prior to the 1940s, medical armamentarium and medical research were limited. World War II marked the beginning of a dramatic expansion of both medical knowledge and federal medical research funding.[1] Prior to the War, federal funding of medical research was almost entirely intramural. That is, federal money was used to fund research in federal labs and few grants were awarded to outside organizations for research projects. Most private not-for-profit research was foundation funded and the amount was not highly significant. Since the late 1940s, a consistently growing program of federally funded grants for medical research outside federal labs occurred. The national priority given to innovations in medical care generated a steadily increasing scientific base for medical practice and a rapidly diversifying technology for application in patient care. Exhibit 1/1 illustrates the growth in federal funding for medical research.

The impact of this extraordinary increase in scientific knowledge on the health care industry was multifaceted. First, the adult lifespan increased about two years per decade during each decade since the 1950s. This represented a significant change because, prior to the 1950s, life expectancy increased as a result of decreases in infant deaths. After the 1950s, in part because of expanded medical knowledge, life expectancy increased because of years added at the end and middle of life.

Second, the growth in medical specialization was likely related to the increasing amount of medical knowledge that had to be mastered initially as well as the substantial continuing education required to remain current in any given specialty. Also, increasing technological options created economically viable specialty areas where none existed previously.[2] In 1950, there were 28 different specialty and subspecialty residency programs in the United States; by 2004, the number had grown to 121.[3]

Finally, data from the Health Care Financing Administration (HCFA) suggested that the increase in medical knowledge contributed to the rapid cost escalation in medical care. The most recent HCFA analysis for fiscal 2000–01 indicated that 46 percent of the 8.7 percent increase in medical care expenditures for that year could be attributed to increased intensity ("changes in the use and kinds of services and supplies") for medical services.[4]

Exhibit 1/1: National Institutes of Health Grants for Medical Research (Dollar Amounts per Year, Selected Years 1940–2000)

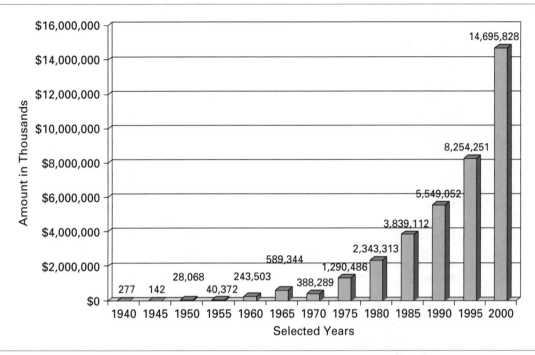

Source: *NIH Almanac 1999*, www.nih.gov/about/almanac/index.html; NIH Office of the Budget, Spending History, http://officeofbudget.od.nih.gov/ui/HomePage.aspx.

Growth in Health Care Spending

The second trend was growth in the percentage of US financial resources allocated to the provision of health services compared with the percentage spent by other developed countries in the world. By 2002, the United States spent about $5,200 per person annually on health care, significantly more than other industrialized nations (see Exhibit 1/2).

Some analysts suggested that the stabilization of expenditure growth relative to gross domestic product (GDP) during the 1990s was a result of the third trend, the changing relationships among health services providers, health care organizations, payors, and patients.[5]

Changing Relationships

Prior to World War II, there was little experimentation with organizational design in the health services industry, resulting in a relatively simple and stable market. After World War II, few new health plan organizations developed,

Exhibit 1/2: Per Capita Health Spending in Industrialized Nations 2002

Austria	$2,220
Belgium	2,515
Canada	2,931
Czech Republic	1,118
Denmark	2,580
Finland	1,943
France	2,736
Germany	2,817
Greece	1,814
Hungary	1,079
Iceland	2,807
Ireland	2,367
Italy	2,166
Luxembourg	3,065
Mexico	553
Netherlands	2,643
New Zealand	1,857
Norway	3,083
Poland	654
Portugal	1,702
Spain	1,646
Sweden	2,517
Switzerland	3,445
United Kingdom	2,160
United States	**5,267**

Source: Organization for Economic Cooperation and Development, http://www.oecd.org/dataoecd/13/53/31963451.xls

covering substantial groups of enrollees. Examples of this type of organization included Group Health Cooperative of Puget Sound and Kaiser Permanente in California. This type of "pre-paid" and "capitated" health plan rather than the traditional "fee-for-service" system was strongly opposed by organized medicine and such plans developed in only a limited number of states.

In capitated systems, providers were prospectively paid a fixed premium per person or per family that covered specified benefits and the payment was independent of the amount of service provided. Fee-for-service was the more traditional method of payment for health care services where a specific payment was made for a specific service rendered. In 1973, the Health Maintenance Organization (HMO) Act was passed by Congress and signed by President Nixon. This law created a set of subsidies and standards that encouraged this capitated or "managed care" form of health care delivery organization to grow. Although encouraged by the legislation, managed care plan enrollment growth was slow during this period.

The factor that spawned more growth in the managed care industry was the rapid health care inflation of the 1980s and early 1990s. For many employers, employee health care costs became their largest single uncontrolled expenditure.

Exhibit 1/3 illustrates the escalation in the cost of health care for employees as a percent of profit for private employers that led to various proposals and programs, including "managing care" to attempt to slow health care costs.

Between 1965 and 1987, employee health benefit spending rose from about 14 percent of after-tax profits to nearly 100 percent of after-tax profits. This situation caused employers to look for ways to stabilize and possibly reduce the cost of health care benefits. Employers began to experiment with and embrace new organizational relationships with their employees (as both payors and clients), health care organizations, providers, and insurors. A diverse array of organizational arrangements evolved, with most of them generally under the rubric of "managed care." These new organizational forms, with their emphasis on efficiency and cost containment, appeared to be succeeding – at least in the short run. During the 1990s, health care cost inflation, as measured as a percent of GDP, stabilized. National health expenditures as a percent of GDP remained between 13 and 14 percent for the entire decade. In 2000, trends began to suggest that this cost-stabilizing effect of managed care might be temporary. By 2002, national health expenditures as a percent of GDP had risen to 14.9 percent. Analysts' projections then suggested increasing proportions of US financial resources would be devoted to health care over the first decade of the twenty-first century.[6]

Exhibit 1/3: Health Service Spending as a Percent of After-Tax Profit; Selected Years 1965–1987

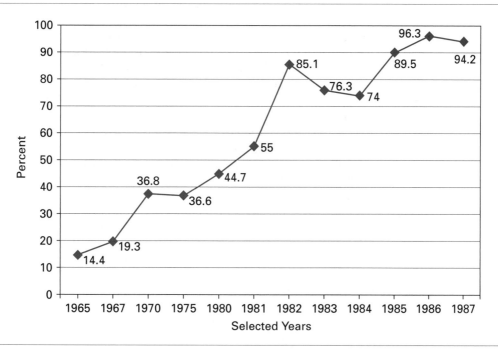

Source: Adapted from D. R. Levit, M. S. Freeland, and D. R. Waldo, "Health Spending and Ability to Pay: Business, Individuals, and Government," *Health Care Financing Review* 10, no. 3 (Spring 1989), Table 5, p. 9.

Significant Events Impacting Health Care Trends

During the past 50 years, many events contributed to these three trends; a handful of them were particularly significant (see Exhibit 1/4).

Economic Characteristics of the Health Services Sector

The overall size of the nation's economy was gauged by the use of gross domestic product statistics. GDP measured the value of all goods and services produced by all sectors of the economy from resources within the United States. The proportion of GDP contributed by the health services sector was rapidly increasing. This has occurred during a period when the GDP itself increased twentyfold from $526.40 billion to $10.48 trillion. Hence, health services have been acquiring an increasingly significant proportion of a rapidly growing US economy. The growth in health expenditures per capita has been dramatic. Per capita health care expenditures between 1960 and 2001 increased nearly thirty-fivefold.

The relationship of the health services component of GDP to other components could be illustrated by considering the sector breakdown in 1950 versus the more recent figures for 2000. In 1950, the health services sector was $4.7 billion of a total GDP of $294.3 billion. Numerous sectors of the economy were larger in dollar terms than health services. For example, the agriculture, forestry, and fisheries sector was four times as large as the health services sector (see Exhibit 1/5). Among the other sectors that were larger than health services were: mining; primary metals manufacturing; machinery manufacturing; food products; transportation; electric, gas, and sanitary utilities; real estate; and the federal government.

By 2000, the situation had changed significantly: health services made up $485.4 billion of a $9.22 trillion GDP. Of those sectors mentioned, the only one that remained larger than health services was real estate. Health services became larger, in GDP terms, than the entire federal government. In addition, the agriculture, forestry, and fisheries sector, that had been almost four times the size of the health services sector, was only about 25 percent of the size of health services in 2000. In 1950, the food products sector was over twice the size of the health services sector. However, by 2000, the food products category was less than one fourth the size of health services. Similarly, real estate, nearly five times the size of the health services sector in 1950, was about twice as large as the health services sector in 2000. The relationship of the health services industry to other sectors of the US economy was significantly altered by the extraordinarily rapid growth in expenditures for health care products. Even rapid growth in other sectors of the economy was no match for the explosive growth in health services.

The growth in health expenditures has not been consistent over time. Up until 1965, growth in health expenditures was moderate. Following the creation of Medicare and Medicaid in 1965, expenditures began to increase rapidly. This rapid growth continued until the 1990s, when expenditures as a percent of GDP

Exhibit 1/4: Significant Health Care Events

1940s – Introduction of antibiotics, penicillin, and sulfonamides gave physicians their first effective therapies for treating infectious diseases. These drugs accelerated the shift from infectious diseases to chronic diseases as the chief source of mortality in the United States.

1946 – Passage of the Hill-Burton Act for Health Facilities Construction stimulated the first major involvement by the federal government in a national program to allocate resources to health services. Over the next 30 years, the program provided billions of dollars in construction subsidies primarily to hospitals. Between 1940 and 1987, community hospital beds per capita increased 25 percent although some areas of the country, such as the East South Central Region, experienced as much as a threefold increase.[a]

1950s – Development of modern anesthesiology, particularly the introduction of synthetic agents for anesthesia, led to significantly reduced risks in surgery, especially for higher-risk patients.

1960s – Extension of the adult lifespan by about two years per decade during each decade subsequent to the 1950s.

1963 – Passage of the Health Professionals Education Assistance Act enabled 41 new medical schools to be opened in the United States (a 48 percent increase).

1964 – Surgeon General's Report on Smoking and Health identified cigarette smoking as one of the primary preventable causes of morbidity and premature death.

1965 – Passage of Medicare and Medicaid (The Social Security Amendments of 1965) marked the first large-scale federal initiative to provide health insurance for major segments of the population. The elderly, and to some extent the poor, became beneficiaries of congressionally mandated health insurance programs. Between 1967 and 1997, total expenditures for Medicare enrollees increased from $4.74 billion to $213.58 billion. During the same period, per capita fee-for-service payments for enrollees increased nearly twenty-fivefold from $217 to $5,314.[b]

1972 – Passage of Social Security Amendments in 1972 created Professional Standards Review Organizations (PSROs), the first direct intervention by the federal government into medical practice by mandating the creation of "standards of care."[c]

1975 – Goldfarb vs. Virginia Bar (421 US 713) was a Supreme Court decision that effectively removed the traditional "learned professions" exemption from antitrust laws. Professional practices were no longer immune from price-fixing restrictions and professional associations could not mandate bans on professional advertising.

1983 – Passage of Social Security Amendments that created the prospective payment system (PPS) for hospital services to Medicare beneficiaries. Financial incentives for hospital care providers were significantly changed.

1992 – Medicare introduced the resource-based relative value scale (RBRVS) system for determining physician payments. Rather than basing payments on reasonable, customary, and prevailing charges in the community, Medicare based its payments to physicians on RBRVS. In addition to Medicare, RBRVS became the leading methodology used by most managed care companies. The system incorporated three basic relative value units (RVUs) to determine the physician's reimbursement: (1) an RVU for physician work time; (2) an RVU for practice expense; and (3) an RVU for malpractice expense.

2000 – Scientists announced they had mapped a first draft of the entire human genome. This achievement created the promise of significant advances in treatment and cure of many genetically based diseases. In addition, it introduced an array of unresolved philosophical and ethical questions for policy makers, health insurors, and health care providers.

2001 – Health Insurance Portability and Accountability Act took effect. The Act, among other things, significantly increased provider and insuror accountability for the privacy and security of patient information. These new responsibilities, with their substantial legal penalties, began to change how members of the medical care community interacted with patients and with each other.

---

[a] National Center for Health Statistics, *Health, United States, 2000* (Hyattsville, MD: US Government Printing Office, 2000), Table 110, p. 156.
[b] Ibid., Table 134, p. 350.
[c] George J. Annas, S. A. Law, R. E. Rosenblatt, and K. R. Wing, *American Health Law* (Boston, MA: Little, Brown and Company, 1990), pp. 526–527.

Exhibit 1/5: Selected Sector Breakdown of GDP, 1950 vs. 2000 (in billions of current dollars)

	1950	2000
Total Gross National Product	294.3	9,224.0
Health Services	4.7	485.4
Agriculture, Forestry, and Fisheries	20.7	125.2
Mining	9.4	95.2
Primary Metals Industries	7.5	57.4
Machinery Manufacturing	7.0	236.0
Gas, Electric, and Sanitary Services	5.5	217.9
Food Products	10.7	118.2
Transportation	16.7	281.1
Real Estate	23.0	1,018.3
Federal Government	18.2	353.0

Source: US Bureau of Economic Analysis, Department of Commerce, Industry Accounts Data, Gross Product by Industry, http://www.bea.doc.gov/ARTICLES/2001/11november/1101gdpxind.pdf

stabilized. Recent data shows that expenditures again began to take a larger proportion of the GDP over the early years of the twenty-first century. (See Exhibit 1/6.)

Of the $ 1,420,700,000,000 spent on health services and supplies in 2001, nearly 75 percent went to five provider categories – hospitals, physicians, other professional services, nursing homes, and drugs. Exhibit 1/7 presents a percentage distribution breakdown for all major components of US national health expenditures in 2002.

Hospitals

Between 1970 and 1990, the hospital sector accounted for approximately 40 percent of total expenditures for health services and supplies. However, the percentage of total expenditures attributable to the hospital sector declined during the past decade. By 2002, the figure stood at 31.3 percent. This expenditure trend was related to a real decline in the use of the inpatient component of the hospital sector. Discharges from nonfederal short-stay hospitals per 1,000 population decreased significantly over the past 20 years. In 1985, there were 151.4 discharges per 1,000 population from nonfederal short-stay hospitals. By 2002, this number decreased to 122.9 discharges per 1,000. During the same period, the actual hospital days of care provided per 1,000 population declined from 997.5 to 541.0.[7] (It should be noted that although hospital discharges have very recently begun to increase, lengths of stay continue to decline and hence total hospital days of care rendered continued to decline.) However, as inpatient utilization of hospitals declined, outpatient utilization increased. Between 1995 and 2002, the number of visits to hospital outpatient departments increased. Total outpatient visits in hospitals increased from 67 million in 1995 to over 83 million in 2002.[8]

Exhibit 1/6: National Health Expenditures, Selected Years 1970–2002

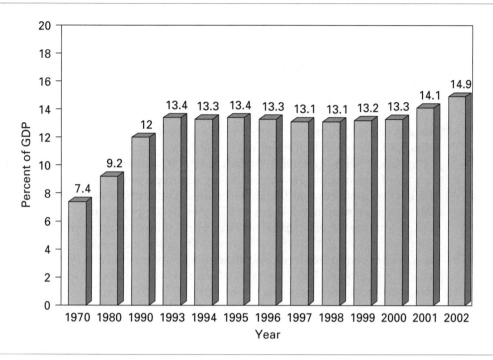

Source: US Health Care Financing Administration, http://www.cms.hhs.gov/statistics/nhe/historical/tl.asp

Exhibit 1/7: National Health Expenditures 2002 (Percent Distribution, Selected Categories)

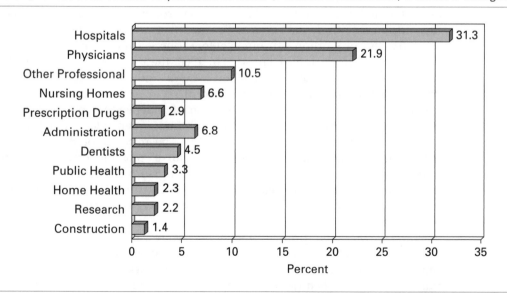

Source: National Center for Health Statistics, *Health, United States, 2004* (Hyattsville, MD: US Government Printing Office 2004), Table 118, p. 329.

Physicians

In terms of national expenditures for health services, physicians made up the largest single professional service component of the health services sector. Payments to physicians accounted for 21.9 percent of total health services expenditures in 2002. Physicians were the only professionals in the health services sector who were broadly licensed to perform any medical procedure. Thus, they had significant influence over the allocation of most health care resources.

Physicians were generally considered to be either doctors of medicine or doctors of osteopathy. However, osteopaths represented only about 5 percent of all active physicians in the United States. The number of active physicians in 2001 was approximately 793,263 or 27.4 per 10,000 population.[9]

Expenditures for physicians' services grew at an average annual rate of about 12.8 percent from 1980 to 1990. However, the following decade saw much slower growth of expenditures in physician services – for most of the 1990s, expenditure growth was around 5 to 7 percent. More recently, physician services expenditures once again grew at an increased rate.[10]

Other Professional Services

In general, the "other professionals" category included chiropractors, optometrists, podiatrists, and licensed medical practitioners other than physicians and dentists.[11] In addition, this category included allied health services, such as kidney dialysis centers and specialty outpatient facilities for mental health and substance abuse as well as ambulance services. Although the proportion of health care expenditures attributable to dental services declined (7.4 percent in 1960 to 4.6 percent in 2001), the proportion attributable to services from other types of health care professionals steadily increased. In 1960, the proportion of the health care dollar spent on other professional services was only 1.5 percent. By 2001, this proportion had increased to about 3 percent.

One reason for this trend was the rise of independent practices by nurse practitioners. Nurse practitioners in full-time independent practice in the United States numbered more than 50,000. The majority of these individuals were family nurse practitioners, adult nurse practitioners, and pediatric nurse practitioners. Forty-six states required nurse practitioners to be certified and data from the American Nurses Credentialing Center (ANCC) suggested that the number of nurses entering private practice each year was increasing.

In 1995, 3,066 family nurse practitioners were certified. By 1997, this figure had risen to 4,577 for that year, and the growth trend in independent nurse practices appeared likely to continue. In 1998, less than 15 percent of all nurse practitioners had decided to operate independent practices.[12] It appeared that many more nurse practitioners could choose to set up independent practices.

Nursing Homes

Nursing home services accounted for 6.6 percent of national health care expenditures in 2002. This was a significant increase over 1960, when nursing home care used 3.2 percent of the health care dollar. During the 1960s and 1970s, there were large increases in average annual expenditures for these services. In that 20-year period, the average annual percentage increase in nursing home expenditures exceeded 15 percent. The rate of annual increase declined during the 1980s to around 11 percent and subsided further during the 1990s to less than 8 percent per year, and in 2002 was 4.1 percent.[13]

Between 1974 and 1999, the number of nursing homes increased from 15,700 to 18,000. In the same period, the inventory of nursing home beds grew from 1.177 million to 1.879 million.[14] However, the availability of beds decreased, as measured by the ratio of nursing home beds to population 85 years of age and over. In 1976, there were 681 beds per 1,000 residents 85 years of age and older. By 1998, that ratio had decreased to 446.9 beds per 1,000.

Drugs

Major international corporations such as Merck, Johnson & Johnson, and American Home Products represented the drug and medical supply industry. Between 1960 and the mid-1980s, the proportion of the domestic health care dollar devoted to products from suppliers such as these actually declined. In 1960, prescription drugs accounted for 10 percent of health care expenditures. By 1980, the proportion decreased to 4.9 percent. However, during the 1990s this trend completely reversed. In 1990, the proportion of the health services dollar devoted to prescription drugs was 5.8 percent, but the proportion was again over 10 percent in 2002.[15]

The elderly purchased the largest share of prescription drugs. By one estimate, people aged 65 and over used three times as many prescription drugs as all other age groups. The 13 percent of the population who were 65 and over accounted for 42 percent of expenditures on prescription drugs in 1998.[16]

Although each of the five components of the health services sector – hospitals, physicians, other health professionals, nursing homes, and drugs – had its own organizations, advocacy groups, and legal and economic structures, it was physicians who largely controlled the allocation of resources on behalf of patients. Obviously, physicians controlled the 22 percent of the health care resources that paid for their services; however, they substantially influenced the allocation of resources in many other components of the health sector as well. For example, hospitals were not licensed to practice medicine. Rather, hospitals approved physicians for a medical staff and the medical staff physicians allocated the 30 plus percent of health care dollars that purchased hospital resources for patient care. Physicians admitted patients to the hospital, discharged patients from the hospital, and made the resource allocation judgments in between. In addition, the influence by physicians on resource allocation was substantial in the prescription drug component and to some degree in the nursing home and home health care components.

Understanding the nature and extent of physician influence over the health sector's resource allocation was important. Regulatory and competitive forces that influenced physician behavior might have resource allocation outcomes that were not immediately obvious. Physician choices, when considered in the aggregate, were strategically important for health care.

Paying for Health Services

In general, health service payor organizations could be dichotomized into those in the private sector and those in the public sector. In 1965, 61.5 percent of all payments for health care goods and services were made directly by private households. By 2000, this percentage dropped to 33.4 percent. For the latest available 14-year period, there was a significant change in the distribution of payments among payor categories in the health services sector – both private sector (household payors, private business payors, and nonpatient revenues) and public sector (federal government payors and state government payors).

Household Payors[17]

Various categories of payment from individual households in the United States made up the largest single payor category until very recently. Within the past few years, public payors (federal, state, and local governments) surpassed individual households as the largest payor category. In 2000, individual households paid out over $418 billion of the $1,255 billion expended on health care goods and services. There were four ways households paid for health services: (1) direct out-of-pocket health spending by individuals; (2) premiums paid by employees and the self-employed into the Medicare hospital insurance trust fund; (3) premiums paid by individuals to the Medicare supplemental medical insurance trust fund; and (4) the employee-paid share of private health insurance premiums and individual health insurance policies. In 1995, the first category – out-of-pocket spending – was nearly half of all dollars expended by households on health services.

Private Business

Payments made by private businesses accounted for 26.6 percent of all expenditures for health care goods and services in 2000. Of this $334.5 billion, employers spent $246.2 billion for private health insurance premiums. These premiums were paid for both traditional indemnity types of insurance and, to an increasing degree, for employer self-insurance programs. In addition, private employers contributed over $61 billion into the Medicare hospital insurance trust fund and another $22.7 billion for workmen's compensation and various forms of disability insurance. A small portion of the private expenditures ($4.2 billion) was made for in-house health services provided by companies at the workplace.

Other Private Revenues

The final category of private payments for health care goods and services was other private revenues. Such revenues accounted for between 4 and 5 percent of health resources. The sources of these revenues included philanthropy and other enterprises for which no patient care services were delivered. Although the dollar amount of such revenue steadily increased, its role in terms of all payments for health care goods and services was becoming less significant. Other private revenue increased from $22.4 billion in 1987 to $53 billion in 2000. However, in terms of the percentage of the total, other private revenue decreased from 4.7 percent in 1987 to 4.2 percent in 2000.

Public Payors – Federal

Public expenditures from all levels of government accounted for 35.8 percent of the payments for health services and supplies in 2000. Among private business, households, and government, governments now paid the most significant portion of health care expenditures. The largest portion of these public payments, $237.1 billion, was from the federal government. The federal government contributed to the health insurance programs for its own employees and expended general tax revenues for various health services programs such as health services for some poor individuals, the health services system of the Veterans Administration, the Indian Health Service (that provided health care services to Native Americans and Alaska Natives), and an extensive military health service operated by the various branches of the US armed services.

Public Payors – State and Local

State and local governments contributed $212.1 billion to total payments for health care goods and services in 2000. In addition to health services programs provided directly by these governmental entities, this figure included state and local government contributions to private health insurance programs for their employees as well as their contributions as an employer to the Medicare hospital insurance trust fund.

Exhibit 1/8 shows expenditures for health services and supplies by type of payor. Exhibit 1/9 shows the changing relationship over time of the major payor organizations. This figure suggests a rationale for why it is difficult to gain a political consensus for substantial changes to the health care system despite rapidly escalating costs.

Exhibit 1/8: Expenditures for Health Services and Supplies, by Type of Payor: United States, Selected Calendar Years 1990–2000 (amounts in $ billions)

		1990	1995	1996	1998	2000
	Total[a]	672.9	957.7	1,005.7	1,111.5	1,255.5
Type of Sponsor						
Private		450.8	607.3	633.4	716.4	806.3
	Private Business	185.8	251.2	265.5	288.1	334.5
	Employer Contribution to Private Health Insurance Premiums	138.4	183.4	194.9	210.5	246.2
	Employer Contribution to Medicare Hospital Insurance Trust Fund[a]	29.5	43.1	45.8	53.6	61.4
	Workers' Compensation and Temporary Disability Insurance	15.7	21.4	21.4	20.2	22.7
	Industrial In-Plant Health Services	2.2	3.3	3.4	3.8	4.2
Households		245.3	314.4	323.2	376.5	418.8
	Employee Contribution to Private Health Insurance Premiums and Individual Policy Premiums	51.3	95.6	96.8	116.1	126.4
	Employee and Self-Employment Contributions and Voluntary Premiums Paid to Medicare Hospital Insurance Trust Fund[b]	35.5	55.9	59.2	68.8	81.5
	Premiums Paid by Individuals to Medicare Supplementary Medical Insurance Trust Fund	10.1	16.4	15.1	17.0	16.3
	Out-of-Pocket Health Spending	148.4	146.5	152.1	174.5	194.5
	Nonpatient Revenues	19.8	41.7	44.7	51.8	53.0
Public		222.1	350.4	372.3	395.1	449.3
Federal Government		115.1	196.6	213.0	214.9	237.1
	Employer Contribution to Private Health Insurance Premiums	9.2	11.3	11.3	11.4	14.3
	Medicaid[c]	55.8	88.1	94.2	101.9	120.8
	Other[d]	61.6	97.2	107.4	101.6	102.0
State and Local Government		107.0	153.8	159.3	180.3	212.1
	Employer Contribution to Private Health Insurance Premiums	33.5	39.8	41.8	45.2	56.9
	Medicaid[c]	41.1	59.2	61.5	73.4	86.1
	Other[e]	38.0	54.7	56.0	61.6	69.1

[a] Excludes Research and Construction.
[b] Includes one-half of self-employment contribution to Medicare Hospital Insurance Trust Fund benefits.
[c] Includes Medicaid buy-in premiums for Medicare.
[d] Includes expenditures for Medicare with adjustments for contributions by employers and individuals and premiums paid to the Medicare Insurance Trust Fund and maternal and child health, vocational rehabilitation, Substance Abuse and Mental Health Services Administration, Indian Health Service, Federal workers' compensation, and other miscellaneous general hospital and medical programs, public health activities, Department of Defense and Department of Veterans Affairs.
[e] Includes other public and general assistance, maternal and child health, vocational rehabilitation, public health activities and hospital subsidies, and employer contributions to Medicare Hospital Insurance Trust Fund.

Source: National Center for Health Statistics, *Health, United States, 2004* (Hyattsville, MD: US Government Printing Office, 2004), Table 123, p. 337.

Exhibit 1/9: Expenditures for Health Services and Supplies by Payor Categories
(percentage distribution, selected years)

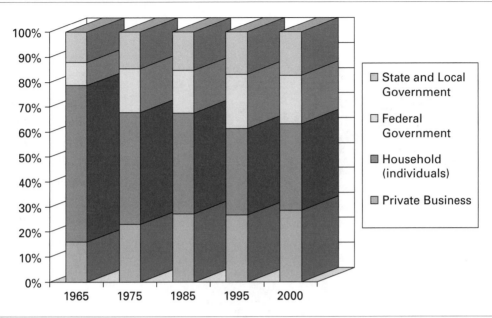

Source: Health Care Financing Administration, Office of the Actuary: Data from the National Health Statistics Group.

Most individuals in the United States had some form of health insurance. Individual out-of-pocket expenditures for health care as a percent of total expenditures declined consistently over time since the mid-1960s. Hence, although health care costs escalated dramatically, the impact on individual households was muted. Government and private business became responsible for increasing proportions of the cost and, therefore, individual households did not feel the entire financial impact of the rapidly increasing costs. From the viewpoint of most households in America, the quality of health care increased, health care providers offered more in terms of palliative and curative services, and the cost increases were moderate. It was difficult to gain a political consensus for change when most Americans maintained positive perceptions about their health services.

Government Public Health Activities

In general, government-provided public health services did not fit neatly into any individual category within the health care sector of the economy. Public health was a provider of personal health services, a regulator of service providers, a payor for services, and a major source of health-related research. Federal, state, and local governments all conducted public health activities and expended resources for

Exhibit 1/10: State Public Health Agency Expenditures by Program Area (percentage distribution, fiscal year 1991)

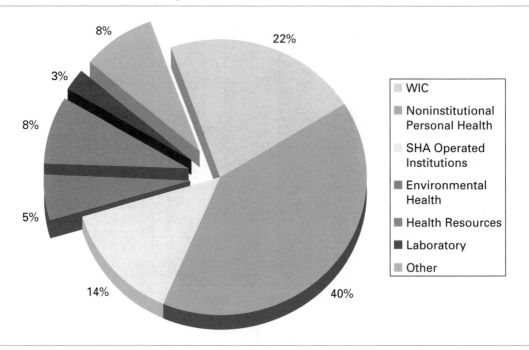

Source: National Center for Health Statistics, *Health, United States, 1996–97* (Hyattsville, MD: US Government Printing Office, 1997), Table 130, p. 264.

public health services. However, the services were highly variable from state to state and from locality to locality within states. These services amounted to 3.3 percent of total health expenditures in 2002.[18] The largest component of this was used to deliver personal health services, often to the medically indigent (see Exhibit 1/10).[19] Although the data in this Exhibit was quite old, no more current data existed on a national level. Anecdotal information from various state health departments indicated that it had not changed much over the past 15 years.

Selected Environmental Trends

Important trends in the health care environment had significant implications for the future of health care in the United States. The external environment essentially created the rules that must be understood for leaders to make sound judgments on behalf of the public's health as well as health care organizations and stakeholders. The ability to explain important environmental trends and their impact on the nation's health represented a fundamental part of being accountable for the decisions made. Numerous environmental trends could be considered when assessing the environment. Three important health care environmental trends serve as illustrations: trends in hospital utilization, in managed care, and in the physician workforce.

Trends in Hospital Utilization

Because the percentage of US health care expenditures devoted to the use of hospital services was declining, the availability of hospital inpatient beds diminished since the mid-1980s. The number of beds taken out of service since 1985 was equivalent to closing seventeen 200-bed community hospitals in every state – a substantial reduction in bed capacity.

The main reason hospitals were taking beds out of service was the declining occupancy rates for in-service beds. There were several reasons for declining use of inpatient hospital service including changes to hospital payment methods that encouraged earlier discharge of inpatients as well as increasing outpatient alternatives to inpatient care. Exhibit 1/11 shows the reductions in the number of inpatient hospital beds over time and the accompanying impact of these bed reductions on the use of the remaining inpatient beds by year. It was evident that the substantial reductions in inpatient beds had little impact on the utilization of the remaining beds. Hospital inpatient bed use was declining as fast as the hospitals took beds out of service.

Hospitals, similar to hotels, must have a reasonable occupancy rate to efficiently utilize available resources. On a typical day in the United States, community hospital beds were approximately 35 percent empty. Hence, a substantial oversupply of hospital beds continued despite the extraordinary closure of hospital inpatient facilities over 16 years. Additional hospital bed closures were likely until hospital inpatient beds achieved an efficient occupancy rate.

Trends in Managed Care

In general, managed care was considered to be any system of health payment or delivery arrangement where the plan attempted to control or coordinate use of health services by its enrolled members to contain health expenditures or improve quality, or both. Managed care was a broad term that encompassed many different types of relationships among health care professionals, health service organizations, payors for health services, and health care clients. Typically, the term managed care organization (MCO) referred to the entity that managed risk, contracted with providers, was paid by employers or patient groups, and handled claims processing.[20]

As previously discussed, the rapid rise of health care costs for private employers during the 1980s encouraged many large employers to adopt some type of managed care arrangement for employee health benefits. This led to a rapid growth of managed care organizations and numbers of enrollees during the 1990s. In more recent years, the number of plans has decreased substantially while the number

Exhibit 1/11: Short-Term Nonfederal Hospitals, Number of Beds and Percent Occupancy, 1985–2002

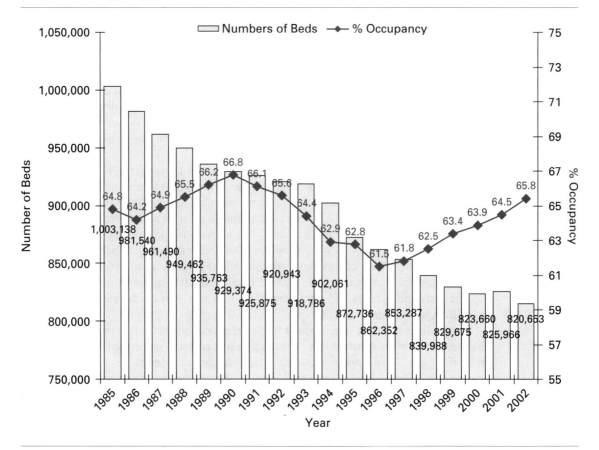

Source: National Center for Health Statistics, *Health, United States, 2004* (Hyattsville, MD: US Government Printing Office, 2004), Table 109, p. 317.

of enrollees has declined to a lesser degree. Between 1990 and 2003, the number of health maintenance organization (HMO, a major type of MCO) plans declined from 572 to 454 while enrollment in HMOs grew from 33 million to 71.8 million.[21]

Government health insurance programs such as Medicare and Medicaid were rapidly moving enrollees into managed care arrangements. Projections suggested that about 25 percent of seniors would be in Medicare HMOs by 2002 and 33 percent would be in such organizations by 2007. Projections for Medicaid, the federal/state health insurance program for the poor, were more dramatic. They suggested that 63 percent of all Medicaid enrollees would be in managed care arrangements within a few years.[22] In fact, such projections were not accurate. By the year 2002, Medicare enrollment in HMOs had actually begun to decline and, while Medicaid enrollment in such plans was still growing slowly, less than one-third of Medicaid recipients were in HMOs.[23]

Exhibit 1/12: HMO Enrollment and Number of Plans, 1987–2003

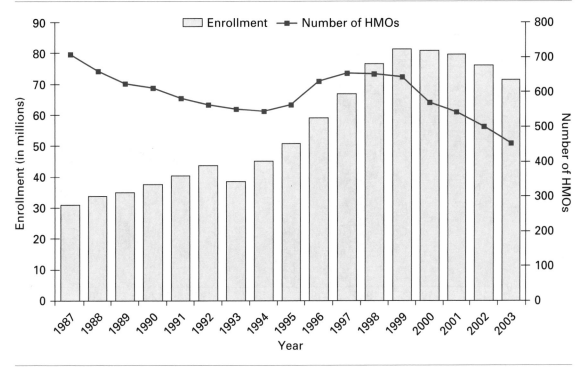

Source: National Center for Health Statistics, *Health, United States, 2004* (Hyattsville, MD: US Government Printing Office, 2004), Table 134, p. 357.

Enrollment in managed care organizations had clearly grown substantially. However, by 2000 it was unclear whether that growth would continue. In addition, the trend relative to the number of managed care organizations themselves was not as clear. The number of HMOs was decreasing (see Exhibit 1/12).

Increased enrollment in HMOs with decreasing numbers of managed care organizations resulted in fewer HMOs with larger numbers of enrollees in each. For example, in 1980 each HMO had an average of 38,723 enrollees. In 1999, with 643 HMOs in existence, each organization had 126,438 enrollees. By 2002, even though the number of HMOs had shrunk to 500, each of these organizations had an average of 152,200 enrollees.[24] Such a trend suggested increasing bargaining power for managed care organizations when they negotiated with providers such as physicians and hospitals. This trend was not going unnoticed by provider organizations. The American Medical Association was pursuing the "Health Care Antitrust Improvements Act of 2003," a House bill that would let doctors "plead their case" to get permission to negotiate collectively with insurors. In addition, the measure called for limiting the amount physicians would have to pay in damages if they were found guilty of violating antitrust laws.[25]

Exhibit 1/13: Population per Active Physician in the United States (selected years)

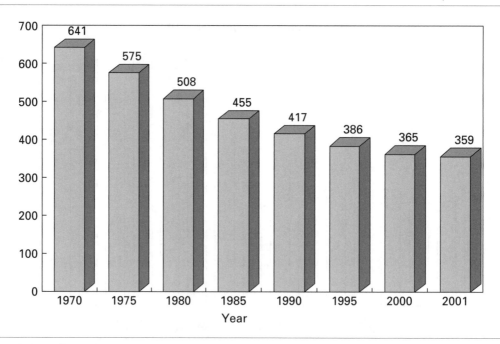

Source: National Center for Health Statistics, *Health, United States, 2004* (Hyattsville, MD: US Government Printing Office), Table 105, p. 312 and http://www.census.gov/popest/states/NST-ann-est.html

Trends in the Physician Workforce

In 1980, there were 427,122 active physicians in the United States. This number for 2001 was projected to be 793,263. On a population basis, the availability of active physicians increased from 190 per 100,000 population in 1980 to 274.3 per 100,000 in 2001.[26]

To consider the strategic importance of this trend, it might be useful to view the physician-to-population ratio differently. Exhibit 1/13 presents population per active physician for selected years between 1970 and 2001. During that period, the number of people available in the United States for each physician, on average, to practice on decreased from 641 to 359.

This trend was primarily because of substantial increases in the number of medical schools and the medical school class sizes in the United States since the passage of the Health Professions Education Assistance Act in 1963. Between 1960 and 1988, the number of first-year enrollees in US medical schools more than doubled. Although a future oversupply of physicians was widely projected, it was unlikely that any medical schools would close or that class sizes would

Exhibit 1/14: Federal and Nonfederal Physicians by Age Group for
Selected Years

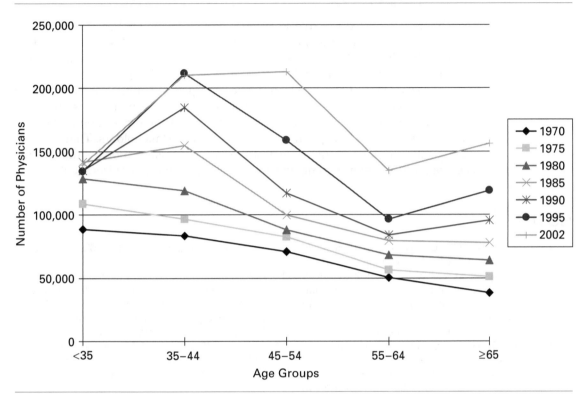

Source: American Medical Association, *Physician Characteristics in the US, 2004*, Table 1.1.

meaningfully decrease. Therefore, an oversupply of physicians was expected to continue, at least for the foreseeable future.

New physicians were entering the workforce at about three times the rate that older physicians were leaving practice.[27] Given the approximately eight-year time lag between a student entering medical school and that student completing training and entering the workforce, this trend was expected to continue for at least a decade.

Exhibit 1/14 presents federal and nonfederal physicians by age group for selected years beginning in 1970. This Exhibit suggests that in the future, the supply of physicians will continue to increase.

Although there are some countervailing trends, such as greater requirements for physician services created by the aging of the US population and increased demands of sophisticated medical technology, it was unlikely that these trends would offset the explosive growth in the supply of physicians. The strategic implications of a substantial oversupply of physicians needed to be carefully considered.

Conclusion

This chapter attempted to provide an introduction to the US health care system as background for the strategic management cases in this book. It should be apparent that the health care system has undergone significant change in the past 50 years and that the future will likely see even more change. Decision making in such an environment required leaders and managers to handle many judgmental challenges. As leaders and managers of health care organizations, decisions made today affect the health of individuals and communities tomorrow. Sound decision making was required to explain decisions to various stakeholders. That decision making must be done in the context of the internal organizational situation, the local competitive environment, and the general health care environment.

NOTES

1. Paul Star, *The Social Transformation of American Medicine* (New York: Basic Books, 1982), pp. 338–339.
2. N. L. Keating, A. M. Zaslavsky, and J. Z. Ayanian, "Physicians' Reports of Focused Expertise in Clinical Practice," *Journal of General Internal Medicine* 15 (2000), pp. 417–420.
3. American College of Graduate Medical Education, http://www.acgme.org/adspublic/reports/program_specialty.asp.
4. National Center for Health Statistics, *Health, United States, 2003* (Hyattsville, MD: US Government Printing Office, 2000), Table 114, p. 308.
5. "By the Numbers: Health Care Costs," *Scientific American* (April 1999), p. 36.
6. Stephen Heffler, Sheila Smith, Sean Keehan, Kent Clemens, Mark Zezza, and Christopher Truffer, "Health Spending Projections Through 2013," *Health Affairs* (February 11, 2004), pp. W4-79 to W4-93.
7. *Health, United States, 2004*, Table 92, p. 289.
8. Ibid., Table 83, p. 274.
9. Ibid., Table 105, p. 312.
10. Ibid., Table 118, pp. 328–329.
11. Covers services provided in establishments operated by health practitioners other than physicians and dentists. These professional services include those provided by private-duty nurses, chiropractors, podiatrists, optometrists, and physical, occupational, and speech therapists, among others. Ambulance services paid under Medicare are also included here. These establishments are classified in NAICS-6213 Offices of Other Health Practitioners or roughly the equivalent of SIC 804-Offices and Clinics of Other Health Practitioners. HCFA website: http://www.cms.hhs.gov/statistics/nhe/quick-reference/.
12. Lynda Flanagan, "Nurse Practitioners: Growing Competition for Family Physicians?" *Family Practice Management* 5, no. 9 (October 1998, http://www.aafp.org/fmp/98100fm/nurse.html).
13. *Health, United States, 2004*, Table 118, p. 328.
14. A. Jones, "The National Nursing Home Survey: 1999 Summary," National Center for Health Statistics, *Vital Health Statistics* 13, no. 152 (June 2002), Table A, p. 2.
15. *Health, United States, 2004*, Table 118, p. 329.
16. "Growth in Drug Spending for the Elderly, 1992–2010," *Families USA* (July 2000), p. 2.
17. *Health, United States, 2004*, Table 123, p. 337.
18. Ibid., Table 118, p. 329.
19. Public Health Agencies, *Inventory of Programs and Block Grant Expenditures* (Washington, DC: Public Health Foundation, 1991).
20. Excerpted from "Glossary of Terms in Managed Health Care," http://www.pohly.com/terms_m.shtml.
21. *Health, United States, 2004*, Table 134, p. 357.
22. Institute for the Future, *Health and Health Care 2010* (San Francisco: Jossey-Bass Publishers, 2000), pp. 43–44.
23. *Health, United States, 2003*, Tables 132 and 137, pp. 339 and 347.
24. Ibid., Table 132, p. 339.
25. Tanya Albert, "Study Hits Physician Collective Bargaining," *AMNews* (August 9, 2004).
26. *Health, United States, 2004*, Table 105, p. 312.
27. Institute for the Future, p. 5.

CASE **2**

Methodist Healthcare: Managing for the Future

A. C. Wharton, chairman of the board of Methodist Healthcare, delivered the news to the management and associates of Methodist Healthcare in a system-wide teleconference on September 26, 2001. "I have the opportunity to come to you along with two individuals who will be leading Methodist Healthcare into the future. As you know, Maurice Elliott made the decision to step out of his role as CEO to become CEO Emeritus effective October 1st of this year. The board appointed Gary Shorb to the position of CEO and President of Methodist Healthcare. Joining Gary at the helm is Cam Welton as executive vice president and chief operating officer."

Wharton continued, "The board is pleased that even as other institutions are losing their best and brightest, Methodist is able to keep this top-level team that has worked so well together for years. Among other things, they have developed a positive and collaborative relationship with physicians, strengthened our ties with The University of Tennessee, moved Methodist into the ranks of the top 50 integrated systems in the country, and made Methodist Healthcare – Memphis Hospitals the third largest hospital in the country, as well as the largest hospital in Memphis and the Mid-South."

Gary Shorb, CEO, began, "The leadership transition is being conducted in a very orderly fashion, thanks to A. C. Wharton and Maurice. Cam Welton and I have been involved with a tremendous

This case was prepared by Mary C. Christy and Gary Shorb, Methodist Le Bonheur Healthcare. It is intended as a basis for classroom discussion rather than to illustrate either effective or ineffective handling of an administrative situation. Used with permission from Mary C. Christy.

amount of detailed planning and now detailed execution. Our primary goal is to work to differentiate Methodist from other health care organizations. We will differentiate Methodist from our competition – not just locally – but regionally as well. And the way we're going to do that is by focusing on our customers; whether they're physicians, or our associates, or our patients and families. We're going to improve our processes so that all of those customers have outstanding experiences when they come to Methodist."

He continued, "Change is on the horizon, and with change is the need to develop a more elaborate strategic management process. I have assembled a leadership team to set the strategic course for the system. We pledge to make the transition as seamless as possible and to strengthen the system by building on our successful past – toward an even brighter future."

System Background

Methodist traced its history to 1918 in Mississippi, but was incorporated as Methodist Healthcare in 1981 for the primary purpose of supporting and extending the health and welfare ministries of the Memphis, North Arkansas, and Mississippi Annual Conferences of The United Methodist Church. Methodist University Hospital (known as Methodist Central until 2002) was located in the downtown Memphis Medical Center on the site of the original Methodist Hospital that opened in 1921 with 72 private rooms. Methodist University Hospital grew according to community needs for over three-quarters of a century. In 1995, Methodist merged with Le Bonheur Children's Medical Center. Methodist Healthcare – Memphis Hospitals ("Methodist Memphis") – owned and operated five acute care hospitals in the Memphis area, including Methodist University, the system's flagship tertiary care hospital. In January 2002, Methodist Memphis had 1,520 licensed acute beds, 44 licensed skilled beds, 55 licensed residential drug and alcohol beds, 63,273 admissions, and more than 6,800 full-time employees at its five hospitals.

Methodist Healthcare – Memphis Hospitals

- *Methodist University* – The hospital that is now known as Methodist University opened in 1918 and completed major construction projects each decade. Methodist University operated with 840 licensed beds, including 58 psychiatric and 44 skilled-nursing beds, and had established Centers of Excellence to provide comprehensive tertiary care for cardiac (Methodist Heart Institute), cancer (Methodist Cancer Center), neurologic (Memphis Neurosciences Center), and obstetric and gynecologic (Methodist Women's Services) care.
- *Methodist South* – Methodist South was opened in 1973 in the area of Memphis known as Whitehaven to serve the fast-growing population in Shelby County and north Mississippi. The hospital was licensed with 174 beds. Over time many ancillary departments were expanded and 26 patient beds added, including six intensive care/coronary care beds. In June 2000, the hospital began providing full cardiac services.

- *Methodist North* – Methodist North was opened in 1978 in the Raleigh/Bartlett area to support the growing needs of north Shelby County and neighboring Tipton County. The hospital was licensed for 174 beds. An obstetrics unit was opened in 1987, adding 20 beds; 14 neonatal intensive care beds were added in 1992, increasing the number of licensed beds to 208. Rapid growth in cardiac and other tertiary services required an expansion of the emergency department and the opening of 26 additional intensive care and intermediate beds in February 2000, bringing the total licensed bed complement to 234.
- *Methodist Germantown* – In 1993, Methodist Memphis purchased a hospital in Germantown, Tennessee (a suburb to the east of Memphis). Built in 1986, the hospital was licensed for 120 beds. Patient volumes at Methodist Germantown increased significantly after Methodist Memphis's purchase, resulting in the need for extensive renovations as well as expansion of obstetric, emergency, outpatient, and ancillary service areas (completed February 1999). Continued growth resulted in the need for another expansion, including 89 additional beds and full cardiac services. In 2002, the total bed complement was 209.
- *Le Bonheur Children's* – In October 1995, Le Bonheur merged into Methodist Memphis. Le Bonheur was the regional pediatric referral center, with 225 licensed beds in its acute care facility located in the downtown Memphis Medical Center. The building was constructed in 1952, with major expansions in 1974, 1979, and 1994. Le Bonheur provided several specialty services, including liver and kidney transplantation, brain tumor resections, cardiothoracic surgery, and invasive and non-invasive cardiac laboratories. In addition, Le Bonheur maintained laboratories where medical scientists performed research in many areas, including neuroscience and infectious and respiratory diseases.

Affiliated Organizations

Methodist began an expansion and acquisition program in 1981 for the purpose of strengthening the referral base to Methodist Memphis and sharing its highly specialized technical and management skills with outlying hospitals in the region. Affiliates of Methodist included eight Tennessee not-for-profit corporations that operated hospitals in the surrounding region outside of Shelby County in western Tennessee. Further, Methodist pursued an agreement with the University of Tennessee.

- *University of Tennessee* – In 2002, Methodist entered into an affiliation agreement with The University of Tennessee (UT) on behalf of the UT Health Science Center at Memphis. Under the agreement, Methodist University Hospital and Le Bonheur became the principal private teaching hospitals for UT in the Memphis area. Also, the parties agreed that any new or expanded UT medical education programs would be located at the Methodist teaching hospitals, and that as a team they would work together to increase clinical research at the Methodist teaching hospitals.
- *Alliance Health Services, Inc.* – AHS provided hospice, private duty nursing, rehabilitative care, infusion, and other related services in the home for Medicare,

Medicaid, and privately insured patients. In addition, the company operated a durable medical equipment business with locations in Memphis and Jackson, Tennessee.

- *Methodist Extended Care Hospital, Inc.* – Methodist Extended Care provided long-term acute care services in its facility located on the campus of Methodist University.
- *Methodist Healthcare Community Care Associates* – Methodist CCA was formed in 1994 for the operation of rural health clinics in Sardis, Robinsonville, and Tunica, Mississippi.
- *Methodist Healthcare Primary Care Associates* – Methodist PCA owned and operated primary care clinics or offices in the Memphis area. It began operations in 1994, with the over 20 physicians involved becoming employees of the system. In 1999, it no longer employed physicians in its operations.
- *Methodist Healthcare West Tennessee Medical Associates* – Methodist WTMA owned and operated primary care clinics and offices in the West Tennessee area.
- *Ambulatory Operations, Inc.* – Ambulatory Operations was the for-profit corporation of Methodist Healthcare that owned and operated: MedLab, Inc., a reference laboratory and pathology services organization with a 150-mile service area; Le Bonheur Ambulatory Services, Inc. (LAS) that provided day-to-day management for various surgery centers; and Memphis Professional Building, Inc. (MPB), mortgage holder for the Memphis Professional Building that housed the corporate and other support area offices.
- *Methodist and Le Bonheur Healthcare Foundations* – The Foundations were devoted to fundraising for both Methodist and Le Bonheur.

Other Partnerships

Methodist was an investor in or member of various other organizations.

- *Health Choice, LLC* – Health Choice was a limited liability company with two members, Methodist and Metro Care, Inc., a not-for-profit corporation formed by physicians practicing primarily at Methodist Memphis. The major function of this joint venture was to market a preferred provider plan to business and industry in the Methodist Memphis service area. Health Choice of West Tennessee marketed similar plans in western Tennessee outside the Memphis area.
- *Germantown Surgery Center, LP; Le Bonheur East Surgery Center, LP; and North Surgery Center, LP* – These for-profit limited partnerships were formed to develop or acquire and operate ambulatory surgery centers in the Memphis area. Methodist Memphis was the general partner for each. Limited partners were physicians on the medical staff of Methodist Memphis.

Methodist, together with its affiliates, was licensed to operate 2,445 beds, including 2,310 for acute care, 44 for long-term skilled-nursing care, 55 for residential drug and alcohol care, and 36 at Methodist Extended Care Hospital. Of the 2,445 licensed beds, 1,805 were in service at the beginning of 2002.

The Management Team

"We have a great group of individuals who collectively have a tremendous amount of experience in health care and within Methodist Healthcare," stated Gary Shorb. (See Exhibit 2/1 for background information on the Methodist Team.) He continued, "It is one of the most talented teams I have ever had the opportunity to work with."

Situational Analysis

Over several months, the strategic process was set in motion. Methodist focused its efforts on reorganizing the leadership team, reviewing and redefining, when necessary, its mission, vision, and values, and restructuring the organization's culture with a strategic mindset.

External Environmental Analysis

Methodist's strategic planning process had consistently been applied to evaluate the system's efficiency and effectiveness against its mission, vision, values, and goals. Goals were set and objectives were identified, prioritized, and analyzed. Action plans were communicated and evaluated. If necessary, goals were revised and set in motion to be consistent with the system's strategic direction. The leadership team understood the need for effective environmental analysis, including the general environment, the health care industry, and competitor analysis.

The General Environment

Shorb spoke to the management team at the beginning of the strategic planning process. He summarized, "Health care trends over the past decade have led hospitals to complex system development with diverse organizational structures and a wide variety of businesses. Some of the businesses have taken on a life and purpose of their own and no longer support the organization's overall mission and strategic direction. Too many boards, companies, and organizations have lacked focus and discipline and drain energy, talent, and resources from the organization's core business. We need to understand the environment to take advantage of the opportunities and avoid the mistakes of others."

Trends/Issues

Nationwide, hospitals were experiencing a shift from inpatient to outpatient procedures, nursing shortages, a decline in federal and state reimbursement programs,

Gary Shorb came to Methodist in 1990 as president and CEO of Methodist Hospitals of Memphis. He had been president and chief operating officer of Methodist Healthcare for 11 years before being appointed president and CEO. Prior to joining Methodist, he served as president and CEO of the Regional Medical Center in Memphis.

Maurice Elliott was CEO Emeritus and had various responsibilities, including working with the Methodist Healthcare Foundation, Corporate Compliance, Internal Audit and Clinical Research. He had served as CEO of Methodist Healthcare from 1990 through 2001. He was executive vice president and COO of the system from 1987 to 1990 and president of Methodist Hospitals of Memphis from 1988 to 1990. Prior to joining Methodist, he served on the administrative staff of Baptist Memorial Hospital (Memphis) for 24 years.

Cam Welton had been with Methodist since 1990 as well. He served in several leadership positions throughout the organization, including vice president of Methodist University Hospital, administrator of both South Hospital and Germantown Hospital, and, most recently, president of Methodist Healthcare's hospitals in Jackson, Mississippi (divested in 1999) and as CEO of Methodist Healthcare – Memphis Hospitals.

Donna Abney became executive vice president of Methodist in 2001, with responsibility for strategic planning and business development, managed care policy, physician services, and marketing and communications. From 1991 up to the 1995 merger with Le Bonheur Children's, she was senior vice president for marketing and planning for Le Bonheur Health Systems, Inc. Between 1983 and 1991 she was vice president and director of marketing for Le Bonheur Children's Medical Center.

Andy Fowler was senior vice president of information systems. Mr. Fowler joined Methodist in 1995 after Methodist merged with Le Bonheur Children's Medical Center, where he served as vice president and chief information officer.

Cato Johnson was senior vice president of corporate affairs at Methodist Healthcare since 1985. Previously, he was vice president of corporate affairs at the Regional Medical Center in Memphis.

Richard McCormick was senior vice president of Methodist Healthcare's west Tennessee operations and the administrator of Methodist Healthcare – Jackson Hospital. Mr. McCormick had been with Methodist since 1990 and had also served as administrator of Methodist Healthcare – Dyersburg Hospital and Methodist Healthcare – McKenzie Hospital.

Chris McLean was senior vice president of finance and chief financial officer of Methodist Healthcare. Prior to that appointment in 2001, he was vice president of finance for Methodist Healthcare – Memphis Hospitals. Mr. McLean rejoined Methodist in 1998 after spending six years as chief financial officer at various hospital systems in East Tennessee. He began his health care career at Methodist in 1984 in corporate finance and had returned to Methodist as vice president of the Mississippi division.

Carol Ross-Spang joined Methodist in 2000 as vice president of human resources. Prior to joining Methodist, she served as director of human resources and community relations at Harrah's Entertainment for 21 years.

Steve West was senior vice president of legal affairs, chief legal officer and assistant secretary. He joined Methodist in 1979 and served as secretary or assistant secretary of Methodist Memphis and each of the affiliates.

Paula Jacobson was president of the Methodist Healthcare Foundation since 2000. Previously, she was executive director of the Jewish Foundation of Memphis.

Larry Spratlin was vice president of finance and treasurer of Methodist since 2001. Mr. Spratlin held the position of vice president of finance, assistant treasurer of Methodist from 1993 to 2001. Mr. Spratlin held a number of positions in financial management at Methodist, beginning in 1982. Previously he held positions in the Southeast consulting division of Ernst & Young, specializing in health care consulting.

and the need to analyze costs system-wide. In addition, it became necessary for health care organizations to decide whether to retain businesses based on their contribution to business performance and mission. Increasingly, health care organizations evaluated business indicators such as market position, financial performance trends, managed care positioning, medical staff commitment, and the level of resources required to be successful in the future.

The Memphis Market

As of January 1, 2002, there were seven short-term acute care hospitals in addition to Methodist Memphis's five hospitals, for a total of 4,104 licensed beds in Shelby County, Tennessee. Four of these facilities, including Methodist University and Le Bonheur, were located in the downtown Memphis area known as the Memphis Medical Center. Exhibit 2/2 shows the distribution of licensed beds in January 2002 among the Shelby County acute care hospitals and the percentage of admissions to each hospital in 1999 and 2000. The distribution of the hospitals is illustrated in Exhibit 2/3. In addition, St. Jude Children's Research

Exhibit 2/2: Distribution of Acute Care Licensed Beds and Admissions: Shelby County, Tennessee

Hospital	Licensed Beds	Percentage of Admissions	
		1999	2000
Methodist Memphis[a]	1,564	40.0	40.5
Baptist Memorial Hospital (Memphis)[b]	706	32.4	30.6
Baptist Memorial Hospital – Collierville[c]	60	0.3	1.0
Baptist Memorial Hospital for Women[d]	140	0.0	0.0
St. Francis Hospital	609	12.6	14.3
Regional Medical Center	620	10.5	9.5
University of Tennessee Hospital	162	2.4	2.3
Delta Medical Center	243	1.8	1.8
Total	4,104	100.0	100.0

[a] Methodist Memphis licensed beds exclude the 55 residential alcohol and drug beds, but include 44 skilled-nursing beds.
[b] Baptist Memorial Hospital (BMH) – Central closed in November 2000. Baptist then changed the name of the BMH – East hospital to BMH and combined the beds under one license. As of December 31, 2001, all of BMH's active licensed beds (706 in the acute care hospital and 140 in the women's hospital) are at the East location.
[c] Baptist Memorial Hospital – Collierville opened in 1999.
[d] Baptist Memorial Hospital for Women opened in May 2001.

Source: 1999 and 2000 Tennessee Joint Annual Reports; excludes well newborns, residential, rehab, and extended care.

Exhibit 2/3: Hospitals in Memphis and Shelby County, Tennessee

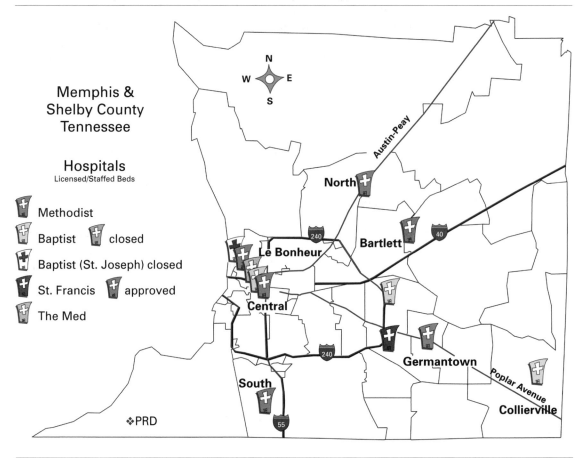

Hospital and a 274-bed Veteran's Administration Hospital, both providing services to specialized populations, were located in the Memphis Medical Center.

Exhibit 2/4 shows the shift in Methodist Memphis's market share for the period 1996 to 2001; it increased from 37.8 percent to 43.9 percent. The shift was largely because of Methodist's merger with Le Bonheur in 1995, the signing of the CIGNA contract in 1996, the merger of St. Joseph's with Baptist and St. Joe's subsequent closure, the closure of Baptist Central in 2000, and the Blue Cross contract obtained in 2000. Methodist positioned itself strongly with the physicians as "partners" in providing care to the community through its development of broad physician networks and the participation of physicians in leadership roles.

In addition to the hospitals in Shelby County, as of January 2002 there were four short-term acute care hospitals (including Methodist Fayette) in the four adjacent counties. Thus, in Methodist Memphis's five-county primary service

Exhibit 2/4: Methodist Healthcare – Memphis Hospitals: Market Share Trends

	1996 (%)	1997 (%)	1998 (%)	1999 (%)	2000 (%)	2001 (%)
Methodist						
University	17.3	17.0	16.6	17.2	17.0	18.5
South	3.6	3.6	3.5	3.5	3.6	4.2
North	6.2	6.5	6.7	6.7	7.3	7.9
Germantown	4.2	4.6	4.8	5.1	5.1	6.3
Le Bonheur	6.5	7.1	6.4	6.5	6.3	6.7
Extended	N/A	0.1	0.2	0.2	0.3	0.3
MHMH	37.8	38.9	38.2	39.2	39.6	43.9
HealthSouth	1.1	1.1	1.1	1.1	1.1	1.2
Baptist						
Central	11.0	9.9	10.1	10.8	9.3	N/A
East	17.8	18.0	18.8	20.8	20.4	20.5
Women's	N/A	N/A	N/A	N/A	N/A	1.8*
Collierville	N/A	N/A	N/A	0.3	1.0	1.8
Rehab	0.8	0.7	0.9	0.9	1.0	0.9
Restorative	N/A	0.1	0.1	0.2	0.2	0.2
BMH	29.6	28.7	29.9	33.0	31.9	25.2
St. Francis	11.9	12.1	12.5	12.5	14.0	14.8
Regional Medical Center	9.6	9.4	9.4	10.2	9.3	10.1
St. Joseph	5.2	5.4	4.4	N/A	N/A	N/A
Univ. Tenn. Bowld	2.5	2.5	2.6	2.3	2.3	2.7
Delta Medical Center	2.3	1.9	1.9	1.7	1.8	2.1
	100.0	100.0	100.0	100.0	100.0	100.0

*Baptist Women's only 5/21/01–9/30/01.

Source: 2001 Tennessee Joint Annual Report of Hospitals.

area there was a total of 4,542 licensed beds. Exhibit 2/5 shows the distribution of licensed beds for the five-county primary service area.

Exhibit 2/6 describes population changes in Memphis's five-county service area. Patients from over 60 counties in Tennessee, Mississippi, Arkansas, Missouri, and Kentucky were referred to Methodist University and Le Bonheur specialists for secondary and tertiary services. The primary service area for Methodist Memphis comprised Shelby, Fayette, and Tipton Counties in Tennessee, as well as DeSoto County, Mississippi, and Crittenden County, Arkansas. In 2000, 71.3 percent of all Methodist Memphis's (including Le Bonheur) discharges were patients who resided in Shelby County. The primary service area population in 2000 was 1,135,614.

Exhibit 2/5: Distribution of Licensed Acute Care Beds and Admissions: Methodist Memphis's Five-County Primary Service Area

Hospital	Licensed Beds	Percentage of Admissions	
		1999	2000
Methodist Memphis[a]	1,564	36.5	37.1
Methodist Fayette	46	0.5	0.4
Baptist Memorial Hospital (Memphis)[b]	706	29.6	27.8
Baptist Memorial Hospital – DeSoto	140	4.0	4.3
Baptist Memorial Hospital – Tipton	100	1.7	1.8
Baptist Memorial Hospital – Collierville[c]	60	0.3	1.0
Baptist Memorial Hospital for Women[d]	140	0.0	0.0
St. Francis Hospital	609	11.5	12.8
Regional Medical Center	620	9.5	8.6
Univ. Tenn. Bowld	162	2.2	2.1
Delta Medical Center	243	1.6	1.6
Crittenden Memorial Hospital	152	2.6	2.5
Total	4,542	100.0	100.0

[a] The Methodist Memphis licensed beds exclude 55 residential alcoholic and drug beds, but include 44 skilled-nursing beds.
[b] Baptist Memorial Hospital – Central closed in November 2000, when its operations were consolidated at its East Campus.
[c] Baptist Memorial Hospital – Collierville opened in 1999.
[d] Baptist Memorial Hospital for Women opened in May 2001.

Source: 1999 and 2000 Tennessee Joint Annual Reports and the 1999 and 2000 AHA Guides. Excludes well newborns, residential, rehab, and extended care.

Exhibit 2/6: Population: Methodist Memphis's Five-County Primary Service Area

County	1970	1980	1990	2000
Shelby (Tennessee)	722,014	777,113	826,330	897,472
Tipton (Tennessee)	28,001	32,930	37,568	51,271
Fayette (Tennessee)	22,692	25,305	25,559	28,806
DeSoto (Mississippi)	35,885	53,930	67,910	107,199
Crittenden (Arkansas)	48,106	49,499	49,939	50,866
Total	856,698	938,777	1,007,306	1,135,614

Source: CACI 2000 Census Data.

West Tennessee Market

Methodist had expanded into the West Tennessee market to strengthen referral lines to Methodist Memphis. Because of long-established physician referral patterns and as a result of managed care, it was a more difficult market to

Exhibit 2/7: Methodist Healthcare: West Tennessee Market Share Trends

County	Hospital	1996 (%)	1997 (%)	1998 (%)	1999 (%)	2000 (%)
Methodist						
Fayette	Fayette	1.3	1.2	1.5	1.2	1.1
Dyer	Dyersburg	6.7	6.0	6.0	6.0	6.0
Haywood	Brownsville	1.9	2.1	1.9	1.9	2.2
Henderson	Lexington	2.3	2.1	1.8	1.9	1.6
Carroll	McKenzie	1.7	1.8	1.5	1.5	1.9
Madison	Jackson			5.4	6.6	7.0
Weakley	Volunteer			4.5	4.4	4.0
McNairy	McNairy			2.3	2.5	2.3
MH		13.9	13.2	24.9	26.0	26.1
Baptist						
Carroll	Huntingdon	3.2	3.1	2.8	2.8	3.0
Lauderdale	Lauderdale	2.0	1.7	1.5	1.5	1.6
Obion	Union City	7.2	7.8	8.1	7.5	7.4
Tipton	Tipton	4.4	3.8	3.8	4.3	4.5
BH		16.8	16.4	16.2	16.1	16.5
Jackson-Madison						
Madison	Jackson-Madison	37.2	38.7	39.8	40.0	38.9
Hardeman	Bolivar General	1.3	1.4	1.1	1.1	1.2
Benton	Camden General	1.1	1.2	1.0	0.8	0.8
Gibson	Gibson General	1.3	1.3	1.3	1.3	1.4
Gibson	Humboldt General	2.3	2.5	2.4	2.2	2.1
Gibson	Milan General	1.5	1.6	1.8	1.5	1.8
JM		44.7	46.7	47.4	46.9	46.2
Others		24.6	23.7	11.5	11.0	11.2
Total		100.0	100.0	100.0	100.0	100.0

Source: Joint Annual Reports of Hospitals.

penetrate. Methodist had steadily increased its market share from 24.9 percent in 1998 to 26.1 percent in 2000, primarily from the lease of Methodist Healthcare – Jackson Hospital ("Jackson"), and Methodist Healthcare – Volunteer Hospital ("Volunteer") in 1998 (see Exhibit 2/7). The inclusion of Jackson and Volunteer expanded Methodist's West Tennessee hospitals to eight. Exhibit 2/8 shows the distribution of the hospitals and related competitors. Selected utilization statistics and demographics as well as primary services are illustrated in Exhibit 2/9.

Jackson-Madison County, Methodist's main competitor, consistently had 46 percent to 47 percent of the market, Baptist had 16 percent, and the remaining county-owned hospitals retained 11 percent of the market.

Exhibit 2/8: Distribution of Hospitals and Related Competitors

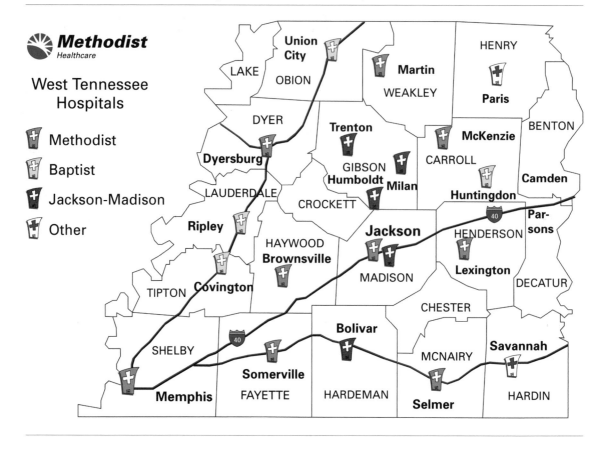

Methodist's strategic goals for the West Tennessee market were as follows:

1. Develop Methodist Jackson into a high-quality tertiary center to serve West Tennessee by improving the mix of high-quality specialists in Jackson and removing barriers to physicians who would like to practice in the Jackson hospital;
2. Tailor rural hospitals to provide those services appropriate to their communities; and
3. Develop a more effective referral network to Methodist hospitals in Jackson and Memphis.

Methodist continued to analyze the effectiveness and efficiency of the West Tennessee market, addressing such issues as capital requirements, success of managed care contracting initiatives, and return on investment. The two hospitals (Jackson and Volunteer) leased from HCA-Healthcare Corporation in 1998 resulted in a 44-year term lease, terminable at Methodist's option in 2007 or 2022 with a termination payment equal to two years' rent, payable in four

Exhibit 2/9: Methodist Healthcare – West Tennessee: Selected Utilization, Service Area, and Primary Services

Fayette Hospital	1999	2000	2001
Licensed Beds	50	49	46
Beds in Service	28	26	10
Patient Days (Inpatient)	3,144	2,920	3,062
Discharges (Inpatient)	799	661	770
Occupancy	30.8%	30.7%	83.9%
Average Length of Stay (Days)	3.9	4.4	4.0
Emergency Room Visits	6,808	6,284	6,353
Ratio of Outpatient to Total Patient Revenue	66.7%	68.9%	68.2%

Inpatient Services:
Family practice specialty.

Outpatient Services:
Ambulatory care center provides family practice, internal medicine, urology, nephrology, orthopedics, ophthalmology, general surgery, cardiology, and podiatry.

Primary Service Area:
The primary service area for Fayette is Fayette and Hardeman Counties, Tennessee. The primary service area population was 56,911 in 2000.

Dyersburg Hospital	1999	2000	2001
Licensed Beds	225	225	225
Beds in Service	105	105	105
Patient Days (Inpatient)	14,205	13,842	14,752
Discharges (Inpatient)	3,603	3,566	3,772
Occupancy	37.1%	36.0%	38.5%
Average Length of Stay (Days)	3.9	3.9	3.9
Emergency Room Visits	17,268	16,732	17,740
Ratio of Outpatient to Total Patient Revenue	50.4%	49.6%	48.9%

Inpatient Services:
General surgery, internal medicine, obstetrics/gynecology, family practice, ophthalmology, pediatrics, nephrology, thoracic surgery, orthopedics, gastroenterology, urology, otolaryngology, pathology, radiology, pulmonology, podiatry, and anesthesiology.

Outpatient Services:
Emergency room and outpatient ancillary services.

Primary Service Area:
The primary service area for Dyersburg was Dyer, Lake and Lauderdale Counties, Tennessee. The primary service area population was 72,334 in 2000.

Exhibit 2/9: *(cont'd)*

Brownsville Hospital	**1999**	**2000**	**2001**
Licensed Beds	62	62	62
Beds in Service	44	44	44
Patient Days (Inpatient)	5,157	4,938	4,791
Discharges (Inpatient)	1,195	1,312	1,288
Occupancy	32.1%	30.7%	29.8%
Average Length of Stay (Days)	4.3	3.8	3.7
Emergency Room Visits	7,353	7,190	7,233
Ratio of Outpatient to Total Patient Revenue	46.3%	46.2%	48.5%

Inpatient Services:
Radiology, laboratory, ultrasound, mammography, CT scanning, respiratory therapy, physical therapy, pharmacy, pulmonary function, and industrial medicine.

Outpatient Services:
Emergency room and multispecialty outpatient clinic providing cardiology, gastroenterology, urology, general surgery, nephrology, podiatry, internal medicine, oncology, and orthopedic services.

Primary Service Area:
The primary service area for Brownsville was Haywood and Crockett Counties, Tennessee. The primary service area population was 34,329 in 2000.

Lexington Hospital	**1999**	**2000**	**2001**
Licensed Beds	52	52	52
Beds in Service	32	32	32
Patient Days (Inpatient)	3,734	3,033	3,432
Discharges (Inpatient)	1,154	930	923
Occupancy	32.0%	26.0%	29.4%
Average Length of Stay (Days)	3.2	3.3	3.7
Emergency Room Visits	11,069	10,273	9,484
Ratio of Outpatient to Total Patient Revenue	57.5%	63.2%	63.7%

Inpatient Services:
General surgery, family practice, otolaryngology, urology, ophthalmology, orthopedics, and obstetrics.

Outpatient Services:
Emergency room, outpatient ancillary services, and a hospital-based home health care agency.

Primary Service Area:
The primary service area for Lexington was Henderson County, Tennessee. The primary service area population was 25,522 in 2000.

Exhibit 2/9: *(cont'd)*

McKenzie Hospital	1999	2000	2001
Licensed Beds	65	65	65
Beds in Service	29	29	29
Patient Days (Inpatient)	2,775	3,332	3,685
Discharges (Inpatient)	938	1,123	1,177
Occupancy	26.2%	31.4%	34.8%
Average Length of Stay (Days)	3.0	3.0	3.1
Emergency Room Visits	5,748	5,669	6,160
Ratio of Outpatient to Total Patient Revenue	61.6%	56.7%	60.1%

Inpatient Services:
General surgery, internal medicine, obstetrics/gynecology, family practice with obstetrics.

Outpatient Services:
Emergency room, outpatient ancillary and ambulance services.

Primary Service Area:
The primary service area for McKenzie was Carroll, Henry, and Weakley Counties, Tennessee. The primary service area population was 77,127 in 2000.

Jackson Hospital	1999	2000	2001
Licensed Beds	154	154	154
Beds in Service	108	127	127
Patient Days (Inpatient)	21,280	21,246	20,725
Discharges (Inpatient)	4,184	4,249	4,361
Occupancy	54.0%	45.7%	44.7%
Average Length of Stay (Days)	5.1	5.0	4.8
Emergency Room Visits	13,973	14,637	14,921
Ratio of Outpatient to Total Patient Revenue	38.7%	38.1%	37.6%

Inpatient Services:
General surgery, internal medicine, cardiology, cardiovascular surgery, diabetes, ENT, family practice, gastroenterology, interventional and conventional radiology, nephrology, obstetrics/gynecology, oncology, ophthalmology, oral surgery, orthopedics, pediatrics, plastic surgery, podiatry, pulmonology, urology, industrial/occupational medicine, physical therapy, and respiratory care.

Outpatient Services:
Emergency room, seniors program, sleep disorders center, and outpatient ancillary services.

Primary Service Area:
The primary service area for Jackson was Madison, Gibson and Chester Counties, Tennessee. The primary service area population was 155,529 in 2000.

Exhibit 2/9: (cont'd)

Volunteer Hospital	1999	2000	2001
Licensed Beds	100	100	100
Beds in Service	65	65	65
Patient Days (Inpatient)	12,100	10,270	11,109
Discharges (Inpatient)	2,793	2,367	2,575
Occupancy	51.0%	43.2%	46.8%
Average Length of Stay (Days)	4.3	4.3	4.3
Emergency Room Visits	9,769	10,005	10,293
Ratio of Outpatient to Total Patient Revenue	47.4%	50.1%	49.9%

Inpatient Services:
General surgery, internal medicine, family practice, obstetrics and gynecology, orthopedics, nephrology, neurology, pulmonology, cardiology, pathology, urology, gastroenterology, pediatrics, and radiology.

Outpatient Services:
Emergency room, Wellness Center, outpatient physical therapy and sports medicine services, and outpatient ancillary services.

Primary Service Area:
The primary service area for Volunteer was Weakley and Obion Counties, Tennessee. The primary service area population was 67,345 in 2000.

McNairy Hospital	1999	2000	2001
Licensed Beds	86	86	86
Beds in Service	48	48	48
Patient Days (Inpatient)	5,836	5,267	4,791
Discharges (Inpatient)	1,499	1,347	1,336
Occupancy	33.3%	30.0%	27.3%
Average Length of Stay (Days)	3.9	3.9	3.6
Emergency Room Visits	9,750	9,837	9,938
Ratio of Outpatient to Total Patient Revenue	53.9%	55.0%	60.5%

Inpatient Services:
General surgery, family practice, obstetrics and gynecology, orthopedics, pediatrics, ophthalmology, cardiology, podiatry, and nephrology.

Outpatient Services:
Emergency room and outpatient ancillary services.

Primary Service Area:
The primary service area for McNairy was McNairy and Hardin Counties, Tennessee. The primary service area population was 25,522 in 2000.

Exhibit 2/10: Methodist Healthcare: Gross Patient Charges by Source

Payor	1999 (%)	2000 (%)	2001 (%)
Medicare	41.6	41.8	40.5
Medicaid/TennCare	18.8	18.2	18.9
Managed Care and Commercial	34.0	34.2	34.7
Self-Pay and Other	5.6	5.8	5.9
Total	100.0	100.0	100.0

installments over the ensuing 24 months. Although market share was on the incline and capital improvements were being made to upgrade the facilities in the West Tennessee market to provide improved patient care, the bottom lines were being evaluated on a tight basis to determine their contribution to the overall system.

Payor Mix

The sources of gross patient charges realized by payor for the fiscal years ended December 31, 1999, 2000, and 2001 are shown in Exhibit 2/10. At 40.5 percent in 2001, Medicare was the system's largest payor, followed by Managed Care and Commercial payors at 34.7 percent and Medicaid/TennCare at 18.9 percent.

MEDICARE

Inpatient acute care services rendered to Medicare beneficiaries were paid at prospectively determined rates per discharge. These rates varied according to a patient classification system that was based on clinical, diagnostic, and other factors. Inpatient nonacute services and certain outpatient services rendered to Medicare beneficiaries were paid based on a cost reimbursement methodology. Defined capital and medical education costs related to services provided to Medicare beneficiaries were reimbursed primarily at prospectively determined rates. Methodist was reimbursed for cost-reimbursable items at tentative rates, with final settlement after submission of annual cost reports by Methodist and audits thereof by the Medicare fiscal intermediary.

MANAGED CARE/COMMERCIAL

Methodist entered into payment agreements with several commercial insurance carriers, health maintenance organizations (HMOs), and preferred provider organizations (PPOs). The basis for payment to Methodist under these agreements included prospectively determined rates per discharge, discounts from established charges, and prospectively determined daily rates.

TennCare

Effective January 1, 1994, the State of Tennessee elected to implement an alternative health care program to Medicaid called TennCare. The State requested and received a demonstration waiver under Section 1115(a) of the Federal Social Security Act to permit this implementation. Tennessee continued to receive the applicable federal subsidies that would have been available to fund the State's Medicaid program; these federal funds were instead dedicated to TennCare. Under the TennCare program, patients enrolled in managed care organizations (MCOs) that contracted with the State of Tennessee to ensure health care coverage to their enrollees. Methodist contracted with the MCOs to receive reimbursement for providing services to these patients. Payment arrangements with these MCOs consisted primarily of discounts from established charges.

Medicaid

Inpatient services rendered to State of Mississippi and State of Arkansas Medicaid beneficiaries were reimbursed primarily at prospectively determined rates per day of hospitalization. Outpatient services rendered to State of Mississippi and State of Arkansas Medicaid beneficiaries were reimbursed at discounts from established charges.

Mission, Vision, Values, and Goals Statement

The management team analyzed Methodist's direction for the future, including an in-depth analysis of the system's mission, vision, values, and goals. The team reaffirmed the Methodist mission and values and they remained the same; the vision statement changed, however, along with the goals and the various strategies to achieve the goals. The new vision statement was:

> Methodist Healthcare
> will be the physicians'
> healthcare system of choice
> by working in partnership
> with them to deliver
> excellent patient care

Five goals were developed to assist the organization in accomplishing its new vision:

1. To clearly differentiate Methodist Healthcare in the market;
2. To implement an information systems strategic plan;
3. To reorganize so that Methodist has the right people in the right places with the focus in the right places;
4. To review financial issues to determine how Methodist will finance the business and changes in the system; and

5. To emphasize Methodist as a learning organization committed to placing resources in and paying a lot of attention to the education of Methodist associates.

To accomplish the goals and move forward with the vision of the organization under the new leadership, Methodist's primary strategy was to become the physician's system of choice. To assist in accomplishing this strategy, a Care Transformation Initiative was created under Care Management to align and integrate all processes and functions that focused on improving patient care. Under one umbrella, the goal of the Care Management team was to establish patient care as the primary focus of Methodist Healthcare and each of its associates, and to cultivate an organizational environment that supported and facilitated the best patient outcomes. The vision statement fostered the strategy of moving Methodist's level of health care from good to great. In addition, the organizational culture of Methodist would be transformed to fully support care that was evidence-based, safe, effective, patient-centered, timely, efficient, and equitable.

The partnership with the physicians focused on defining the best processes to move patients smoothly through the system. A series of strategic meetings was scheduled with the physicians to learn what the physicians valued, what they wanted, and what they preferred in a facility. The ultimate goal was to improve patient care and to become partners with the physicians in caring for patients.

Internal Environmental Analysis

While the partnership with the physicians further developed, the management team focused its efforts on identifying the strengths and weaknesses within the organization. Every aspect of Methodist, including organizational culture, finance, information systems, and human resources, was reviewed to determine the strategies to be developed for the future.

Organizational Culture

The leadership team started a "Senior Executive Walkaround" program to assess a variety of issues from the customer perspective – patients, physicians, and associates. Although the team applauded successes, they realized that there needed to be some changes in attitudes. Associates were hesitant to ask for or expect the resources they needed to deliver excellent service. Those resources would make the difference between acceptable customer service and stellar customer service. Leaders were challenged to move quickly to inform associates of Methodist Healthcare's commitment to service excellence. Urgency was the call for the day; not a moment could be wasted.

To facilitate change in the organizational culture, Shorb challenged the directors to:

1. have the right people in the right places;
2. have a strong resolve for action and results, and clearly share expectations;

3. communicate and let associates know their role in making changes for the better, solving problems, and giving great customer service; and
4. be accountable.

He knew the associates could make it happen and charged them to "Just do it!"

Information Technology

The goal of transforming the delivery of care at Methodist was the guiding force for the implementation of state-of-the-art patient information technology. The IT package called *Cerner Millennium* had been selected to provide the solution to many of the initiatives identified for the Methodist organization. Standardization of the systems was important. Decreased variation in processes would lead to increased clinical accuracy and efficiency. The primary goal of the initiative was to improve the quality of care at Methodist by:

1. Measurably improving patient safety and outcomes;
2. Making it easier for physicians to practice at Methodist by standardizing access to information, terminology, and policies/procedures within and across facilities and by consolidating all duplicative functions;
3. Reducing variance in clinical processes and outcomes;
4. Eliminating or reducing paper-based processes wherever possible; and
5. Improving operational efficiency, particularly for nursing and other clinical staff.

Enhanced quality of care and provider productivity were in direct support of the refined vision of making Methodist Healthcare the physicians' health care system of choice.

Financials

Exhibits 2/11 and 2/12 summarize the consolidated balance sheets and financial results of operations for the years ended December 31, 1999, 2000, and 2001. Methodist's consolidated "net patient service revenues" increased $75.1 million from 2000 to 2001. The net increase was primarily attributable to an increase of $67.8 million at Methodist Memphis, where patient discharges and outpatient volumes increased by 8.6 percent and 8.0 percent, respectively.

"Salaries and benefits" plus "supplies and other expenses" grew by $57.5 million between 2000 and 2001. These increases were driven by volume increases at Methodist Memphis and increased pay rates for associates in nursing and certain clinical areas. "Provision for bad debts" increased $9.6 million, primarily at Methodist Memphis, where an increase of $7.2 million was attributable to the combined impact of increases in patient volumes and increases in gross charges.

Exhibit 2/11: Methodist Healthcare and Consolidated Affiliates: Condensed Consolidated Balance Sheets

	Year Ended December 31,		
Assets	**1999**	**2000**	**2001**
		(Dollars in Thousands)	
Current Assets:			
Cash, Cash Equivalents, and Short-Term Investments	172,070	175,964	234,238
Accounts Receivable Net – Patient, Third Party, Other	198,256	200,632	172,169
Inventories	17,183	16,910	18,920
Prepaid Expenses and Other Current Assets	6,033	4,259	5,563
Assets Limited as to Use – Current Portion	8,461	11,090	14,215
Total Current Assets	402,003	408,855	445,105
Assets Limited to Use, Less Amounts Required to Meet Current Obligations	20,642	21,443	20,992
Property, Plant and Equipment, Net	387,915	371,117	372,985
Unamortized Debt Issue Costs	4,889	4,379	3,845
Other Assets	25,347	29,584	37,546
Total Assets	840,796	835,378	880,473
Liabilities and Net Assets	**1999**	**2000**	**2001**
Current Liabilities:			
Accounts Payable and Accrued Expenses	52,634	48,162	56,119
Accrued Payroll and Payroll Taxes	29,470	30,936	37,342
Accrued Interest	4,385	4,248	4,033
Due to Medicare and Medicaid Programs	–	–	7,778
Long-Term Debt Due Within One Year	10,361	10,592	14,660
Total Current Liabilities	96,850	93,938	119,932
Long-Term Debt, Less Amounts Due Within One Year	254,580	242,540	238,418
Accrued Pension and Other Long-Term Liabilities	26,554	29,905	37,448
Minority Interest	2,164	2,229	2,365
Total Liabilities	380,148	368,612	398,163
Net Assets:			
Unrestricted	448,176	453,357	467,031
Temporarily Restricted	12,472	13,409	15,279
Total Net Assets	460,648	466,766	482,310
Total Liabilities and Net Assets	840,796	835,378	880,473

"Excess of revenues and other support over expenses" showed a favorable improvement of $12.4 million from 2000 to 2001, mostly because of increased volume levels at Methodist Memphis.

"Cash, cash equivalents, and short-term investments" increased in 2001, primarily because of improvements in collection of accounts receivable as indicated by a reduction of $28.5 million in net accounts receivable. "Other assets"

Exhibit 2/12: Methodist Healthcare and Consolidated Affiliates: Summary Consolidated Financial Results of Operations

	Year Ended December 31,		
	1999	**2000**	**2001**
	(Dollars in Thousands)		
Unrestricted Revenues and Other Support:			
Net Patient Service Revenues	798,445	800,253	875,363
Other Revenues	55,048	47,137	48,162
Gain on Sale of Hospital Facilities	7,792	–	–
Equity in Net Income of Unconsolidated Subsidiaries	3,560	3,351	2,825
Net Assets Released From Restrictions Used for Operations	1,062	5,366	6,803
Total Unrestricted Revenues and Other Support	865,907	856,107	933,153
Expenses:			
Salaries and Benefits	421,192	421,595	456,179
Supplies and Other Expenses	299,012	299,839	322,753
Provision for Bad Debts	64,123	70,404	80,036
Depreciation and Amortization	50,475	47,085	46,808
Interest	15,054	13,232	10,990
Total Expenses	849,856	852,155	916,766
Excess of Revenues and Other Support Over Expenses	16,051	3,952	16,387
Minority Interest	(1,485)	(1,505)	(1,597)
Other Changes in Unrestricted Net Assets:			
Change in Net Unrealized Gains and Losses on Investments	(3,269)	2,734	(1,116)
Discontinued Operations	(7,994)	–	–
Extraordinary Gain on Early Extinguishment of Debt	1,458	–	–
Increase in Unrestricted Net Assets	4,761	5,181	13,674
Temporarily Restricted Net Assets:			
Restricted Contributions	1,071	6,303	8,673
Net Assets Released From Restrictions	(1,062)	(5,366)	(6,803)
Increase in Temporarily Restricted Net Assets	9	937	1,870
Increase in Net Assets	4,770	6,118	15,544
Net Assets at Beginning of Year	455,878	460,648	466,766
Net Assets at End of Year	460,648	466,766	482,310

increased $8 million in 2001 from a $12.5 million note receivable created in the financing of a Memphis professional office building. "Accounts payable and accrued expenses" increased by $8 million because of increases in end-of-year accounts payable accruals. Proposed Medicare/Medicaid cost report liabilities were recorded at $7.8 million. "Accrued payroll and payroll taxes" increased in 2001 by $6.4 million from the timing of the year-end payroll processing cycles. "Accrued pension and other long-term liabilities" increased by $7.5 million in 2001 from the increase in the reserve for professional and general liability claims of $5.9 million.

Exhibit 2/13: Methodist Healthcare and Affiliates: Net Income (Loss)

	1999	2000	2001
		(Dollars in Thousands)	
Methodist Healthcare-Memphis Hospitals:			
University	1,465	(5,804)	(2,870)
South	455	1,293	1,843
North	4,592	7,546	4,941
Germantown	5,255	5,997	10,369
Le Bonheur	12,611	15,144	16,420
Total	24,378	24,176	30,703
MH of Fayette	(1,004)	(644)	(434)
WT Operations:			
MH of Dyersburg	1,276	81	99
MH of Brownsville	(447)	(175)	(374)
MH of Lexington	235	(29)	130
MH of McKenzie	(65)	(161)	(238)
MH–Volunteer Hospital	194	(2,251)	(669)
MH–Jackson Hospital	(2,737)	(2,363)	(5,421)
MH–McNairy Hospital	(102)	(469)	(140)
West Tennessee Medical Associates	(2,512)	(1,623)	(1,660)
Total	(4,158)	(6,990)	(8,273)
Mississippi Operations:[a]			
Methodist Medical Center	15,052	–	–
MH of Middle Mississippi	(4,742)	–	–
Central Mississippi Medical Associates	(3,173)	–	–
Total	7,137	–	–
Methodist Primary Care Associates	(2,880)	(4,086)	(1,963)
Methodist Community Care Associates	(1,747)	(2,195)	(1,330)
Methodist Extended Care Hospital	(370)	(608)	(231)
Alliance Health Services	5	1,308	1,144
Ambulatory Operations, Inc.	(9,716)	(1,655)	(1,195)
Corporate Financial Services	(6,767)	(5,022)	(4,527)
MH Foundations	(108)	1,834	1,650
Total	(21,583)	(10,424)	(6,452)
Combined Total	4,770	6,118	15,544

[a] Near the end of 1999, Methodist Medical Center was sold to Health Management Associates, Inc.; MH of Middle Mississippi transferred assets to the University of Mississippi Medical Center Hospitals and Clinics; and Central Mississippi Medical Associates was sold to Premier Practice Management, Inc.

The breakout of the net income (loss) by organizational operation is illustrated in Exhibit 2/13 for the same period. Although Methodist Memphis had expanded many of its tertiary services, Methodist and its affiliates had also experienced the dissolution of assets and operations as follows.

SALE OF MISSISSIPPI OPERATIONS

Methodist Healthcare – Jackson Hospitals (Methodist Medical Center) transferred its lease of a 473-licensed bed hospital and sold other assets in Jackson, Mississippi, to Health Management Associates, Inc. in April 1999. In February 2000, Methodist Healthcare – Middle Mississippi Hospital transferred its 83-licensed bed hospital in Lexington, Mississippi, to the University of Mississippi Medical Center Hospitals and Clinics, and in October 1999 Methodist Healthcare Central Mississippi Medical Associates sold its Kosciusko Clinic to Premier Practice Management–Jackson, Inc. Following the dispositions, Methodist's operating assets in Mississippi were limited to two primary care clinics located south of Memphis in Tunica and Robinsonville as part of its Methodist Healthcare Community Care Associates operations.

WITHDRAWAL FROM PHYSICIAN PRACTICES

Like many other hospital systems, Methodist determined that its affiliates' ownership and operation of physician practices in primary care clinics needed to be discontinued in many cases. In addition to the closing of the Kosciusko Clinic, Methodist Healthcare Community Care Associates ceased operating a clinic located in Sardis, Mississippi, in February 2001, and continued to consider reducing or eliminating operations of its remaining clinics. Similarly, Methodist Healthcare Primary Care Associates had terminated its physician employment contracts in connection with its Memphis area primary care clinics and offices. Methodist Healthcare West Tennessee Medical Associates continued to evaluate its 14 physician employment contracts, which were the only remaining primary care physician contracts with Methodist or its affiliates.

Although the combined operations resulted in net income of $4.8 million, $6.1 million and $15.5 million for 1999, 2000 and 2001, respectively, the margins needed to be stronger to finance future capital needs and the implementation of an information systems strategic plan with an estimated cost of nearly $100 million over the next ten years. The information systems plan involved the replacement of all applications relating to pharmacy, pathology, radiology, scheduling, transcription, patient management and accounting, and order entry/results with an integrated system that required new hardware and software licenses. When implemented, the system was expected to enable Methodist and its affiliates to track clinical procedures and results and to bill and account for services provided throughout the Methodist system. According to Chris McLean, senior VP of finance and CFO, "A critical part of the formula to pursue the vision is a prudent financial plan that enables us to meet our day-to-day requirements, while also funding our strategic initiatives." To accomplish this goal, all business lines, including the West Tennessee division, remaining Mississippi operations, and programs within the system that were not part of the strategic priorities, needed to be reviewed and decisions had to be made about the future. For Methodist Le Bonheur Healthcare to meet its goals, it was important to focus financial and human resources on priorities.

Human Resources

The system leadership had made a renewed commitment to hiring and retaining the right people who shared the "Methodist Way" values of quality, fairness, service, and integrity. Having the right people to pursue the vision was imperative, and Shorb thought that the formula for success was in analyzing the results of the *Associate Feedback Survey*. He commented, "Communication of the results of the survey is the key driver to the future success of the organization in reducing voluntary turnover and retaining excellent, customer-focused associates."

According to Carol Ross-Spang, the VP of human resources, "The survey results indicate that associates find their work satisfying, they are personally committed to the future success of Methodist, they would recommend Methodist as a good place to work, and they would recommend Methodist services to family and friends. At the other end of the spectrum, it looks as though we could do a much better job in asking for suggestions from associates." Associates themselves were extremely valuable in providing information about why processes did or did not work effectively. The survey results showed that the perception of Methodist Healthcare as a place to work was good, but there was room for improvement. Shorb added, "Our ability to move our organization to the next level of excellence requires a focused discipline to understand and resolve the issues that create barriers for our associates' satisfaction and performance. With management, associates, and physicians all working together we can make Methodist great."

For its associates, Methodist made a commitment to develop educational programs in health care management and leadership. As part of this commitment and in honor of Maurice Elliott's years of service in leading Methodist Healthcare, the Maurice Elliott Leadership Institute (MELI) was established to further the education of Methodist associates. In collaboration with the University of Memphis Department of Health Administration and through a $1 million grant funded by Le Bonheur Health Services, Inc. (the former parent holding company turned grant-making organization following the 1995 merger of Methodist and Le Bonheur), MELI focused on middle managers because they often held the key in translating the vision of a company to employees.

The University Medical Center Initiative

According to Dr. Henry Herrod, Dean of the College of Medicine at the University of Tennessee at Memphis, "Research shows that the best medical centers in the country are academic medical centers." Although Methodist was reviewing its internal processes for improvement, the system was simultaneously working as part of the University Medical Center Coordinating Council (UMCCC) that included The Regional Medical Center at Memphis (The Med), the Veterans Affairs Medical Center (VA), and University of Tennessee Bowld Hospital (UT Bowld). The goals of the council were to improve quality of medical care, achieve financial savings, and foster a smoother working relationship among the medical center hospitals. The affiliation agreement signed in early 2002 between

Methodist Healthcare and The University of Tennessee Health Science Center set the strategic course for the delivery of medicine in Memphis and the Mid-South. Through the new learning environment, the best and brightest physicians from private practice were merged with the greatest minds among academic physicians and educators.

As part of the process of building the University Medical Center into a major center for treatment, research, and education, Methodist entered into discussions with the UT Bowld Hospital to assume management of UT Bowld with the objective of strengthening transplant and chronic disease programs at Methodist University Hospital. According to Shorb, "A strong transplant program is key to building the University Medical Center, and the transition of the management of UT Bowld to Methodist will ensure its continued success."

What's Next?

It had been almost a year since Gary Shorb was appointed CEO. He met with his leadership team to discuss the future of Methodist Healthcare based on the results of their analysis. He stated, "The future looks exciting for Methodist. Together we are moving the organization toward greatness. We have a number of successes, such as the launch of the Care Transformation initiatives, including plans for Cerner Technology, a stronger affiliation with the UT Health Science Center leading to exciting physician partnerships, the possibility of moving UT Bowld Hospital to Methodist management, the involvement in Medical Center initiatives through the UMCCC, record participation in the *Associate Feedback Survey*, and improved financial performance. There are challenges on the horizon, but I am confident that with committed and competent associates, each challenge will be met."

He continued, "I am asking each of you to evaluate the future strategic direction of Methodist Healthcare. How would you answer the following questions?

- How should we proceed with our remaining clinics in Mississippi?
- What are your thoughts on the strategic direction of our West Tennessee Division?
- We're headed in the right direction with UT Bowld and moving Methodist University Hospital toward academic medical center status, but will we have enough capital to proceed?
- How can we continue to improve our customer satisfaction – physicians, patients, and associates? Are we on track?
- Have our associates become 'service fanatics?' Are we continuing to raise the bar? Are our associates accountable?"

Shorb summed up: "The quest for excellence in clinical quality, service, and financial performance is something we must work at every day – we owe it to our patients. Getting better never stops. Together, we're looking forward to the future. Thanks to each of you for giving Methodist the chance to reach for a big vision and a big dream. We all can savor our successes as we head into an even brighter future."

Community Blood Center of the Carolinas: Donations, Donations, Donations

Tom Hassett, group vice president for Carolinas Healthcare System, was responsible for studying the laboratory service line for his hospital system in 2002 (one of 17 service lines with escalating costs). He recalled, "Our costs were actually going down from vendors who were working with us in a very tight time for health care in general and hospitals specifically. But blood costs kept increasing. In just one year, our cost for blood doubled! Discussions with the Red Cross – which was the dominant supplier of blood in our area – went nowhere. I think there were a couple of reasons for that. Charlotte is headquarters for a blood services region for the Red Cross and one of eight national blood testing labs is located here, but all business decisions are made in St. Louis and they don't appreciate our problems since they have problems of their own. They're trying to cover the costs for all the activities required by the consent decree. The St. Louis guys told us if we didn't like their prices we should get our blood elsewhere. That's when we really got serious about an independent blood center."

This case was written by Linda E. Swayne, The University of North Carolina at Charlotte and Thomas Hassett, Group Vice President for Carolinas Healthcare System. It is intended as a basis for classroom discussion rather than to illustrate either effective or ineffective handling of an administrative situation. Used with permission from Linda Swayne.

Discussions Begin

"We began to talk with hospitals in our immediate area about their experiences and found them to be similar to our experience. As informal word got around, more hospitals called to express their interest in looking at an alternative. Then we discovered America's Blood Centers – a national group serving as the umbrella organization for some 75 independent community blood centers spread around the country. When we approached them, ABC suggested that we contact two or three members about their centers and their willingness to help our group look at how we might set up an independent community blood center," Hassett explained.

He continued, "We then found out some interesting things. The Red Cross had a blood center in Springfield, Missouri that the hospitals there were not very happy with. When discussion began about a community blood center in Springfield, the Community Blood Center of Greater Kansas City was contacted for assistance. Don Thomson, CEO of the Red Cross center was hired to become the executive director of the Springfield area center, named the Community Blood Center of the Ozarks. Not long afterward, almost the entire staff of the Red Cross resigned and moved to the Community Blood Center of the Ozarks. This caused such a wrangle that the Red Cross filed lawsuits against the Ozarks and brought in a Red Cross executive by the name of Bob Carden. After an unfruitful battle against the community blood center, Bob resigned from the Red Cross, switched sides, and became the executive director at Virginia Blood Services, a community blood center in Richmond, Virginia.

"With the Ozark group's experience in mind, we pulled together the 22 hospitals that had indicated interest in a community blood center and asked these two gentlemen to speak to our group. Certainly, the event in Springfield became a model for what could happen with the start-up of a new center – both positively and negatively. Shortly thereafter, the North Carolina Hospital Association became interested in what was going on. At a meeting they organized for the state, some 60 hospitals attended to hear these same speakers, as well as Bill Coenen, the CEO of Community Blood Center of Greater Kansas City."

Although a statewide effort did not emerge, ten Charlotte-area hospitals committed to work together to develop a community-based blood organization. It was the first time that there had been such collaboration. Hassett recalled, "The hospitals worked extremely well together to resolve a common problem. The rising cost of blood was an issue for us all and blood is critical to all hospitals' operations. Although there is pretty intense competition among some of us, we had a common need and blood was neutral territory."

Charlotte Area Hospitals Agree to Investigate

Hassett continued, "Although the Red Cross says it has 'national pricing,' Premier did a study that documented the variation in the cost of blood across the United States. The lowest costs were in places where there was competition. We decided that we needed the competition in the Charlotte area and, despite some misgivings over tackling the Red Cross, we decided to investigate an independent blood center."

The hospitals' leadership group commissioned Astraea, Inc., parent company of Virginia Blood Services (VBS) in Richmond, Virginia, to evaluate the feasibility of starting an independent blood center to serve the Charlotte region. The VBS study showed that more than 1.5 million people lived in the region and if 60 percent of the population was eligible and able to donate blood, there were 900,000 potential donors in the area. Typically, about 5 percent of the population actually donated (75,000 people).

CBCC Begins

Community Blood Center of the Carolinas, the first community blood center in North Carolina, was the result of the collaboration by the hospitals. Because licensing generally takes three years to complete and the hospitals were anxious to begin operations, CBCC began by working under Virginia Blood Center's US Food and Drug Administration blood license. CBCC focused on serving the needs of blood donors, patients, and health care providers in the Charlotte region. (See Exhibit 3/1 for an overview about blood and blood collection.)

Exhibit 3/1: Blood: The River of Life

Using human blood to treat disease and trauma began in France in 1667 when Jean-Baptiste Denis documented a direct human blood transfusion. These early direct donor-to-patient transfusions were often unsuccessful because it was not possible to predict donor–recipient blood type compatibility. In 1901, a German scientist, Dr. Karl Landsteiner, discovered that there were different blood groups. Since he found that all humans fall into one of these groups, the ABO system provided an answer to the puzzle of why some transfusions had worked and others failed.

Blood had no substitute. Individuals who donated blood literally saved lives – more than 4.5 million American lives each year. Someone needed blood every three seconds. One pint (unit) of donated blood could save three lives. One out of ten hospital patients needed blood. Car accident and blood loss victims often needed transfusions of 50 pints or more of red blood cells. Bone marrow transplant patients needed platelet donations from about 120 people and red blood cells from about 20 people. Severe burn victims typically needed 20 units of platelets during their treatment.

The amount of blood in the body of an average adult was ten pints. Blood made up about 7 percent of a person's body weight. Sixty percent of the US population was eligible to donate blood but only 5 percent did so. About 32,000 pints were used each day in the United States.

When patients had organ transplants, cancer treatments, gastrointestinal disease, trauma, aneurysms, anemia and clotting disorders, accidents, open heart surgeries, burns, and so on, blood was required. However, blood from anyone would not necessarily be what the patient required.

BLOOD TYPES
Blood came in four different types – A, B, AB, or O – and differed by Rhesus factor (RH) as either positive or negative (approximately 15 percent of the population had negative blood). Nearly half of the blood "ordered" by hospitals was O– because it was the universal donor, meaning that everyone could safely receive O– type blood. Patients with any of the positive blood types could safely

receive O+ blood, but only O– could be used safely with all blood types. The most common type of blood was O+ (37.4 percent of the population) and the least common was AB– (0.6 percent).

Blood types in the population were as follows:

Type	Percent of the population
AB–	0.6
B–	1.5
AB+	3.4
A–	6.3
O–	6.6
B+	8.5
A+	35.7
O+	37.4

Blood type compatibility was as follows:

Type	Could be transfused to patients with blood type:
O+	O+, A+, B+, AB+
A+	A+, AB+
B+	B+, AB+
AB+	AB+
O–	O+, A+, B+, AB+, O–, A–, B–, AB–
A–	A+, AB+, A–, AB–
B–	B+, AB+, B–, AB–
AB–	AB+, AB–

THE PROCESS

Volunteers were screened to determine whether they were likely to be successful blood donors. The screening process became far more arduous after the emergence of HIV/AIDS and the discovery that numerous patients were infected from blood transfusions and organ transplants. Volunteer donors used to answer about 15 questions. After belatedly understanding that HIV was carried in transfusions, screening intensified. With the advent of mad cow disease, SARS, and West Nile virus, the number of questions increased to 50 or more, covering health, travel, and sexual history.

Blood was withdrawn from the volunteer to fill several vials and a one pint plastic bag (each marked with a unique bar code to match a particular donor's record and to track it electronically until the pint was delivered to a hospital and administered to a patient). The actual blood donation only took about 10 to 20 minutes, although the entire process took from 45 minutes to an hour. The blood was kept refrigerated until it reached a lab, where the unique bar code was read into the computer for tracking and monitoring of test results. The vials were used to type the blood (O, A, B, AB, plus RH factor) and to determine whether there were any transmissible diseases present. Fourteen tests (11 for infectious diseases) were performed on each unit of donated blood.

The pint of blood was separated into its components: leukocytes (white blood cells), red blood cells, platelets, and plasma. (Some patients required whole blood, but some did not. By separating the blood into these components, as many as three patients' lives could be saved from one donated unit.) Then the blood was stored under refrigeration until the test results were received. Testing generally took 12 to 16 hours and the results were returned electronically, enabling the blood to be distributed for use generally within 24 hours. Hospital professionals transfused the blood (or blood components) to the patient.

Exhibit 3/1: (cont'd)

Blood Components

Patients seldom required all the components of whole blood. The request for blood transfusion was specified based on the blood component needed for the patient's condition or disease. Thus, several patients benefited from a single pint of donated blood.

Apheresis, an increasingly common procedure, was the process of removing a specific component of the blood, such as platelets, and returning the remaining components, such as red blood cells and plasma, to the donor. This process allowed more of one particular part of the blood to be collected than could be separated from a unit of whole blood. Apheresis was also performed to collect red blood cells, plasma (liquid part of the blood), and granulocytes (white blood cells). The apheresis donation procedure took longer than the 45–60 minutes for whole blood donation; an apheresis donation might take between one to two hours. Not only were blood components different in the benefits they offered to patients, they had different shelf lives.

Red blood cells – Red blood cells had a shelf life of 21 to 42 days and could be treated and frozen for up to ten years. Red blood cells were particularly needed by patients who had chronic anemia, malignancies, gastrointestinal bleeding, and those with major blood loss from trauma.

Patients scheduled for surgery might be eligible to donate blood for themselves, a process known as autologous blood donation. In the weeks before nonemergency surgery, an autologous donor could have blood drawn that was stored until the surgical procedure.

White blood cells (leukocytes) – White blood cells protected the body from invasion by bacteria and viruses but they were also a factor in making some patients intolerant to blood transfusions. Therefore, much whole blood was filtered to remove leukocytes. The filtration had to occur within 48 hours of donation. However, for immunosuppressed patients, one type of white blood cells – granulocytes – were used to attempt to improve resistance to infection. Granulocytes were collected through apheresis donation or through centrifuging whole blood. White blood cells had to be transfused within 24 hours.

Plasma – Plasma was 90 percent water and contained albumin (protein), fibrinogen (helps with clotting), and globulins (antibodies). Although it looked like dirty river water, plasma maintained blood volume and pressure, supplied critical proteins for blood clotting and immunity, and provided a medium of exchange for vital minerals. This liquid component of blood was frozen soon after donation and could be stored for up to one year.

Platelets – Platelets helped to clot blood (stop the bleeding). They were collected by apheresis (or plateletpheresis) and through centrifuging whole blood. Platelets could be stored for up to five days at room temperature, provided that temperature was maintained at 72°F and the platelets were kept moving to avoid sticky clumps.

Blood Testing

Blood was tested for a variety of diseases that were determined to be transmitted (or theoretically could be transmitted) through blood donation. Prior to identification of the HIV/AIDS virus, blood was tested for syphilis and hepatitis B. During the 1980s, a number of tests were added: HIV/AIDS antibody tests (starting in 1985, with additional tests in 1992, 1996, 1999), hepatitis C (with additional tests for hepatitis A in 1986 and hepatitis B in 1987), human T-cell, and human lymphotropic virus. During 2000, blood tests and screening questions were added for SARS; in 2003, tests were added for West Nile virus.

The tests were performed to maintain a safe blood supply, but many blood collection organizations were concerned that the increased number of deferrals (healthy individuals who are not permitted to donate because of their travel or place of residence) would decrease the number of blood donors and endanger the blood supply.

As a blood center, CBCC gathered blood donations – the raw material for its operations – from people in the community and after breaking down the whole blood into red cells, plasma, platelets, and other components and testing for safety, the blood was returned to the community that donated it. CBCC planned to serve residents in York, Chester, and Lancaster counties in South Carolina; and Anson, Cleveland, Cabarrus, Catawba, Gaston, Iredell, Lincoln, Mecklenburg, Rowan, Stanly, and Union counties in North Carolina (Exhibit 3/2 maps the service area). Residents in these counties were served by the ten hospitals that originally developed the plans to establish CBCC (see Exhibit 3/3 for a brief description of the hospitals). The CBCC partner hospitals had 2,985 beds and used about 62,000 units of red blood and about 6,000 platelet doses annually.

Exhibit 3/2: Map of CBCC's Service Area

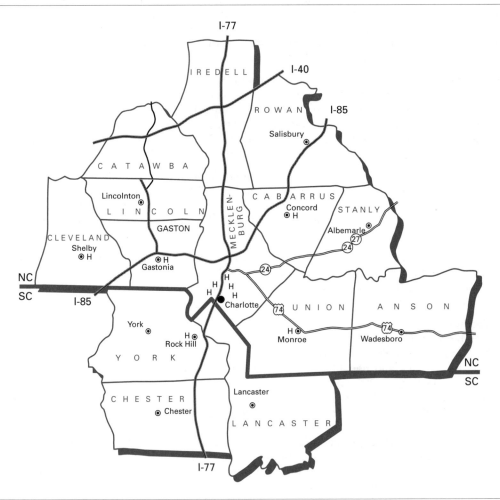

Exhibit 3/3: Hospitals that Formed CBCC

Ten hospitals came together to form the Community Blood Center of the Carolinas.

Carolinas Healthcare System, a not-for-profit, self-supporting organization, was the largest health care system in the Carolinas and one of the largest publicly owned systems in the nation. CHS was a vertically integrated system that owned and managed hospitals, nursing homes, physicians' practices, and physical and radiation therapy facilities in both North and South Carolina. It was comprised of more than 4,900 beds and employed more than 23,000 people. Its physicians' network included approximately 640 primary care doctors and other providers. The flagship hospital, *Carolinas Medical Center*, was named in *US News & World Report's* 2002 America's Best Hospitals list. *CMC Mercy Hospital, CMC – University*, and *CMC – South* were three partner hospitals to Carolinas Medical Center, the region's only Level 1 Trauma Center.

Gaston Memorial Hospital, with 1,543 employees, was operated by CaroMont Health and located in Gastonia, North Carolina (to the west of Charlotte). The 442-bed, independent, not-for-profit hospital was recognized nationally as one of the 100 top hospitals in the country. The growth of specialty services, such as the CaroMont Heart Center, the Comprehensive Cancer Center, and Women's and Children's Services, along with the addition of state-of-the-art surgical and treatment options, underscored Gaston Memorial Hospital's commitment to meeting the region's health care needs.

NorthEast Medical Center was established in 1937. This private, not-for-profit medical facility offered state-of-the-art services in affiliation with Duke University School of Medicine and Johns Hopkins. Offering a broad scope of services, 457 licensed beds, 275 skilled physicians and 3,500 employees, NorthEast Medical Center was a leading health care facility located in Kannapolis, North Carolina (in the north Charlotte region).

As one of the 118 hospitals owned by Tenet Healthcare, *Piedmont Medical Center*, located in Rock Hill, South Carolina, prided itself in keeping health care affordable, accessible, and effective for all families. With a staff of 1,400 employees combining advanced technology and highly skilled doctors, Piedmont provided a comprehensive care facility offering a wide variety of programs including cardiac surgery, neonatology services, emergency medical care, a cancer center, and a sleep disorder center.

Based in Charlotte, Presbyterian Healthcare was in the Southern Piedmont Region of Novant Health, the largest private, not-for-profit health care system in North Carolina. Presbyterian was comprised of four hospitals, *Presbyterian, Presbyterian Matthews, Presbyterian Orthopaedic Hospital* (one of the top 100 orthopedic hospitals in the nation), and *Presbyterian North* (opened in fall 2004). Novant's Southern Piedmont Region had 581 licensed beds and 5,772 employees, a skilled-nursing facility, physician division, and ancillary services.

The Organization

Gregory A. Ball was hired as the first executive director in November 2002 to start the Center. A native of Gastonia, he had worked for the American Red Cross for 26 years before doing consulting work in the blood industry. At the Red Cross he was credited with starting one of the first automated platelet-collection programs in the industry and building four local offices or manufacturing facilities. He had managed eight different Red Cross business units around the country. As a consultant, Ball worked with Astraea, Inc. (Virginia Blood Services) to develop the feasibility study for CBCC. He was then hired as the first executive director responsible for start-up, from identifying a local board of directors and a medical advisory board to finding a facility and beginning production.

In November, Ball stated his goals: "I need to hire 50 people necessary to staff CBCC, find the Center's first Charlotte collection facility, draw the first unit of blood by spring 2003, raise the percentage from the typical 5 percent of the population donating in Charlotte to 9 percent, and bring in revenues of $3.4 million in the first year."

In addition to Greg Ball, CBCC was led by a group of local business people who served as its board of directors and advised about the organization's business decisions – the products offered, where those products were to be sent, and how much they would cost. A medical advisory committee, comprised of local professionals, counseled the directors about medical concerns. Experts on this team – business and medical – were entrusted as stewards of local health care resources and were responsible for ensuring that the community received the most value possible for its health care dollars. (Exhibit 3/4 lists the 2004 board of directors and the medical advisory board.)

Start-Up

Temporary housing for the Center was in Presbyterian Hospital. The Center handled its first unit of blood on August 15, 2003. Ball estimated that a facility of 20,000 sq. ft. was needed initially, but 32,000 sq. ft. would be needed when CBCC was collecting 60,000 units per year – the community's annual need for blood. A 30,000 sq. ft. facility was found on South Boulevard, a major artery near Charlotte's city center, less than five miles from the two major hospitals in Charlotte and with easy Interstate access for the other hospitals. Leased for seven years, the price was $3.50 per sq. ft. in the first year and escalated over the period of the lease to $7.00 per sq. ft. (Exhibit 3/5 has a schematic of the facility.)

Ball stated at a September 19, 2003 open house for the new facility, "My requirements are two: compliance and customer service. Compliance requires that we have the size and the capabilities to keep the blood supply protected. Customer service has enabled us to have one to three blood drives a day with about one-third of the donors not having participated in a drive previously."

CBCC became a member of America's Blood Centers (ABC) because the group subscribed to the same philosophy as CBCC – community-focused blood banking – meaning that community donors knew that the blood they gave stayed in the community to help family members, friends, and neighbors. Only excess supply was shared with other communities when needed. CBCC was a member of the American Association of Blood Banks (AABB) as well. (Exhibit 3/6 contains an overview of these organizations.)

CBCC Mission

CBCC's mission was to provide local control of the blood supply, ensuring that local needs were met first. This local control provided greater choice for blood

Exhibit 3/4: CBCC Board of Directors and Medical Advisory Committee

Each of the five hospital systems involved with CBCC had a permanent seat on the board of directors. The remaining CBCC directors were elected to represent the communities served. These volunteer members of the board were business leaders and medical experts who made decisions to benefit the patients and donors in the greater Charlotte community. Board members included:

Jennifer Appleby – President and Chief Creative Officer, Wray Ward Laseter Advertising Agency.
Steven Burke – Vice President, Ancillary Services, Presbyterian Hospital* and CBCC Board Chair.
Jeffrey Canose, MD – Vice President, Medical Services Division, Gaston Memorial Hospital.*
Bob Carden – President/Chief Executive Officer, Virginia Blood Services.
John Cox – Chief Executive Officer, Cabarrus Regional Chamber of Commerce.
Scott Gollinger – Vice President, Clinical Services, NorthEast Medical Center.*
Mark Keener – Regional Chief Financial Officer, Carolinas Healthcare System.*
Edward Lipford, MD – Carolinas Pathology Group.
Kim McMillian – Vice President, Marketing/Public Relations, Allen Tate Realty Co.
Mark Patafio – Vice President, Small Business Sales Leader, Wachovia Bank.
Jeff Smyre – Senior Manager, Pricewaterhouse Coopers CPA.
Joseph Stough – Vice President, Piedmont Medical Center.*
*System permanent seats.

The CBCC medical advisory committee advised the board on medical matters. The medical advisory committee members were:

Linda Boggs – Transfusion Medicine Section Chief, Presbyterian Hospital.
Pam Clark, MD – Medical Director, Community Blood Center of the Carolinas.
Beth Curtis – Blood Bank Specialist, NorthEast Medical Center.
Rita Duffy – Blood Bank Supervisor, Gaston Memorial Hospital.
Stephen D. Harris, MD – Presbyterian Pathology Group.
Philip Leone, MD – Leone Pathology, Gaston Memorial Hospital.
Ned Lipford, MD – Carolinas Medical Center Laboratory.
Barbara McElhiney – Manager, Transfusion Services, Carolinas Laboratory System, Carolinas Healthcare System.
Beth Prichard, MD – NorthEast Medical Center Department of Pathology.
Rita Tate – Technical Director, Community Blood Center of the Carolinas.
Rob Thomas, MD – Piedmont Medical Center.
Kelly Ware – Transfusion Services Team Leader.
Jennifer Carpenter – Laboratory Director, Piedmont Medical Center.

products and services. Local doctors could select products and services that best met the needs of their patients. And for the first time in the region, donors had a choice of where they gave blood. CBCC was a customer-focused organization, and its service philosophy was to exceed expectations.

Ball said, "Control and choice lead to lower costs. CBCC is committed to offering services of the highest quality at more affordable and predictable pricing. Lower costs reduce patient charges and help our hospitals to control costs, become better stewards of resources, and improve patient care." CBCC emphasized regulatory

Exhibit 3/5: Plan of the CBCC South Boulevard Facility

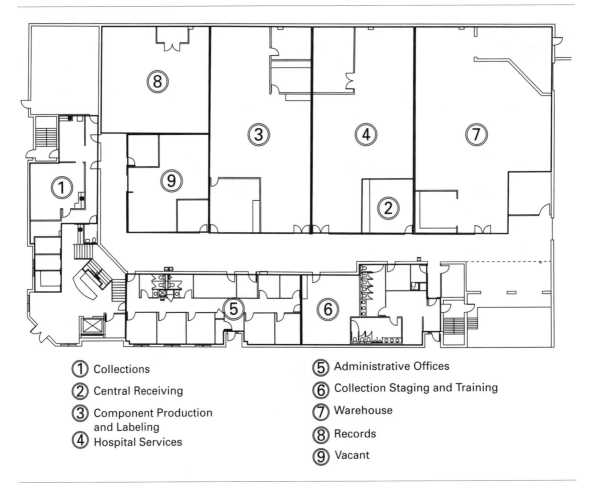

① Collections

② Central Receiving

③ Component Production
and Labeling

④ Hospital Services

⑤ Administrative Offices

⑥ Collection Staging and Training

⑦ Warehouse

⑧ Records

⑨ Vacant

Exhibit 3/6: Blood Banking Organizations

AMERICAN ASSOCIATION OF BLOOD BANKS
Founded in 1947, the American Association of Blood Banks (AABB) was organized to support and encourage continued blood research, promote exchange of scientific information, and develop standards of practice for blood banks. The AABB was an international association of blood banks, including hospital and community blood centers, transfusion and transplantation services, and individuals involved in activities related to transfusion and transplantation medicine. The AABB supported: high standards of medical, technical, and administrative performance; scientific investigation; clinical application; and education. It was dedicated to encouragement of voluntary donations of blood and other tissues and organs through education, public information, and research. The AABB member facilities were responsible for collecting virtually all of the nation's blood supply and transfusing more than 80 percent.

The AABB's mission statement was to establish and promote the highest standard of care for patients and donors in all aspects of: blood banking; transfusion medicine; hematopoietic, cellular, and gene therapies; and tissue transplantation. The AABB International's mission statement was to coordinate and promote improvements in blood banking and transfusion safety internationally by supporting: (1) the development of national and/or regional standards in blood banking; transfusion medicine; hematopoietic, cellular, and gene therapies; tissue transplantation; and (2) the development of mechanisms for assessing compliance with those standards.

More than 2,200 institutions (community and hospital blood banks, hospital transfusion services, and laboratories) were AABB members (AABB accreditation was a requirement for institutional membership). More than 8,500 individuals were members of the AABB (anyone interested in or actively involved in transfusion medicine and related biological therapies was eligible for individual membership, including physicians, scientists, administrators, medical technologists, blood donor recruiters, and public relations personnel). Members were located in all 50 states and 80 foreign countries. The AABB's active membership provided direction to the Association through its elected board of directors and more than 30 committees of volunteer professionals.

Accreditation

The AABB Accreditation Program strove to improve the quality and safety of collecting, processing, testing, distributing, and administering blood and blood products. The Accreditation Program assessed the quality and operational systems in place within the facility. The basis for assessment included compliance with Standards, Code of Federal Regulations, and federal guidance documents. This independent assessment of a facility's operations helped the facility to prepare for other inspections and served as a valuable tool to improve both compliance and operations. Accreditation was granted for: collection, processing, testing, distribution, and administration of blood and blood components; hematopoietic progenitor cell activities; cord blood activities; perioperative activities; parentage testing activities; immunohematology reference laboratories; and specialist in blood bank schools. Since 1957, the AABB has been a leader in the development of standards for voluntary compliance in blood bank blood component collection, processing, and transfusion. *Standards for Blood Banks and Transfusion Services* was developed by experts in blood banking and transfusion medicine. Standards were based on good medical practice and, when available, scientific data, principles associated with good manufacturing practices and quality assurance that were consistent with FDA regulations. These standards, along with the requirements specified in the *Accreditation Information Manual* provided the basis for the AABB Accreditation Program.

AMERICA'S BLOOD CENTERS

In 1962, seven community-based blood centers came together with the help of local hospitals, physicians, and civic groups to establish America's Blood Centers (ABC). Medical expertise, customer service, and a community-first blood banking philosophy were the founding principles of America's Blood Centers. The community-based blood banking philosophy meant that community donors knew that the blood they gave stayed in that community first – helping family members, friends, and neighbors. Any excess supply was shared with other communities that needed it most.

America's Blood Centers became an international network of 76 community-based blood centers around the United States and Canada. ABC members collected 7.5 million units of whole blood in 2003 – nearly half of the United States as well as 25 percent of the Canadian blood supply. ABC members yearly provided more than 10 million blood components (including red blood cells, platelets, and plasma) to hospital customers.

ABC members supplied a majority of the nation's tissue, bone marrow, stem cell, and transfusion services. In addition, America's Blood Centers members received the majority of blood-related NIH research funds. Fifteen members managed cord blood banks for transplantation. The New York Blood Center operated the largest cord blood bank in America.

ABC's national office provided members with support for national awareness campaigns, lobbying with the government, information on medical issues of concern to the blood banking community, blood resource sharing, group purchasing, educational programs, fund-raising support, blood center quality management issues, and federal regulation training programs.

Six ABC centers were located in South Carolina; Community Blood Center of the Carolinas was the only one in North Carolina.

and quality assurance standards to help make certain that only the highest quality blood products were collected and used, and ensured that the safety and well-being of donors and patients were protected. Residents of the region had an alternative to the Red Cross.

The American Red Cross[1]

Clara Barton and a circle of acquaintances founded the American Red Cross (ARC) in Washington, DC on May 21, 1881. Barton first heard of the Swiss-inspired International Red Cross Movement while visiting Europe following the Civil War. After returning home, she campaigned for an American Red Cross Society and for ratification of the Geneva Convention protecting the war-injured. She was successful on both.

Prior to World War I, the ARC introduced first aid, water safety, and public health nursing programs. With the outbreak of war, ARC staffed hospitals and ambulance companies, and recruited 20,000 registered nurses to serve the military. Additional Red Cross nurses came forward to combat the worldwide influenza epidemic of 1918. As a member of the International Federation of Red Cross and Red Crescent Societies, which it helped found in 1919, the American Red Cross joined more than 175 other national societies in bringing aid to victims of disasters throughout the world.

After World War I, ARC focused on service to veterans and enhanced its programs in safety training, accident prevention, home care for the sick, and nutrition education. In addition, it provided relief for victims of major disasters such as the Mississippi River floods in 1927 and severe drought and the Depression during the 1930s.

The Red Cross provided extensive services once again to the US military, Allies, and civilian war victims during World War II. It enrolled more than 104,000 nurses for military service. At the military's request, the Red Cross initiated a national blood program that collected 13.3 million pints of blood for use by the armed forces. After World War II, the Red Cross introduced the first nationwide civilian blood program that supplied nearly 50 percent of the blood and blood products in the United States. In addition, the Red Cross expanded its role in biomedical research and entered the new field of human tissue banking and distribution.

ARC's Biomedical Services[2]

The biomedical services division of the Red Cross comprised blood services, tissues services, plasma services, and research. Blood Services was the most visible of ARC's Biomedical Services Divisions and collected about 50 percent of the blood donated in the United States through 36 blood services regions. The Red Cross estimated that the United States needed 38,000 units of blood per day (over 13 million units annually). In fiscal year 2003, 6.42 million units were collected through the Red Cross – a decrease of 2.6 percent compared with fiscal 2002.

ARC Blood Services Division Has Its Problems

Although the Red Cross was known for its disaster relief as well as its blood products, it was the blood services division that caused its headaches.

BLOOD SAFETY[3]

The Red Cross had been under a court-supervised consent decree since 1993 to eliminate safety problems in its blood program. In the 1993 consent decree, the Red Cross agreed to establish clear lines of managerial control over a newly established, comprehensive, quality assurance program in all regions; to enhance training programs; and to improve computer systems, records management, and policies for reporting problems, including adverse reactions.

In February 1999, the ARC had completed its "Transformation," a $287 million program that reengineered its Blood Services' processing, testing, and distribution system and upgraded its computer system for tracking blood products (among other management activities). As a result of this investment, the ARC's Biomedical Services had:

- a single, standardized computer system that efficiently maintained its blood donor database;
- a network of eight national testing laboratories;
- a biomedical institute that provided training and other educational resources to Red Cross Blood Services' personnel;
- a quality assurance/regulatory affairs department to assure compliance with FDA regulations; and
- a centrally managed blood inventory system to ensure the availability of blood/blood components throughout the country.

Poor donor screening, the release of mislabeled blood, collecting blood from disqualified donors, flawed procedures aimed at keeping unsuitable blood in quarantine, falsified records, retaliation against employees who reported problems, poor inventory controls, computer errors in tracking blood, and failing to ask donors about risky health practices were some of the issues that the FDA had identified over time in various ARC facilities or its home office in Washington, DC. An FDA inspection of the Red Cross headquarters in December 2002 revealed that the ARC failed to correct deviations from the last inspection, that the ARC's lack of quality assurance oversight led to the release of unsuitable blood products, and that the lack of inventory control led to the unknown disposition of blood products. Thus, the FDA was ready to sue for a revised consent decree.

The revised consent decree stemmed from "FDA concerns arising from inspections over the past 17 years revealing persistent and serious violations of blood safety rules." The revised consent decree included the following fines if the ARC failed to comply with blood safety rules and the revised requirements:

- $10,000 per event for any violation of the ARC's standard operating procedures (FDA mandated and approved written procedures designed to help ensure product quality), the law, or consent decree requirements and timeline.
- $50,000 for the preventable release of each unit of blood if the FDA determined that there was a reasonable probability that the product might cause serious adverse health consequences or death, as well as $5,000 for the release of each unit that might cause temporary problems, up to a maximum of $500,000 per event.
- $50,000 for the improper re-release of each unsuitable blood unit that was returned to inventory.
- $10,000 for each donor inappropriately omitted from the National Donor Deferral Registry, a list of all unsuitable donors.

In February 2004, the FDA informed the ARC of its intention to assess fines because the ARC's Problem Management Standard Operating Procedures, submitted October 2003, did not meet the terms of the Amended Consent Decree. The Red Cross issued a statement that it "continues to share with the FDA the steadfast commitment to the safety and availability of the blood supply" and was "working diligently to review and implement satisfactory SOPs" that would bring it to "swift regulatory compliance." In addition, the Red Cross stated that it had made provisions within its operating funds to cover the cost of the penalties and that "no monetary donations will be used to pay these penalties."[4]

September 11, 2001: Attacks and Discarded Blood Units[5]

According to *The Washington Post*, the General Accounting Office reported that the vast amount of blood collected from new donors was not needed by victims of the terrorist attacks – fewer than 280 units were used of the approximately 572,000 additional pints collected. In the end, one in every three pints was thrown away – about 208,000 pints. The *Los Angeles Times* reported that critics had faulted the Red Cross for its "unrelenting call for blood donors after September 11th resulting in more than 250,000 pints being discarded because it was too old to use."[6]

The Red Cross was criticized for continuing to collect tens of thousands of pints after it was clear the blood would not be needed by the victims of the September 11 attacks and after many members of America's Blood Centers had halted collections rather than accept surplus blood. The Red Cross defended its actions and said it continued collections because it needed to build inventories in case of future attacks and wanted to enable Americans to do something for their country. In addition, the Red Cross said it planned to freeze more than 100,000 pints for future emergencies, but ended up freezing about 9,000 units.

Because of the bad publicity over the discarded blood, a backlash occurred, resulting in apathy toward donating. These first-time donors did not return. The Red Cross had 276,423 first-time donors within weeks of the attacks, but fewer than one in 20 returned.

Red Cross Research

The Red Cross national research program was established to make contributions to biomedical science, blood safety, plasma-derived therapeutics, and transfusion technology. Red Cross scientists were engaged in research to develop the next generation of blood products and services. Each year, the Red Cross invested more than $25 million in research projects seeking to improve the safety, purity, and efficacy of blood.

Recent examples of research results were the actions taken for leukocytes and cellular therapy. Ordinarily, leukocytes (white blood cells) help fight off foreign bodies, such as bacteria, viruses, and abnormal cells, to avoid sickness or disease; however, when transfused to another person, these foreign leukocytes in whole blood were often not tolerated well by some patients and have been associated with transfusion complications. Although not required by many patients, the Red Cross moved to a system-wide, pre-storage leukocyte reduction to improve patient care. Within 48 hours of donation, all blood was filtered to remove leukocytes, adding about $65 to the cost of processing each unit of blood.

Cellular therapy involved collecting and treating blood cells from the patient or another blood donor. The treated cells were then returned to the patient to help revive normal cell function; to replace cells that were lost as a result of disease, accidents, or aging; or to prevent illnesses. Cellular therapy might prove to be helpful for patients undergoing treatment for cancer, because researchers hoped that treated cells would battle cancerous cells.

ARC's Carolinas Blood Services Region[7]

Headquartered in Charlotte, North Carolina, Carolinas Blood Services was established to serve a population of more than 6 million people from 82 counties in North Carolina and parts of South Carolina, Georgia, and Tennessee. In addition, Charlotte was the location for one of eight Red Cross national testing laboratories. The Red Cross estimated that more than 1,500 units of donated blood were needed daily in the Carolinas region; between 1,500 and 1,600 blood products were distributed daily to more than 100 hospitals. Blood was collected from ten permanent sites (Asheville, Cary, Charlotte, Durham, Greensboro, North Raleigh, Raleigh, Wilmington, and Winston-Salem in North Carolina and Johnson City, Tennessee) and more than 10,000 blood drives each year involved businesses, churches, schools, shopping malls, and so on. In 2002, individuals donated more than 400,000 units of whole blood and more than 50,000 apheresis products. The Carolinas Blood Services Region led the nation in collections from 1997 through 2003.

Additional services offered by the Carolinas Blood Services Region included: two reference labs (operated 24/7); frozen units of rare blood (the American Red Cross maintained the National Rare Blood Registry); therapeutic apheresis; perioperative autologous salvage (recycling of a patient's blood during surgery); and bone marrow, stem cell, and sickle cell programs (typing for matching, and so on).

Blood Challenges

ARC collected about 45 percent of the blood supply, ABC-related organizations collected about 45 percent, and hospitals collected about 10 percent. Estimates were that approximately 32,000 units of blood were needed daily in the United States.

Number of Donors

The major challenge in blood banking was to increase the number of donors as well as increase the number of donations made by each individual donor. A healthy person could donate blood every 56 days (six times per year). Only 5 percent of the population donated blood. During the late 1990s and the early years of the new millennium, the advent of mad cow disease, SARS (severe acute respiratory syndrome), and the West Nile virus severely impacted the number of potential donors.

Donors had to be at least 17 years old, 110 pounds or more, and meet the requirements of the screening process. As the number of screening tests performed and the restrictions on donors increased, blood donors decreased. Screening for HIV/AIDS and hepatitis had been done for some time, but new tests were required for mad cow disease, SARS, and West Nile virus.

SCREENING FOR MAD COW DISEASE

In 2002, because of mad cow disease, the FDA enacted restrictions on blood donations from anyone who lived in the United Kingdom for three months or more between 1980 and 1996; spent five years or more in Europe since 1980; spent six months or more from 1980 to 1990 on a military base in Belgium, the Netherlands, Germany, Spain, Portugal, Turkey, Italy, or Greece; or who received a blood transfusion in the UK since 1980.

SCREENING FOR SARS

The first SARS case was identified in November 2002 and in April 2003 the FDA recommended guidelines for donations:

- Individuals who had traveled to high-risk areas for SARS (People's Republic of China, Hong Kong, Hanoi, Vietnam, Singapore, Taiwan, and Toronto, Ontario) were deferred from giving blood for 14 days after returning even if they showed no symptoms of infection.

* Individuals who had close contact with someone who had SARS were deferred for 14 days following the last close contact.
* Individuals who had SARS or were suspected of having SARS were deferred for 28 days after complete symptom resolution and termination of medical treatment.
* Recent donors who experienced a SARS related exposure were encouraged to report the information up to 14 days after donation.

SCREENING FOR WEST NILE VIRUS

The first West Nile virus cases in the United States occurred in 1999. Over the three years till 2001 there were 18 deaths. Then, in 2002, the number jumped to over 4,000 cases and 284 deaths. At least 23 people were infected by the virus through blood transfusion and four more through organ transplants. Nucleic acid amplification tests (NATs) of collected blood were required by the FDA as of July 1, 2003. Although donors were specifically asked if they had experienced fever with headache during the seven days prior to donation, only about 20 percent of individuals who had been exposed to the virus actually developed symptoms (flu-like, with headache, fever, and muscle aches). Individuals were deferred for 14 days after the last occurrence of symptoms (headache and fever) or if the NAT identified the presence of the virus.

Cost of Blood

Although donated blood is free, there are significant costs associated with: collecting, testing, preparing components, labeling, storing, and shipping blood; recruiting and educating donors; and quality assurance. As a result, processing fees are charged to recover costs. Hospitals charge for any additional testing that may be required, such as cross matching, as well as for the administration of the blood. When CBCC began operations in 2002, the Red Cross charged about $200 per unit and CBCC charged $150. For CBCC hospitals, the difference amounted to a $3 million saving. In 2004, the differential remained about the same.

Demand Exceeding Collections

The blood supply level fluctuated throughout the year. During holidays and in the summer, supplies tended to fall because donations declined, but demand remained stable or even increased. Persons 69 years and older accounted for approximately 10 percent of the population, but they required 50 percent of all whole blood and red blood cells transfused, according to the National Blood Data Resource Center. Using current screening and donation procedures, a growing number of blood banks found blood donation by seniors to be safe and practical.

Reality Sets in for CBCC

Trouble in collection volume became apparent in October 2003. Ball's estimates for blood collection were not being met (700 units collected versus 1,400 projected per month) and costs were considerably higher than budgeted. In November 2003, CBCC was required to undergo some "rightsizing." The board replaced Ball with an interim executive director, Linda O'Neal, who was director of marketing and strategic planning at Virginia Blood Services. O'Neal traveled to Charlotte each week from November to May, when chairman of the board, Tom Hassett, became the interim director.

Hassett had been intimately involved with CBCC since its inception. He flatly stated, "The critical success factors for CBCC are donations, donations, donations. The regulatory part is critical but it's a given. We need to be as near perfect as humanly possible. But if we don't have donations, it doesn't matter."

He continued, "When the budget was so bad, the board reduced the staff from 50 to 31. Blood requires a highly specialized staff and if they are not kept busy, we can't reduce the time they work per week because they will quit and go elsewhere – and there are plenty of places that will hire them."

One concern in particular to Hassett was that the board found it necessary to wipe out the marketing budget at a time when it was so necessary to get CBCC's name out to the community. He went on to describe other cost-cutting measures: "We have two apheresis machines that lease for $4,000 per month. We are not using those machines sufficiently and I'm trying to get out from one of the leases until we build the number of apheresis donors. In addition, several of the hospitals wanted us to do autologous blood collection at the hospital. We had three set up with that capability but it really made more sense for us to centralize that process. Now we have autologous collection, apheresis collection, and whole units collected at the Center."

Hassett expressed some frustration in CBCC's inability to attract donors. He commented, "The Red Cross is really entrenched here. They have had drives at companies and churches for years. We were warned that it would be challenging for CBCC to get started, but I don't think any of us realized how hard it would be. That's why we put back some marketing money in our tight budget. We began the '100 Sponsors in 100 Days' campaign that ran from April to August 5, 2004." Exhibit 3/7 shows one of the ads that ran in local newspapers.

Hassett summarized, "We ended up with 112 new sponsors, bringing the total number to 285 organizations. We are trying to contact new organizations that do not have pre-set ideas about only donating to the Red Cross. We are happy when anybody gives blood because it saves lives – but we would like more donors to give through CBCC. We've had some success going to high schools. Kids have to be over 17 to donate, but there are a good number of seniors who are. Targeting them is really a long-range strategy because we hope that over their lifetime they will continue to donate to CBCC."

He continued, "We collected about 1,000 units a month – by fiscal year end 2004. In 2004–05, CBCC is satisfying 70 percent of the need for blood in the region

Exhibit 3/7: 100 in 100 Ad

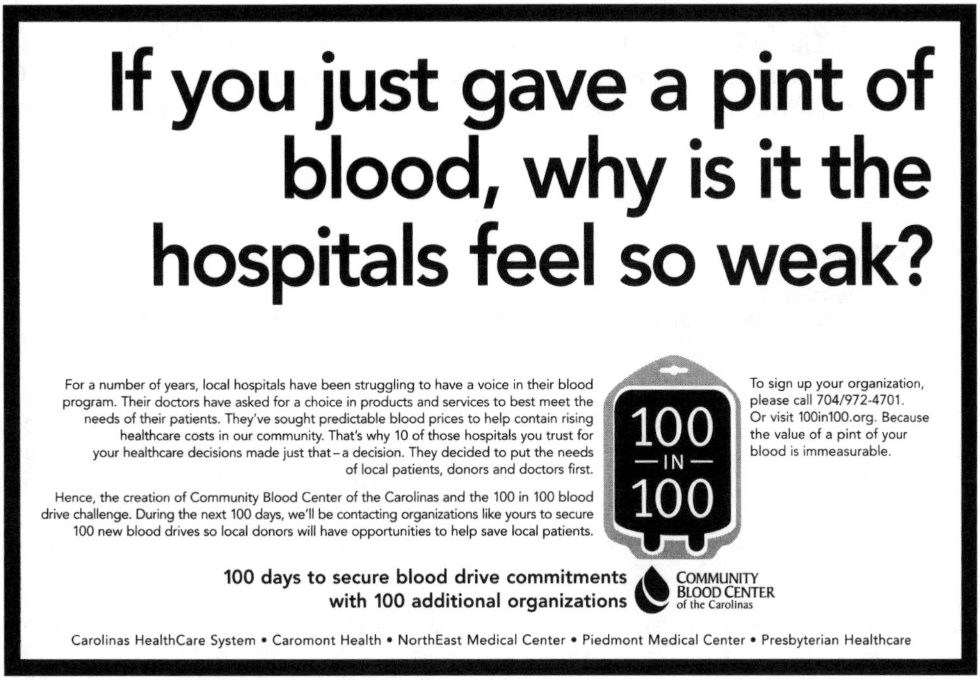

– from what we draw [local donations] and from other independent centers that are ABC members. Charlotte area hospitals need about 60,000 units a year. With CBCC collections nearing 14,000 this fiscal year, and increasing help from other centers, we are well on our way to supplying the entire blood need in just a few years. It is important to the hospitals we serve to do that."

Some ABC blood centers were fortunate enough to collect more blood than they regularly use. CBCC contracted with some of them for excess blood for one year; contracts with others were by the quarter. Because it was excess blood for the centers, the price was reduced. Hassett said, "We don't want to rely on blood from other centers, but for now it is an effective bridge to help us get where we need to be."

Financial Concerns

"We have three crews that handle our drives," explained Hassett. "We need to keep them and the Center staff busy to lower our costs of production. We have also been talking with hospitals in western North Carolina and Greensboro that might start community blood centers and ship blood to us for processing. It seems logical that we don't all need processing facilities and ours is certainly large enough.

I don't know if we can make that work, but it is an interesting scenario. Right now our hands are full managing our operations and building the number of donors.

"Our original budget (see Exhibit 3/8) was optimistic. When we didn't hit the numbers, we were fairly drastic in 'rightsizing.' We cut staff – from 50 employees to 31 – and reviewed all ways to manage more efficiently. Despite the

Exhibit 3/8: Initial Budget

A: Forecasted Collections

FY 2003 (April through September)

	Oct.	Nov.	Dec.	Jan.	Feb.	Mar.	Apr.	May	Jun.	Jul.	Aug.	Sep.	Total
Collections													
Whole Blood							400	400	600	700	700	800	3,600
Autologous								150	150	150	150	150	750
Apheresis										25	50	75	150
Total							400	550	750	875	900	1,025	4,500

FY 2004

	Oct.	Nov.	Dec.	Jan.	Feb.	Mar.	Apr.	May	Jun.	Jul.	Aug.	Sep.	Total
Collections													
Whole Blood	700	800	900	1,000	1,100	1,200	1,350	1,400	1,450	1,500	1,500	1,600	14,500
Autologous	75	75	75	75	75	75	75	75	75	75	75	75	900
Apheresis	10	10	20	30	40	40	40	50	50	50	50	50	440
Total	785	885	995	1,105	1,215	1,315	1,465	1,525	1,575	1,625	1,625	1,725	15,840

B: CBCC Summary P&L (Forecasted) ($)

	FY 2003	FY 2004		FY 2003	FY 2004
Revenue			Education	7,200	0
Blood Products			Public Relations	153,330	104,000
Red Blood Cells (RBCs)	513,000	2,493,909	Services Purchased	448,365	711,785
RBCs Leukoreduced	0	4,743,920	Utilities	45,000	85,325
RBCs-Auto's	168,750	200,475	Business Expense	54,690	27,700
Random Donor Platelets	54,530	272,655	Insurance	39,328	146,122
Fresh Frozen Plasma	98,800	1,060,245	Depreciation	70,487	123,680
Recovered Plasma	24,273	0	Interest Expense	68,956	100,380
Apheresis Platelets	20,000	230,400	Duplication Expense	59,618	4,460
Total Revenue	**879,353**	**9,001,604**	Building Repair	0	0
			Renovations	0	0
Operating Expenses			Shipped-in-Blood	0	5,107,544
Salaries	1,338,480	1,882,440	Postage	11,250	6,000
Salaries O/T	88,316	55,680	Contributions	0	0
Bonus	0	0	Freight	32,528	28,992
Benefits	285,359	327,341	Taxes	20,000	0
Professional Services	391,360	503,100	Lease/Rent	128,749	207,479
UNCAP Equipment	16,862	1,500	Purchase Expense	6,270	0
Equipment Rentals	17,472	48,000	**Total Operating Expense**	**3,498,696**	**9,819,008**
Equipment Repair	27,364	15,925			
Supplies	187,712	331,555	**Net Income (Loss)**	**(2,619,343)**	**(817,404)**

loan guarantees from the hospitals that created CBCC, projections were that we might run out of cash by September."

Hassett's task during the summer of 2004 was straightforward:

- Increase cash flow to keep the Center alive.
- Increase the number of donors and sponsors.
- Increase the level of customer service.
- Hire a highly talented and energetic executive director.

CASH FLOW

With a projection of running out of credit in September, the hospitals agreed to institute a fast-pay program – CBCC submitted invoices daily and was paid weekly. Consequently, days in accounts receivable were significantly reduced and the Center was positioned to stay alive while the other cost-reduction strategies were implemented.

SPONSORS AND DONORS

The "100 in 100" campaign was given major focus with a very positive outcome of signing 112 new sponsors in 100 days. Because of new sponsors, future donations would increase because of the relationships being built.

CUSTOMER SERVICE

Every drive needed to be as near perfect as possible. Collecting blood was nearly identical no matter whether it was the Red Cross or a community blood center because the process was so heavily regulated by the FDA. The difference would be seen in donor satisfaction and sponsor satisfaction. Survey instruments were implemented so that CBCC could score and track satisfaction. The reports pointed out where improvement could be made and provided positive feedback to the collection and support staff. Satisfaction scores increased to the level of between "very satisfied" and "extremely satisfied."

EXECUTIVE DIRECTOR

With cash flow in order, the number of sponsors significantly increased, and donor satisfaction high, it was time to recruit a permanent executive director. First, the board defined the qualities desired in CBCC's top executive. A proven track record of success in a sales-oriented business was considered to be of utmost importance. Secondly, the individual's personality would need to exhibit passionate energy for the community role and success of CBCC. Thirdly, it would take someone who could manage operations well. Because of the expertise of Virginia Blood Services regarding all regulatory and quality functions, the board felt that the executive director did not have to be an expert in the science of blood banking but he or she would certainly have to have a healthy respect for the need to be outstanding in the areas of quality and regulation and to assure compliance.

What's Next?

Challenges remained for CBCC. Although the budget for the Center called for breakeven operations by September 2005, it also called for a 40+ percent increase in the number of collections. It was considered doable, but challenging. The largest companies and government agencies in the region had a long history of sponsorship with the Red Cross; it continued to fight to maintain its market share despite 70 percent of the blood collected in the Charlotte area being sold across the country. CBCC had to earn its way to increased blood drive sponsors by proving over and over its commitment to the local community and telling its story by every avenue possible.

After an extensive search, Martin Grable was hired as executive director in September 2004 (see Exhibit 3/9 for the news release announcing the appointment). In accepting the position, he stated, "It's all about donor development – there is nothing else. CBCC is meeting the quality and service standards. Clearly we have to build the donor and sponsor base."

He continued, "The fiscal year has just started. Three days after I arrived one of the recruiting managers resigned. We can't get behind the curve in October

Exhibit 3/9: News Release

CBCC APPOINTS NEW EXECUTIVE DIRECTOR

Charlotte, NC – Community Blood Center of the Carolinas' Board Chair, Steven Burke, announces the appointment of Martin A. Grable of Charlotte as Executive Director. Mr. Grable has 17 years of experience delivering consulting, financial, and professional services to large corporations. Most recently, he was cofounder, president and CEO of Matrix Absence Management, Inc. of San Jose. Founded in 1985, Matrix is a national benefits administrator providing professional services to many of the Fortune 500 companies – a number of which have remained with the company since its beginnings. The first seven Matrix clients – Philips Semiconductor, University of the Pacific, Amdahl, LSI Logic, National Semiconductor, Sun Microsystems and Intel Corporation – have remained as clients. He sold the company in 1998 to Delphi Financial Group and agreed to remain as President and CEO for three years.

In 2002, Martin Grable had the good fortune to travel and reflect on the opportunities that might lie ahead. He did an exhaustive search for the right community for his family – one that was growing, with a diverse economic base, in a good location with a great climate and a major airport, and a strong sense of community. After many visits to a number of locations, he became a Charlottean by choice.

His interest in doing something different that would make a difference led Grable to apply for the position of Executive Director at CBCC. Grable stated, "I came to CBCC because I recognized the importance and value a community blood center brings to the community. The blood supply is a community asset, best managed locally, with the interests of the local community as the top priority." CBCC was established in 2003 through the collaborative efforts of ten area hospitals to better provide for the blood needs of the communities in the Charlotte area. Steven Burke, CBCC Board Chair said, "The Board is really excited that Martin Grable is bringing both his concern for the community and his entrepreneurial spirit to assist in meeting the blood needs for our community."

Grable was born and raised in Kansas and attended the University of Kansas. He is married to Cathy and they have three children: Lauren 20, Nicole 26, and Heather 30.

because the months of November and December are traditionally slow months for donations. I have to figure out what to do now – the immediate plan. Then, determine a mid-range plan for the next two quarters, followed by a longer term strategic plan . . . But, they all have to work together or there will be a mixed message to donors and sponsors and that won't help us at all."

He concluded, "I like the odds. We'll have a few bumps in the road, but I like the geometry of the hospitals, the community, and the blood center. We are a service to the community and we will develop that sense of community."

NOTES

1. This section is taken from "A Brief History of the American Red Cross," http://www.redcross.org/museum/history/brief.asp, accessed July 10, 2004.
2. Information in this section is from "Biomedical Services," http://www.redcross.org/services/biomed/, accessed July 10, 2004.
3. "American Red Cross Agrees to Revised Consent Decree to Improve Blood Safety," *FDA News* at http://fda.gov/bbs/topics/NEWS/2003/NEW00891.html, accessed September 18, 2004.
4. "American Red Cross Statement on FDA Adverse Determination Letter of Feb. 6, 2004," http://www.redcross.org/pressrelease/0,1077,0_314_2271,00.html, accessed September 18, 2004.
5. Gilbert M. Gaul and Mary Pat Flaherty, "Troubled Times for Red Cross; Blood Bank Faces Shortages, Dispute over Safety Violations," *The Washington Post* (September 16, 2002), p. A-2.
6. Charles Ornstein, "FDA Cites Concerns over Red Cross' Handling of Blood," *Los Angeles Times* (December 11, 2001), p. A-44.
7. This section is adapted from "About Us," American Red Cross Carolinas Blood Services Region at http://www.redcrossblood.org/about.htm, accessed on July 10, 2004.

4 *CASE*

ASPIRE^2 in Arkansas

In 1995, members of the senior staff and the health officer of the Arkansas Department of Health (ADH) were increasingly concerned about changes taking place in public health nationally and within the state. The programs at professional meetings were packed with public health experts warning of the dire consequences of managed care and increasingly aggressive competition from the private health sector. The news media bombarded all public agencies with legislative demands for accountability. A sense of anxiety, insecurity, and uncertainty was growing among the staff.

How soon would this new environment materialize? Did the Department have time to prepare for the changes and perhaps convert what appeared to be threats into new opportunities for public health in Arkansas? Would the most vulnerable clients of the Department suffer from the changes? Would employees have jobs in this new health environment painted by the futurists? The senior staff and the health officer knew it was their responsibility not only to ask the questions but also to create the capacity within the Department to lead rather than merely react to the changes taking place.

Thinking strategically about the future of public health in Arkansas would require the time, talents, and energy of many people. It was important that people in the field as well as people in the central office be involved in the strategic thinking. All were

This case was written by Peter M. Ginter and W. Jack Duncan, University of Alabama at Birmingham, and Linda E. Swayne, The University of North Carolina at Charlotte. It is intended as a basis for classroom discussion rather than to illustrate either effective or ineffective handling of an administrative situation. Used with permission from Pete Ginter.

Appreciation is expressed to Ms. Gail Gannaway and Ms. Cathy Flanagin for their participation in the preparation of this case.

busy people who had full-time jobs seeing patients, collecting health statistics, tracking diseases, promoting health, and hundreds of other activities. The future was too important, however, and the opportunity to influence the Department's destiny was compelling.

ASPIRE

In July 1996, the Arkansas Department of Health initiated a comprehensive strategic thinking process known as ASPIRE (Arkansas Strategic Planning Initiative for Results and Excellence). The formal planning process required a year to complete, but ASPIRE continued in Arkansas because strategic thinking became a way to lead this large and complex organization. During the time of the initiative, the governor of the state changed, the health officer changed, and public health in Arkansas struggled with limited resources and higher standards of accountability. The Department's commitment was based on the dedication of the leaders and employees – all colleagues – to put the public health of Arkansas above personal agendas, make difficult decisions, respect the dignity of individuals adversely affected by change, and provide the most secure environment possible in turbulent times.

Strategic leaders, faced with the uncertainty created by environmental chaos, had two choices regarding their future. They could close themselves off into bureaucratic cocoons and deny the reality of change, becoming progressively more irrelevant and, ultimately, contributing to their own demise. Or, they could choose to influence the direction of change where possible and reinvent themselves to better cope with turbulence and chaos. The Arkansas Department of Health decided to do what it could to influence its future.

The ADH completed its first strategic plan – ASPIRE – in 1997. Colleagues from all parts of the Department were involved in assessment of the external and internal environments, development of mission and vision statements as well as guiding principles, goal setting, and action plans.

Dr. Fay Boozman was appointed director for the Arkansas Department of Health in February 1999 (Exhibit 4/1 provides a brief biographical summary). When Dr. Boozman was named, the usual amount of uncertainty arose among the employees because it was unclear what his view would be regarding ASPIRE. Would he have another approach to management that he found successful and more suited to his leadership style? Would he associate ASPIRE with the past and prefer to dismantle it, regarding it as a useful exercise but not the program to take the Department into the future?

The planning and policy staff as well as the Steering Committee attempted to inform the new director about the accomplishments of ASPIRE and the tasks that remained to be accomplished. Dr. Boozman endorsed ASPIRE, complimented the vision it created, and committed himself to reenergizing the strategic management process.

The director began traveling around the state and talking to people in local health units as well as the central office regarding all matters, including ASPIRE. He

Exhibit 4/1: Fay Boozman, MD, MPH: Biographical Summary

Fay Boozman was an ophthalmologist, former Arkansas state senator, Republican nominee for the US Senate, husband, father, and grandfather. On February 9, 1999, he assumed another role: Director of the Arkansas Department of Health. Dr. Boozman was born in Ft. Smith, Arkansas, and received the MD degree from the University of Arkansas Medical Center where he completed residencies in pediatrics and ophthalmology. He engaged in private medical practice for more than 20 years. Soon after his appointment as director, Dr. Boozman entered the Master of Public Health Program at Tulane University and completed the degree in 2001.

Dr. Boozman stated that one of his primary responsibilities was to help local communities become public health minded. During the two years he spent traveling as a US Senate candidate, he developed an appreciation for community relations. He described himself as a "hands-on person" who enjoyed face-to-face communication and gave high priority to spending time with local health units, community representatives, colleagues, and civic clubs. When he accepted the director's job he said, "This is a great opportunity. There are few jobs in your life where you can really make a difference and impact people's lives in a positive way."

stressed, "Arkansas is one of the most unhealthy states in the nation and that is unacceptable." In May 1999, a comprehensive review session was conducted, at which time Dr. Boozman left no doubt about his commitment to change public health in Arkansas and his commitment to strategic management in general and ASPIRE in particular. Dr. Boozman, in open letters to colleagues and in public statements, continued to emphasize his commitment to "absolutely change the way we do public health by removing barriers to excellence." He committed to move ASPIRE and the ADH to the next level of excellence.

To change public health in Arkansas, the reenergized initiative became known within the Department as ASPIRE². Dr. Boozman wanted to strengthen the focus on improving customer and colleague satisfaction and more effectively use Department resources. He wanted to employ strategic management and create the future for public health in Arkansas.

Organization of the Process

Although the ADH had a long history of systematic program planning, the agency had not previously engaged in strategic management. From the beginning, broad participation in the strategic management process was believed to be essential. Employees from all functional specialties and organizational levels were included. A task force structure with six working groups was developed to accomplish the important tasks of strategic management. (The task forces and their general responsibilities are presented in Exhibit 4/2.) Each group was composed of approximately 20 members, with the exception of the Communications Task Force that had 10 members. More than 100 colleagues were involved in the process. Task force members were encouraged to solicit the assistance of other colleagues with special skills that would contribute to the efficiency and effectiveness of the group. The Steering Committee facilitated more than 200

Exhibit 4/2: Arkansas Department of Health Strategic Management Structure

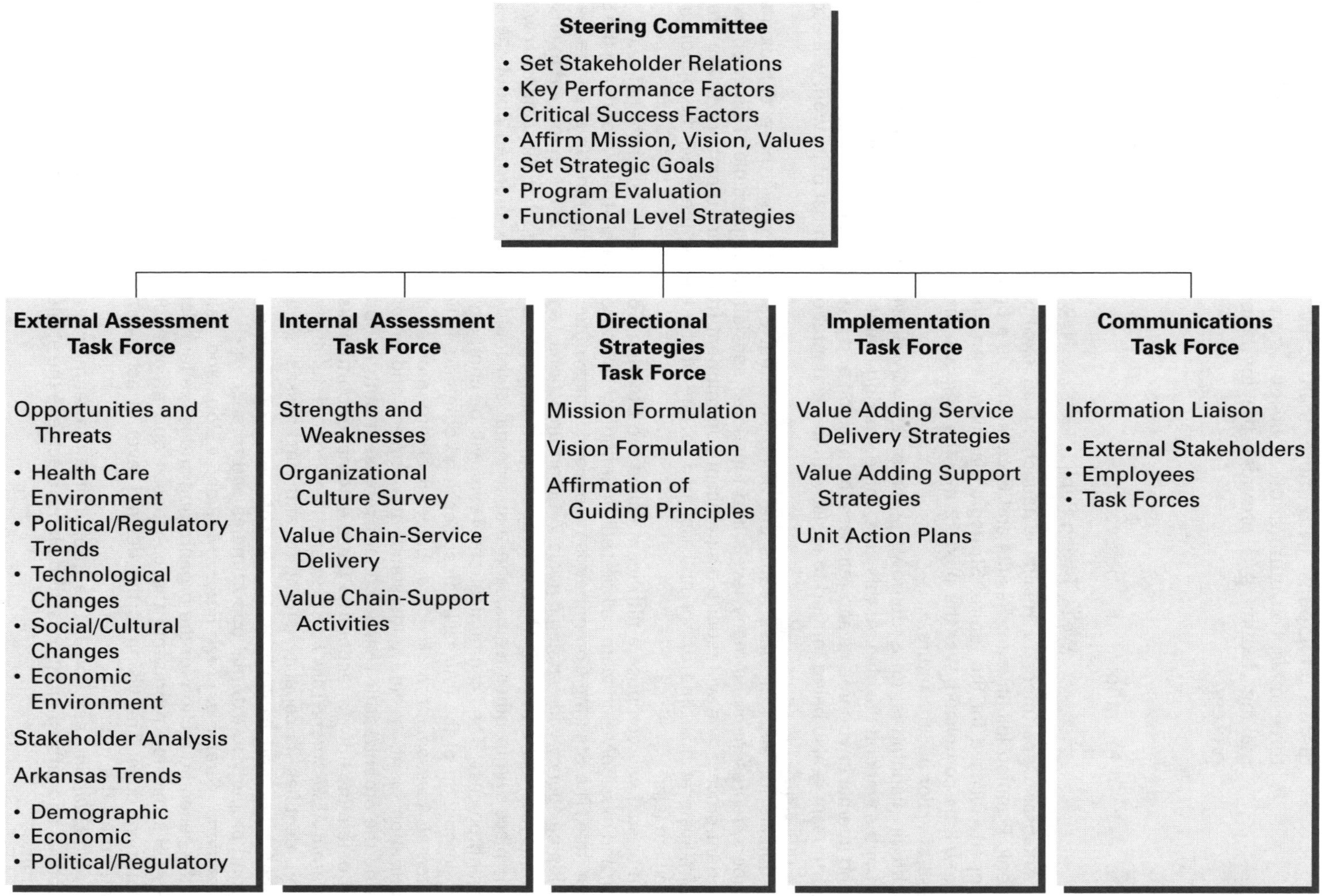

Steering Committee

- Set Stakeholder Relations
- Key Performance Factors
- Critical Success Factors
- Affirm Mission, Vision, Values
- Set Strategic Goals
- Program Evaluation
- Functional Level Strategies

External Assessment Task Force

Opportunities and Threats

- Health Care Environment
- Political/Regulatory Trends
- Technological Changes
- Social/Cultural Changes
- Economic Environment

Stakeholder Analysis

Arkansas Trends

- Demographic
- Economic
- Political/Regulatory

Internal Assessment Task Force

Strengths and Weaknesses

Organizational Culture Survey

Value Chain-Service Delivery

Value Chain-Support Activities

Directional Strategies Task Force

Mission Formulation

Vision Formulation

Affirmation of Guiding Principles

Implementation Task Force

Value Adding Service Delivery Strategies

Value Adding Support Strategies

Unit Action Plans

Communications Task Force

Information Liaison

- External Stakeholders
- Employees
- Task Forces

discussion groups with more than 2,500 colleagues to obtain feedback in three areas: communication, colleague growth and development, and decision making. Exhibit 4/3 provides the invitation for participation in the ASPIRE process.

Exhibit 4/3: An Invitation to Participate

We're Taking Public Health to New Heights!

The Arkansas Department of Health is launching an exciting new project! ASPIRE – Arkansas Strategic Planning Initiative for Results and Excellence – is a process to ensure that the Department is properly focused for the future. Strategic planning is an ongoing interactive process. The initial phase will be completed over the next 12 months and will provide the Department with a specific course of action for the future.

Strategic planning is not a top-down process; it involves everyone in the agency. Employees do much of the work on the plan. At this time, three working teams are being formed to assess the external and internal environments and reassess the mission and vision. Their work will begin next month. A fourth team is also being formed to assist with implementation, so most of its work will occur later in the process.

Volunteers for each of these teams are being solicited. Each team will have approximately 20 members, representing as many levels and functional specialties as possible. This is an extremely important process and will require a significant commitment from team members. If you are unable to participate at this time or are not assigned to one of the teams, there will be opportunities to participate later.

Senior staff will compose a fifth team called the Steering Committee. The external team, internal team, and mission/vision team will present their findings in approximately three months to the Steering Committee. The Steering Committee is responsible for synthesizing the reports of all the teams and developing agency-wide strategic goals. A Communications Team is also being formed to ensure that all employees are aware of what is happening in strategic planning, that all teams know what is taking place within other teams, and that external stakeholders are informed about the strategic planning process. The Communications Team will be composed of specialists in the Department. A brief description of the four task forces seeking volunteers is listed below.

External Assessment Task Force. External environmental analysis is the process by which an organization identifies and understands the current and emerging issues and trends taking place outside the organization. These changes represent both opportunities and threats. The Department must determine how to respond to these external opportunities and threats to succeed in the future.

Internal Assessment Task Force. Internal environmental analysis is the process by which an organization identifies its capacity (strengths and weaknesses) so as to specifically relate its resources, competencies, and capabilities to the changes taking place in the external environment and to respond properly to external opportunities and threats.

Directional Strategies Task Force. Mission, vision, and values formulation is the process that sets the general direction for the organization and is the foundation on which the strategic plan rests. The ADH's mission represents the consensus and articulation of the understanding of what the Department does. The vision is the desired level of achievement that the Department believes is optimum for the future.

Implementation Task Force. The implementation team has the responsibility to develop specific objectives and implementation action plans to achieve the strategic goals established by the Steering Committee.

As an additional aid in organizing the process, a milestone chart was developed to help everyone visualize the entire process and the interrelationships of the individual elements. The milestones highlighted priorities and the appropriate sequence for accomplishing the required tasks.

Arkansas – The Natural State

Arkansas was one of the most scenic states in the United States, with 3 national forests, 45 state parks, 13 major lakes, 2 mountain ranges, and 9,000 miles of rivers and streams. Tourism was one of the state's major industries and Arkansas ranked fourth nationally in the percentage of retirees. *Governing* magazine ranked Arkansas eleventh lowest overall in terms of tax rates, energy costs, and labor costs. The labor force was recognized for its work ethic and during the 1990s it grew 13.9 percent, when the nation's labor force as a whole grew only 11.5 percent. The cost of living index for Arkansas in 1998 was 91.0. The business climate was favorable, with business and health services growing by more than 40 percent during the 1990s.

The market within a 550-mile radius of Arkansas contained over 100 million people, or 42 percent of the population of the United States. There were more than 200 cultural institutions located in the state, including community and professional theater and ballet groups, symphonies, museums, galleries, and a nationally respected arts center. Exhibit 4/4 contains more information about the state.

Exhibit 4/4: General History and Information on Arkansas

In 1541, the Spanish explorer Hernando De Soto was the first European to set foot in Arkansas. Arkansas became a territory in 1819 and the twenty-fifth state in 1836. The scenic beauty of Arkansas prompted the adoption of "The Natural State" as its official nickname.

Economic Base

Advancements in farming, lumbering, manufacturing, tourism, and government gained Arkansas an increasing role in global markets. Arkansas was located in the south-central region of the nation. It ranked fourteenth among states in harvested acreage. Nationally, it ranked number one in rice and poultry production; number five in sorghum grain; number six in cotton; and number eight in soybeans and grapes.

Although Arkansas was primarily an agricultural state, it was the home of a number of major companies, including Jacuzzi, Tyson Foods, Riceland Foods, Sam Walton's Wal-Mart, Maybelline, Dillards Department Store, and J.B. Hunt Transport Company. Other major manufacturers in the state included Whirlpool Corporation, International Paper, American Greetings, and Georgia Pacific. Although not a manufacturer, Stephens Incorporated, in Little Rock, was the largest off-Wall Street investment firm in the country. Arkansas was a producer of petroleum, natural gas, and coal. The state led the nation in the production of bauxite, quartz crystal, silica stone, and bromine (number one in the world). Arkansas had the only active diamond mine in America, and the only public diamond mine in the world – Crater of Diamonds State Park in Murfreesboro. In 1998, per capita income had increased to $20,346, moving the state to a ranking of forty-sixth.

Exhibit 4/4: (*cont'd*)

Population and Government

With a population of 2.3 million, Arkansas ranked thirty-third in terms of population (projected to be 3.1 million in 2025). Most cities in the state were small; only 29 had populations of more than 10,000. Little Rock, the capital, was the largest city, with a population of 190,000.

Arkansas had 7 Constitutional officers, a 35-member state Senate and a 100-member House of Representatives. The State had 75 counties with headquarters in the county seats. For the convenience of county residents, 10 rural counties had 2 county seats. In the most recent Gubernatorial election, almost 60 percent of the state voted Republican. In 1998, total state general expenditures were $9.6 billion. Of this amount, $3.2 billion was spent on education, $1.6 billion was spent on public welfare, $876 million on health and hospitals, and $823 million on highways.

Education

Arkansas had 1,097 public schools: 618 elementary, 138 junior high/middle, and 341 high schools. Arkansas had 10 state and 10 independent four-year colleges; 10 state two-year colleges; 23 state vocational/technical schools; and many specialty colleges. In 1998, nearly 77 percent of Arkansans were high school graduates and 16.2 percent had graduated from college.

Health

The ten leading causes of death (ranked by incidence per 100,000 population) in Arkansas were as follows. Heart disease was the leading cause (332.26), followed by cancer (234.4) and cerebrovascular disease (92.3). The fourth leading cause of death was accidents, including motor vehicle collisions and other misadventures (51.1), followed by chronic obstructive pulmonary disease (48.7), pneumonia and influenza (43.2), diabetes mellitus (25.4), nephritis and nephrosis (15.5), septicemia (14.1), and suicide (13.6).

Infant mortality in Arkansas increased from 8.7 deaths per 1,000 live births in 1997 to 9.2 in 1998. The Arkansas rate remained higher than the national average of 7.2 per 1,000 live births in 1998. The infant mortality rate among African-Americans increased from 11.5 per 1,000 live births in 1997 to 12.8 in 1998. The death rate for all Arkansans was 10.8 per 1,000 population compared with the national average of 8.6. The following table provides some Arkansas vs. United States comparison data on selected sociodemographic indicators.

Indicator	Arkansas	United States
Population Density (per square mile)	48.7	76.4
Percent Below Poverty Level	19.7	13.3
Percent Rural Population	46.5	24.8
Percent White Population	82.7	82.5
Percent Nonwhite Population	16.1	16.9
Divorce Rate per 1,000 Population	6.4	4.2
General Fertility Rate per 1,000 Women (15–44)	67.5	51.1

Source: US Census Bureau, *Statistical Abstract of the United States: 1999–2000*, 119th edn (Washington, DC: US Census Bureau, 2001); Arkansas Center of Health Statistics, *Arkansas Department of Health*, *Arkansas 1998*, Volumes on "Mortality Statistics," "County Trends," "Vital Statistics," and "Maternal and Child Health Statistics." General information about Arkansas located on state website at www.sosweb.state.ar.us

Arkansas Department of Health

The Arkansas Department of Health was one of 21 department-level units in state government. The director was appointed by and served at the pleasure of the governor. As the chief executive officer, the director, Dr. Fay Boozman, was responsible for overall leadership of the Department. When ASPIRE was initiated, the ADH was organized according to a traditional public health model (illustrated in Exhibit 4/5), with six bureaus reporting to the director. The director was assisted in completing the overall management of the ADH by the senior staff (the director's executive-level staff and the directors of the six bureaus).

The structure of the ADH appeared to be decentralized, with 10 area offices and 95 local health units. In reality, the structure was highly centralized, with much of the decision-making authority concentrated in Little Rock. Moreover, the simultaneous presence of area (regional) and local (county) administrators and professional authority (professional discipline) for nursing, social work, nutrition, health promotion, and so on, in the central office caused confusion. More than 3,000 people worked within the ADH and the Department provided 140 separate ADH service and support programs (see Exhibit 4/6).

External Environmental Analysis

If the ADH was to know what it *should* be doing, it had to understand the external environment, as the external opportunities and threats represented the fundamental issues that would spell success or failure. The specific objectives that guided the External Assessment Task Force were to:

- classify and order information generated outside the Department;
- identify the most important stakeholders of the Department;
- identify and analyze current important issues that affected the Department;
- detect and analyze the weak signals of emerging issues that would affect the Department;
- speculate on the likely future issues that would have significant impact on the Department;
- provide organized information for the development of the Department's mission, vision, guiding principles (values), goals, and strategy; and
- foster strategic thinking throughout the Department.

The external analysis was carried out in two phases. First, stakeholders were identified. Second, the Department used trend/issue identification and analysis to focus on the issues considered to be most important. Stakeholders were used to assist in the issue identification and in the validation of the issues identified.

Exhibit 4/5: Organizational Chart of the Arkansas Department of Health, 1996

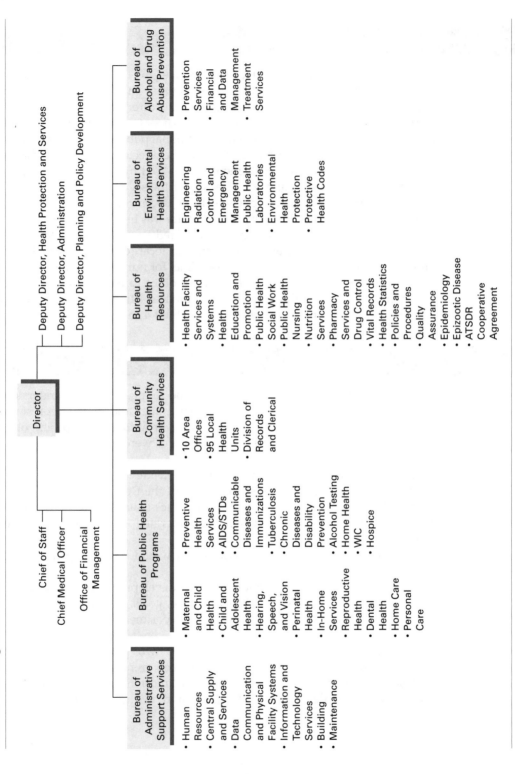

Exhibit 4/6: List of Programs for Priority Setting

Programs

1. Legal Services
2. Planning and Policy Development
3. Media Response
4. Minority Health
5. Financial Management – Budget
6. Financial Management – Funds Control
7. Financial Management – Grants
8. Financial Management – Payroll
9. Financial Management – Cost Allocation/Accounting
10. Financial Management – Purchasing
11. Financial Management – Accounts Payable
12. Alcohol & Other Drug Education & Prevention
13. Alcohol & Other Drug Information – Safe & Drug Free
14. Alcohol & Other Drug Training
15. Alcohol & Other Drug Treatment Services
16. Common Ground/Youth Violence
17. Drugs Won't Work
18. Regional Alcohol and Drug Detoxification
19. Copy Center
20. Garage
21. Mail Room
22. Print Shop
23. Supply Distribution/Shipping & Receiving
24. DP: Communication Network Develop., Support, & Train.
25. DP: Support/Training – Large Data Bases & Mainframe
26. DP: Support/Training – Personal Computers
27. Employee Training & Quality Management
28. Human Resources
29. Maintenance & Physical Plant Supply
30. Records & Clerical Services/Professional Supervision
31. Environmental Revenue & Billing
32. Geographic Information Systems (GIS)
33. Consumer Product Safety
34. FDA Contract
35. Food Protection
36. General Sanitation
37. Individual Sewage Disposal
38. Lead Abatement & Testing
39. Marine Sanitation
40. Milk & Dairy
41. Septic Tank Cleaners
42. Swimming & Recreational Facilities
43. Tattoo Inspection & Certification
44. Cross Connection Control
45. Community Public Water Supply Protection
46. NonCommunity Public Water Supply Protection
47. Plan Review
48. Water Operator Testing & Licensing
49. Wellhead Protection
50. CLIA/Quality Assurance
51. Clinical Chemistry
52. Clinical Microbiology
53. Food Chemistry
54. Immunology
55. Inorganic Chemistry
56. Organic Chemistry
57. Radiochemistry
58. Sanitary Bacteriology
59. Lab: TB & Mycology
60. Heating, Ventilation, AC, & Refrig. Regulation
61. Plumbing & Natural Gas Protection
62. Chemical Stockpile Emergency Prepare
63. Emergency Communications Center
64. Emergency Response
65. Mammography
66. Naturally Occurring Radioactive Materials
67. Nuclear Planning & Response
68. Radioactive Materials
69. Radiological Protection Systems
70. Radon
71. Registration & Compliance
72. EMS and Training Systems
73. Environmental Epidemiology
74. General Epidemiology
75. Epizootic Disease
76. Technical Assistance/Professional Supervision
77. Support/Resource Library
78. CLIA Certification
79. Medicare Certification
80. State Licensure
81. Utilization Review
82. Health Statistics
83. Medical Waste Regulation
84. Nursing Services – Professional Supervision
85. Nutrition Services – Professional Supervision
86. Pharmacy Services
87. Policies & Procedures
88. Primary Care
89. Quality Assurance
90. Rural Health
91. Social Work/Professional Supervision
92. Vital Records
93. ADH Information Management System
94. AIDS/STD: HIV/AIDS Community Planning
95. AIDS/STD: HIV/AIDS Medical Care
96. AIDS/STD: HIV/AIDS Prevention
97. AIDS/STD: HIV/AIDS Surveillance/Seroprevalance
98. AIDS/STD: HIV/AIDS STD Services
99. Alcohol Testing
100. Breastfeeding Services
101. Adolescent Health
102. Child Health Clinic Services
103. Child Health Support Services
104. EPSDT
105. Newborn Screening
106. SIDS
107. School Health
108. Breast & Cervical Cancer Control
109. Cancer Registry
110. Diabetes
111. Injury/Disability Prevention
112. Tobacco Prevention & Control
113. Adult Immunization
114. Child Immunization
115. General Communicable Disease
116. Immunization Registry
117. Dental Health: Dental Health Education
118. Dental Health: Fluoridation
119. Hearing & Speech Clinical Services
120. Newborn Hearing Registry
121. Vision & Hearing Screening
122. Home Care
123. Home Health
124. Hospice
125. Maternal Infant Program
126. Personal Care
127. Targeted Case Management
128. Medicaid Outreach & Education Project
129. Campaign for Healthier Babies
130. Lay Midwife Licensing
131. Maternity Medical Services
132. Maternity Support Services
133. MCH Health Line
134. Nurse Midwife Project
135. Pap Smear Follow-up
136. Family Planning Services
137. Medical Services
138. Tuberculosis Registry
139. Third-Party Reimbursement
140. WIC

Stakeholders

The stakeholder task group identified five major categories of stakeholders. These were politicians, associations and providers, other state agencies, consumers, and taxpayers. Exhibit 4/7 provides some examples of important stakeholders under each category. As a matter of convenience and to keep the

Exhibit 4/7: External Stakeholders

Political and Regulatory Stakeholders

- Arkansas State Legislators
- Association of Arkansas Counties
- Municipal League
- University of Arkansas School of Medicine
- Department of Human Services
- Provider Groups (Medical Society, Hospital Association)
- Third Party Payors (Blue Cross, Prudential)
- Arkansas Children's Hospital
- Community Health Centers
- AHECs
- Livestock and Poultry
- Pollution Control and Ecology
- Plant Board
- Health Services Agency
- Consumer advocacy groups (AARP, Disability Coalition, Rain, Cancer Society)
- Foundations (Arkansas Policy Foundation, Winthrop Rockefeller Foundation)

Technology Stakeholders

- Arkansas Science and Technology
- University of Arkansas School of Medicine
- Complete Computing
- University of Arkansas at Little Rock
- Systematics
- USDA
- CDC
- EPA
- Pollution Control and Ecology
- Medicaid
- DCS Telecom
- Department employees involved in technology

Social Issues Stakeholders

- Department employees
- Patients
- Ministers
- School administrators
- Health care providers
- Civic groups
- Industry representatives

Economic/Demographic Stakeholders

• Hospital CEO:	Washington Regional Medical Center
• County Judges:	Washington County Lee County Jefferson County
• State Senators:	Washington County Lee County
• State Representatives:	Lee County St. Francis County Washington County
• Economist:	University of Arkansas at Little Rock
• Insurance Co. CEO:	Blue Cross, Blue Shield

Health Care Environment/Marketplace Representatives

- Home Health Association in North Central Arkansas
- Private home health agency
- University of Central Arkansas professor from Graduate School of Nursing
- Rural health clinic in Marshall County
- Hospital administrator in Van Buren County
- Department Core Team in Area 10
- Van Buren County Judge
- AHH
- V. P. Sparks Regional Medical Center

stakeholder analysis consistent with the issues analysis, the various stakeholder groups were divided into political/regulatory stakeholders, technology stakeholders, social issues stakeholders, economic/demographic stakeholders, and health care stakeholders.

A sample of stakeholders was selected for interviews to evaluate the Department as well as identify the most important issues facing public health in Arkansas. Another sample of stakeholders was used to validate the issues identified.

Environments

The External Assessment Task Force was subdivided into five task groups corresponding to the five "environments" that the ADH believed represented the major classifications of the public health environment in Arkansas. These were health care, economic/demographic, political/regulatory, technological, and social. Each task group was given the responsibility of gathering information, using internal/external and personal/nonpersonal sources of data to identify key trends and issues within its area of responsibility.

The *health care task group* interviewed providers, hospital administrators, insurance companies, and other health professionals and experts inside and outside the Department. In addition, the group surveyed the literature and reviewed statistical data in external databases and information provided by the ADH Center for Health Statistics to identify the health care issues and trends that were most likely to affect the Department.

The *economic/demographic task group* interviewed experts inside and outside the Department as well as key stakeholders. In addition, the group reviewed and analyzed published research and statistical data to determine which economic and demographic trends were most likely to impact Arkansas in the future.

The *political/regulatory task group* looked at three types of stakeholders. These were: (1) organizations that provide input to the ADH; (2) organizations that compete or have overlapping regulatory oversight; and (3) those organizations that have a particular interest in how the ADH functions. Personal interviews and focus groups with key stakeholders were completed and journal articles, news reports, and related information were reviewed to determine those factors most likely to impact the Department.

Members of the *technological task group* interviewed ADH staff with knowledge of or need for technology and individuals outside the agency with particular technological expertise. Further, the group conducted an Internet search and reviewed newsletters, published articles, and papers before constructing its list of significant issues.

Finally, the *social issues task group* interviewed ADH employees, patients, and members of the community at large in developing a list of the most significant social issues. See Exhibit 4/8 for the various trends and issues that were identified by the different groups.

Exhibit 4/8: Trends/Issues by External Environmental Classification

Health Care Environment	Economic/Demographic Environment	Political/Regulatory Environment	Technological Environment	Social Environment
Reductions in Medicaid and Medicare funding	Immigration – Number of Hispanics served by WIC and immunizations	Public pressure to reduce tax burden and reduce size of government	Increases in telecommunication technologies	Early sexual activity
Growth of outpatient care and corresponding reduction of inpatient care	Increased competition from managed care organizations	Pressure to remove ADH from direct care services	Increases in biotechnologies and applications	Increases in communicable diseases
Advances in medical technologies	Federal and state tax cuts	Pressure to ensure ADH fills voids in areas of health education and public awareness	Increases in access to information by all people	Changes in family structure
Women continue to grow in number as primary medical decision maker	Block grants		Automation of equipment for analytical testing and analysis	
Continued push to "do more with less" to control health care costs	Increase in unemployment with corresponding increase in welfare recipients	Quality assurance and utilization responsibility to increase	Miniaturization and portability of electronic equipment and devices	
Growth in home care	Welfare reform and social tensions caused by attempts to reduce welfare roles	Public insistence on ADH ensuring access to health care for all citizens		
Growth in alternative medicine	Aging of the Arkansas population			
Competition continues to make survival of small hospitals difficult	Increasing diversity of Arkansas population			
Increase in the number of uninsured in the state	Emphasis on improvement of public education			
Increase in the number of physician assistants and nurse practitioners – particularly in rural areas				
Increase in the placement of foreign trained health professionals in rural areas				

Exhibit 4/9: Classifications for the Health Care Environment

Issue Strength	Scope of Issue		
	National	State	County
Current	Reductions in Medicaid and Medicare funding	Continued push to "do more with less" to control health care costs	Increase in number of physician assistants and nurse practitioners in rural areas
Emerging	Women continue to grow in number as primary health care decision makers	Growth in home health	Increase in the placement of foreign-trained health professionals in rural areas
Speculative	Growth in alternative medicine		Competition continues to make survival of small hospitals difficult

Strategic Issues

After the initial data-gathering activity, the External Assessment Task Force decided that the trends and issues identified by the various task groups should be classified by (1) scope (national, state, or county issues) and (2) strength (current, emerging, or speculative issues). To illustrate the classifications, an example from the health care environment is shown in Exhibit 4/9.

Using this approach, each task group – health care, economic/demographic, political/regulatory, technology, and social issues – identified over 50 national, state, and county, current, emerging, and speculative issues (more than 250 total). However, the groups concluded that some of the issues were trivial or would have little direct impact on the Department. Furthermore, only the most important issues ultimately could be addressed by the strategic plan. Therefore, each group reduced the list of trends/issues by assessing the importance of the impact on the ADH. Subsequent discussions and the combination of some trends resulted in a total of 33 environmental issues. These issues were subjected to a forced ranking technique that resulted in the identification of the top ten external environmental issues facing the ADH (Exhibit 4/10).

The comprehensive analysis of the external environment provided leaders at the ADH with the important external issues that must be considered in strategic decision making and provided information on what the Department should be doing for the citizens of Arkansas. The second strategic question that had to be answered in the situational analysis was "What *can* the ADH do?" To address this question, it was necessary to assess the internal environment.

Exhibit 4/10: Most Important External Environmental Issues Facing the ADH

Issue/Trend	Rationale	Opportunity for Action	Threat of Inaction
Welfare Reform	Welfare reform is expected to have a major impact on health of citizens of Arkansas Medicaid coverage for groups such as children, women, immigrants, and the elderly who no longer receive cash benefits from welfare may lose all ties to Medicaid. Many will be forced to take low-paying jobs with no health insurance. ADH must ensure these individuals get the necessary health services	Long-range planning for needed services, levels of staffing, approaches to delivery of services, and redefining those who qualify for services	Reductions in funding will continue with unnecessary spending of government money. Fraud will increase and the quality of care will deteriorate
Growth in Managed Care	Managed care is expected to become the primary form of health care in the US. Health care access will continue to be a problem in rural and inner city areas where private companies find it hard to make a profit	Health care can be made available to more people at lower cost. An increase in the quality of care can take place if industry growth is carefully monitored and regulated	Managed care will continue to prosper but access issues will increase in rural areas and inner cities where profits are hard to make. Quality of care could diminish and the cost of health care for the entire state could continue to rise
Federal and State Tax Cuts	Tax cuts mean decreasing revenues. Agencies that rely on public funds will be adversely affected. There will be less money to go around. Herein lies the push for "doing more with less"	Fewer dollars will be available for health care, making it important to prioritize services and spend every dollar wisely	With managed care, welfare reform, and immigration there will be a demand on the ADH to provide certain services. If planning and prioritizing has not occurred there will be insufficient funds and personnel to provide these services
Growing Elderly Population	Currently 15 percent of Arkansas' population is aged 65 or older. By 2030 this percentage will increase to 25, requiring more home care, case management, and emphasis on chronic diseases	Aging population increases the demand for home health services. More demand is created for rural health clinics and preventive services Elderly patients require case management	More chronic illnesses in the future will result in increased health care costs
Information and Communications Technology	ADH has responsibility for health related data collection and analysis. New communication technologies have created new demands for sharing data. Confidentiality issues are increasing	Reduction in time and expense for holding meetings. Facilitate communication among individuals, agencies, and programs. Extend the reach of health care providers. Facilitate communication among patients, families, and caregivers. Speed up turnaround on reports Increased ability to develop targeted programs based on data	ADH will not be able to access the information that is critical to its mission ADH will not have the ability to share data with other stakeholders. Problems will develop if technology is adopted without adequate technical support

Exhibit 4/10: (cont'd)

Issue/Trend	Rationale	Opportunity for Action	Threat of Inaction
Early Sexual Activity	Arkansas' teen fertility rate is about 30 percent higher than the national average. Early sexual activity increases the incidence of STD, HIV, and teen pregnancy. Adolescents who engage in high-risk behavior such as drinking and drug use may also be more likely to be sexually experienced	Increased need for early intervention and prevention services. Increased need for evaluation of lifestyle, decision making, self-esteem, refusal skills. Increased need for prenatal services. Greater demand for social work. Every investment of $1 in family planning reduces health and welfare costs by $4	Increases in STD, HIV, which will spread rapidly. Increase in unintended pregnancies leading to more problems. Emotional and mental problems such as isolation, loneliness, lowered self-esteem, lowered academic achievement, can keep the vicious circle of early sexual activity going
Push to "Do More With Less"	Mentioned under decreased tax revenues, efforts to reduce costs will result in a number of implications for ADH. Outsourcing is on the rise, especially in nonrevenue producing functions. Dangers exist in the area of quality control as the focus falls on cost cutting	Could require more focus on priorities and reduce attempt to be everything to everyone	Quality of care could deteriorate. There will be fewer resources so fewer services will be provided while the demand for services increases
Growth in Home Health	Home health increased 27 percent from 1990 to 1995 in the state and 134 percent in HHS Region VI, which includes Arkansas, Louisiana, Oklahoma, Texas, and New Mexico. As a cost-effective alternative to hospital and other forms of institutional care, the upward trend is likely to continue	Increase in business for the provider divisions of ADH Increased need for home health inspectors	Fraud and abuse of the system will increase. More private competition will make it harder for ADH to maintain paying patients, which will mean providing fewer services to nonpaying patients
Growth in Immigration and Minority Populations	Increased immigration and the growth of minority populations creates the need for more maternal and child health and primary care services Communication and cultural barriers hinder public health initiatives	More need for maternal and child health. More need to ensure immunizations. More need for bilingual employees. Create need for culturally sensitive services, programs, and service delivery	With the increase in immigrant and minority populations inaction will make us increasingly irrelevant. More low birth weight babies can be expected and higher infant mortality
Communicable Disease	Diseases such as STD, HIV, and AIDS have great social costs in addition to financial costs. STDs are more easily transmitted to women and more difficult to detect. STDs are particularly dangerous since women can transmit diseases to children during pregnancy	Increased need for health education. Increased need for early intervention and preventive services. Increased need for contact notification, social work, and home health	Increasing numbers of communicable diseases Increased health care costs Threat to large numbers of people if not controlled

Internal Environmental Analysis

The general objective of the Internal Assessment Task Force was to provide the Steering Committee with an assessment of the strengths and weaknesses of the various components of the value chain. However, the focus of the strategic planning process at the ADH was state level and with few exceptions public health services were delivered by local health units in Arkansas. The state-level ADH value adding opportunities were primarily in the support activities. Therefore, attention was directed toward strengths and weaknesses relative to organizational culture, organizational structure, and strategic resources.

The specific objectives of the Internal Assessment Task Force were to:

- analyze the results of the organizational excellence questionnaire administered to all members of the Department;
- identify the key value chain components that collectively determined the strategic capacity of the ADH;
- isolate the relevant components of the value chain and analyze the strengths and weaknesses associated with each;
- identify specific strengths and weaknesses of the Department relative to each value chain component and classify them as resources, competencies, and capabilities;
- recommend, based on the findings of the analysis, actions for maintaining strengths and eliminating weaknesses; and
- foster strategic thinking throughout the Department.

The Internal Assessment Task Force decided to form task groups to cover three areas – organizational culture, organizational structure (including communication networks), and strategic resources (including finance, facilities and equipment, information systems, and human resources).

Assessing the Organizational Culture

The *organizational culture task group* assessed the culture of the ADH with the aid of a self-administered survey form provided to every employee. The questionnaire was designed to obtain the opinions of the Department's 3,000 employees regarding seven different areas: mission/vision, service and managerial innovation, leadership and employee orientation, responsiveness to external change, teamwork, external and internal customer/client orientation, and quality. Colleagues on this task force thought that these areas would provide insights into the shared assumptions, values, and behavioral norms.

The general conclusions of the culture survey were summarized in terms of strengths and weaknesses. Strengths included commitment to the importance of the work they performed and commitment to the mission of the ADH. Behavioral norms emphasized a focus on quality of services provided and service to the public. Employees valued anticipation of and responsiveness to change. Weaknesses were found in the lack of understanding of the vision, behavioral norms that emphasized policies and procedures over employees and customers, and a lack of appropriate appreciation for internal customers.

Organizational Structure

Issues regarding the organizational structure of the ADH emerged in several places during the *organizational structure task group*'s assessment process. Although it was considered an internal issue, surveys and interviews conducted by the External Assessment Task Force indicated concerns about the organizational structure. In addition, the organizational culture survey and other internal assessment task groups collected information regarding the structure of the agency.

The more important strengths included the statewide network of clinics, centralization of appropriate areas such as vital records and quality assurance, and an effective governance structure. Important weaknesses were identified as inadequate delegation of authority to program managers, lack of freedom to recruit and hire appropriate staff, and outdated organizational structure and management style.

Strategic Resources

The *strategic resources task group* focused on facilities and equipment, finances, information technology, and human resources. Internal surveys were conducted concerning facilities and equipment. In addition, financial resources and the administration of financial resources were examined. In the case of finance, sources and uses of funds for public health in Arkansas were compared with two similar southern states – Alabama and Louisiana. In the area of the administration of financial resources, the group evaluated the budgetary development and monitoring system, reporting system, financial technical support, payment process, and general resource management. Information was obtained from a survey of employees with financial responsibilities, including bureau directors, associate bureau directors, bureau budget coordinators, area managers, and division directors.

Data regarding information systems resources were collected by means of a survey that was sent to a random sample of ADH employees who were asked questions about the adequacy of information technology resources. Finally, a survey regarding human resources issues was sent to a sample of employees, equally divided between local health units and central office personnel, asking opinions about various aspects of human resources operations.

Exhibit 4/11 includes the identified strengths and weaknesses from the organizational culture task group, the organizational structure task group, and the strategic resources task group.

Exhibit 4/11: Strengths and Weaknesses by Value Chain Component

Strength and Weakness	Description	Classification
	Organizational Culture	
Strengths	Employees believe their job is important and take pride in what they do	Capability
	Employees believe the Department places great importance on quality	Capability
	Employees understand the mission of the Agency	Capability
	Individual work areas are supportive of new and improved ways of providing services	Capability
	Management staff is aware of employee needs	Capability
	Agency leadership tries to anticipate change	Capability
	Agency is responsive to needs of citizens of Arkansas	Capability
	Employees believe serving the public is the most important part of their jobs	Capability
Weaknesses	Employees do not believe ADH rewards individual excellence	Resource
	Most employees do not understand the ADH vision	Capability
	Employees do not think ADH supports creativity	Capability
	Employees think Agency leadership puts policies and procedures before people	Capability
	Agency has no systematic way of dealing with change	Capability
	Employees believe Agency leadership puts policies and procedures before service to public	Capability
	More communication is needed regarding satisfaction of internal customers	Resource
	Central Office less satisfied with internal customer service than local health units	Capability
	Employees do not believe groups work as teams	Capability
	Organizational Structure	
Strengths	Statewide network of clinics	Resource
	Centralization of vital records and quality assurance	Capability
	Governance structure with diverse Board of Health	Resource
Weaknesses	Program managers do not have latitude to do their jobs	Capability
	Directors need more freedom to hire and terminate staff	Capability
	Decision-making authority needs to be delegated to local level	Capability
	ADH management style is outdated	Capability
	Organization structure is barrier to change	Capability
	Strategic Resources	
Strengths	Work sites are well maintained, parking facilities adequate, and security is good	Resource
	Materials and supplies are adequate and obtainable in reasonable time	Resource
	Appropriate property control systems	Capability
	Inventories are up to date	Resource
	Expense reimbursements made in reasonable time	Competency
	Financial personnel are knowledgeable	Competency
	Agency is in compliance with all financial reporting requirements	Capability
	Employees are confident that information is reliable and accurate	Capability
	Employees have information needed to do their jobs	Resource
	Information systems personnel respond to requests in reasonable time	Competency
	Adequate communication links between local health units and central office	Resource
	Employees are encouraged to obtain job-related training	Capability
	Agency human resources system complies with state system	Capability
	Human resources personnel are knowledgeable	Competency
Weaknesses	Space is inadequate and physical layout does not promote efficiency	Resource
	Telephones, cellular phones, email, and voice mail inadequate or unavailable	Resource
	Inadequate notification when inventory stockouts occur	Capability
	Lab specimens are often rejected, lost, or received late	Competency
	Financial management personnel are not proactive in finding out what internal customers need	Capability
	Program managers do not have adequate control over budgets	Capability
	Purchasing not responsive to needs of work units, contractors, or vendors	Capability
	Financial system not user friendly	Capability
	Assistance not available from financial staff in a timely manner	Resource
	Reports are not provided on a timely basis	Resource
	Agency not maximizing current funding or revenue sources	Capability
	Program managers do not have necessary flexibility in utilization of resources	Capability
	Agency does not use most effective or appropriate technology	Resource
	Employees do not know enough about the services available from information technology	Capability
	Information is not distributed equally to all locations	Resource
	Telephone system problems exist	Resource
	Personnel action requests not processed in timely manner	Capability
	Employees do not think job grades and classifications are always equitable	Capability
	Agency pay and benefits not adequate to compete in labor markets	Resource
	Agency not aware of personnel needs at local levels	Competency
	High-tech knowledge is not classified properly or paid for adequately	Capability

Directional Strategies

The development of directional strategies (mission, vision, values, and strategic goals) enabled an organization to address the third strategic question, "What does the Department *want* to do?" The ADH determined early in its strategic planning process that the formulation of directional strategies, similar to assessment of the external and internal environments, had to come from consensus-building among as many employees (managerial and nonmanagerial) as possible. Therefore, the Steering Committee included a task force to address the formulation of the Department's mission, vision, values, and goals. Prior to the beginning of the strategic management process, the ADH had committed itself to a total quality management program and had dealt extensively with the development of a statement of guiding principles (values). These are shown in Exhibit 4/12.

The Directional Strategies Task Force focused on the formulation of the mission and vision statements. Its objectives were to:

Exhibit 4/12: Guiding Principles (Values) of the Arkansas Department of Health

Dedication to the Public. We are committed to serving the public health needs of Arkansas. The needs of those we serve will drive our actions. We will treat all individuals with understanding and respect.

Responsiveness. We will identify the changing public health needs of Arkansans and adapt our programs and services appropriately. We will respond promptly to requests and concerns identified by those we serve.

Appreciation of Employees. We value all our employees and recognize that we need each other to do our jobs. All employees will be given equal opportunity and encouraged to achieve their potential. We will maintain an atmosphere in which initiative and diversity are valued and employees are respected and appreciated for their contributions.

Open Communication. We are committed to open and honest communication in an atmosphere that fosters individual thinking and new ideas. We will share information in an honest, complete, and timely way.

Quality. We will strive for excellence in everything we do and continually pursue strategies that improve our services and performance.

Accountability. We will be good stewards of public funds and uphold the public trust through adherence to the law and to Department policies, standards, and guidelines. We will be results-oriented and will focus our resources to accomplish our goals in the most effective and efficient way.

Innovation. We will provide an environment in which innovation and originality are encouraged and reasonable risks are accepted as necessary for progress. We will apply creative, sound, and practical solutions to public health challenges.

Leadership. We will be a visible, active, and continuing advocate for the health of the people of Arkansas. We will be a guiding force in the development of science-based health policies that further the mission of public health. We will work with other organizations and groups that share our goal of a healthier future for Arkansans.

- generate and develop consensus for a clear, concise statement of the Department's mission through consideration of primary clients, principal services, geographical domain, philosophy, and desired public image;
- reach a consensus on a challenging, exciting, and inspiring statement of vision (hope) for the ADH; and
- foster strategic thinking throughout the Department.

To accomplish the objectives, the task force decided to divide into two groups. One group was to focus on the development of the mission statement and the second was to focus on the development of a vision statement.

Mission Statement

The *mission statement task group*'s desire was to create a living document whereby colleagues could easily relate their jobs to the accomplishment of the ADH's mission and see immediately how they fit into the larger organization. The group researched the academic and applied literature on mission statements, reviewed the Institute of Medicine's report, *The Future of Public Health*, examined a position paper from the National Governors' Association, and reviewed documents on core public health functions before beginning the mission statement formulation process.

In addition to the external information, the group sponsored a series of brainstorming sessions where subgroup members traveled across the state to gather input from colleagues. Five of the ten public health management areas were selected and each area manager identified 20 employees to participate in the sessions. In addition, sessions were conducted with central office employees. Participants represented a broad cross-section of employees from different organizational levels and functional disciplines.

To assist in developing the ADH mission statement, the group decided to use a working template to devise key words as adapted to the ADH (see Exhibit 4/13). The subgroup realized that dealing with issues relating to philosophy, desired self-image, and external image would overlap excessively with the work already done in the development of guiding principles, so it decided to focus primarily on the definition of the customer, services provided, and geographic domain as the most productive route to the determination of the Department's distinctiveness.

Vision Statement

The *vision statement task group* used a similar process in its work. To ensure broad input, members of this group visited the five public health management areas not visited by the mission group and conducted brainstorming sessions with groups of 20 employees in each location as well as central office personnel. In each of the sessions, a short motivational video was reviewed and participants discussed futuristic issues. Members of the vision group interviewed senior staff members

Exhibit 4/13: Strategic Thinking Map for Writing the ADH Mission Statement

Component	Key Words Reflecting Component		
1. Target Customers and Clients: *The individuals and groups we attempt to serve are . . . Do not be limited to only the obvious.*	individuals	communities	institutions
2. Principal Services Delivered: *The specific services or range of services we will provide to our customers are . . .*	enforce laws	enforce regulations	prevent disease
	health promotion	community assessment	service delivery
3. Geographical Domain of the Services Delivered: *The geographical boundaries within which we will deliver our services to our customers are . . .*	Arkansas	outside state in cases	
4. Specific Values: *Specific values that constitute our distinctiveness in the delivery of our services to customers are . . .*	covered in guiding principles		
5. Explicit Philosophy: *The explicit philosophy that makes us distinctive in our industry is . . .*	covered in guiding principles		
6. Other Important Aspects of Distinctiveness: *Any other factors that make us unique among competitors are . . .*	covered in guiding principles		

in the Department and asked what their hopes were for the agency over the next five years. Exhibit 4/14 identifies the key words that were assembled.

Guiding Principles (Values)

The ADH had worked on a set of guiding principles or values prior to the initiation of ASPIRE[2]. Over 300 people in the Department participated in the process.

Exhibit 4/14: Strategic Thinking Map for Writing the ADH Vision Statement

Component	Key Words Reflecting Component		
1. Clear Hope for the Future: *If everything went as we would like it to go, what would our organization look like five years from now? How would we be different/better than today?*	leader	responsive	guardian
2. Challenging and About Excellence: *When stakeholders (patients, employees, owners) describe our organization, what terms would we like for them to use?*	dedicated / customer-focused	resources / compassionate	knowledgeable / motivated
3. Inspirational and Emotional: *When we think about the kind of organization we could be if we all contributed our best, what terms would describe our collective contributions?*	caring	professional	efficient
4. Empower Employees First: *How can we ensure that employees understand and are committed to the vision? What needs to be done to achieve buy in?*	communicate	role modeling	reward support
5. Memorable and Provides Guidance: *What types of words should be included to ensure all organizational members remember and behave in accordance with the vision?*	pride	partners	excellence

The purpose of determining the guiding principles was to identify qualities that were valued by all colleagues in the ADH. Then participants were asked to indicate values the ADH needed to strengthen. Of the eight guiding principles, five were determined to need improvement: accountability, appreciation of employees, innovation, leadership, and open communication. Five working groups, composed of approximately 125 volunteers representing all levels and all areas of the Department, were created to develop recommendations to better integrate these five principles into daily operations.

Critical Success Factors

To address common issues, the Steering Committee reclassified the recommendations under the headings of communications, human resources, management system, need for data, and miscellaneous. The Steering Committee evaluated each recommendation and committed to take action in the following categories: (1) activities that were being done; (2) activities that can be done immediately; (3) activities that need to be developed through a work group; (4) activities that need a strategic plan; and (5) other activities that the agency does not control or would require extensive research.

The Steering Committee looked at all the information it collected and developed a list of service category (public health) critical success factors – those things the Committee thought were absolutely essential to the success of the Department. In thinking about the meaning of critical success factors, the ADH decided that more meaningful terms should be used in light of the agency's history and previous planning initiatives. In place of service category critical success factors the ADH substituted the term "key performance areas." Key performance areas were defined as those factors that make a difference relative to success in the public health arena.

The term "critical success factor" was used to represent those areas believed to be required for success with regard to the ADH's internal operations. Thus, for ADH, key performance factors were external and critical success factors were considered to be internal. The identified factors are listed in Exhibit 4/15.

The Steering Committee Meets

The different task forces had each presented formal reports to the Steering Committee. It was time to begin finalizing the hard work of the many people who had contributed to the process. The Steering Committee objectives were to:

- review and confirm the external opportunities and threats and internal strengths and weaknesses;
- finalize and approve the mission, vision, and guiding principles;
- specify the set of programs and services that would achieve the mission and vision;
- operationalize a select number of internal critical success factors and key performance areas through the development of clear and concise strategic goals for ADH and to provide guidance for departmental operations;
- coordinate the development of the adaptive strategies;
- coordinate the development of program implementation objectives; and
- foster strategic thinking throughout the Department.

Expectations were high for the Steering Committee to finalize the work that had been done for development of the directional strategies (mission and vision)

Internal Critical Success Factors

Human Resources
Adequate number of appropriately prepared employees is critical to the success of ADH

Financial Resources and Stewardship
Adequate and appropriate levels of stable financial resources and stewardship of the public funds and trust placed in our agency are critical to the success of ADH

Organizational Structure and Responsiveness
The agency's organizational structure is critical to its future success and should provide for effective and efficient management of resources and provide for employee and public trust

Information, Equipment and Technology
Access to and availability of information systems, medical equipment, and support systems are critical to ADH attempts to accomplish its mission

Customer Focus
It is the many and varied customers of the ADH who best judge the success of our efforts; therefore, recognizing their needs and providing customer satisfaction is critical to the success of ADH. Respect for our customers is essential. Responding to their needs is inherent in our philosophy

Quality Emphasis and Continuous Improvement
With a changing environment, our ability to improve our processes and efficiencies become critical in determining ways to do more with less. The quality of our services is judged by our customers and other important stakeholders

Communication
Employees spend more of their life in our workplace setting than any other single place
Employees deserve to be informed about the goals of the organization and how they are part of accomplishing them. Effective, two-way communication ensures the agency's success by providing employees with the information they need and allowing them to query for enhanced understanding

Public Image
A critical success factor for the agency is the image it has in the minds of its many stakeholders. Thus, its corporate identity statewide should be consistent and not based solely on personal interactions

Key Performance Areas

Disease Prevention
Contribute to the reduction of premature death and morbidity

Ensuring Compliance with Public Health Laws and Regulations
Promote, monitor, and enforce laws and regulations that have been entrusted to our administration

Community Health Assessment
Aid and assist in the assessment of the public health needs in our communities

Health Promotion
Provide information and education as a means of preventing premature death and disease and improving the quality of life

Service Delivery
Assure that quality health services are accessible

Development of Public Health Policy
Provide leadership in the development of public health policy based on information, experience, and expertise

and develop strategic goals for the ADH. In setting the strategic goals, the Steering Committee wanted to limit the number of goals to provide focus, but, at the same time, provide enough generally stated goals that all programs could anchor their unit objectives to one or more of the strategic goals. The goals selected were to address internal critical success factors and external key performance areas that were determined to be essential in moving the ADH in a direction that would accomplish its mission.

In addition, the Steering Committee carefully examined the information acquired in the situational analysis to ensure that the strategic goals addressed important external issues; capitalized on a strength or corrected a weakness; were consistent with the mission, vision, and guiding principles; and contributed to the achievement of an external key performance area or internal critical success factor. Members of the Steering Committee knew that their decisions would set the future course of the ADH.

5

CASE

Can This Relationship Be Saved? The Midwestern Medical Group's Integration Journey

Introduction

On a snowy January evening, the Midwestern Medical Group (MMG) management team held a retirement party for Judith Olsen, MMG president. During the evening, Olsen reflected back on the years she had worked for MMG with mixed feelings about her experience. Over the course of their eight-year integration journey within the Midwestern Health System (Midwestern), the MMG management team experienced many encouraging moments, achievements, and successes as well as many struggles, disappointments, and conflicts. She was scheduled to meet with the board chair the next day to talk about the major issues her

This case was written by Rhonda Engleman and Jisun Yu under the supervision of Professor Andrew H. Van de Ven of the Carlson School of Management at the University of Minnesota. We also appreciate the editorial assistance of Julie Trupke and useful comments of Gyewan Moon and Margaret Schomaker. We gratefully acknowledge Stuart Bunderson, Shawn Lofstrom, Russel Rogers, Frank Schultz, and Jeffery Thompson who assisted in collecting data during this eight-year longitudinal study of MMG's integration journey. The case was prepared to promote class discussion and learning. It was not designed to illustrate either effective or ineffective management. Used with permission from Rhonda Engleman.

Exhibit 5/1: Major Midwestern Health System and MMG Events

Date	Event
1994	Health Systems Corporation and Midwest Health Plan merged to become Midwestern Health System (Midwestern)
1994	Midwestern established three divisions – Delivery Services, Professional Services, and Health Plan
1994	Midwestern established the Midwestern Medical Group (MMG), with 20 primary care clinics
1995–1996	MMG expanded by acquiring 30 additional primary care clinics
July 1997	Patrick, the original MMG president, was promoted to System vice president of Clinical Services, and Erickson was appointed the new MMG president
Fall 1998	MMG decided to hire an ophthalmologist to expand clinic services; Midwestern protested decision; MMG ordered to cancel hiring negotiations
February 1999	Johanson, Midwestern CEO, announced a new organizational structure, moving from three divisions to two, the Hospitals & Clinics division and the Health Plan division; the new divisions were charged to select and organize around market business segments (MBSs), focusing on specific customer groups to be determined by the divisions
Spring 1999	MMG decided to hire a spine surgeon; Midwestern hospital protested decision; MMG ordered to cancel hiring negotiations
Mid-1999	Hospital & Clinics division selected six market business segments – three metropolitan hospitals, regional hospitals, MMG, and home care
Summer 1999	Johanson commissioned a benchmarking study to compare MMG with benchmark medical groups; MMG compared favorably to benchmark group performance standards
Fall 1999	MMG decided to hire a general surgeon; Midwestern hospital protested decision; MMG ordered to cancel hiring negotiations
Spring 2000	Midwestern System board commissioned a study to evaluate the appropriateness and value of MMG referrals to Midwestern hospitals; the study demonstrated appropriateness and significant financial value of MMG referrals to Midwestern hospitals
Spring 2000	Johanson announced planned retirement in summer 2001; Novak promoted from president of Midwest Health Plan to Midwestern COO to prepare to take over System CEO position
May 2000	MMG began negotiations to expand clinic services with one Midwestern hospital's assistance; specialists affiliated with another Midwestern hospital protested the decision and threatened to leave the System to establish a competitive practice if negotiations continued
May 2000	Johanson requested Erickson's resignation in aftermath of conflict between Midwestern hospitals and specialists
June 2000	Midwestern executive council reviewed options to restructure MMG, including status quo, establishing MMG as a separate MBS, full divestiture, partial divestiture, and hiring outside management; council ruled out divestiture and separate MBS options, but deferred a decision on other options
June 2000	Midwestern initiated a national search for a new MMG president
August 2000	MMG management team presented list of demands to Midwestern board, including demands to maintain a single MMG, increase MMG representation in System leadership, acknowledge contributions of MMG to the System, and clarify expectations and accountabilities of System members

Exhibit 5/1: (cont'd)

Date	Event
September 2000	Erickson officially retired; Olsen selected as interim MMG president
Early 2001	Novak commissioned Deloitte & Touche to evaluate hospitals and MMG to identify potential costs savings and revenue enhancement; Deloitte & Touche found that the MMG was performing better than benchmark clinic groups
March 2001	MMG president search committee interviewed two candidates and rejected both
Spring 2001	Novak commissioned group to evaluate eight models for restructuring the MMG
April 2001	MMG sent out request for proposals for radiology services
June 2001	Novak suspended search for MMG president
July 2001	Novak left Midwestern; several other Midwestern executives left the System; Norton appointed chair of Midwestern board
Fall 2001	MMG selected radiology providers; Midwestern hospitals protested decision; MMG ordered to reverse its selection decision and utilize services of Midwestern hospital-affiliated specialists
October 2001	Johanson retired; Norton appointed as interim CEO of Midwestern
June 2002	Olsen presented an MMG break-even plan to Midwestern board; board passed plan unanimously
October 2002	Olsen announced plan to retire in January 2003
January 2003	Olsen officially retired and Midwestern initiated a new national search for a president of MMG

successor would need to address as president of MMG. Knowing this might be her last contribution to MMG before she retired, Olsen wanted to provide the board chair with helpful advice to pass on to her successor.

Olsen pondered the historical events in MMG's integration journey as she thought about what to say in that meeting. (See Exhibit 5/1 for major Midwestern and MMG events.)

Background

Midwestern Health System (Midwestern) was established in July 1994 through the merger of Health Systems Corporation and Midwest Health Plan, making it the largest health care organization in its region. Health Systems contributed hospitals, clinics, nursing homes, a home health agency, and other health care services while Midwest Health Plan contributed health insurance products and relationships with physician groups. The vision guiding Midwestern's development was to "offer an integrated health care system to affordably enhance the health of people living and working in communities we serve." This vision implied two priorities: the commitment to build an integrated health care system and the goal to improve community health.

MMG was founded in 1994 with an initial network of 340 employed physicians working in 20 clinics previously owned by Health Systems Corporation hospitals at the time of the merger with Midwest Health Plan. Hal Patrick was selected as the first MMG president. Under Patrick's leadership, MMG grew rapidly during its first two years, acquiring 30 additional primary care clinics in strategic locations across Midwestern's geographic market. By mid-1996, MMG's management attention shifted from growth by acquisition to management and organizational development of its 50 clinics with 450 physicians and over 3,000 employees. MMG experienced many challenges during these formation and establishment periods within the Midwestern Health System. System integration processes proved complex, involving many interdependent change initiatives. The initiatives included: (1) creating a large integrated group medical practice from formerly small independent physician clinics; (2) transitioning the identities and roles of physicians from being principals of private clinical practices to becoming agents and employees of health care companies; (3) building an organizational culture that aligned incentives and strengthened the commitment of clinicians with MMG and Midwestern while maintaining their commitment to the medical profession; and (4) developing an integrated system of health care for patients by linking MMG's clinical and business services with other Midwestern units, including the hospitals and the Midwestern Health Plan.

In July 1997, Patrick was promoted to System vice president of clinical services for Midwestern. Midwestern leaders appointed Lief Erickson as the new MMG president. Erickson represented a strong voice for MMG physicians and patient care and had worked as an MMG manager since its formation. Despite continuous hardships in both finances and operations, Erickson led MMG as the group rebounded from a record loss of $41 million in 1996, decreasing losses to $22 million in 1997 and $20 million in 1998. MMG was on track to improve its financial performance in 1999 by decreasing its losses to $17 million; still far from ideal but movement in the right direction (see Exhibit 5/2). Under Erickson's leadership, MMG developed a solid management team of administrative and physician leaders as the Group shifted from a culture of survival to a culture of performance. MMG had faced many challenges since its formation in 1994, but Erickson and his management team weathered the storm to establish MMG as an integral part of the Midwestern Health System. The MMG management team still faced many tensions in their relationships with others in the Midwestern system, but Erickson was confident that his team had demonstrated MMG's value to Midwestern and would continue their journey to lead MMG to even better results in the future.

Arranged Marriage of Equals

The Midwestern Health System experienced escalating financial pressures in 1998 and 1999. Since Midwestern's formation, the system had not achieved its overall financial performance goals. Johanson, CEO of Midwestern, anticipated that the system would experience reductions of $50 million in Medicare

Exhibit 5/2: MMG Annual Operating and Financial Performance, 1994–2002

	1994	1995	1996	1997	1998	1999	2000	2001	2002
Revenue									
Gross Charges	119,380	164,524	204,739	204,491	218,612	259,454	271,470	331,821	390,166
– Discounts	24,393	38,732	58,346	53,756	63,779	77,181	74,041	116,135	150,596
Net Patient Revenue	94,987	125,792	146,393	150,735	154,833	182,273	197,429	215,686	239,570
Other Income	4,277	5,310	4,642	5,913	7,508	10,478	13,255	14,972	18,363
Net Revenue	99,264	131,102	151,035	156,648	162,341	192,751	210,684	230,658	257,933
Expenses									
Physician Comp. & Benefits	43,210	54,943	71,533	66,086	62,688	72,939	68,776	73,681	74,404
Other Comp. & Benefits	37,681	52,406	60,180	61,178	65,651	77,254	97,082	104,397	112,537
All Other Expense	41,794	52,633	60,769	51,733	51,732	59,089	87,936	100,445	108,813
Total Expenses	122,685	159,982	192,482	178,997	180,071	209,282	253,794	278,523	295,754
Net Income (Loss)*	(23,421)	(28,880)	(41,447)	(22,349)	(17,730)	(16,531)	(43,110)	(47,865)	(37,821)
Key Statistics									
# Patient Visits	1,149,096	1,717,288	1,954,693	1,892,141	1,865,120	2,137,005	2,168,890	2,161,563	2,149,040
Charges per Visit ($)	103.89	95.80	104.74	108.07	117.21	121.41	125.17	153.51	181.55
Discount Rate (%)	20.43	23.54	28.50	26.29	29.17	29.75	27.27	35.00	38.60
Net Revenue Per Visit ($)	86.38	76.34	77.27	82.79	87.04	90.20	97.14	106.71	120.02
Physician FTEs	313	324	380	356	327	374	387	385	382
Support FTEs	1,107	1,573	1,913	1,913	1,898	1,895	2,156	2,207	2,170

*Annual net income is not comparable because formulas and policies on corporate subsidies to MMG changed in 1995, 1996, 1997, and 2000.

reimbursement over the next five years because of changes in the program made by the Balanced Budget Act of 1997. Reimbursement rates from other commercial payors were also declining. Johanson feared that Midwestern could not survive without major system-wide changes to improve the organization's financial performance in patient care services.

Meanwhile, Midwest Health Plan had achieved stellar results with the Market Business Segment (MBS) business model. In 1997, Midwest Health Plan experienced significant financial losses, but then it adopted the MBS business model, moving from a structure with staff organized by major functions (such as marketing, member relations, and product development) to a structure with staff organized around Midwest Health Plan's major customer segments (such as government payors, small business, and other commercial payor groups). The move to the MBS business model allowed Midwest Health Plan leaders to streamline the organizational structure and develop products and pricing systems tailored to customer needs in each business segment. As a result, Midwest Health Plan improved its financial performance, moving from a significant financial loss before the MBS restructuring to a sound financial gain after its implementation. Johanson decided to extend the MBS business model to the rest of the Midwestern system, anticipating that the hospitals and MMG could achieve financial results similar to Midwest Health Plan's and enable Midwestern to improve the performance of all its individual units.

In February 1999, Johanson officially unveiled the plan to implement the MBS business model in the Midwestern hospitals and MMG. Johanson announced that in the MBS business model, Midwestern would move from three divisions – Hospitals, MMG, and Health Plan – and reorganize as two divisions – the Health Plan division and the Hospitals & Clinics division (see Exhibits 5/3 and 5/4). Midwest Health Plan would continue with the MBS business model as previously defined and implemented. The Hospitals & Clinics division, including the Midwestern hospitals and MMG, would define and organize around its own market business segments. These two divisions would be assigned accountability and responsibility to become the leader in their chosen market business segments.

Johanson stated that the MBS model signaled a short-term move away from system-wide integration. The old Midwestern business model assumed that individual units shared one customer and attempted to provide a single "Midwestern experience." The MBS model acknowledged that the old view was inadequate because each division served unique customer groups. Midwest Health Plan's customers were health plan members, corporations, other purchasers, and insurance brokers. MMG's primary customers were patients. The Midwestern hospitals' primary customers were physician specialists. Although the mission and vision of Midwestern would remain the same, the system would back off from tight integration and pursue high-impact integration in a few selected areas to meet the unique customer needs of each division. Johanson charged each division to maximize financial and patient care performance within certain "rules of the game," including open communication between divisions and "no tolerance for badmouthing other parts of the organization." Johanson declared

Exhibit 5/3: Midwestern Health System Organization Chart (January 2000)

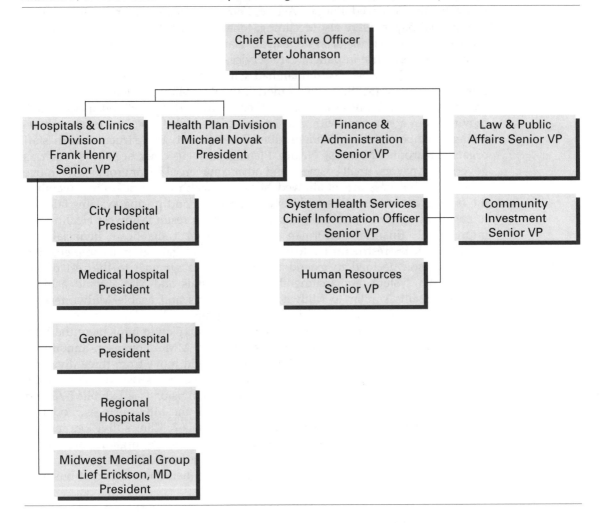

1999 as the year of "freedom to act." He expected the units within each division to coordinate their activities, but each division would be free to define and manage its own unique set of market business segments.

Johanson purposely designed the MBS business model to force the hospitals and the MMG to resolve their tensions and conflicts by combining them into a single division. According to Johanson, "We're learning more about integration. We used to assume that if we put them all together, they'd see the need to talk and automatically coordinate. They don't; it's not natural. Our new model acknowledges that and encourages integration more directly." Johanson expected and looked forward to watching these tensions unfold and play out between the hospitals and MMG in the move to the MBS model.

Exhibit 5/4: MMG Organization Chart (January 2000)

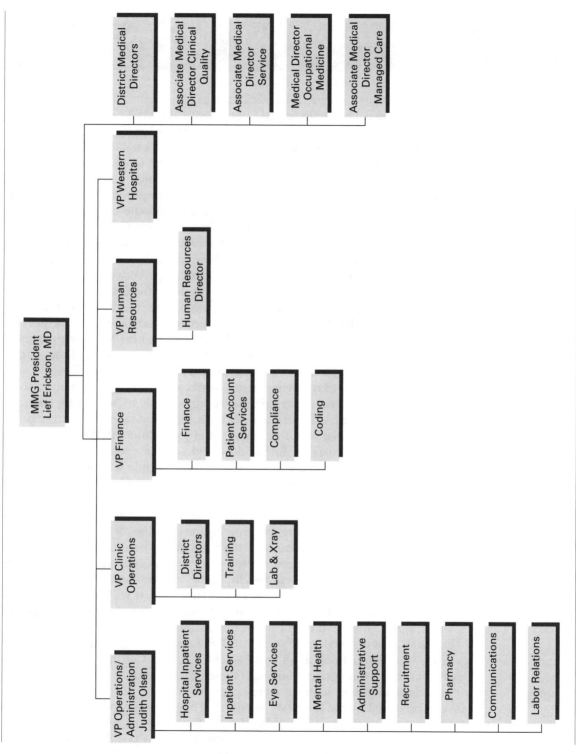

We Don't Know How This Will Go, But Let's Hope For the Best

After the announced restructuring, Erickson expressed mixed feelings about the MBS model when he discussed the change with his MMG management team. Erickson expected that MMG would have an equal voice in the MBS implementation process, with representation on a new board established to govern the Hospitals & Clinics division. He welcomed the freedom to act that Johanson had given to the hospitals and to MMG to establish their own business market segments. Johanson promised that if MMG decided that improving patient care was one of their most important goals, then his expectation would be that MMG would outperform their competitors in that area. Erickson reported, "Then he will go away, and wait for me to come back and tell him how MMG did. That's different, isn't it! They're not going to tell us how to do it." Erickson hoped that the MBS model would help to improve relationships between MMG and the Midwestern hospitals. He felt that this really would be the first time that the hospitals and MMG had a chance to test integration. The hospitals and the MMG had not yet been able to work together to prove what they could achieve in combination to improve patient care. Erickson reassured his MMG management team, "There is a lot of instability and uncertainty. I'm convinced, though, that the strategy is right to focus more on customers and relationships."

At the same time, Erickson wondered if MMG and the hospitals could resolve the differences in their customer groups and approaches to health care delivery. "The structure by itself will not do away with those fundamental market activities that make us see the world differently and to be different. When they think of a customer, they look out the window and see the specialist building; my customer is this region because at some time those people will eventually wind up in the hospital. For MMG, the customer is across the table. They simply have a different customer set. It's funny how you won't face what you have to face. Hospitals say they have patients and referring doctors, as on an equal plane. When you really look at it, though, the referring doctor is on the top of the priority list. . . . In MMG, the patient is center, and it's relationship based. We see customers and markets differently. And now you say you've got to get together in a 'market-based segment?' Hang on! It will be OK, but it will be another game; all those market dynamics are still in place. If we can survive it, it will be good. No matter how good a new model is, if you make a change like this, the bridge in between is tough. I don't think we've got many more shots at this thing."

Erickson went on to note, "If you're the CEO and you say, 'I expect you to outperform your competition at all costs' – which is a part of this market segment idea – but then I put you in a box with these other groups, who have the ability to impede you, you're sending a very complex message. Every day, the clinics are compromised by the hospitals' needs. . . . They have a good theory, but if it's not carried out well, it's not a good theory. But, anyway, we're going to try." Erickson urged his MMG management team to send a positive message about the new MBS business model to the staff and physicians working in their clinics:

"No matter which way we go, we're partners with the hospitals; we've got to coordinate, and the future's about relationships. . . . As we sell this to our clinics and our partners, we want to make it positive and build hope."

The Children Get Separate Rooms

Johanson appointed Frank Henry as senior vice president of the Hospitals & Clinics division. Henry formed a division management team of representatives from each unit to review options for selecting market business segments. The team explored three options. First, the group considered the status quo option, with MMG as one business segment and each of the three hospitals as a separate business segment. Second, the group explored the implications of establishing two business segments – hospital services and ambulatory care services. Finally, the group considered creating a regional model, with each metro hospital forming the anchor of three separate MBSs and the clinics organized geographically around these hospitals. After discussing the pros and cons of each option, the team decided to maintain the status quo, with a few additions by selecting six market business segments for the Hospitals & Clinics division: three metropolitan hospitals, regional hospitals, MMG, and home care.

MMG as the Problem Child

In early 1999, Johanson asked the Midwestern financial management staff to compare MMG's performance to a best-practice model developed by a national consulting group. In a study of seven health system-sponsored primary care groups, the consulting group concluded that financial losses were inevitable in such groups because of costs associated with system membership, including high practice acquisition costs, additional system overhead, increased employee benefit costs, new information systems expenses, and loss of ancillary revenues to hospital affiliates. The consulting group developed a model of realistic performance expectations for health system-sponsored primary care groups given such limitations.

The finance staff found that MMG gross revenues were lower than the benchmark, but that MMG compared favorably in net revenue, expenses, and loss per RVU[1] when compared with the best-practice standards. MMG also compared favorably in productivity, producing 6,428 RVUs per physician in 1998 compared with best-practice benchmarks of only 6,100. Erickson summarized the significance of these findings, "What's important is that it should eliminate the notion that MMG can gradually move to a zero loss."

Erickson presented MMG's favorable benchmark comparisons to the Midwestern board. The board expressed a new appreciation for MMG, its performance, and its value to the larger Midwestern system. They reported that this study gave them a better understanding of how to measure MMG's financial and operational performance, how to set benchmarks for its performance, and the need to recognize the value that MMG contributed to the Midwestern system.

Despite the board's affirmation of MMG's value to Midwestern and recognition that its financial performance exceeded expectations, MMG leaders heard repeated comments by other Midwestern leaders that there must be something wrong with the management team of a unit that consistently lost money. For example, when an MMG vice president presented an analysis of MMG's financial losses to a group of other Midwestern leaders, one of the hospital vice presidents in the audience taunted her, saying: "It pretty much sucks to be you, doesn't it?" When she made the same presentation to MMG's own physician advisory group members, many of whom had sold their practices to MMG, "They went off the deep end on it. Their mindset was, 'No, we used to at least break even. Something's wrong if we lose $17 million!'"

One Midwestern hospital administrator summarized the hospital leaders' views on the "MMG problem" this way: "Looking at MMG's bottom-line losses, the hospital leaders started thinking that they must not be very good managers and resented having to subsidize MMG. . . . They were making money before they became part of Midwestern and now they were getting fat and lazy. . . . The move to the MBS only reinforced that 'what's your problem?' mentality, regardless of the data that showed MMG being set up to lose money. The data became almost irrelevant. There was no view that we were in this together."

These negative reactions affected the MMG management team morale. The perception by other Midwestern leaders that MMG was a financial drain on the system was clearly felt by MMG leaders. The MMG financial manager acknowledged the view that, "MMG's been looked down on – if it weren't for us, the hospitals would have more capital to spend." In one MMG leadership meeting when the group reviewed a report showing that MMG's losses were far lower than budget, one MMG manager lamented, "If we're doing so great, how come we are not feeling better?" Another manager replied, "It's because we're in a lousy business. No matter what we do, we lose money." In another meeting, one MMG physician manager urged, "We need to stop presenting that awful $20 million loss figure. That turns us into the no-joy club. We should be talking instead about how we compare to best practice clinic groups." Searching to bolster his team's morale, Erickson asserted that, "MMG is a very important piece of the Midwestern Health System, and we are not underperformers."

In addition to concerns about MMG's financial losses, some Midwestern hospital administrators expressed concern that MMG failed to honor its responsibility to other system members by inappropriately referring patients to non-Midwestern hospitals. In Spring 2000, the Midwestern board commissioned another study to quantify the value and appropriateness of MMG referrals to Midwestern hospitals. Erickson felt that this new study was another example of, ". . . some guys in the board room occasionally waking up and wondering, 'why do we have this clinic, again?'" This MMG valuation study provided evidence that MMG stabilized and increased referrals to Midwestern-owned facilities plus affiliated specialists, and provided a large and geographically well-located clinic group to strengthen Midwestern's position in contract negotiations with payors. In addition, this study showed that MMG clinics contributed more than $500 million in net revenue and about $250 million in contribution margin to the

Midwestern hospitals annually. Overall, the MMG valuation study once again affirmed MMG's value to the larger Midwestern system, despite its individual unit losses.

The Midwestern system and hospital leaders were not entirely impressed by the results of the MMG valuation study. When the MMG leaders presented the MMG valuation study findings to the Midwestern executive committee, members initially responded that the results "couldn't be this good." They sent MMG back to check their numbers and review their findings with Midwestern's chief financial officer. This additional review confirmed the original results. The MMG leadership team found the hospital administrators' interpretations of the MMG valuation study results interesting. While the study showed that MMG contributed $250 million to the hospitals, Olsen summarized the hospital leaders' attitudes toward this news as, "We would have gotten those referrals anyway, so sit down and shut up."

Family Squabbles in the Hospitals & Clinics Division

Midwestern held the individual market business segments accountable for their individual revenue and expense statements. As its own MBS within the Hospitals & Clinics division, MMG continued to experience significant financial losses. MMG attempted several strategies to improve its financial performance. One promising strategy was to expand MMG services to the community by hiring specialists because their services are typically reimbursed at a higher rate than primary care services. The MMG leaders engaged in their "freedom to act" within the general guidelines set out for them by Johanson in the MBS rollout. They committed to hire outside specialists only if Midwestern hospital-affiliated specialists could not meet their needs. However, MMG's efforts to hire specialists led to several squabbles with other members of the Hospital & Clinics division.

In late 1998, MMG decided to hire an ophthalmologist to provide outpatient laser surgery in an MMG clinic near one of Midwestern's hospitals. The ophthalmologists practicing at that hospital perceived this MMG decision as promoting unfair competition within their service area. According to the hospital administrator, MMG made the decision to hire an ophthalmologist unilaterally without consulting with him or his ophthalmologist group. The ophthalmologists affiliated with this Midwestern hospital said, "To heck with that. We've been taking ER calls in the middle of the night and MMG doesn't do that." This group of ophthalmologists resigned and established a new independent practice. Midwestern hospital lost patient volume to this new competitor and had to find another group to provide emergency room coverage for ophthalmology services. According to the hospital administrator, "It was a good business decision for MMG, but it was a dumb decision for Midwestern."

In early 1999, MMG learned that Midwestern had developed a formal specialty strategy. In a strategy presentation to a management group, a Midwestern leader cited MMG's plan to recruit an independent spine surgeon as a prime example of this strategy in practice. MMG leaders were excited to see their strategy moving forward and receiving acceptance and support from the Midwestern leadership group. A week later, MMG learned that Midwestern system leaders had made a commitment to a group practicing at one of the Midwestern hospitals and decided that all Midwestern business related to spine surgery should go to them. MMG was forced to comply with this new contract by working with the Midwestern hospital group to provide spine surgery services and had to retract their previous employment offer to the independent surgeon.

Later in 1999, MMG hired a general surgeon to practice at another of its clinics. According to Erickson, "It's got the whole damn city up in arms. The official policy, though, is that we, when we can, should work with existing specialists. If they can't meet your needs to out-compete the market, then you can get your own. In this clinic, there's a stodgy old surgeon group who won't meet our needs in our new great facility, so we're going outside to hire." Once again, Midwestern system leaders had other ideas. They demanded that the MMG leaders retract their plan to hire the general surgeon originally selected and instead work with the local Midwestern hospital's surgeon group.

Johanson blamed Erickson for these conflicts with Midwestern hospital-affiliated specialists. According to Johanson, "It was so painfully obvious to me that Erickson needed to get key players together to hash out issues, but he simply wasn't getting to the issues." Johanson went on to note that, "Erickson falls into the trap of seeing our need for information and coordination as questioning respect; he refuses at times to admit he needs help and discussion. . . . On this specialty issue, he didn't get the big picture about implications for the whole organization and the ripple effects he might be creating. There's a 'lack of learning' problem."

Erickson viewed these conflicts as evidence to support his suspicion that the Midwestern hospitals wanted to regionalize MMG. His management team tried to follow the expectation that MMG would work with Midwestern hospital-affiliated specialists and only go outside the system when they could not meet MMG's needs. Even so, the MMG leaders were handcuffed in their attempts to improve MMG financials and expand services by hiring specialists. Erickson and the MMG management group were discouraged by the lack of a coherent specialty strategy at the Midwestern system level. One MMG manager expressed frustration "because you start going down a path, and then it gets pulled out from under you. And then you find out that there was never really a strategy to begin with."

MMG Moves Along With Its Work

Despite difficulties implementing the MBS business model in the Hospitals & Clinics division, MMG continued to move on with its work in 1999. The MMG management team focused on fine-tuning their systems, structures, and working procedures across clinics as well as developing patient-focused quality improvement initiatives. A 1998 billing practices audit report showed that MMG billing practices were often inaccurate and patient care documentation was sometimes incomplete.

MMG leaders worked hard in 1999 to implement standardized patient care documentation and billing practices to assure that MMG was in compliance with the government's billing and documentation standards. Improving these systems also provided an excellent opportunity to increase revenues by collecting payments for previously unbilled and underbilled services.

While they were trying to improve such administrative issues, the MMG management team also initiated several programs to enhance their patient care quality. One program of focus was the Clinical Care Improvement (CCI) initiative. The MMG management team believed that MMG could produce measurable improvement in clinical care and transfer successful experience from one clinic to another. Thus, the MMG managers established a CCI cross-functional team to lead MMG on clinical care improvement initiatives. The CCI cross-functional team set out to prioritize health care services where MMG could have a strong impact on community health improvement such as diabetes care, elderly care, and smoking cessation. The team identified methods that MMG clinics could use to improve their services and established incentives to motivate clinics to improve their patient care outcomes in these areas. The MMG leaders hoped that their work would provide an example to other Midwestern system units by demonstrating the benefits of continuous care improvement in action. These continuous improvement efforts paid off. Early in 1999, at an executive leadership retreat, one of Midwestern's executive officers stated that, "MMG really is the cornerstone of any meaningful changes we make." He explained that MMG could demonstrate best practices and clinical care improvements and urged the other units to follow their example.

Is the Family Going to Stay Together?

Despite the positive results of the benchmarking study, the MMG valuation study, and improvements within the MMG, the Midwestern executive council began to reconsider MMG's future in the Midwestern system. Concerns about MMG's financial losses continued, and squabbles with Midwestern hospitals and specialists indicated to the executive group that some change was needed. In their June 2000 meeting, the executive council reviewed seven options for restructuring MMG's role in the Midwestern system:

1. Status quo, with MMG as one MBS within Hospitals & Clinics division;
2. Separate MMG as its own division;
3. Regionalize MMG by placing clinics under Midwestern hospital management;
4. Divest MMG;
5. Partial sale of selected MMG clinics or programs;
6. Hire an outside group to manage MMG; and
7. Transfer ownership of MMG to a community trust.

The executive council decided to keep MMG within the Midwestern system and rejected the divestiture option. The group also rejected the option to regionalize

MMG or establish it as a separate division but deferred a decision on any of the other options, fearing that any decision would be premature.

Erickson expressed frustration with the executive council's decision-making process to determine MMG's future status in the Midwestern system. When asked by his MMG management team about his sense of Midwestern's direction, he replied, "I should know, but I don't. MMG is not at the table. Johanson doesn't meet with me, and Henry's met with me twice in six months. . . . We've been systematically excluded from all that activity. The experience we've had in this division is the most ridiculous thing we've gone through. Midwest Health Plan and the hospitals have come up with a grand scheme, perhaps, on delivery, and they're keeping it from us. . . . I don't have an answer." Erickson went on to note that, "On the down side, there is apparently no willingness, no openness to think about an MBS structure where we're cut loose from the division, which is where I think we need to go. People in the organization are saying that the two divisions are constantly fighting, so why would we want three? I'm saying that we had far less turmoil with three."

While Midwestern leaders and MMG were trying to clarify MMG's future in the Midwestern system, some of the MMG clinics began to make their own decisions about their future. A Midwestern competitor approached the physician leaders of one MMG clinic with an offer to expand the facility if they would associate with the competitor's system. If they chose not to, then the competitor warned the MMG clinic physicians that they would build new clinics in the area to compete with MMG. The Midwestern system executives conceded to the sale, believing that this MMG clinic was not large enough to withstand the potential competition. They decided that it was better to cut their losses and negotiated the sale of that clinic to the competitor. After watching this sale transpire and wondering about their own future in the Midwestern system, other MMG clinics also threatened to defect. According to Erickson, the executive council wanted much more clarity about its direction on some of the MMG clinics that could try to leave the system. "They're realizing that when a medical group wants to leave, it leaves. . . . It took one clinic to get their attention, but I think it will get bigger with other clinics."

Maybe Uncle Novak Will Take Care of Us

In Spring 2000, Johanson announced his plan to retire in Summer 2001. Johanson selected Michael Novak as his heir apparent. Novak had led Midwest Health Plan's turnaround effort. In preparation for taking over the reins, Novak changed his role as president of the Midwest Health Plan to the Midwestern chief operating officer. Olsen summarized the MMG's reactions to Novak's appointment, saying: ". . . he's my hope. What he says about his values is encouraging. Two things about him give me hope. First, he's visiting the facilities, using his time as an understudy to get to know the organization from a front-line perspective. Second, he'll be very clear about the direction of the organization. He'll be clear, and follow through on what he will and will not tolerate."

Olsen was heartened by a statement that Novak made in a meeting with the MMG leaders. "We asked you to pull together 50 clinics and make them into one. You actually did it, and we never said thanks. Now we've tried to make you the scapegoat for the fact that we don't know what to do with it now that you've succeeded." Olsen was impressed with the changes Novak had implemented in Midwest Health Plan. Although some described how Novak handled Midwest Health Plan's turnaround as "scorching the earth" because he had let many of the original management staff go, Olsen believed that many who left Midwest Health Plan really did need to go. "Midwestern needs somebody who can see that and act on it." Novak confirmed with the MMG managers that he would be very clear in his expectations for Midwestern managers, using phrases like, "I won't drag anyone along." At the same time, Olsen was confident that Novak would emphasize paired physician–executive leadership. "Novak doesn't think anyone can be everything to everyone, and he'll put strong physicians with strong managers."

Erickson Shunned For Misbehaving One Too Many Times

In May 2000, another contentious conflict exploded between MMG and Midwestern hospital-affiliated specialists. Erickson asked the pulmonary specialist group associated with Midwestern's City Hospital for help in implementing a Healthy Lung program at the Wellview Clinic by extending the clinic's smoking cessation and early heart disease detection services. The City Hospital pulmonary group declined the invitation to work with this program. When he learned of MMG's difficulties in working with City Hospital, the chief medical officer from Midwestern's General Hospital facilitated a relationship with MMG so it could provide the program and contract negotiations began. The chief medical officer at City Hospital heard of these plans and demanded that Erickson stop MMG negotiations with the General Hospital group well after they had begun. The pulmonary group based at City Hospital also had an office at General Hospital. They were angered by the proposed relationship between General Hospital and MMG and closed their General Hospital office after this conflict erupted. They also threatened to leave City Hospital and set up an independent practice to compete with the Midwestern system if Erickson did not agree to work with them on the Healthy Lung program at Wellview. The City Hospital pulmonary group sent a letter to Johanson and the Midwestern board demanding Erickson's resignation for causing this conflict.

The conflict culminated in Johanson conceding to the City Hospital pulmonary group's demands by asking for Erickson's resignation. Reflecting on the events leading to this decision, Johanson acknowledged Erickson's success in providing internal leadership of MMG. "The problem is when you get out of the sandbox in managing relationships with other parts of the system. I am not saying that Erickson was wrong; only that he has not been able to handle them well and prevent problems from growing to high visibility crisis situations." Johanson went on to say that Erickson's "building of the MMG silo may be at the expense of the undoing of the Midwestern system. Erickson has not been willing to bring the Midwestern mission into MMG." Johanson suggested that Erickson had taken MMG as far as he could and should retire while he was at the peak of his career. "I have known Erickson for a long time; he came from a primary care clinic, and he has been in front of the business in the development of primary care. Now he is in the middle of managing relationships with specialists, which is causing him trouble." Johanson initially suggested to Erickson that he resign in July 2001. Johanson later decided to move up the timetable for Erickson to transition out of MMG by the end of 2000. Johanson reported that he had talked with the MMG board and district medical directors, who said they recognized Erickson's strengths and weaknesses, and they wanted to make sure there was an orderly transition in leadership and the right leadership for MMG.

Henry agreed with Johanson's view that Erickson had made great strides in molding MMG into one entity. "Now we need to put MMG into better alignment with the Midwestern hospitals. Erickson has not agreed with this strategy; nor is it part of his skill set." Henry cited concern that Erickson participated in senior management team meetings only to pull back later and do his own thing on billing and other simple things. Henry supported the call for Erickson's resignation saying, "We need to stop working at cross-purposes. Erickson has simply not bought into our strategy and has been unwilling to work toward consensus with a division team."

The Midwestern hospital administrators supported the call for Erickson's resignation. One administrator summarized her views on Erickson and MMG's role within Midwestern: "We act like a classic dysfunctional family. In a dysfunctional family, there is always a problem child. MMG is the classic child that acts out in the Midwestern family. Erickson played that part well; in fact, he seemed to be born to it. One way to act out is to take money from the specialists and that starts a lot of conflict." Another Midwestern hospital administrator agreed, saying: "Erickson just loved to mix it up. He was their guy, take out the word ophthalmology and insert any number of other specialties. If I'm never disciplined for stepping over an organizational line, then I'm doing the right thing. . . . We ought to be Midwestern leaders first and work this out. We've got to always think of the big picture."

Erickson acknowledged two reasons for his forthcoming resignation. First, he cited Johanson's response to a "group of thugs . . . who are writing letters to the board and Johanson, and being successful at it." Erickson stated that a second and deeper issue was the MBS business model. "I don't believe in it and do not want to put MMG in with the hospitals. The more I challenged this issue the more peripheral I became. The vertical structure and hierarchy of the company does not permit conflict, and this is foreign to my horizontal conflict management approach." Later in the year, he appeared to have come to terms with his pending resignation, saying: "I am happy to be leaving because I no longer trust the values of top management. I recognize I do not fit in this organization." Erickson ultimately attributed his demise to a classic case of failed leadership. Erickson believed that Midwestern executives failed to implement the MBS strategy because power and control stayed in the hands of a few people who were unwilling to leave their power and allow the system to establish market business segments. Instead, the Midwestern leaders tried to regionalize the system around the three metro hospitals. "The strategy was to have a collaborating set of divisions, each of which would compete fiercely in the market for their customers. They turned around and said that's not what they meant; instead, they said be subservient to the hospitals. The soul has gone out of the company." Erickson summarized his sense of betrayal, saying: "When introducing the market business segments strategy, the company told us that we would be judged by our ability to implement the strategy. They left unspoken that if you get others upset, we will kill you."

MMG Leaders Rally to Defend Their Rights

The MMG management team was alarmed at the potential implications of Erickson's ousting to the future of MMG. They felt that Johanson had violated his previous assertions that Erickson would be evaluated based on MMG's financial and clinical performance, reflecting a lack of integrity in the Midwestern system leadership. One MMG physician manager noted, "If the company treats Erickson this way, then it may happen to the next person or yourself." The MMG management team feared that the call for Erickson's resignation was a sign that the system intended to break up or sell MMG.

During his transition period, Erickson urged the MMG management team to step up to the plate to keep Midwestern from tearing MMG apart. Working with Erickson, the MMG management team generated a list of demands for the Midwestern board to clarify MMG's future role in the Midwestern system:

1. Maintain a single MMG with physician executive leadership;
2. Give MMG increased representation at the division and system tables;
3. Acknowledge the contributions of MMG to the system;
4. Develop a realistic plan to attract and retain physician leaders; and
5. Expectations, accountabilities, and roles must be clarified.

The MMG management team presented these demands to the Midwestern board in August 2000. The board listened to their presentation, and Novak said he would get back to them on the issues they presented. Novak came to an MMG management team meeting in October 2000 to respond to the demands. He hedged on the demand to have a single MMG. "I have no idea how this will play out, but whatever we decide to do, it will be to improve patient care. I think there is value in having MMG together, but there is also value in regional efforts." He affirmed that Midwestern was searching for a physician executive as the future MMG leader, a person with 15 years of clinical and operational experience. "I don't need to tell you that that's a lot to ask. That makes for a very small pool of candidates; finding someone with a career combining both is rare. We don't want to put that person in position to fail. We need to find someone who fits the profile. We are looking for a physician right now; we'll see how we do."

Regarding MMG presence on the executive council, Novak stated that until the new MMG president was selected, Henry would represent MMG in operational matters and the Midwestern chief medical officer would represent MMG physician interests on the executive council. He stated that he was not ready to include the MMG president as part of the executive council. When the MMG management team noted concern about their lack of involvement at the executive council level, Novak replied that it was a temporary arrangement, and "What I can tell you is that the only constant for MMG and Midwestern overall will be change. I'm not sure what the ultimate structure will be."

Novak expressed confusion about the MMG demand to have a representative on the Midwestern board because he believed that MMG had a representative. Olsen noted that people do not see the person appointed to represent MMG as a true MMG representative. She added, "I think our major concern is about being consumed by hospitals; that's not the best way to take care of patients. I think what we are saying is that we want to have a voice in whatever strategy is decided for how to organize MMG and how it relates to the rest of Midwestern." Novak acknowledged this concern and committed to maintaining a continued dialogue with MMG involvement in such decisions, whether through the board, the executive council, or other channels.

When the discussion turned to how to better reflect the value of MMG to Midwestern, Novak stressed that, "What I want to get to is the role for MMG; how we account for it in the books is not really important to me. I think that it's more important how we decide where we're going. I will be working with the board on the strategic planning process." One manager pointed out that Novak should understand that MMG had been "put under the gun about our numbers and that's why we are so sensitive about that." Novak replied, "I'm not saying that the numbers are not important, but that discussion won't take us anywhere." He framed the problem as finding an economic model that fits the current economic realities facing Midwestern and MMG. "I want you to know that the numbers are not important to me. The more time I spend in MMG, the more I believe that this is Midwestern's crown jewel."

Novak went on to acknowledge that recruiting and retaining physician leaders were major challenges for Midwestern. The system had lost many talented physician leaders, and many who remained expressed frustration with their limited ability to impact the organization. Novak informed MMG that the physician resources committee of the board was taking this issue seriously, making it their top priority.

Novak heartedly agreed with the MMG demand to clarify roles and accountabilities in the Midwestern system. "We can be about financials, but I think for our employees it's more about feeling valued than the bottom line. I believe that organizations that have clarity around purpose and values do better than organizations that are focused on the bottom line. The number one thing we can do to improve bottom line is to have clarity of purpose. The other is to take responsibility. Having those two things is essential to having a healthy organization." Olsen noted that she and other MMG leaders had often been confused about decision-making authority. "We get very confused with knowing whether we have the ability to make decisions or whether someone else has the power to make our decisions for us." Novak agreed with this concern. "Who's on first, who is in charge, that's a problem. We have a lot of people working on committees and no one knows who is in charge; it's wasted time. We need to be willing to let someone be in charge. That person needs to understand the organization's needs. I'm working to try to get a handle on these things; we need to keep having conversations about this issue."

Who Is Going to Lead Us Now?

With Erickson's resignation imminent, Johanson appointed Henry to lead a national search for a new president of MMG. Henry explained the search process to the MMG management group in June 2000. A selection committee of Midwestern system leaders was appointed to make the hiring decision. The committee would include one MMG representative, yet to be determined. The committee planned to develop a new MMG president job description and would have better-defined position requirements in 30 days. He stated that the committee would like to have a candidate in place by the end of 2000, but a national search could take longer to complete.

One MMG manager pointed out that, "It sounds like you have a good process in place, but I think it's important to do a good bit of soul searching to figure out what failed this time and how to make it work the next time." Olsen added, "I think you have to understand that we are mourning a loss here. Many of us are feeling that there is a certain disconnect here. We have an excellent leader, and it's not clear to us what exactly went wrong." Another manager added, "There are many things about Erickson that have been very successful, and we need to keep those things and build on the others. If we don't do that, the environment and relationship pieces won't be successful." Henry agreed and expressed openness to feedback from the entire group on how to improve the success of the new MMG president. "It's no secret that we have a poor track record with physician leaders. Is it preparation, culture, fit, selection?" Henry assured the group that the search committee would consider this issue seriously in the recruitment process.

The MMG management team assumed that Olsen was the most logical choice to lead MMG in the interim following Erickson's resignation. Olsen had served as senior vice president of MMG since 1997. In that role, she had provided leadership on several major initiatives. However, weeks passed after Johanson's call for Erickson's resignation in May 2000 and Olsen was bewildered by Henry's silence regarding a plan to manage the MMG leadership transition. The absence of any contact about this made Olsen wonder if she would not be invited to stay on with MMG. Olsen also wondered if this lack of succession planning communication was a further indication that the Midwestern leaders intended to sell MMG or split it up by regionalizing clinics with the hospitals. She felt that the option to replace Erickson and keep MMG intact was not behaviorally apparent since no efforts had been made to communicate with the MMG top management team to keep it intact.

In July 2000, Olsen talked briefly with Henry after a large management meeting. Olsen told Henry that she had heard a rumor that Erickson was leaving on September 1st. She asked if that was true and could people begin talking about it and making plans? Henry was shocked and shushed Olsen saying that people weren't supposed to know; he had only told one or two people. Olsen asked, "Well, if it's true, who will run MMG with Erickson gone?" This question appeared to catch Henry off guard. "Um, well, you are doing a good job right now," he replied. Olsen informed him that she did not want to do the job just by default. Olsen was disturbed by Henry's lack of communication with her and other MMG management staff on the MMG leadership transition outside of sidebar conversations. Henry assured her that he would set up a time very soon to talk with her formally.

Weeks went by again until Henry finally called Olsen to ask if Erickson had told people about his leaving in September. Olsen replied: of course, many people knew by then. Henry was flustered and said that he needed to send out a memo announcing Erickson leaving, Olsen taking over, and other management changes. Olsen replied, "Wait. Hold on. You need to talk to me about this first. The memo can't go out today; you need to talk to me and not just take this as a natural default move."

Henry finally set up a meeting with Olsen in mid-August 2000. Olsen asked him to describe exactly what the MMG interim president position entailed. Henry replied, "Well, it's just running MMG, you know." Olsen asked for clarification of her role within Midwestern, such as what decision-making authority she would have in MMG versus decisions that would be made by Henry and other system executives. Henry hadn't thought about those issues. By October 2000, when asked about how the transition from Erickson was working, Olsen reported that the transition was going well by that time. At first people were sad to see Erickson go but, after a time, the grieving subsided. However, Olsen and the rest of the MMG management team remained concerned that this interim MMG leadership period might be used to justify breaking up and parceling out MMG clinics. Olsen's role and MMG's role within Midwestern had not yet been clarified, but Olsen was determined to hold the MMG management team together despite this.

MMG Continues to Move Along With Its Work

Despite leadership transitions at the system and MMG levels, MMG continued to move on with its work in 2000. MMG leaders pushed forward with their clinical quality improvement initiatives. In addition, they established a new initiative focusing on patient safety and drug interactions. They established a safety committee to implement a mechanism for reporting safety issues and medical errors in MMG clinics. To support this effort, they emphasized the need to create a "blameless culture" in which clinic staff and physicians could feel safe to report issues without fear of reprisal. The MMG management team initiated a project to implement same-day scheduling in MMG clinics. This initiative improved patient satisfaction with the scheduling process and allowed the MMG clinics to improve quality of care by addressing patient needs on a more timely basis. The MMG management team also improved patient care by implementing new patient education programs. The MMG medical leaders established a Council of Evidence-Based Medicine to set priorities for evaluating and implementing clinical best-practice standards in MMG clinics.

The MMG management team implemented changes in its employee recruitment and compensation systems as well. MMG was suffering from increased employee turnover rates as staff left MMG for better-paying positions with other organizations. MMG's compensation rates had been kept lower than market rates for many positions, and annual salary increases had not kept pace with inflation. Also, some MMG clinics found that to recruit new staff, they had to offer higher compensation to new employees than more tenured employees, creating an equity problem in staff compensation. MMG needed to address these issues to retain its workforce. The MMG management team successfully lobbied for the approval and additional funding needed from Midwestern to address these recruitment and compensation issues.

Continued Family Squabbles

In her interim MMG president position, Olsen experienced continued conflicts with hospital-affiliated specialists. In April 2000, MMG had sent out a request for proposals for radiology services in MMG clinics when the contracts with the groups providing these services were about to expire. In September 2000, MMG reviewed the proposals received, chose to offer the groups currently providing services first right of refusal for new contracts, and sent them all a letter verifying this decision. These new contracts established service and quality expectations and clarified the MMG–radiology group relationship overall.

After the fact, some of the Midwestern hospital leaders protested MMG's decision. For example, under MMG's decision, the Wellview Clinic would retain its current radiology provider, Central Radiology. The chief medical officer at Midwestern's City Hospital demanded that Wellview replace Central Radiology with City Hospital's radiology provider, Allied Radiology. Responding to such complaints by Midwestern hospital leaders, Henry informed Olsen that MMG should be following "the guiding principle" in their contracting. Olsen replied that she had no idea what this guiding principle was, or when it was decided that MMG was supposed to be following it. Henry explained that the guiding principle referred to a decision made by the executive team that MMG should give preference to specialist relationships that had been established in the local Midwestern hospital when contracting for specialist services. He explained that if a Midwestern hospital used a certain radiology group, the local MMG clinic should give their radiology contract to the same group. In the Wellview Clinic, this would mean replacing the current provider, Central Radiology, with the City Hospital provider, Allied Radiology.

Olsen explained to Henry that following this "guiding principle" could wreak havoc in MMG. MMG had contracts with various specialists where, in return for covering some of the rural, less desirable clinics, a specialist group was given some of the urban, more desirable sites, like Wellview. Olsen explained that following this new "guiding principle" might accomplish the hospitals' objectives of giving their specialists the MMG sites they wanted, but that this would mean severing relationships with providers that had established, long-standing relationships with a given site. She pointed out that if a specialist group loses one of the urban sites to a Midwestern hospital-affiliated group, they would have no incentive to cover MMG's rural sites. Olsen feared that implementing the "guiding principle" could result in some MMG clinics losing specialist services entirely, which could, in turn, compromise patient care quality.

Henry ignored Olsen's concerns, negated MMG's radiology vendor decision, and forced MMG to use the local Midwestern hospital radiologists. Henry's plan was more expensive than the plan MMG had originally developed. As vendors were moved out of MMG clinics, they took their equipment with them, forcing MMG to purchase replacement equipment. Technical support staff also transitioned, and MMG incurred additional recruitment and training costs to hire replacement staff. In addition, Henry's plan put the organization at risk of legal action for breach of contract from the radiologists originally selected to provide services to the MMG clinics.

Tell Me Again, Why Is MMG Such a Problem Child?

In late 2000, Novak hired Deloitte & Touche to conduct a benchmarking study of the individual MBS units in the Hospital & Clinics division. Deloitte & Touche reviewed MMG's performance in the areas where they had typically found opportunities for improvement in other primary care physician networks. They found that MMG compared favorably to other groups in productivity, compensation, number of support staff, ancillary revenues, billing practices, and referrals provided to other system members. Deloitte & Touche found that the most significant factor contributing to MMG's financial losses was excessive system overhead costs assigned to the group by the Midwestern system. MMG was carrying far more system overhead than the average medical group – $110,000 per physician compared to a Deloitte & Touche benchmark of $50,000 per physician. Further, MMG was forced to provide staff benefits to match benefits provided by the hospitals, benefits that most independent groups did not provide. In addition, MMG had incurred technology costs that did not create operational improvements, technology imposed on the group by other Midwestern system members. Just like the earlier benchmarking analysis and the MMG valuation project, the Deloitte & Touche analysis once again reaffirmed that MMG did provide value to the Midwestern system and was performing as best it could given the constraints placed on it by the Midwestern system.

Is the Family Going to Stay Together? – Round Two

In Spring 2001, despite Deloitte & Touche's findings and reaffirmation of MMG's value to Midwestern, Novak commissioned a group to investigate how to retain the benefits of MMG while minimizing its financial losses. This group analyzed the potential of eight models to achieve this objective:

1. Sell MMG to an outside party;
2. Spin off MMG by selling the clinics back to the physicians;
3. Form a holding company in which MMG would become its own separate Midwestern division;
4. Use a hospital-centered approach, with MMG clinics managed to maximize hospital benefit;
5. Move to a regional model, with the hospitals and clinics reporting to a regional executive;
6. Merge MMG and Midwest Health Plan;
7. Form a Midwestern ambulatory company with all ambulatory services across Midwestern managed under one umbrella; and
8. Maintain status quo, with MMG as one MBS within the Hospitals & Clinics division.

The group rejected the option to merge MMG and Midwest Health Plan, fearing that this could have negative financial effects on the Midwestern hospitals. The group rejected the option to form a Midwestern ambulatory company as an essentially unmanageable change. Novak decided to present the status quo, sell, spin off, holding company, and a combination of the hospital-centered/regional models to the board to make a final decision. According to Olsen, selling MMG seemed unlikely since this would likely result in significant loss in hospital volumes, although it would bring Midwestern an immediate $75 to $100 million in capital from the sale. Spinning off MMG via selling it back to the physicians seemed unlikely to Olsen because MMG physicians were hesitant to assume the financial management responsibility. Forming a holding company seemed unlikely because this would require significant changes in current leadership and high transition costs. Some combination of the hospital-centered/regional models seemed the most likely board choice of the change options, but it would require transition costs and probably additional layers of management. Olsen felt that the current state was adequate, and "if the loss bothers you, restate the financials."

Olsen Remains at the MMG Helm by Default

In March 2001, the MMG president search committee interviewed two candidates for the permanent MMG president position. However, the search committee determined that neither candidate fitted the needs of the position and extended the search process. Olsen had been evaluating her role and was not interested in being a perpetual interim. Olsen wondered if she laid low and stayed quiet, she just might end up getting the job by default.

In June 2001, Novak officially suspended the search for an MMG president. He made an announcement at the Midwestern leadership council saying that, given the strategic planning work the board was doing that would likely alter the MMG role in Midwestern, recruiting top talent would be difficult. Because of these issues, Novak announced that Olsen would remain the MMG interim president through the end of 2001 or early 2002. Olsen was surprised by this announcement and found it demeaning – it was as if they were saying they had to scrape the bottom of the barrel and had no choice but to leave her in the position. Olsen spoke to Novak before the next board meeting and discussed the tone of the message with him. The message Novak gave the board was much more positive. Overall, Olsen felt like the top leaders were "patting her on the head." She found the way Novak and other leaders were communicating about her role as strange. Novak was including her now in top leadership meetings and the executive council. But, the other Midwestern leaders talked about her participation as if she was merely sitting in on the meetings, not like she was a true participant.

Changes at the Top

Although Novak had intended to take the remaining options to restructure the MMG to the Midwestern board in July 2001, these plans were placed on hold indefinitely when the system leadership fell apart. Novak left the organization unexpectedly in July 2001. Johanson retired in October 2001. Henry also retired and several other Midwestern executives left the organization. Timothy Norton was appointed chair of the Midwestern board and interim CEO of Midwestern when Johanson retired. Midwestern initiated a national search for a new CEO. In March 2002, Norton formed the "Office of the Chief Executive Officer" with Norton as interim CEO, Mark Jepson as chief operating officer of Midwestern's hospitals and MMG, and Steven Flander as chief administrative officer supervising system support functions, including accounting, finance, human resources, and legal services. Norton decided that the hospitals and clinics would continue to be managed as a single division.

During this interim system leadership period, Norton and the remaining Midwestern leadership team focused on addressing Midwestern's financial performance. Midwestern had experienced record losses in 2001. While restructuring MMG was still on the table, the system needed to take immediate short-term actions to bolster Midwestern's bottom line. What to do with the "MMG problem" slipped off the top management team priority list while the system leaders focused on other issues of more immediate concern.

And MMG Continues to Move Along in Its Work

Despite the distractions from these new leadership transitions, system perform-ance issues, Olsen's interim status, and continued questions about MMG's role in Midwestern, the MMG management team continued to move on with its work in 2001. The group continued implementing the same-day scheduling system in MMG clinics. The Council of Evidence-Based Medicine continued by developing a formal charter and appointing MMG medical leaders to the group. The CCI program expanded its quality improvement initiatives, including a project to improve congestive heart failure services and a tobacco cessation counseling initiative. MMG established a new service endeavor to improve the physician–patient relationship, developing a service resource manual and holding an MMG conference focused on educating physicians on how to improve their commun-ications with patients, including improving courteousness, listening skills, and involving patients in their treatment decisions. The MMG management team also developed strategies to improve physician productivity by developing mentor-ing relationships for new physicians and addressing other organizational barriers that constrained physician productivity. MMG conducted a clinic benchmarking study to better understand the variance in financial and clinical performance across MMG clinics and develop strategies for implementing best practices in low-performing clinics.

MMG Exercises Its Right to Self-Determination

While the Midwestern system leaders struggled to decide about MMG's future in the system, several more clinics left MMG and others were threatening to leave. Olsen and her team decided not to sit still and be "plucked to death like a duck." They felt that before they lost all of their clinics by default, they needed to do something to establish a sense of direction for MMG in the absence of a system strategy. Olsen pulled together an MMG team in Fall 2001 to develop a vision for MMG's future. The team focused on three main scenarios. First was complete divestiture of MMG. The group determined that it would cost Midwestern about $86.4 million to close down MMG. They estimated an approximate 50 percent down-stream loss to Midwestern hospitals depending on who bought MMG. Second was the enterprise model. In this model, MMG would go to the Midwestern hospitals and ask which clinics they wanted and which they wanted to close. If a Midwestern hospital wanted to keep a clinic because it generated substantial referrals to the hospital, then the hospital would be charged with supporting the clinic's financial losses. The third option Olsen's team explored was the multi-specialty practice model. This would involve developing a hub-and-spoke clinic system, with large multispecialty clinics such as Wellview in the center and other primary care clinics as spokes that would refer to those hubs. Clinics that could not generate enough contribution to the hubs would be closed.

In addition, Olsen and her group developed a plan to address the needs of clinics in rural areas of Minnesota, referred to by the team as the "Greater Midwest strategy." In some areas, a local non-Midwestern hospital received the majority of referrals generated by these clinics. In those areas, MMG planned to negotiate joint venture relationships with the local hospitals to share support of those clinics. Olsen envisioned that her team would pursue the Greater Midwest strategy in conjunction with the restructuring model ultimately selected.

While Olsen and her management team were moving along with their MMG visioning process, Norton contacted Olsen and instructed her to develop an additional plan for MMG. He instructed Olsen to not worry about politics but to put together a plan to bring MMG to a break-even position or better in three years. He gave Olsen three weeks to complete this plan, which she did. This plan included elements that would allow MMG to hire specialists in direct competition with some of the Midwestern hospital-affiliated specialists, develop ancillary services within MMG (such as laboratory services, which previously had been directed to the hospitals), and carry out other potentially controversial strategies. But, the plan clearly demonstrated that, if allowed to engage in practices that made sense for MMG from a business perspective, MMG could clearly break even or even make a profit within three years.

In May 2002, Olsen presented the results of her team's MMG visioning process and the break-even plan to Norton, Jepson, and Flander. Jepson and Flander were uneasy with some of the elements of the break-even plan, particularly those that would allow MMG to compete with the Midwestern hospitals and affiliated specialists. Nonetheless, Norton supported the break-even plan, and Olsen presented it to the Midwestern board in July 2002. The board unanimously approved the plan.

Several issues surfaced as Olsen moved forward to implement the approved MMG break-even plan. Some Midwestern board members later said that they did not really intend to pass the plan, but felt that they could not speak up in the meeting to voice their objections. In subsequent board meetings, Olsen noted that MMG budget projections her team had calculated based on the break-even plan were not reflected in 2003 to 2005 budget figures presented to the board's finance committee. Figures presented in these meetings reflected the previous projections, showing sustained MMG losses according to budget assumptions made before the break-even plan was approved. Olsen voiced concern about this to the board's finance committee and asked that the MMG budget figures presented be changed to reflect the new MMG plan. One Midwestern executive told Olsen, "You couldn't really think that you would be allowed to move ahead with the plan." She was hearing the same old message, to shut up and stop making trouble.

Outside the boardroom, some Midwestern executives questioned whether Olsen was "playing fair" with this new break-even MMG plan. One Midwestern executive felt that Olsen was being disingenuous in "pushing" her break-even plan through with Norton. Jepson, Flander, and other members of the Midwestern executive team saw Norton as the type of person who often failed to follow chain of command. In their perspective, Olsen took unfair advantage of

Norton's management style. Since Norton asked Olsen to develop a break-even plan for the MMG and she included tactics that would reignite old conflicts with Midwestern hospitals, some Midwestern executives felt that Olsen was wrong to take Norton's approval at face value and proceed. They felt that Olsen should have discussed these strategies with them before including them in her plan for the MMG.

Olsen seemed undeterred by these criticisms. She and the MMG management team proceeded to implement the MMG break-even plan. Olsen and her team broke the plan into three phases. Phase One involved moving forward with the Greater Midwest strategy to develop joint venture relationships with non-Midwestern hospitals to share support for MMG clinics that provided them substantial referrals. This phase involved developing partnerships to share financial and management support of some MMG clinics with Midwestern hospitals and negotiating improved contracts with various payors. Phase One projects were expected to have immediate impact on improving MMG financials. Phase Two involved projects that would be implemented with impact from 2003 to 2005. Phase Two projects included the expansion of laboratory services and additional hospital–MMG clinic partnerships. Phase Three involved strategic planning to expand MMG services in promising outpatient markets. By October 2002, the MMG management team had met most of its Phase One goals and was developing detailed action plans to move into Phase Two.

Olsen Says Goodbye

In mid-October 2002, Olsen announced her plan to retire in January 2003. Olsen felt that she could say goodbye knowing that she was leaving MMG in good hands and headed in the right direction. But, she still had to decide what to tell the board chair the following day. How could she summarize the key issues that her successor would face in managing MMG? What actions should she recommend to address these issues?

NOTE

1. RVU stood for relative value unit. An RVU was a physician productivity measure calculated by using a multilevel factor system to assign a set value to each clinical service based on the complexity of the patient visit. More complex services were assigned higher RVUs than less complex services to reflect the additional work performed in providing these services.

6 CASE

Vietnam International Hospital: What Now?

Introduction

In early October 1999, Mr. Simond Lee, an Australian industrialist, was preparing to fly from Sydney to Hanoi, Vietnam, to preside over a meeting of the board of directors of Vietnam International Hospital (VIH). He, along with the hospital's managing director, Ms. Ann Mitchell, had decided to call the meeting to review VIH's options. The hospital had sustained heavy losses throughout its first year of operations and they felt it was time to reassess the situation. The need to talk things over had been given added impetus by the board's receipt of an unsolicited offer from a French firm to buy the facility, though at a considerable loss. As Lee reflected on the situation, he wanted very much to get a handle on what the viable options were for VIH. Regardless of which way the board went, it appeared the status quo was unacceptable.

History of Vietnam International Hospital

The 1990s saw tremendous changes in the economic structure of Vietnam. With the collapse of its primary sponsor, the former Soviet Union, the poverty that had gripped the country since the nation's reunification in 1975 grew even worse. The government, realizing that the country's economy had to change or collapse,

This case was written by Mark J. Kroll, Louisiana Tech University; Barbara Ross Wooldridge, University of Tampa; and Nguyen Viet Anh, Vietnam National University. It is intended as a basis for classroom discussion rather than to illustrate either effective or ineffective handling of an administrative situation. © Mark J. Kroll, Barbara Ross Wooldridge and Nguyen Viet Anh, and the North American Case Research Association. Reprinted by permission from the Case Research Journal. All rights reserved.

took its cue from so many other former satellites and allies of the USSR and began an economic liberalization program. One of the key elements of this reform effort was to open Vietnam to direct foreign investment (DFI), oftentimes structured as joint ventures (JVs) between foreign firms and Vietnamese state-owned enterprises. As a result of these JVs, many foreign nationals – known as expatriates (expats) – moved to Hanoi, Vietnam's capital.

This program of economic reform and opening was given the name "Doi Moi." Through 1997, Doi Moi resulted in tremendous growth in GDP in Vietnam, albeit from a very small base. So, while in 1995 (when the vision of VIH was first conceived) the Vietnamese economy was not that large and robust, the growth trajectory was very encouraging. Even more important, the government was promising more of the same economic efforts. It pledged more free market reforms and more moves to curb government corruption and smooth the way for private sector initiatives and direct foreign investment.

During the years of Doi Moi an extensive infrastructure had been put in place to cater to the needs of the expat community and their families. Given their unique foreign tastes and expense accounts, the expats wanted and were able to afford products and services that Hanoi had previously not provided. Everything from western-style restaurants to up-market hotels, apartments, and private clubs sprang up to fill the void and bring a little bit of home to Hanoi. Oftentimes these projects were undertaken with the expectation that the Vietnamese economy would continue to attract more expats and that while the expat market was not yet large enough to support all the projects underway, it would grow large enough to do so. VIH was intended to be the exclusive medical services provider for what was hoped would be the ever-growing expat community. The investors hoped that by entering the market early, they would establish a customer base and achieve a first-mover advantage. It was anticipated that most of these newcomers to Vietnam would, for the most part, be from modern industrialized countries, and would be accustomed to state-of-the-art medical care. Unfortunately, Vietnam's state-run medical system offered very substandard care when compared with that available in more developed countries. An example of the differences in expectations can be found in Exhibit 6/1, which relates an American expat's experience of visiting a state hospital.

The problem of substandard medical care first caught the attention of Dr. Eric Tan, a leading Australian surgeon, during a visit to Vietnam in 1995. On his return to Australia he approached Simond Lee, an acquaintance and fellow Australian of Chinese ancestry, about bringing better health care to the expat community in Vietnam. Though not one to seek notoriety, Mr. Lee was widely recognized as a multimillionaire industrialist with major investments in Australia and various Southeast Asian countries. In Vietnam, Mr. Lee's investments already included major stakes in the country's leading steel producer as well as a leading producer of finished steel sheet goods. In addition, he was exploring the possibility of building a new steel mill in Hai Phong, Vietnam, a major port city of 2 million people.

Based on their personal observations concerning the lack of modern medicine in Hanoi, and expectations of an even larger expat community there, the two men concluded there was a need for a health care facility outside the state system. Such a facility would offer the same quality of care that could be found in either Singapore

Exhibit 6/1: An Expatriate's Horror Story at a Vietnamese Hospital

In 1996, I was working in Hanoi as a consultant for a rural water project. In March, I came down with a very serious cold, which turned into the flu, then bronchitis, then finally pneumonia. I had experienced this problem before, so I was pretty sure what was wrong even without a doctor's diagnosis. I was lying around in bed trying to breathe, thinking it would be much easier just to die. My wife then insisted that I see a doctor.

She called my interpreter at the office where I worked, who decided that I needed to go visit "the best hospital in Hanoi." This turned out to be the facility reserved for government and high Communist Party officials. I could not believe it when I got there. It was something out of an old horror movie. The place was dirty and ancient looking. Everything was run-down and disorganized. After talking with someone who seemed to be a doctor or something, I was escorted down one level to a kind of underground area where I was supposed to get a chest X-ray. When I finally saw the old machine I was really scared. I was wondering what the exposure to too much or the wrong kind of X-rays would do to my life expectancy. Going back home and waiting to die didn't seem to be such a bad idea.

Anyway, I went through with the procedure, then waited in a very uncomfortable wooden chair in a dirty room. I tried to have a conversation with a Japanese man who was having heart trouble. He was really in bad shape. He told me he was the head of one of the Japanese automobile companies that was trying to set up an operation in Vietnam. No wonder he was having heart trouble! After what seemed to be an eternity, the "doctor" came back and told me that I had bronchitis and pneumonia, which I had already figured out.

Since they had no good medicine available, he asked me if I had any antibiotics at home, which I did. So I went home and took my own medicine. I cannot really say that I experienced any "value added" from the visit, and it certainly wore me out going through the ordeal. It was not that the Vietnamese staff didn't try, but rather they seemed to lack the necessary training, equipment, and money to do the job at an international standard. When I learned a year later that someone was going to try to build an international hospital in Hanoi, I thought, "It's about time!"

Source: Interview with an American expatriate living in Hanoi.

or Australia. In early 1997, Mr. Lee in concert with Dr. Tan decided to found Vietnam's first privately owned hospital in Hanoi. According to Mr. Lee, the hospital's original mission was to provide health care to the growing expat community in Hanoi and save them the worry, stress, and great expense of having to be evacuated from Vietnam in the event of serious illness. Additionally, the hospital would provide its clients with a full range of outpatient medical services. The plan called for offering a fairly limited list of medical services initially, but later expanding services to encompass the full range of procedures performed in large western hospitals.

To facilitate the authorization and launch process and cement the hospital's position in Hanoi, the Australians brought into the project Bach Mai Hospital, a major state-owned facility located in Hanoi. The initial capitalization of the hospital was US$10.5 million. Dr. Tan provided $1 million, Simond Lee provided $6.5 million, and Bach Mai Hospital provided land and a used building, valued at $3 million. This arrangement obviously left Mr. Lee in control of the project. The funds were used to renovate and equip the building, as well as provide initial operating capital. Mr. Lee and Dr. Tan envisioned VIH quickly establishing itself as the only real option for expats seeking quality health care in Hanoi.

Service Offerings

The facility that Mr. Lee and Dr. Tan envisioned would be staffed and managed by foreign doctors and administrative personnel, as well as Vietnamese professionals. The technology available was to be comparable to that found in a smaller, less-comprehensive health care facility in Australia or the United States. Additionally, while the building used would not be new, it would be completely renovated and have the "feel" of a modern, high-quality health care facility. They initially conceptualized the project as consisting of two phases. The first phase was to renovate the building provided by Bach Mai Hospital into a 56-bed facility with surgical and laboratory space, as well as an outpatient care department. The second phase, to be undertaken after the phase 1 facilities became more or less fully utilized, involved the addition of another 200 beds and facilities that would permit VIH to offer more comprehensive medical services. Exhibit 6/2 lists

Exhibit 6/2: Vietnam International Hospital's Medical and Professional Staff
(Operating Year 1998)

Expatriates
Dr. Laurie Haywood (Australian): General Practitioner (GP) and Director of Medical Services
Dr. Bruno Wauters (Belgium): GP
Dr. Ingo Neu (German): GP, Anesthesiology
Dr. Paul Camelo (Italian): GP
Dr. Kerry Griffin (Australian): GP
Dr. Lorna Mercado (Filipino): Dentistry, Orthodontia
Mr. Brad Simmons (Australian): Chief Radiographer
Ms. Lynn Stannus (Australian): Clinical Nurse Supervisor, Midwife
Ms. Sue Prest (United Kingdom): Clinical Nurse Supervisor, Midwife
Mr. James Kurtz (USA): Clinical Nurse Supervisor

Vietnamese
Dr. Nguyen Thi Tuyet Minh: GP, Cardiology
Dr. Nguyen Thi Tan Sinh: Obstetrics, Gynecology
Dr. Nguyen Thi Thuong: Obstetrics, Gynecology
Dr. Doan Thien Huong: GP, Endoscopy
Dr. Vu Manh: Surgery
Dr. Tran Thi Kim Quy: GP, Anesthesiology
Dr. Nguyen Trung Ha: Pediatrics
Dr. Bui Thu Oanh: General Dentistry
Dr. Bui Huu Quang: Opthalmology and Optometry
Dr. Nguyen Thi Kim Loan: Pathology
Dr. Vu Quang Huy: Pathology
Mr. Nguyen Ngoc Thanh: Pharmacy
Ms. Thanh Huong: Pharmacy

Note: The observant reader will see that many of the staff at VIH have the same last name of "Nguyen." However, none of them is related. Very large numbers of Vietnamese have Nguyen as part of their names.
Source: Internal documents of Vietnam International Hospital.

the names and nationalities of the initial professional staff. The available hospital facilities under phase 1 and the medical services initially offered by the hospital are shown in Exhibit 6/3.

The Medical Alternatives Available in Hanoi

As VIH was intended to be the only medical facility of its kind in Vietnam, it was thought that it would essentially have no direct competitors in its market. The only other hospitals in Vietnam were owned by the government and were part of the state-sponsored health care system. Physicians at VIH and in the state system recognized that both the quality of care provided by the state hospitals

Exhibit 6/3: Facilities and Services Offered at Vietnam International Hospital

Facilities
- 24-Hour Comprehensive Emergency Care Center
- Outpatient Surgery Suite
- One Fully Equipped Operating Theater
- X-Ray Room and Ultrasound Room
- On-Site Laboratory and Blood Bank
- Pharmacy
- Four General Outpatient Examination Rooms
- Two Obstetrics/Gynecology Outpatient Examination Rooms
- Two Birthing Suites
- One Fully Equipped Dental Clinic
- One Fully Equipped Eye Examination Clinic
- One Pediatric Outpatient Examination Room
- One ECG Stress Test Room
- 56 Inpatient Beds of Various Types (single room, twin shared room, VIP, pediatric, maternity, intensive care, intermediate care)

Services Offered
- Primary and Emergency Medical Care
- Pharmacy
- Radiology
- Pathology
- Internal Medicine
- Elective and Emergency Surgery (General Surgery; Orthopedics; Ear, Nose, and Throat; Neurosurgery; Pediatric Surgery; Urology)
- Dental and Orthodontic Care
- Psychology and Counseling
- Ophthalmology and Optometry
- Family Health Care (Obstetrics and Gynecology, Pediatrics)
- Critical Care
- Evacuation and Repatriation Services
- Referral Network to Specialized Clinics in Thailand and Singapore

Source: Vietnam International Hospital brochure.

and the breadth of services and procedures available were perceived by the expat community to be so inferior to those available in their home countries as to not be considered as viable sources of medical care.

Rather, VIH administrators saw their major competition in the form of a "substitute good," that being medical evacuation to Singapore, Australia, or the United States for quality medical care. The owners and managers of VIH believed their most important marketing task was to convince their target market, expat patients, as well as their medical insurance providers, that VIH represented a high-quality, much less expensive and stressful alternative to medical evacuation. With medical evacuation ranging in cost from $5,000 to $6,000 for those patients who could sit upright to $10,000 to $15,000 for those who had to be transported on a gurney, the economics seemed quite attractive.

The leading provider of evacuation services both around the world and in Vietnam was AEA International SOS. AEA operated primary care clinics throughout the world, but its major service was medical evacuation. AEA had contracts with over 800 health care insurors worldwide. In Hanoi, AEA operated a small clinic staffed by two expat physicians who could handle minor out-patient cases. Cases requiring anything more than basic care were evacuated to Singapore or to the patient's home country if the patient's policy permitted. Although the cost of such evacuation was quite high, many expats living in Hanoi had medical evacuation coverage.

In addition, there were two other very small outpatient clinics located in Hanoi. They were staffed by expat physicians and marketed themselves to the expat community. Though fairly complete in terms of on-site facilities, offering limited in-house lab work and basic radiology services, neither was in a position to offer anything more than nonacute care.

Initially, international health insurance companies did not recognize VIH as a legitimate health care alternative for their expat clients. However, as the first full year of operation progressed, the compelling economics of paying for treatment at VIH versus medical evacuation began to win over converts. Many insurors had annually negotiated contracts with AEA and could not make a change until that contract expired.

The Economy Sours and Expatriates Go Home

The opening of the economy to DFI-financial projects brought with it the prospect of Vietnam becoming home to expatriate business persons, managers, and technical personnel. Unfortunately, for Vietnam as well as all of Southeast Asia, the party that began after the Soviet Union's collapse came to an end in the summer of 1997. That summer Thailand's monetary unit, the baht, came under intense pressure from international money speculators. The perception that the Thai currency was grossly overvalued, given the economic policies of the Thai government, soon became the reality as it plummeted in value versus the US dollar. In short order, the currencies of neighboring countries such as Malaysia and Indonesia also came under pressure and a severe economic downturn quickly followed. Vietnam's economy fell victim to the same economic shocks. Proposed joint ventures were canceled and DFI started to dry up.

At the same time, at least to many in the foreign business community, the feeling began to take root that the Vietnamese government's commitment to real economic liberalization was more imagined than real. For many foreign firms, the complexity and costs of securing government approval for new ventures remained burdensome and often excessively complex and corrupt. These difficulties led to higher start-up and operating costs than many foreign firms had first imagined, and made profitability, especially during a region-wide recession, elusive. As a consequence, while in 1997 it was estimated there were close to 9,000 expats at work in Hanoi, by 1999 that number had been cut in half. Given that a key part of VIH's original mission was to cater to the medical needs of the Hanoi expat community, when that community stopped growing and started shrinking, it became obvious VIH was in serious trouble.

By the end of 1998 the hospital had lost money both on a cash flow basis and a net income basis every month it had been open. As demonstrated by the financial data presented in Exhibit 6/4, the good news was that it appeared VIH was getting closer to at least having a positive "Earnings Before Depreciation, Amortization, Interest, and Taxes" (EBDAIT) figure. However, it was a long way from profitability on a traditional "net income" basis. This was owing to the very high depreciation charges incurred as a result of the extremely capital intensive nature of hospital operations.

Given the continuous losses, the original investors, especially Mr. Lee, were compelled to continue to supply funds to VIH in order to keep it afloat; however, instead of making contributions in the form of new equity investments, the investors loaned the hospital additional funds. The hospital also used supplier credit to cover its shortfalls in between infusions from the investors.

VIH's Managed Care Plan

In the first quarter of 1998 the hospital's management and board decided to bring in a consultant who could take a look at VIH's approach to its market and offer some suggestions for more effectively positioning the facility as the Southeast Asian economy soured. The board felt it was critical to broaden the hospital's base beyond the expat community and start attracting upper-income Vietnamese.

After examining the current customer base of the hospital, the potential for expanding that customer base, and looking into the issue of availability of health care insurance to cover private care in Vietnam, the consultant came to two conclusions. First, while there was talk of private European health insurance firms entering the Vietnamese market, the products these firms were considering would be slow in coming and very expensive by Vietnamese standards. Second, Vietnamese consumers did not have a history of being willing to spend heavily for health care. When one very wealthy Hanoi native was approached by a VIH representative with regard to using VIH, he asked about the daily room rate. When informed it was at that time $400 per day, the VIH representative reported

Exhibit 6/4: Vietnam International Hospital – Financial Data for 1998 (in US dollars)

	Jan.	Feb.	March	Apr.	May	June
Income Statement Items						
Revenue						
Inpatient Revenue	51,285	49,786	47,160	59,995	42,345	32,598
Discount on Inpatient	0	(213)	(635)	(7,194)	(14,858)	2,374
Outpatient Revenue	38,841	51,666	62,449	80,774	83,037	71,744
Discount on Outpatient	0	(1,908)	(5,785)	(7,175)	(6,858)	0
MCP Revenue	0	0	0	0	0	0
Total Revenue	90,126	99,331	103,189	126,400	103,666	106,716
Expenses						
Salaries & Wages	(177,690)	(177,247)	(156,858)	(156,478)	(164,060)	(167,713)
Other Operating Expenses	(49,503)	(80,924)	(76,934)	(68,580)	(129,910)	(112,623)
EBDAIT	(137,067)	(158,840)	(130,603)	(98,658)	(190,304)	(173,620)
Depreciation Expenses	(206,633)	(204,756)	(203,038)	(201,571)	(200,039)	(198,285)
EBIT	(343,700)	(363,596)	(333,641)	(300,229)	(390,343)	(371,905)
Balance Sheet Items						
Current Assets	340,147	430,453	343,292	478,504	468,551	551,084
Fixed Assets	12,397,995	12,285,369	12,182,290	12,094,287	12,002,317	11,897,109
Total Assets	12,738,142	12,715,822	12,525,582	12,572,791	12,470,868	12,448,193
Current Liabilities	665,667	701,221	749,823	725,133	921,560	990,913
Noncurrent Liabilities	0	200,000	200,000	480,000	480,000	679,985
Total Liabilities	665,667	901,221	949,823	1,205,133	1,401,560	1,670,898
Equity	12,072,475	11,814,601	11,575,759	11,367,658	11,069,308	10,777,295
Total Liabilities & Equity	12,738,142	12,715,822	12,525,582	12,572,791	12,470,868	12,448,192

	July	Aug.	Sep.	Oct.	Nov.	Dec.
Income Statement Items						
Revenue						
Inpatient Revenue	53,849	44,341	53,543	55,084	80,647	59,778
Discount on Inpatient	(7,529)	(7,921)	(12,464)	(13,649)	(20,283)	(15,840)
Outpatient Revenue	74,291	73,092	66,184	80,374	100,557	79,129
Discount on Outpatient	(7,429)	(7,561)	(7,835)	(5,878)	(9,151)	(8,836)
MCP Revenue	0	0	0	453	755	1,095
Total Revenue	113,182	101,951	99,428	116,384	152,525	115,326
Expenses						
Salaries & Wages	(180,091)	(118,914)	(113,408)	(92,250)	(84,663)	(107,318)
Other Operating Expenses	(40,370)	(65,681)	(72,273)	(27,807)	(123,952)	(46,583)
EBDAIT	(107,279)	(82,644)	(86,253)	(3,673)	(56,090)	(38,575)
Depreciation Expenses	(195,929)	(196,154)	(194,353)	(192,853)	(191,216)	(189,798)
EBIT	(303,208)	(278,798)	(280,606)	(196,526)	(247,306)	(228,373)
Balance Sheet Items						
Current Assets	451,013	503,487	446,540	463,486	444,705	518,209
Fixed Assets	11,755,710	11,769,250	11,661,178	11,571,176	11,472,990	11,387,880
Total Assets	12,206,723	12,272,737	12,107,718	12,034,662	11,917,695	11,906,089
Current Liabilities	819,043	844,728	870,499	904,999	849,433	682,947
Noncurrent Liabilities	830,000	980,000	980,000	980,000	1,080,000	1,380,000
Total Liabilities	1,649,043	1,824,728	1,850,499	1,884,999	1,929,433	2,062,947
Equity	10,557,680	10,448,010	10,257,219	10,149,662	9,988,261	9,843,142
Total Liabilities & Equity	12,206,724	12,272,737	12,107,718	12,034,661	11,917,695	11,906,089

Source: Financial statements for Vietnam International Hospital.

his response was that "for that much, in a state hospital, he could hire 50 nurses to dance around his bed all day. They probably would not be qualified to treat him, but would be very entertaining." In light of these realities, the consultant recommended that VIH launch its own managed care program that would offer, by western standards, modest amounts of coverage for relatively modest premiums. After undertaking a limited research effort that attempted to explore consumer preferences, VIH's consultant developed the VIH Managed Care Plan (MCP).

In July 1998, Vietnam International Hospital's management introduced the MCP program, a set of four plans it hoped would help build a steady patient flow. Although the program was billed as "managed care," in effect what the hospital offered was a set of fairly traditional fixed-amount "hospitalization" or "major medical" policies. However, unlike such policies sold in the West, the policies were only valid when used at VIH. The MCP consisted of four grades of coverage:

1. *Red Star Plan:* provided total coverage amounting to no more than $5,000 per year. Items included in this plan were:
   - Hospital accommodations, meals, and admission fees;
   - Accident and emergency care on either an inpatient or outpatient basis;
   - All nursing, medical, surgical, and anesthesia fees;
   - Diagnostic and medical imaging procedures;
   - Surgical facility fees; and
   - Drugs and surgical items used during a hospital stay.
   The plan made no provision for nonemergency outpatient care, routine gynecological visits, or annual check-ups. In addition, the plan did not cover any treatment beyond the competence and scope of VIH, medical evacuation costs, or hospital stays related to maternity; nor was it available to those 65 years of age and older. Cost: $300 per person, per year.
2. *Silver Star Plan:* provided essentially the same benefits and exclusions as the Red Star Plan, but also provided one complete annual check-up. Cost: $400 per person, per year.
3. *Gold Star Plan:* provided the same benefits and exclusions as the Red Star Plan up to an annual maximum of $6,000 per year. It also provided unlimited outpatient clinical visits, including eye and dental care. Cost: $650 per person, per year.
4. *Diamond Star Plan:* provided the same benefits and exclusions as the Gold Star Plan up to an annual maximum of $7,000 per year. In addition, it provided for one complete annual check-up. Cost: $720 per person, per year.

For couples with children, a 25 percent discount was offered on the first child, and a 50 percent discount was provided for additional children.

After some analysis, the consultant who had developed the plans observed, given the fact the hospital was operating so far below capacity, the key to the MCP program was that, on average, for every dollar of services provided, only about 20 cents represented true marginal or additional out-of-pocket costs for the hospital. Given that so much of VIH's costs of providing care were fixed, and with the vast majority of costs required to provide the services billed through MCP likely to be incurred anyway, care provided through the MCP program would represent little added burden to the hospital.

VIH's Search for a New Patient Base

As a result of the collapse of the expat market and the string of monthly losses, in October 1998 VIH's management decided to take two major steps. First, the hospital cut its staff from 230 employees to 120 and closed off the upper floor of the two-story facility. This move reduced its bed count from 56 beds to about 10. Second, the decision was made to undertake a marketing effort designed to turn the situation around. Ms. Thy Anh was hired as marketing director.

Marketing Comes to VIH

Thy Anh previously worked in the marketing department for a major international soft drink company. She immediately set about the task of repositioning the hospital as one not only for expats but also for high-income Vietnamese families seeking world-class medical care. She built a marketing staff that consisted of four sales representatives in addition to herself and a secretary. Her analysis of the market led her to the following conclusions:

- Among the population of Hanoi (and all of Vietnam for that matter) there was a latent preference for all things not Vietnamese. The general perception was that products manufactured outside the country were inherently better than those built within the country. For example, the label on cans of Raid insect spray announced that it is the leading brand in the USA. Honda motorcycles assembled outside of Vietnam were more coveted and sold for higher prices than Honda motorcycles built in Vietnam. The same kind of latent belief probably existed that western health care was superior to that available in the state hospitals.
- The younger generation of professional Vietnamese couples was well aware of the inadequacies of the state-run health care system, and wanted access to better quality care for themselves and their children. Although the hospital's previous marketing focused almost exclusively on expats, almost half of inpatient volume was from Vietnamese. Exhibit 6/5 provides a census of inpatient admissions by nationality and sex.
- Although the state hospitals were at least ostensibly free, patients were expected to pay small bribes and gratuities to obtain treatment. Based on Ms. Anh's estimates, VIH's charges were at least ten times greater than what it would cost a Vietnamese patient to go to a state hospital and pay the gratuities necessary to ensure that they received the best care the state-owned hospital could provide. (A sample of VIH's prices can be seen in Exhibit 6/6.) Other than the state-owned hospitals, there was no other facility in Hanoi that provided the comprehensive services offered by VIH.
- There were two very damaging rumors circulating in the marketplace. One was that, in light of the recent layoffs, VIH was about to close its doors. The second rumor circulating was that VIH was not interested in treating Vietnamese.

Exhibit 6/5: Inpatient Report by Nationality and Gender (Operating Year 1998)

Nationality	Total	Percent	Male	% Male	Female	% Female
Australian	13	4	7	4	6	3
British	14	4	6	4	8	4
Canadian	8	2	1	1	7	4
Chinese	8	2	6	4	2	1
Filipino	7	2	5	3	2	1
French	39	11	23	14	16	8
German	8	2	6	4	2	1
Indian	10	3	4	2	6	3
Japanese	19	5	12	7	7	4
Korean	14	4	8	5	6	3
US	9	2	7	4	2	1
Vietnamese	157	43	61	36	96	49
Other	59	16	24	14	35	18
Totals	365	100	170	47	195	53

Source: Vietnam International Hospital internal report.

Exhibit 6/6: Schedule of Prices

	Price (US$)	Notes
Medical Consultation		
• w/General Practitioner	35*	→ Normal/Short (1/2 hour)
or Pediatrician or	60*	→ Long (1 hour)
Ophthalmologist/	10*	→ Follow-up
Optometrist		
• w/Dentist-Orthodontist	30*	→ Short (Oral Examination)
	50*	→ Long (Oral Examination)
• w/Obstetrician-Gynecologist	50*	→ Ante/Post-Natal Initial
	20*	→ Obstetric Follow-up
	40*	→ Gynecology Initial
	10*	→ Gynecology Follow-up (Charges vary on other procedures)
• w/Senior Consultants	60*	→ Initial
(inpatient's acceptance)	35*	→ Follow-up
Accident and Emergency		
• Within the city	60*	→ Doctor's attendance at the hospital
	100*	→ Doctor call-out with ambulance to patient's place
• Outside the city	From 150*	→ Depending on certain cases
Elective/Emergency Surgery		
• Procedures (Band A to Band X)	From 130*	Each costs individually on the basis of the complexity involved, utilizing the Australian Hospital Procedural Bands and Australian Hospital Operation Levels
• Operations (Level A to Level X)	From 300*	

	Price (US$)	Notes
Hospital Accommodation		
• For a patient (including meals, laundry, dressing, standard medical care by doctors and nurses; excluding medications, tests, blood transfusion, communication costs . . .)	**50*** **250** per night **150*** per night	→ Day stay (less than 8 hours) → Single room → Shared room/maternity room/pediatric room
• For a visitor of patient (excluding meals)	**800** per night **400** per night **30*** per night **Free**	→ Intensive Care Unit → Intermediate Care Unit → Meals and accommodation for one person accompanying under-12-year-old patient are offered free of charge
Medical Imaging		
• X-ray & Ultrasound (On-site)	**20** to **80**	→ Depending on types
• CT Scan	**120**	
• MRI	**350**	
Pathology		
• Onsite (depending on types)	**5** to **180***	→ Our laboratory subscribes to the Australian Quality Assurance Programme managed by the National Association of Testing Authorities (NATA)
• Sending overseas – Extra charge	**50**	→ Courier fee
Immunizations		
• Vaccines (Anti-Rabies, BCG, Chickenpox, Hepatitis A/B, Japanese Encephalitis B, MMR, Meningococcus A/C, Pneumococcus, Polio, Tetanus, Typhoid . . .)	**0.78** to **80*** **10*** to **355***	→ Vaccine charge (depending on types) → Injection charge (w/doctor's check-up) → Scheduled immunizations package for baby up to 12-months old
Health Checks		
• Basic Health Check (includes a GP Consultation, Chest X-ray, Urine Labstick, Full Blood Count)	**80***	Other health check package can be tailored for specific requirements (adoption, marriage, pre-employment, etc.)
Maternity Package		

• Full-term Maternity Package
  For non-Vietnamese
  For Vietnamese
	
	 2,000 or **2,500**
	 1,500 or **1,900**
		→ Including antenatal visits, tests, ultrasound + costs for normal delivery/Cesarean section + hospital stay + antenatal class + post-natal check-up for mother and baby

• Delivery Package
  For non-Vietnamese
  For Vietnamese
	
	 900 or **1,700**
	 550 or **1,000**
		→ Including one antenatal visit, tests, ultrasound + costs for normal delivery/Cesarean section + hospital stay

Medical Membership		
• The Managed Care Package (MCP)	**300** to **750**	Depending on options selected (Red Star/Silver Star/Gold Star or Diamond Star), financial cap and policies attached

Note: * means 30 percent discount available for all Vietnamese.

Source: Vietnam International Hospital internal document.

• Although the top managers and professionals employed by the Vietnamese government or working for state-owned enterprises might have wanted to access VIH, and were able to afford the kind of health care VIH provided, they were unable to do so. This was owing to the adverse political consequences of word getting out that they preferred the foreign facility to a state facility.

These facts led Ms. Anh and the VIH management to conclude that they had three important marketing tasks. First, they had to dispel the damaging rumors about the hospital. Second, they had to launch some form of program aimed at employers of both expats and Vietnamese that would generate traffic. Third, they had to create the perception of lower prices at VIH.

Her response to the first two challenges was the introduction of a "Priority Service Agreement" (PSA) for employers. Under the terms of the agreement, expat employees of a firm which adopted the PSA got a 5 percent discount on all medical care costs incurred at VIH, while Vietnamese nationals got a 30 percent discount off list prices. Under the plan the hospital would bill the employer for all costs incurred by its employees, and it was the responsibility of the employer to collect from their employees. In effect, the employer became the guarantor of all payments due from its employees. After six months of marketing the PSA program only nine small firms had joined, representing about 250 employees.

To respond to the pricing issue, Ms. Anh proposed that the hospital lower its prices across the board. While, for accounting and billing software reasons, this recommendation was not fully implemented, she did get the price of a private room lowered from $400 to $250 and a semiprivate room cut from $250 to $150.

Armed with these new products and prices, Ms. Anh and her team of four sales representatives aggressively pursued the market. After about six months of effort, traffic through the hospital was increasing, but profitability remained elusive. Exhibits 6/7 and 6/8 provide outpatient and inpatient data for all of 1998 and the first ten months of 1999. Exhibit 6/8 provides pharmacy department volume figures for the same period. Exhibit 6/9 provides case activity data for the Accident and Emergency Clinic, Laboratory, and Radiology Department. Although not being able to achieve profitability was worrisome for Ms. Anh, more disappointing was the failure to generate any significant volume with either the PSA or MCP products. In early 1999, after about six months on the job, Ms. Anh announced her departure.

A New Marketing Manager with New Ideas

With Ms. Anh's departure, VIH's management turned to Mr. Nguyen Viet Anh (no relation to Thy Anh), who had previously worked in a number of marketing positions, though outside of health care. He too came to the conclusion that VIH would have to attract more Vietnamese nationals – and did not believe that the products available would do it. Additionally, he felt there was the possibility of building a referral network in the city that could funnel significant numbers of patients, both Vietnamese and expats, to VIH. He made the following observations:

Exhibit 6/7: Outpatient Monthly Volumes

1998 Outpatient Monthly Volume Report

Month	General Practice	Dental	Pediatric	Obs. & Gyn.	Psych.	Optometry	Ear, Nose, & Throat	Monthly Total
Jan.	242	79	63	99	4	17	3	507
Feb.	273	74	67	117	6	11	6	554
Mar.	312	81	88	149	11	32	21	694
Apr.	407	107	117	245	3	31	19	929
May	485	98	113	178	11	33	21	939
Jun.	434	110	70	169	0	30	31	844
Jul.	386	103	99	222	0	32	14	856
Aug.	369	66	96	189	0	37	21	778
Sep.	399	62	157	180	1	35	5	839
Oct.	487	73	172	250	25	41	16	1,064
Nov.	382	82	171	226	9	34	33	937
Dec.	398	83	141	208	16	26	14	886
Total	**4,574**	**1,018**	**1,354**	**2,232**	**86**	**359**	**204**	**9,827**

1999 Outpatient Monthly Volume Report

Month	General Practice	Dental	Pediatric	Obs. & Gyn.	Psych.	Optometry	Ear, Nose, & Throat	Monthly Total
Jan.	432	89	153	233	18	30	19	974
Feb.	316	86	105	181	7	17	7	719
Mar.	407	119	155	179	12	31	9	912
Apr.	523	135	179	197	16	38	28	1,116
May	449	93	161	291	12	28	33	1,067
Jun.	439	91	164	271	20	35	34	1,054
Jul.	461	90	163	341	32	38	17	1,142
Aug.	462	79	167	301	31	83	27	1,150
Sep.	581	133	225	348	35	74	25	1,421
Oct.	426	73	197	295	18	42	12	1,063
Total	**4,496**	**988**	**1,669**	**2,637**	**201**	**416**	**211**	**10,618**

Source: Vietnam International Hospital internal document.

- VIH needed to do a better job of getting the word out to foreign travelers, new expat arrivals, and local Vietnamese about the hospital.
- The majority of expats continued to use AEA or one of the two clinics targeted at expats. VIH was going to have to do a better job of providing medical evacuation services to reassure expats that, if the need arose, they would be evacuated to a more comprehensive facility.
- The products thus far developed by VIH (MCP and PSA) simply were not attractive to potential Vietnamese patients.

Exhibit 6/8: Inpatient and Pharmacy Report

Inpatient Monthly Report

1998 Night Occupancy

Month	General Ward	High-Dependency Unit	Maternity	Pediatric	Monthly Total
Jan.	26	22	36	2	86
Feb.	41	31	13	7	92
Mar.	111	7	7	9	134
Apr.	135	6	18	9	168
May	56	10	14	7	87
Jun.	87	5	22	4	118
Jul.	145	5	12	19	181
Aug.	81	0	37	66	184
Sep.	100	0	18	38	156
Oct.	124	24	18	15	181
Nov.	147	23	15	23	208
Dec.	87	12	12	26	137
Total	**1,140**	**145**	**222**	**225**	**1,732**

1999 Night Occupancy

Month	General Ward	High-Dependency Unit	Maternity	Pediatric	Monthly Total
Jan.	89	8	33	14	144
Feb.	85	11	20	60	176
Mar.	119	25	16	47	207
Apr.	103	9	26	67	205
May	100	1	34	14	149
Jun.	126	6	16	42	190
Jul.	80	10	28	18	136
Aug.	126	2	36	27	191
Sep.	116	7	23	26	172
Oct.	107	1	28	17	153
Total	**1,051**	**80**	**260**	**332**	**1,723**

Pharmacy Monthly Volume Report

1998

Month	Outpatient Script	Inpatient Script	Staff Script	Discharged Script	Monthly Total
Jan.	138	37	5	7	187
Feb.	525	126	50	13	714
Mar.	654	69	28	28	779
Apr.	688	169	54	49	960
May	670	118	40	50	878
Jun.	634	108	52	34	828
Jul.	762	1	65	69	897
Aug.	702	0	35	52	789
Sep.	783	0	19	64	866
Oct.	814	2	28	44	888
Nov.	896	3	22	63	984
Dec.	959	4	22	37	1,022
Total	**8,225**	**637**	**420**	**510**	**9,792**

1999

Month	Outpatient Script	Inpatient Script	Staff Script	Discharged Script	Monthly Total
Jan.	845	3	22	75	945
Feb.	653	2	39	80	774
Mar.	944	0	42	73	1,059
Apr.	908	0	66	82	1,056
May	1,033	0	192	95	1,320
Jun.	1,251	0	216	114	1,581
Jul.	996	0	89	88	1,173
Aug.	1,260	0	54	85	1,399
Sep.	1,181	1	52	103	1,337
Oct.	1,073	1	61	79	1,214
Total	**10,144**	**7**	**833**	**874**	**11,858**

Source: Vietnam International Hospital internal document.

Exhibit 6/9: Accident and Emergency, Laboratory, and Radiology Volumes

Accident & Emergency Monthly Volume Report (Cases Handled)			Laboratory Monthly Volume Report (Tests Run)	
Month	1998	1999	1998	1999
Jan.	49	126	700	1,515
Feb.	67	125	791	1,485
Mar.	115	137	1,187	1,960
Apr.	106	200	1,200	1,742
May	143	164	1,138	1,427
Jun.	135	169	903	1,652
Jul.	152	216	863	1,363
Aug.	160	219	1,130	1,527
Sep.	145	219	1,339	1,654
Oct.	147	140	2,249	1,243
Nov.	163		2,362	
Dec.	114		1,336	
Total	1,496	1,715	15,198	15,568

Radiology Monthly Volume Report (Procedure and Patient Counts)

Month	1998			1999		
	X-ray	Ultrasound	Patients	X-ray	Ultrasound	Patients
Jan.	69	17	77	169	97	234
Feb.	49	17	60	117	95	179
Mar.	127	49	148	206	82	254
Apr.	100	88	168	161	90	213
May	136	79	191	130	108	199
Jun.	108	75	166	144	124	234
Jul.	83	72	137	140	88	198
Aug.	94	77	153	155	111	228
Sep.	125	73	181	130	106	202
Oct.	174	104	252	154	91	214
Nov.	136	108	217			
Dec.	125	105	190			
Total	1,326	864	1,940	1,506	992	2,155

Source: Vietnam International Hospital internal document.

In response to these problems Mr. Nguyen undertook three separate initiatives. Each initiative was intended to attract a separate segment of the market to the hospital.

First, to build traffic from travelers and recent arrivals to Vietnam, Mr. Nguyen and his sales team launched a referral system for local hotels, mini-hotels, travel companies, and local private Vietnamese clinics. Each of these organizations contacted was told that for each referral they made to the hospital, they would receive a 5 percent referral fee on all outpatient billings generated by the referral, and a flat $25 referral fee for each inpatient they referred to the hospital. With literally hundreds of hotels, clinics, and travel companies operating around Hanoi, Mr. Nguyen anticipated considerable volume might be generated. He also thought referrals might be obtained from hotels and clients located in Hai Phong. Hai Phong, the north's major port city, was located about 60 miles east of Hanoi and had no medical facility comparable with VIH. Quite a number of light manufacturing facilities had opened outside Hai Phong as well as along the highway between Hai Phong and Hanoi in recent years.

His second step was to more aggressively go after the existing expat market. To do this he wanted to position VIH as a clear alternative to AEA in terms of evacuation services. Although the hospital had previously advertised itself as a provider of evacuation services, the focus had always been on treating patients in the hospital rather than evacuating them. To instill greater confidence in expats that they would be evacuated if needed, he felt he had to build a credible evacuation service. However, the hospital's management and board were slow to completely embrace the need for such an effort. Board members expressed anxieties about VIH becoming so much of an evacuation service that its hospital facilities would be too often bypassed.

Third, to build the Vietnamese traffic through the hospital, he launched a new minor-medical health insurance product with which he could approach private employers and individual Hanoi residents to get them to at least consider using VIH. He called the new product "Health Care Membership 21," or "HC 21" for short. It was only available to Vietnamese nationals. The sole purpose of HC 21 was to make increasing numbers of Vietnamese patients more comfortable with using the facility and, thereby, conditioned to expecting a higher standard of care than that available at Vietnamese state-run facilities. HC 21 essentially offered unlimited access to general practice consultations as well as eye and dental check-ups for US$55 per year, per person. It also provided a 35 percent discount for all additional services provided by the hospital. After six months of marketing HC 21, Mr. Nguyen and his staff had managed to sell 171 memberships, over half of which were for children.

In addition to these three steps, he decided, as had Ms. Anh, that VIH had to address the cost issue. He concluded, and was able to convince the board, that VIH's prices were simply out of line with the market it sought to serve, especially if they were going after the Vietnamese market. Rather than going through the hospital's accounting software and pricing codes and making individual adjustments, it was decided to simply state prices in Australian dollars rather than US dollars. As the Australian dollar was worth about 65 percent of the US dollar, by making this change, VIH effectively discounted all of its services by 35 percent without having to change its software and pricing codes.

With a full complement of different programs to promote, along with the medical services themselves, the VIH marketing team again mounted a sales effort. In the course of the next nine months, Mr. Nguyen and his staff contacted 2,500 businesses and organizations in an attempt to sell MCPs, PSAs, and HC

Exhibit 6/10: MCP and HC 21 Sales Volumes

MCP Sales Volume

	Quarter 4/98	Quarter 1/99	Quarter 2/99	Quarter 3/99
Diamond	2	1	1	2
Gold	13	5	3	6
Silver	2	9	5	1
Red	15	13	12	19
Total	32	28	21	28

HC 21 Sales Volume

	July '99	August '99	September '99
HC 21	64	63	49

In the first three months of 1999 51 percent of total sales were for children (less than 12 years old). In October and November 1999, no effort was made to sell HC 21 policies.

Source: Vietnam International Hospital internal document.

21s, as well as annual check-ups, vaccination packages, and maternity packages. In addition, the team contacted over 2,000 individuals, both upper-income Vietnamese and expats. Upper-income Vietnamese were identified through a credit card holder list purchased from the local issuing bank, because only the wealthy in Vietnam held credit cards. To identify newly arriving expats, a contact was made with the Vietnamese customs service. This fed the hospital's marketing staff the names and local addresses of all arrivals at the airport who came in with visas for six months or longer.

Mr. Nguyen continued his predecessor's efforts and sold the various MCP packages. The results of these efforts are presented in Exhibit 6/10. The MCP program as of mid-1999 had not been deemed a significant success. In October 1999, VIH discontinued the MCP program. Mr. Nguyen believed the board took this action for the following reasons. First, the plan generated very small numbers and never fulfilled management's or the board's aspirations. Given the small numbers, they probably felt inclined to simply forget the whole thing. Second, a couple of relatively expensive cases (expensive in terms of billable services) occurred, which frightened the board in terms of what the hospital's potential liability might be (in terms of revenues forgone) when assuming the worst. As a result of these large expenses, the board became frightened by the potential liability of the MCP program, especially if it were to expand. Mr. Nguyen concluded they were mistaken because, as he observed, the MCP program appeared to be profitable when the total costs of providing the services were estimated, and especially when only out-of-pocket costs were considered. Exhibit 6/11 provides an analysis of the revenues and costs associated with the MCP program from its inception.

On the positive side, however, by mid-1999 VIH was operating tantalizingly close to cash flow break even and was just about able to cover all of its direct costs of operations (see Exhibit 6/12 for selected financial data for January to May, 1999).

Exhibit 6/11: MCP Program Performance Summary

Total MCP premiums paid-in from program inception to termination:	US$43,380
Revenues from MCP patients for services not covered by the MCP from inception to termination:	US$10,422
Total Revenues Generated by MCP	**US$53,802**

Revenues forgone (based on ordinary charges) by providing care under the MCP by type:	
Accidents (1 case)	US$ 2,314
Cesarean sections (2 cases)	US$ 1,561
Hospitalizations – Pediatric (13 cases)	US$ 9,597
Hospitalizations – Adult (2 cases)	US$ 965
Total Revenues Forgone	**US$14,437**

Estimated marginal (variable) costs associated with providing MCP covered care ($14,437 × 20%):	US$ 2,887.40*

*It will be recalled from earlier in the case that, given most of VIH's costs are fixed and the facility is underutilized, the actual marginal or out-of-pocket costs of additional services were estimated to be only about 20 percent of such revenues.

Source: Various Vietnam International Hospital internal documents.

Exhibit 6/12: Vietnam International Hospital Financial Data (January to May, 1999 in US dollars)

	January	February	March	April	May
Income Statement Items					
Revenue					
Inpatient Revenue (before discount)	62,082	53,406	60,207	55,251	42,826
Outpatient Revenue (before discount)	78,818	69,565	93,731	89,548	79,417
MCP Revenue	1,478	1,890	1,947	2,328	2,461
Total Discount	(15,548)	(9,271)	(6,552)	(12,700)	(13,071)
Total Revenue	126,830	115,590	149,333	134,427	111,633
Expenses					
Salaries and Wages	(74,508)	(78,105)	(76,388)	(79,926)	(78,275)
Other Operating Expenses	(62,794)	(56,909)	(80,662)	(84,819)	(56,176)
EBDAIT	(10,472)	(19,505)	(7,717)	(30,318)	(22,818)
Depreciation Expenses	(188,231)	(186,596)	(184,618)	(183,013)	(181,370)
EBIT	(198,703)	(206,101)	(192,335)	(213,331)	(204,188)
Balance Sheet Items					
Current Assets	593,234	507,762	640,648	653,454	609,626
Fixed Assets	11,293,854	11,195,754	11,077,083	10,980,768	10,882,215
Total Assets	11,887,088	11,703,516	11,717,731	11,634,222	11,491,841
Current Liabilities	779,975	723,356	651,602	705,566	693,483
Noncurrent Liabilities	1,380,000	1,380,000	1,580,000	1,580,000	1,580,000
Total Liabilities	2,159,975	2,103,356	2,231,602	2,285,566	2,273,483
Equity	9,727,113	9,600,159	9,486,128	9,348,656	9,218,357
Total Liabilities & Equity	11,887,088	11,703,515	11,717,731	11,634,222	11,491,841

Source: Vietnam International Hospital financial statements.

Choices

Mr. Lee and the board had some difficult choices to make in October 1999. Mr. Lee, after months of lending money to the hospital, had decided he had put all he could afford into the venture and was going to discontinue the loans. Given its financial history, it was unlikely that VIH was going to be able to borrow from anyone else. On the positive side, the hospital was almost in a position to avoid the need for additional outside borrowing, as its revenues were nearly sufficient to cover all out-of-pocket costs.

Very recently, however, Mr. Lee and the other owners were presented with a way out, albeit not without considerable pain. A French medical services firm had approached them about the possibility of taking the hospital off their hands. The French firm was prepared to pay $5.6 million to the owners for their 70 percent of the hospital, leaving Bach Mai Hospital with its 30 percent stake still intact. In addition, the French firm required that Mr. Lee forgive the loans he had made to the hospital. The investors and board had to now decide whether the situation could be salvaged, or whether it was time to take their medicine and move on.

7 CASE

Indian Health Service: Creating a Climate for Change

"As an enrolled member of the Laguna Pueblo in New Mexico, I am a member of the Sun Clan and have the name of my great grandfather, Osara, meaning 'the sun'," Dr. Michael Trujillo told the United States Senate Committee on Indian Affairs in 1994 during his confirmation hearing as Director of the Indian Health Service (see Exhibit 7/1). He told the committee that he had known the remoteness of Neah Bay at the northwest tip of Washington on the Makah reservation, lived in the Dakotas, and experienced the winters and geographic barriers to health care in Eagle Butte, Rosebud, and Twin Buttes. He had come before them, he also told them, "as the President's nominee for the Director of a national health care program that is essential to the well-being of 1.3 million American Indians and Alaska Natives belonging to more than 500 federally recognized tribes."

Three years later, Trujillo was in front of the same Committee discussing the fiscal year 1998 budget request for the Indian Health Service (IHS). For the fourth consecutive year, the IHS would receive no after-inflation increase in its budget allocation. But what Trujillo said in 1994 was still true: "We, who are involved in Indian health care, are facing a changing external environment with new demands, new needs, and a shifting political picture. The changing internal environment demands increased efficiency, effectiveness, and accountability."

This case was written by Robert J. Tosatto, US Public Health Service; Terrie C. Reeves, University of Wisconsin, Milwaukee; W. Jack Duncan, University of Alabama at Birmingham; and Peter M. Ginter, University of Alabama at Birmingham. All quotes are taken from statements made before committees of Congress or the houses of Congress by the person quoted. Used with permission from Terrie Reeves. Copyright © by Robert J. Tosatto, Terrie C. Reeves, W. Jack Duncan, and Peter M. Ginter and the North American Case Research Association. Reprinted by permission from the *Case Research Journal*. All rights reserved.

Exhibit 7/1: Dr. Michael Trujillo: Chief Advocate for Indian Health

Dr. Michael H. Trujillo was named Director of the Indian Health Service on April 9, 1994. His appointment was noteworthy for two reasons: (1) he was the first IHS Director appointed by the President of the United States and confirmed by the Senate; and (2) he was the first full-blooded American Indian to be appointed Director of the IHS. Dr. Trujillo was a member of the Sun Clan in the Laguna Pueblo in New Mexico. His parents were elementary school teachers for the Bureau of Indian Affairs and were active in the political life of the pueblo. His grandfather was a governor of the pueblo and was instrumental in drafting the first Laguna Pueblo constitution. From an early age, Dr. Trujillo had been taught and shown by example to feel an obligation to the Indian people.

The first American Indian to graduate from the University of New Mexico School of Medicine, Dr. Trujillo received both his undergraduate and medical degrees from that institution. Family practice and internal medicine were his specialties but he was also chosen for a clinical fellowship in preventive medicine at the Mayo Clinic. In addition, he received an MPH in Public Health Administration and Policy from the University of Minnesota School of Public Health.

Dr. Trujillo had numerous assignments within the IHS prior to becoming Director. As an IHS physician, he worked with many tribes in diverse locations. As an IHS administrator, he was Deputy Area Director and Chief Medical Officer for the Phoenix, Aberdeen, and Portland areas, as well as a Clinical Specialty Consultant to the Bemidji area. He initiated nationwide quality assurance programs and a medical provider recruitment program for urban Indian health centers.

Shortly after being sworn in as Director, Trujillo released his vision for the Indian Health Service. He envisioned a new IHS: one that adapted to the challenges it faced, yet continued to be the best primary care, rural health system in the world; one that recognized the contributions and dedication of employees, as well as the active participation of tribal members; one that was redesigned to be more effective, efficient, and accountable. Trujillo cautioned that any change must be accomplished in such a way that the Indian people noticed only improved quality of care.

Trujillo's position as IHS Director allowed him to be a strong advocate for Indians in all matters regarding health. Not only did he want to improve IHS, but he also wanted improvement for the entire Indian health care system. IHS leadership and direction would provide the course the agency would take in making these improvements.

Dr. Trujillo knew that in order to accomplish the agency's mission, IHS must honor past treaties as well as respect the beliefs and spiritual convictions of the various tribes. The need to respect local traditions and beliefs was formally recognized in Indian self-determination.

The Indian peoples had always managed with very scarce resources. However, Dr. Trujillo was concerned. IHS had not developed an adequate third-party payor billing system, it faced difficulty recruiting professional staff, and it served a population whose health status was below that of the rest of the United States.

IHS was considered a discretionary agency in the congressional budget process. Dr. Trujillo recognized the need to increase the health status of IHS's population in order to gain continued congressional funding and support. He needed to answer some difficult and complex questions. How could Indian self-determination be implemented? What should be IHS's role in the future? How should IHS change to best serve the self-determination of the Indian peoples?

Dr. Trujillo knew that his most difficult task was to provide additional, much needed health services to a growing and needy population when there was little prospect of increasing resources. Simultaneously, he had to ensure that local health needs were recognized and addressed.

Indian Self-Determination

In January 1994, Dr. Trujillo told the same Committee that the local tribes and communities needed to be more involved in the decision-making process to facilitate Indian self-determination, the process by which the Indian people may choose to assume some degree of the administration and operation of their health services. The Indian Self-Determination and Education and Assistance Act was passed by Congress in 1975 and gave federally recognized tribes the option of staffing, managing, and operating the IHS programs in their communities. Dr. Trujillo was on record as fully supporting greater self-determination of all tribes as a means of enabling Indian people to operate their own health care systems. He emphatically stated that "During my tenure, there is going to be continued emphasis throughout the agency and in our interactions with other health partners for complete recognition of the Indian self-determination process."

Dr. Trujillo knew that self-determination was far from complete. Although IHS still had many important functions to fulfill, putting health care back into the hands of the tribes was proving to be difficult. Each tribe had different concepts of health, and it was difficult to accommodate such variety in a government agency. Moreover, in the face of scarce resources there was always an inclination to centralize rather than decentralize decision making, and Dr. Trujillo knew that if the IHS created the impression that it could fulfill all the needs of local communities, it would contribute to false expectations and disappointment.

Historical Perspective

IHS had a clear mandate: to provide high-quality health services to American Indians and Alaska Natives (AI/ANs). The basis for this responsibility was established and confirmed by numerous treaties, statutes, and executive orders. The first treaty between the US government and an American Indian tribe was signed in 1784 and promised that the federal government would provide physician services to members of the Delaware Nation as partial payment for rights and property ceded to the United States. Treaties were signed with many individual tribes and periodic appropriations were made by Congress to control specific diseases such as smallpox and tuberculosis and to educate the tribes about disease. Recurring appropriations were not made until the Snyder Act of 1921, which authorized health care services for AI/ANs by an act of Congress.

Health care for Native Americans was originally the responsibility of the Bureau of Indian Affairs; however the services provided were, in general, very poor. Despite the employment of field nurses, the building of hospitals for Native Americans, and the addition of dental services, the health status of AI/ANs remained far behind that of the general population. For example, Indian infant mortality was more than double that of the general population and life expectancy for Indians was ten years less than that of the rest of the United States.

The major health problems found in the Native American population became evident during World War II when thousands of Indians volunteered for service in the US armed forces. The poor health of many Indian volunteers was noted during induction physical examinations. Citing the AI/AN health statistics, various state, medical, and professional groups began a push to put the US Public Health Service (USPHS) in charge of health care for Native Americans. They argued that the Bureau of Indian Affairs could not run a quality health care system because health was only one of its many concerns. Years of debate and political maneuvering followed. Finally the IHS officially became a division of the USPHS on July 1, 1955. The Transfer Act stated "that all functions, responsibilities, authorities, and duties relating to the maintenance and operation of hospital and health facilities for Indians, and the conservation of Indian health shall be administered by the Surgeon General of the United States Public Health Service."

Although the overall health status of AI/ANs did not improve immediately, much progress appeared over the longer term. Since 1973, infant mortality among AI/ANs had decreased 60 percent and death due to tuberculosis dropped 80 percent. During the same period, life expectancy for AI/ANs increased by more than 12 years; life expectancy for AI/ANs was just 2.6 years below that of the general population in the early 1990s.

Over the years after the transfer, the IHS developed a model for the provision of high-quality, comprehensive health services. A major component of this model was the involvement of the tribes in the provision of health services to their people. This provision had a "snowballing" effect. As the health status of their tribes improved, more tribal members began to get involved in the provision of health care which, in turn, allowed the tribes to provide even more services.

Congress followed up the Indian Self-Determination and Educational Assistance Act with the Indian Health Care Improvement Act in 1976 and attempted to elevate the health status of AI/ANs to a level equal to that of the general population. This Act gave IHS a larger budget, allowed expanded health services, and provided for new and renovated medical facilities and construction of safe drinking water and sanitary disposal facilities. In addition, it established scholarship and loan payback programs to increase the number of Indian health professionals. IHS was elevated to agency status within the USPHS in 1988. This reflected the improving reputation of IHS as an institution, as well as the growth of support for Indian self-determination and the IHS mission. See Exhibits 7/2 and 7/3.

The Service Population: American Indians and Alaska Natives

Traditional AI/AN beliefs concerning wellness, sickness, and treatment were different than the modern public health approach or the medical model. American

Exhibit 7/2: Timeline of Key Events In IHS History

1784	First treaty between the US government and an American Indian tribe signed.
1849	Bureau of Indian Affairs transferred from War Department to Department of the Interior. Physician services extended to Indians.
1880s	First federal hospital built for Indians.
1908	Professional medical supervision of Indian health activities established with position of chief medical supervisor.
1921	The Snyder Act authorized Indian health services by the federal government (under control of the Bureau of Indian Affairs).
1955	The Indian Health Service officially became a division of the United States Public Health Service (USPHS).
1975	Congress passed the Indian Self-Determination and Education Assistance Act.
1976	Congress passed the Indian Health Care Improvement Act.
1988	IHS was elevated to agency status within the USPHS. IHS was allowed to bill third-party payors where applicable.
1994	Dr. Michael Trujillo appointed as Director of the Indian Health Service.
1995	Preliminary recommendations of the Indian Health Design Team (a task force composed of Tribal leaders and IHS employees) published.
1997	Final recommendations of the Indian Health Design Team published.

Exhibit 7/3: IHS Mission

The mission of the Indian Health Service, in partnership with American Indian and Alaska Native people, is to raise their physical, mental, social, and spiritual health to the highest level.

Indians' and Alaskan Natives' beliefs included close integration within family, clan, and tribe; harmony with the environment; and a continuing circle of life–birth, adolescence, adulthood, elder years, the passing-on, and then rebirth. Individual wellness was conceived of as the harmony and balance among mind, body, spirit, and the environment. Effective health services for AI/ANs had to integrate the philosophies of the tribes with those of the medical community.

Of the more than 2.4 million AI/ANs in the United States, approximately 1.4 million belonged to the 545 federally recognized Indian tribes. All American Indian tribes were sovereign nations. Therefore, AI/ANs were citizens of both their tribes and of the United States. This meant that AI/ANs had a unique relationship with the federal government. Based on the "treaty rights" established between most tribes and the United States, the federal government had a "trust responsibility" to these tribes that entitled the Indian people to services such as education and health care. However, because not all tribes signed treaties with the United States, less than two-thirds of all people with an Indian heritage were eligible to participate in the federal programs. Since October 1978, the Bureau of Indian Affairs had received 215 letters of intent and petitions for

Exhibit 7/4: Service Population

Area	1990 (Census) Population	1997 (Estimated) Population
Aberdeen	74,789	94,313
Alaska	86,251	103,713
Albuquerque	67,504	78,851
Bemidji	61,349	79,930
Billings	47,008	55,630
California	104,828	119,976
Nashville	48,943	73,042
Navajo	180,959	215,232
Oklahoma	262,517	297,888
Phoenix	120,707	140,969
Portland	127,774	148,791
Tucson	24,607	27,612
All Areas	1,207,236	1,435,947

Exhibit 7/5: Age Distribution (by percentage of total population)

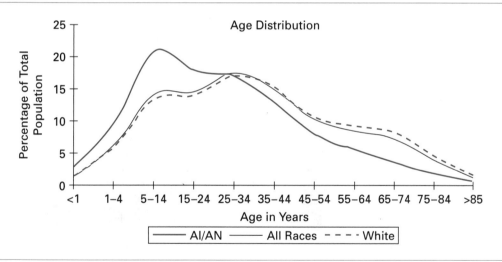

Source: Adapted from *Trends in Indian Health 1996.*

federal recognition. Forty-one of these petitions have been resolved with 21 "new" tribes being recognized.

The total number of AI/ANs eligible for IHS services in 1997 was approximately 1.43 million and increased about 2.2 percent each year. Selected demographics of the service population are shown in Exhibits 7/4 through 7/10. Tribal members lived mainly on reservations and in rural communities in 34 states.

Similar to the nation's health care system, IHS operated in an environment of increasing health care costs, growing numbers of beneficiaries, and excess demand

Exhibit 7/6: Median Household Income (1990 Census)

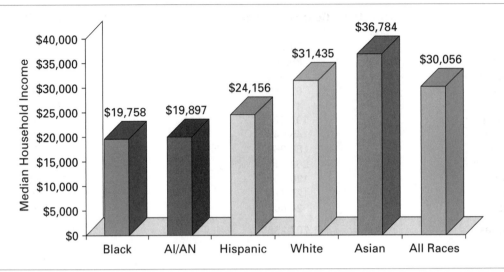

Source: Adapted from *Trends in Indian Health 1996*.

Exhibit 7/7: Percent of Total Population Below Poverty Level

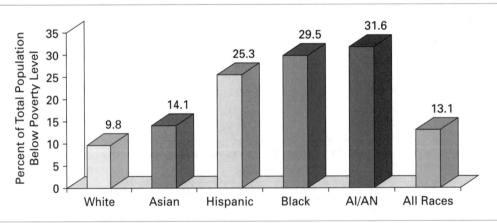

Source: Adapted from *Trends in Indian Health 1996*.

for services. The shift in disease patterns (from acute to chronic diseases) and the increasing elderly population played an important role in health planning for the IHS as well. As with the Veterans Administration, IHS was a health care provider within the US governmental system – though unlike the VA, the IHS was not a Cabinet department and had no voice in policy making at the White House. Unlike *any* other health care system in the country, IHS was subject to both the mandates of Congress and the approval of more than 540 sovereign Indian Nations.

Exhibit 7/8: Infant Mortality Rates

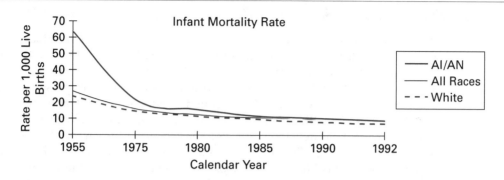

Source: Adapted from *Trends in Indian Health 1996*.

Exhibit 7/9: Overall Measures of Health

	AI/AN	All Races	White
Life Expectancy at Birth (Years)	73.5	75.5	76.3
Years of Productive Life Lost (Rate per 1,000 population)	83.0	55.6	49.9
Age-adjusted Mortality Rate (per 100,000 population)	598.1	513.7	486.8

Source: Adapted from *Trends in Indian Health 1996*.

Exhibit 7/10: Leading Causes of Death, Hospitalization, and Outpatient Visits

Leading Causes of Death

Heart Diseases
Accidents (Motor Vehicle and Other)
Chronic Liver Disease and Cirrhosis
Pneumonia and Influenza
Chronic Obstructive Pulmonary Diseases

Cancer
Diabetes Mellitus
Cerebrovascular Disease
Suicide
Homicide

Leading Causes of Hospitalization

Obstetric Deliveries and Complications
  of Pregnancy
Injury and Poisoning
Genitourinary System Diseases
Endocrine, Nutritional, and Metabolic Disorders

Respiratory System Diseases
Digestive System Diseases
Circulatory System Diseases
Mental Disorders
Skin Diseases

Leading Causes of Outpatient Visits

Respiratory Diseases
Endocrine, Nutritional, and Metabolic Disorders
Musculoskeletal System Diseases
Complications of Pregnancy and Childbirth

Nervous System Diseases
Injury and Poisoning
Skin Diseases
Circulatory System Diseases

Source: Adapted from *Trends in Indian Health 1996*.

IHS Today: A Key Component of the Indian Health Care System

Health care for AI/ANs was delivered through a system of interlocking programs. The system was composed of the IHS, the Tribal Programs, and the Urban Programs. IHS programs, called service units, were those projects and facilities that were directly staffed, operated, and administered by IHS personnel. As of October 1995, there were 68 IHS-operated service units that administered 38 hospitals and 112 health centers, school health centers, and health stations. Tribal programs were those developed through the process of Indian self-determination. Administered through 76 tribal-operated service units were 11 tribal program hospitals and 372 health centers, school health centers, health stations, and Alaska village clinics. Urban programs were relatively new, but were expected to face a future of brisk demand because of the relocation of significant Indian populations from reservations to urban settings. The urban programs ranged from information referral and community health services to comprehensive primary health care services. As of October 1995, there were 34 Indian-operated urban programs.

IHS headquarters and the IHS area offices had ties to the tribal governments as well as to the Indian-operated urban projects. The Indian and Alaskan tribal governments had input into the decisions of IHS-operated Service Units. This interrelation between the federal government, tribal governments, and urban Indian groups was a key component of Indian health care management. Exhibit 7/11 shows various features of the Indian health care system.

Exhibit 7/11: Elements of the Indian Health Care System

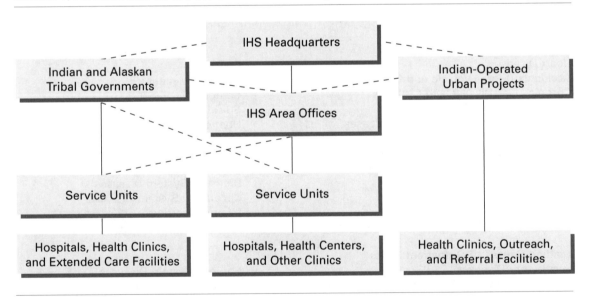

Note: Solid lines reflect formal relationships; dashed lines (-----) reflect important but less formal relationships.

Source: Adapted from *Trends in Indian Health 1996.*

Exhibit 7/12: Executive Branch Organizational Chart

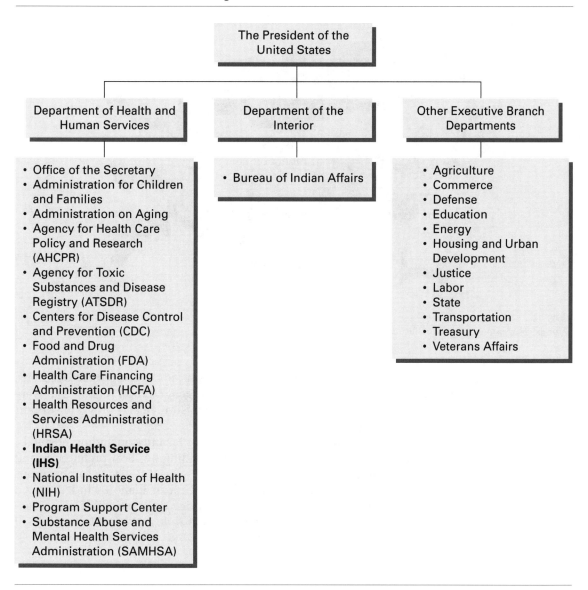

To further complicate the organizational structure, IHS was an Operating Division within the Department of Health and Human Services (DHHS). Exhibit 7/12 shows the position of the IHS (in bold) on the organizational chart of the executive branch of the federal government.

Within IHS, the organizational structure consisted of three levels: headquarters, area offices, and service units. IHS headquarters, located in Rockville, Maryland,

Exhibit 7/13: IHS Area Offices

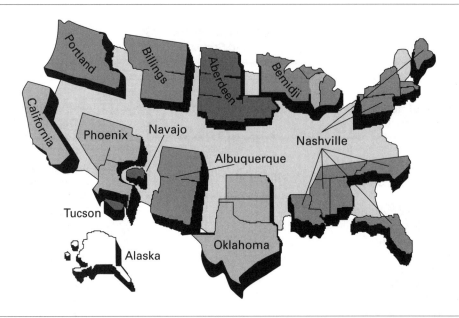

Source: IHS Homepage (www.ihs.gov).

was ultimately responsible for all policy, operations, and management decisions. The 12 area offices (see Exhibit 7/13) represented geographical regions and were responsible for performing various roles in administrative and program support for the local service units.

Service units were composed of several types of facilities, including hospitals, health centers, health stations, and clinics. Depending on local preferences and circumstances, these service units could exist as single entities or as combinations of facilities. For example, the Fort Hall Service Unit in Idaho included only a single health center, whereas the Pine Ridge Service Unit in South Dakota consisted of a hospital in Pine Ridge, health centers in Kyle and Wanblee, and small health stations in Allen and Manderson.

IHS Programs and Initiatives

In many (but not in all) cases, IHS provided comprehensive health care services to eligible AI/ANs. To be eligible for services, AI/ANs had to be members of federally recognized tribes with whom the United States had treaty agreements. Services were provided through various programs and initiatives administered by the IHS, covering a full range of preventive health, behavioral health, medical care, environmental health, and engineering services. The initiatives focused on timely issues such as care of the elderly, women's health, AIDS, traditional

Exhibit 7/14: IHS Programs and Initiatives

IHS Services and Programs

Preventive Health:
Prenatal and Postnatal Care
Well Baby Care
Immunizations
Family Planning Services
Women's Health Program
Nutrition Program
Health Education Program
Community Health Representative Program
Accident and Injury Reduction Program

Medical:
Inpatient Hospitalization
Outpatient Services
Emergency Services
Pharmacy Program
Laboratory Program
Nursing Program
Contract Health Services

Behavioral Health:
Mental Health Program
Social Services
Alcohol and Substance Abuse Program
Diabetes Program

IHS Initiatives:
AIDS Initiative
Traditional Medicine Initiative
Indian Youth Initiative
Maternal and Child Health Initiative
Sanitation Facilities Initiative
Indian Women's Health Initiative
Injury Prevention Initiative
Elder Care Initiative
Otitis Media Initiative
State Initiative

Environmental Health and Engineering:
Water and Waste Treatment
Food Protection
Environmental Safety and Planning
Pollution Control
Insect Control
Occupational Safety and Health
Facility Construction and Maintenance

medicine practices, and injury prevention, as shown in Exhibit 7/14. However, in some locations, the IHS did not have the necessary equipment or facilities to provide comprehensive services. In these instances, services which were not readily accessible to AI/ANs could be provided under contracted health services with local hospitals, state and local health agencies, tribal health institutions, and individual health care providers.

In its relatively short history, the IHS had contributed to tremendous improvements in the health status of its service population. Some of the many reasons for these status improvements included increased primary medical care services, sanitation facility construction, and community health education programs. The IHS was often instrumental in the infrastructure changes. Exhibit 7/15 shows some of the more impressive accomplishments of the IHS.

IHS Personnel

The Indian Health Service employed a workforce of approximately 15,000 people. Of these, more than 62 percent were of American Indian or Alaska Native

Exhibit 7/15: Program Accomplishments

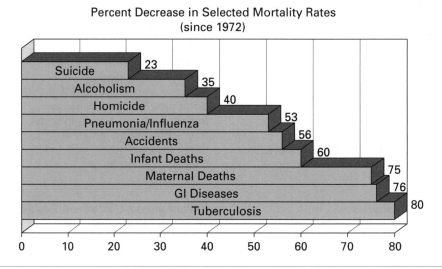

Percent Decrease in Selected Mortality Rates
(since 1972)

Source: Adapted from *Trends in Indian Health 1996.*

Exhibit 7/16: Percentage of Outpatient Visits by Type of Provider

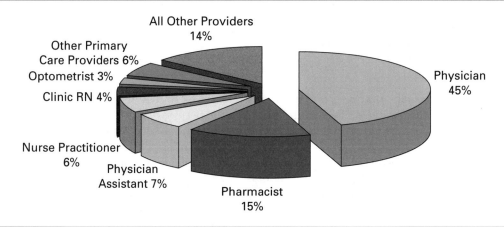

Source: Adapted from *Trends in Indian Health 1996.*

heritage. IHS personnel consisted of nearly every discipline involved in the provision of health, social, behavioral, and environmental health services. The IHS clinical staff was composed of primary care professionals and other providers, as well as clinical technicians and assistants. Primary care providers included physicians, physician assistants, dentists, nurse practitioners, and nurse midwives. Other providers included pharmacists, optometrists, public health nurses, clinic nurses, physical therapists, and dietitians (see Exhibit 7/16). Over several years, because

Exhibit 7/17: IHS Staffing Trends

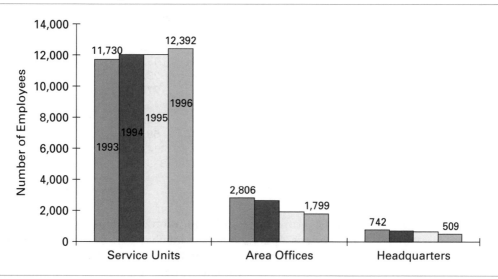

Source: Adapted from *Trends in Indian Health 1996.*

of the "Reinventing Government" initiative of the Clinton Administration result-ing from a national preference for moving government decision making closer to "the people," as well as the IHS redesign process initiated by Dr. Trujillo, the trend in IHS staffing was towards an increase in personnel at the service unit level and decreases at the area and headquarters levels (see Exhibit 7/17).

An ongoing personnel problem concerned the recruitment and retention of dedicated, qualified professionals. Most IHS sites were remote and many lacked adequate schools, stores, and amenities. To compensate for some of these quality-of-life imbalances, IHS offered financial incentives in the form of scholarships, loan payback agreements, and summer employment to selected health care professionals. For most professionals, however, the pay scales continued to lag behind those in the private sector.

Further exacerbating the personnel recruitment and retention problems, many employees were concerned about the changes that were occurring within the IHS. Federal employees at the service unit level wondered how long they could remain in their positions once the local tribes assumed responsibility for health services. Area and headquarters employees were concerned about the future of their careers because there were so many cuts being made in these programs. All such issues concerning the organizational changes were addressed often by IHS leaders in memorandums, reports, and speeches. Information technology resources, particularly the Internet and electronic mail, were also used to disseminate information. Upper management felt that it was imperative to keep the lines of communication open and to involve IHS personnel at all levels of the change process, but the uncertainty could not be eliminated.

Exhibit 7/18: Tribal Contract and Compact Funding (in millions of dollars)

Fiscal Year	Contracts	Compacts	Total
1987	$200.9	$9.8	$210.7
1988	217.2	13.1	230.3
1989	306.6	23.5	330.1
1990	320.7	27.4	348.1
1991	410.1	40.1	450.2
1992	511.6	50.9	562.5
1993	491.5	59.9	551.4
1994	648.1	114.5	762.6
1995	297.5	335.0	632.5

Source: Adapted from *Trends in Indian Health 1996.*

The Indian Self-Determination and Education Assistance Act gave federally recognized tribes various options for their involvement in staffing. The original Act allowed tribes to contract with the federal government. These contracting tribes could redesign and assume responsibility for any aspect of their health care services. Some tribes made the choice to contract all of their health care services. A limitation of the contracting process was that IHS had to approve and allow all redesign proposals.

Amendments to the Act removed this limitation by creating the Tribal Self-Governance Demonstration Project. This project allowed selected tribes to compact their health care services; that is, they took over complete responsibility without the need for IHS approval or oversight. The project originally called for 30 tribes to be selected for inclusion, but by 1997 there were already 34 participating tribes with several more anticipating their inclusion. The number of tribes choosing to deliver at least some portion of their own health care had increased steadily. Although contracts and compacts accounted for only an estimated 22 percent of the total IHS budget in 1987, these obligations grew to over 32 percent by 1995, and were expected to reach 50 percent by 2000. Exhibit 7/18 shows the trend in funding for tribal contracts and compacts.

IHS Funding

Sources of funding for IHS included appropriations from the federal budget and collections from third-party billing. Congress passed the Indian Health Care Amendments of 1988, which authorized the IHS to bill third parties for both inpatient and outpatient services. Medicaid, Medicare, and other insurance payors were all defined as third-party payors and these were considered the only new revenue source for IHS programs. IHS did not collect the co-payments or deductibles that were required with some policies, and those eligible individuals who did not have insurance coverage were not charged for the services they received. Although collections from third-party payors were increasing, there were still many concerns over the inability of IHS to bill and collect

Exhibit 7/19: Trend in IHS Budget Appropriations

IHS Budget (FY87–FY98)

Category	FY 1987	FY 1988	FY 1989	FY 1990	FY 1991	FY 1992	FY 1993	FY 1994	FY 1995	FY 1996	FY 1997	FY 1998
Services:												
Clinical[a]	$748	$817	$883	$1,031	$1,235	$1,276	$1,252	$1,325	$1,370	$1,418	$1,452	$1,468
Preventive Health	66	70	73	78	90	65	70	75	77	78	81	82
Other[b]	56	60	63	70	85	90	204	246	260	264	274	285
Total Services	$869	$947	$1,019	$1,179	$1,410	$1,431	$1,526	$1,646	$1,707	$1,760	$1,807	$1,835
Facilities	71	62	62	72	166	274	334	297	253	239	248	287
Total Appropriations	$940	$1,009	$1,081	$1,251	$1,576	$1,705	$1,860	$1,943	$1,960	$1,999	$2,055	$2,122

[a] All values are dollars ($) in millions.
[b] Other services include urban health, Indian health professions, Tribal health management, direct operations, self-governance, and contract support costs.

Source: Adapted from *Trends in Indian Health 1996.*

Exhibit 7/20: Trend in Third-Party Collections

Category	FY 1988	FY 1989	FY 1990	FY 1991	FY 1992	FY 1993	FY 1994	FY 1995	FY 1996
Medicare/Medicaid	$66	$75	$88	$94	$122	$141	$160	$162	$177
Private Insurance	–	–	3.5	8	12	18	23	31	34
Total Collections	$66	$75	$91.5	$102	$134	$159	$183	$193	$211

Note: All values are dollars ($) in millions.

Source: Adapted from *Trends in Indian Health 1996.*

adequately for all of the services that it provided. In fact, a 1995 review published by the Office of the Inspector General of the Department of Health and Human Services estimated that the IHS underbilled by about $8.5 million each quarter because of untrained staff, shortage of staff, or lack of controls.

Because the IHS was considered a discretionary program within the confines of the federal budget and because any attempts to balance the federal budget would involve cuts in discretionary programs, stakeholders of IHS were very concerned about the level of funding that the organization received from the federal government. The term "discretionary" referred to funds controlled by the annual appropriations process. This included most of the regular operating funds for the federal agencies, as well as funds for the thousands of large and small programs that have no binding legal obligations to their beneficiaries. Estimates were made that many IHS programs were underfunded by 30 to 40 percent, although some went as low as 70 percent below their level of need. Exhibits 7/19 and 7/20 show the trends for these funding sources. The 1998 budget request allowed no fund increases to account for inflation, population growth, or newly recognized tribes. Exhibits 7/21 and 7/22 show the financial position of IHS for fiscal year 1996 and fiscal year 1997.

The shift from direct federal funding to state block grant funding of health care programs (such as a Medicaid managed care program) was another great concern of IHS and tribal leaders. It was a common occurrence for states to overlook or ignore Indian concerns when developing programs. Many state governments had the misconception that Indian tribes had relationships only with the federal government and were not eligible for state resources, when in fact AI/ANs were entitled to the same privileges and resources as any other state citizen. In response to these concerns, a state initiative workgroup was created by the IHS to focus on the social, economic, legal, and policy issues pertaining to state health reform initiatives and Indian health programs.

Also, a strategic business plan was being developed by a workgroup composed of tribal leaders, IHS personnel, and private sector consultants. This plan would focus on revenue generation, cost control, internal business improvements, and allocation of tribal shares. Although the business plan was still in the development stage, this committee represented the IHS commitment to a new style of leadership, one that focused not only on the efficient and effective use of resources, but also on the partnership with the Indian people.

Exhibit 7/21: Statement of Financial Position

	(in millions)	
	1996	**1997**
Assets		
Entity Assets:		
Fund Balances with Treasury	$1,172	$1,108
Investments	–	–
Accounts Receivable, Net:		
From Federal Agencies	19	6
From the Public	4	16
Interest Receivable	–	–
Advances:		
To Federal Agencies	13	–
To the Public	10	40
Inventories	13	15
Property and Equipment, Net	497	647
Non-Entity Assets:		
Accounts Receivable, Net:	–	–
Total Assets	$1,728	$1,832
Liabilities		
Funded Liabilities:		
Payables:		
Due Federal Agencies	$24	$26
Due the Public	42	48
Advances:		
From Federal Agencies	47	64
From the Public	–	–
Accrued Payroll and Benefits	29	30
Unfunded Liabilities:		
Annual Leave	60	60
Workers' Compensation Benefits	44	45
Other Liabilities	1	2
Pensions	–	–
Total Liabilities	247	275
Net Position		
Unexpended Appropriations	991	954
Invested Capital	511	662
Cumulative Results of Operations	84	48
Future Funding Requirements	(105)	(107)
Total Net Position	1,481	1,557
Total Liabilities and Net Position	$1,728	$1,832

Source: DHHS website (http://www.hhs.gov).

Exhibit 7/22: Statement of Operations and Changes in Net Position

	(in millions)	
	1996	**1997**
Revenues and Financial Sources		
Appropriated Capital Used:		
General Appropriations	$1,991	$2,135
Matching Contributions	–	–
Employment Taxes	–	–
SMI Premium Collected	–	–
Interest Revenue	–	–
Sales of Goods and Services	310	415
Imputed Financing	–	71
Other Revenue and Financing	–	–
Total Revenue and Financing Sources	$2,301	$2,621
Expenses		
Operating:		
Personnel Costs	$745	$755
Travel and Transportation	46	48
Rent, Communications and Utilities	43	40
Printing and Reproduction	2	1
Contractual Services	738	851
Supplies and Materials	80	180
Grants	516	605
Insurance Claims and Indemnities	–	1
Other Operating Expenses	81	–
Depreciation and Amortization	24	24
Imputed Personnel Costs	–	71
Other Non-Operating Expenses	–	1
Total Expenses	$2,275	$2,577
Excess of Revenues and Financing Sources	$26	$44
Net Position, Beginning Balance	$1,464	$1,481
Adjustments	–	178
Net Position, Restated Beginning Balance	1,464	1,659
Excess of Revenues and Financing Sources	26	44
Non-Operating Changes	(9)	(146)
Net Position, Ending Balance	$1,481	$1,557

Source: DHHS website (http://www.hhs.gov).

The Future of the IHS

Dr. Trujillo knew that the IHS was a very dynamic organization, that it was staffed by professional personnel, that the AI/AN populations were unique, and that tribal cultures, values, religions, and traditions must always be considered and respected when delivering health services to them. In addition, he knew that the IHS was at a crucial juncture in its existence. Stakeholders in Indian health were calling for major changes in the organization. Various economic changes were signaling the need for new and innovative ways to fund programs. Tribes were asking for more control over the health care for their members. At the same time that the IHS was constrained by treaties, it was also considered a discretionary agency of the United States.

Dr. Trujillo was committed to Indian self-determination and knew that the spirit of self-determination required local assessment and definition of health service requirements. At the same time, he was responsible for improving the health status of the American Indians and Alaska Natives to the highest level possible. Although there was no inherent conflict between self-determination and improvements in health status of all the Indian peoples, in the face of scarce resources Dr. Trujillo knew there were limits to the services that could be provided to any single community. He needed to carefully manage the expectations created by self-determination while not discouraging local communities from becoming involved in their own health affairs. The creation of false expectations could be as damaging as not involving tribes in local health affairs. Balancing expectations with local support required some serious thinking about the future mission and role of the IHS.

REFERENCES

Kendrick, T. (1997). *A Future of Possibilities for Health, Indian Health, and Indian Health Leaders*. Available: http://www.ihs.gov

Trujillo, M. H. (January 27, 1994). *Confirmation Hearing Statement Before the United States Senate Committee on Indian Affairs*. Available: http://www.ihs.gov

Trujillo, M. H. (May 11, 1995). *Opening Statement Before the Interior Subcommittee of the Senate Appropriations Committee*. Available: http://www.ihs.gov

Trujillo, M. H. (November 28, 1995). *Time of Change . . . Time for Change: The State of the Indian Health Service* (presented at the National Indian Health Board 13th Annual Consumer Conference). Available: http://www.ihs.gov

Trujillo, M. H. (February 20, 1996). *Challenges and Change: The State of the Indian Health Service*. Available: http://www.ihs.gov

Trujillo, M. H. (December 1996). "Message From the Director: Looking to the Future of the Indian Health Service," *IHS Primary Care Provider* 21, no. 12, pp. 157–160.

Trujillo, M. H. (March 1997). *The Future Indian Health Care System*. Available: http://www.ihs.gov

8 CASE

Dr. Louis Mickael: The Physician as Strategic Manager

Industry Background

In the early 1900s, hospitals were perceived by the majority of the population in the United States as places where very sick people went to die. However, in the past five decades, rapid progress in medical technology, knowledge base, and expertise enhanced professional capability, and the public then demanded high levels of health care services.

In 50 years, many demographic changes occurred. The population, longevity, and standard of living continued to increase. To address the needs of this changing population, government health care insurance programs for the older and needy segments of society were instituted. Private insurance companies proliferated, and although workers had begun to expect employers to share with them the financial responsibility for their health service needs, employers were searching for less expensive ways to provide such care. The government was also attempting to reduce costs associated with the insurance programs it sponsored.

By the early 1980s, costs to provide these health care services reached epic proportions; and the financial ability of employers to cover these costs was being stretched to breaking point. In

This case was written by C. Louise Sellaro, Youngstown State University. It is intended as a basis for classroom discussion rather than to illustrate either effective or ineffective handling of an administrative situation. The names of firms, individuals, locations, and financial information have been disguised to preserve the organization's desire for anonymity. Presented and accepted for the Refereed Society for Case Research. All rights reserved to the author and SCR. Copyright © 1992 by C. Louise Sellaro. Used with permission of Louise Sellaro.

addition, new government health care regulations had been enacted that have had far-reaching effects on this US industry.

The most dramatic change came with the inauguration of a prospective payment system. By 1984, reimbursement shifted to a prospective system under which health care providers were paid preset fees for services rendered to patients. The procedural terminology codes that were initiated at that time designated the maximum number of billed minutes allowable for the type of procedure (service) rendered for each diagnosis. A diagnosis was identified by the *International Classification of Diseases, Ninth Revision, Clinical Modification*, otherwise known as *ICD-9-CM*. The two types of codes, procedural and diagnosis, had to logically correlate or reimbursement was rejected.

Put simply, regardless of which third-party payor insured a patient for health care, the bill for an office visit was determined by the number of minutes that the regulation allowed for the visit. This was dictated by the diagnosis of the primary problem that brought the patient into the office and the justifiable procedures used to treat it.

These cost-cutting measures initiated through the government-mandated prospective payment regulation added to physicians' overhead costs because more paperwork was needed to submit claims and collect fees. In addition, the length of time increased between billing and actual reimbursement, causing cash flow problems for medical practices unable to make the procedural changes needed to adjust. This new system had the effect of reducing income for most physicians, because the fees set by the regulation were usually lower than those physicians had previously charged.

Almost all other operating costs of office practice increased. These included utilities, maintenance, and insurance premiums for office liability coverage, workers' compensation, and malpractice coverage (for which costs tripled in the late 1980s and early 1990s). This changed the method by which government insurance reimbursement was provided for health care disbursed to individuals covered under the Medicare and Medicaid programs. Private insurors quickly adopted the system, and health care as an industry moved into a more competitive mode of doing business.

The industry profile differed markedly from that of only a decade earlier. Hospitals became complex blends of for-profit and not-for-profit divisions, joint ventures, and partnerships. In addition, health care provided by individual physician practitioners had undergone change. These professionals were forced to take a new look at just who their patients were and what was the most feasible, competitively justifiable, and ethical mode of providing and dispensing care to them.

For the first time in his life, Dr. Mickael read about physicians who were bankrupt. In actuality, Dr. Charles, who shared office space with him, was having a financial struggle and was close to declaring bankruptcy.

January 6, 1994

The last patient had just left, and Dr. Lou Mickael ("Dr. Lou") sat in his office thinking about the day's events. He had been delayed getting into work because a patient telephoned him at home to talk about a problem with his son. When he arrived at the office and before there was time to see any of the patients waiting for him, the hospital called to tell him that an elderly patient, Mr. Spence, admitted through the emergency room last night had taken a turn for the worse.

"My days in the office usually start with some sort of crisis," he thought. "In addition to that, the national regulations for physician and hospital care reimbursement are forcing me to spend more and more time dealing with regulatory issues. The result of all this is that I'm not spending enough time *with* my patients. Although I could retire tomorrow and not have to worry financially, that's not an alternative for me right now. Is it possible to change the way this practice is organized, or should I change the type of practice I'm in?"

Practice Background

When Dr. Lou began medical practice the northeastern city's population was approximately 130,000 people, most of whom were blue-collar workers with diverse ethnic backgrounds. By 1994, suburban development surrounded the city, more than doubling the population base. A large representation of service industries were added, along with an extensive number of upper and middle managers and administrators typically employed by such industries.

Location

Dr. Lou kept the same office over the years. It was less than one-half mile from the main thoroughfare and located in a neighborhood of single-family dwellings. The building, constructed specifically for the purpose of providing space for physicians' offices, was situated across the street from City General, the hospital where Dr. Lou continued to maintain staff privileges. Three physicians (including Dr. Lou) formed a corporation to purchase the building, and each doctor paid that corporation a monthly rental fee, which was based primarily on square footage occupied, with an adjustment for shared facilities such as a waiting room and rest rooms.

Office Layout

One of the physicians, Dr. Salis, was an orthopedic surgeon who occupied the entire top floor of the building. Dr. Lou and the other physician, Dr. Charles, were housed on the first floor. Total office space for each (a small reception area, two examining rooms, and private office) encompassed a 15' × 75' area (see Exhibit 8/1). The basement was reserved for storage and maintenance equipment.

The reception area and each of the other rooms that made up the office space opened on to a hallway that Dr. Lou shared with Dr. Charles. The two physicians and their respective staff members had a good rapport; and because the reception desks opened across from each other, each staff was able to

Exhibit 8/1: Shared Office Space of Dr. Mickael and Dr. Charles

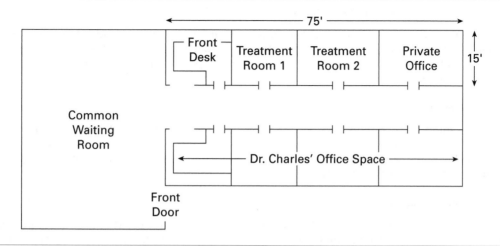

provide support for the other by answering the phone or giving general information to patients when the need arose.

The large, common waiting room was used by both physicians. After reporting to their own doctor's reception area, patients were seated in this room, then paged for their appointment via loudspeaker.

Dr. Charles was in his mid-forties and in general practice as well. His patients ranged in age from 18 to their mid-eighties, and his office was open from 10:00 A.M. until 7:30 P.M. on Mondays and Thursdays, and from 9:30 A.M. until 4:30 P.M. on Tuesdays and Fridays; no office hours were scheduled on Wednesday. He and Dr. Lou were familiar with each other's patient base, and each covered the other's practice when necessary.

Staff and Organizational Structure

Dr. Lou's staff included one part-time bookkeeper (who doubled as office manager) and two part-time assistants. The assistants' and bookkeeper's time during office hours was organized in such a way that one individual was always at the reception desk and another was "floating," taking care of records, helping as needed in the examining rooms, and providing office support functions. There were never more than two staff people on duty at one time, and the assistants' job descriptions overlapped considerably (see Exhibit 8/2 for job descriptions). Each staff member could handle phone calls, schedule appointments, and usher patients to the examining rooms for their appointments.

Although Dr. Lou was "only a phone call away" from patients on a 24-hour basis, patient visits were scheduled only four days a week. On two of these days (Monday and Thursday) hours were from 9:00 A.M. to 5:00 P.M. The other two were

Exhibit 8/2: Job Descriptions for Dr. Mickael's Office Staff

Job Description: Bookkeeper/Office Manager

In addition to responsibility for bookkeeping functions, ordering supplies, and reconciling the orders with supplies received, this person knows how to run the reception area, pull the file charts, and usher patients to treatment rooms. In addition, she can handle phone calls, schedule appointments, and enter office charges into patient accounts using the computer.

Job Description: Assistant 1

The main responsibility of this position is insurance billing. Additional duties include running the reception area, pulling and filing charts, ushering patients to treatment rooms, answering the phone, scheduling appointments, entering office charges into patient accounts, and placing supplies received into appropriate storage areas.

Job Description: Assistant 2

This is primarily a receptionist position. The duties include running the reception area, pulling and filing charts, ushering patients to treatment rooms, answering the phone, scheduling appointments, entering office charges into patient accounts, and placing supplies received into appropriate storage areas.

"long days" (Tuesday and Friday), when office hours officially were extended to 7:00 P.M. in the evening, but often ran much later.

The fifth weekday (Wednesday) was reserved for meetings, which were an important part of Dr. Lou's professional responsibilities because he was a member of several hospital committees. He was one of two physicians residing on the ten-member board of the hospital, and this, along with other committee responsibilities, often demanded attendance at a variety of scheduled sessions from 7:00 A.M. until late afternoon on "meetings" day. Wednesday was used by the staff to process patient insurance forms, enter patient data into their charts and accounts receivables, and prepare bills for processing.

When paperwork began to build after the PPS regulations came into effect in the 1980s, patients had many problems dealing with the forms that were required for reimbursement of services received in a physician's office. It was the option of physicians whether to "accept assignment" (the standard fee designated by an insurance payor for a particular health care service provided in a medical office). A physician who chose to *not* accept assignment must bill patients for health care services according to a fee schedule ("a usual charge" industry profile) that was preset by Medicare for Medicare patients. Most other insurances followed the same profile. Dr. Lou agreed to accept the standard fee, but the patient had to pay 20 percent of that fee, so the billing process became quite complicated.

In 1988, Dr. Lou decided that he needed to computerize his patient information base to provide support for the billing function. He investigated the possibility of using an off-site billing service, but it lacked the flexibility needed to deal with regulatory changes in patient insurance reporting that occurred with greater and greater frequency. Dr. Charles was asked if he wished to share expenses and develop a networked computer system. But the offer was declined; he preferred to take care of his own billing manually.

An information systems consultant was hired to investigate the computer hardware and software systems available at that time, make recommendations for programs specifically developed for a practice of this type, and oversee installation of the final choice. After initial setup and staff training, the consultant came to the office only on an "as needed" basis, mostly to update the diagnostic and procedure codes for insurance billing.

Computerization was an important addition to the record-keeping process, and the system helped increase the account collection rate. However, at times problems would arise when the regulations changed and third-party payors (insurance companies) consequently adjusted procedure or diagnosis codes. For example, there was often some lag time between such decisions and receipt of the information needed to update the computer program. Fortunately, the software chosen remained technologically sound, codes were easily adjusted, and vendor support was very good.

Although the new system helped to adjust the account collection rate, fitting this equipment into the cramped quarters of current office space was a problem. To keep the computer paper and other supplies out of the way, Dr. Lou and his staff had to constantly move the heavy boxes containing this stock to and from the basement storage area.

January 8, 1994 (Morning)

On Dr. Lou's way in that day, the bookkeeper told him that something needed to be done about accounts receivable. Lag time between billing and reimbursement was again getting out of hand, and cash flow was becoming a problem (see Exhibits 8/3 through 8/6 for financial information concerning the practice).

Cash flow had not been a problem prior to PPS, when billing for the health care provided by Dr. Lou was simpler, and payment was usually retrospectively reimbursed through third-party payors. However, as the regulatory agencies continued to refine the codes for reporting procedures, more and more pressure was being placed on physicians to use additional or extended codes in reporting the condition of a patient. Speed of reimbursement was a function of the accuracy with which codes were recorded and subsequently reported to Medicare and other insurance companies. In part, that was determined by a physician's ability to keep current with code changes required to report illness diagnoses and office procedures.

Cathy, the receptionist, had a list of patients who wanted Dr. Lou to call as soon as he came in. She also wanted to know if he could squeeze in time around lunch hour to look at her husband's arm; she believed he had a serious infection resulting from a work-related accident. The wound looked pretty nasty this morning, and Cathy thought maybe it should not wait until the first available appointment at 7:00 P.M.

Exhibit 8/3: Trial Balance at December 31

	1991	1992	1993
Debits			
Cash	$15,994	$9,564	$8,666
Petty cash	50	100	100
Accounts receivable	19,081	25,054	28,509
Medical equipment	11,722	11,722	11,722
Furniture and fixtures	3,925	3,925	3,361
Salaries	117,455	124,608	132,325
Professional dues and licenses	1,925	1,873	1,816
Miscellaneous professional expenses	1,228	2,246	3,232
Drugs and medical supplies	2,550	1,631	2,176
Laboratory fees	2,629	524	1,801
Meetings and seminars	2,543	838	3,880
Legal and professional fees	5,525	2,057	5,400
Rent	16,026	16,151	18,932
Office supplies	4,475	3,262	4,989
Publications	1,390	406	401
Telephone	1,531	1,451	2,400
Insurance	8,876	9,629	11,760
Repairs and maintenance	3,547	4,240	5,352
Auto expense	1,009	1,487	3,932
Payroll taxes	3,107	2,998	3,780
Computer expenses	846	938	1,905
Bank charges	438	455	479
	$225,872	$225,159	$256,918
Credits			
Professional fees	$172,281	$172,472	$204,700
Interest income	992	456	210
Capital	46,122	43,137	40,117
Accumulated depreciation (furniture and fixtures)	1,692	2,151	2,796
Accumulated depreciation (medical equipment)	4,785	6,943	9,095
	$225,872	$225,159	$256,918

Exhibit 8/4: Gross Revenue and Accounts Receivable

	December 31	
	1979	1986
Gross revenue	$116,951	$137,126
Accounts receivable	15,684	32,137

Exhibit 8/5: Statements of Income for the Years Ended December 31

	1991	1992	1993
Operating Revenues			
Professional fees	$172,281	$172,472	$204,700
Interest income	992	456	210
Total revenues	173,273	172,928	204,910
Operating Expenses			
Salaries (Dr. Mickael, Staff)	117,455	124,608	132,325
Professional dues and licenses	1,925	1,873	1,816
Miscellaneous professional expenses	1,228	2,246	3,232
Drugs and medical supplies	2,550	1,631	2,176
Laboratory fees	2,629	524	1,801
Meetings and seminars	2,543	838	3,880
Legal and professional fees	5,525	2,057	5,400
Rent	16,026	16,151	18,932
Office supplies	4,475	3,262	4,989
Publications	1,390	406	401
Telephone	1,531	1,451	2,400
Insurance	8,876	9,629	11,760
Repairs and maintenance	3,547	4,240	5,352
Auto expense	1,009	1,487	3,932
Payroll taxes	3,107	2,998	3,780
Computer expenses	846	938	1,905
Bank charges	438	455	479
Total operating expenses	175,100	174,794	204,560
Net Income (Loss)	($1,827)	($1,866)	$350

"I'm just starting to see my patients, and I've already done a half-day's work," Dr. Lou thought when he buzzed his assistant to bring in the first patient. He was 45 minutes late.

Patient Profile

When Dr. Lou walked into Treatment Room 1 to see the first patient of the day, Doris Cantell, he was thinking about how his practice had grown over the years. His practice maintained between 800 and 900 patients in active files. In comparison to other solo practitioners in the area, this would be considered a fairly large patient base.

"Well, how are you feeling today?" he asked the matronly woman. Doris and her husband, like many of his patients, were personal friends.

In the beginning years of practice, Dr. Lou's patients had been primarily younger people with an average age in the mid-thirties; their average income was approximately $15,000. Their families and careers were just beginning, and it was not unusual to spend all night with a new mother waiting to deliver a baby.

Exhibit 8/6: Balance Sheets at December 31

	1991	1992	1993
Assets			
Capital equipment			
Medical equipment	$11,722	$11,722	$11,722
Furniture and fixtures	3,925	3,925	3,361
Less-accumulated depreciation	(6,477)	(9,094)	(11,891)
Total capital equipment	9,170	6,553	3,192
Current assets			
Cash	15,994	9,564	8,666
Petty cash	50	100	100
Accounts receivable	19,081	25,054	28,509
Total current assets	35,125	34,718	37,277
Total assets	$44,295	$41,271	$40,467
Liabilities			
Current liabilities			
Income taxes payable	($639)	($653)	$122
Dividends payable	1,158	1,154	1,154
Total current liabilities	519	501	1,276
New income	(1,188)	(1,213)	228
Less dividends	1,158	1,154	1,154
Retained earnings	(2,346)	(2,367)	(926)
Capital	46,122	43,137	40,117
Total owner's equity	43,776	40,770	39,191
Total liabilities and owner's equity	$44,295	$41,271	$40,467

Although often dead tired, he enjoyed the closeness of the professional relationships he had with his patients. He believed that much of his success as a physician came from "going that extra mile" with them.

Many things had changed. Today all pregnancies were referred to specialists in the obstetrics field. His patients ranged in age from 3 to 97, with an average of 58 years; their median income was $25,000. Most were blue-collar workers or recently retired, and their health care needs were quite diverse.

Approximately 60 percent of Dr. Lou's patients were subsidized by Medicare insurance, and most of the retired patients carried supplemental insurance with other third-party payors. Three types of third-party payors were involved in Dr. Lou's practice: (1) private insurance companies, such as Blue Cross and Blue Shield; (2) government insurance (Medicare and Medicaid); and (3) preferred provider organizations.

Preferred provider organizations and health maintenance organizations were forms of group insurance that emerged in response to the need to cut the costs of providing health care to patients, which resulted in the prospective payment system. Both types of organizations developed a list of physicians who would accept their policies and fee schedules; using the list, subscribers chose the doctor from whom they preferred to obtain health care services.

Contrary to reimbursement policies of most other major medical third-party payors, PPOs and HMOs covered the cost of office visits, and the patient might not be responsible for any percentage of that cost. Although the physician had to accept a fee schedule determined by the outside organization, there was an advantage to working with these agencies. A physician might be on the list of more than one organization, and a practice could maintain or expand its patient base through the exposure gained from being listed as a health service provider for such organizations.

Those patients who were working usually had coverage through work benefits. Some were now members of a PPO. Dr. Lou was on the provider list of the Northeast Health Care PPO; only a few of his patients were enrolled in the government welfare program.

"How's your daughter doing in college?" Dr. Lou asked. He had a strong rapport with the majority of his patients, many of whom continued to travel to his office for medical needs even after they moved out of the immediate area. "Are you heading south again this winter, and are you maintaining your 'snowbird' relationship with Dr. Jackson?"

It was not unusual for patients to call from as far away as Florida and Arizona during the winter months to request his opinion about a medical problem, and Doris had called last year to ask him to recommend a physician near their winter home in the South. Because of this personal attention, once patients initiated health care with him, they tended to continue. Dr. Lou had lost very few patients to other physicians in the area since he began to practice medicine. The satisfaction experienced by his patients provided the only marketing function carried out for the practice. Any new patients (other than professional referrals) were drawn to the office through word-of-mouth advertising.

Dr. Lou: Profile of the Physician

Dr. Lou had grown older with many of his patients. His practice spanned more than three generations; a lot of families had been with him since he opened his doors in 1961. Caring for these people, many of whom had become personal friends, was very important to him. However, as the character of the health care industry was changing, Dr. Lou was beginning to feel that he now spent entirely too much time dealing with the "system" rather than taking care of patients.

Eighty-year-old Mr. Spence was a good example. Three weeks before, he was discharged from the hospital after having a pacemaker implanted. He had been living at home with his wife, and although she was wheelchair bound, they managed to maintain some semblance of independence with the assistance of part-time care. Lately, however, the man had become more and more confused. The other night he wandered into the yard, fell, and broke his hip. His reentry to the hospital so soon meant that a great deal of paperwork would be needed to justify this second hospital admission. In addition, Dr. Lou expected to receive calls from their children asking for information to help them determine the best alternatives for the care of both parents from now on. He had never charged a fee for such consultation, considering this to be an extension of the care he normally provided.

"Things are really different now," he thought. "Under this new system I don't have the flexibility I need to determine how much time I should spend with a patient. The regulations are forcing me to deal with business issues for which I have no background, and these concerns for costs and time efficiency are very frustrating. Medical school trained me in the art and science of treating patients, and in that respect I really feel I do a good job, but no training was provided to prepare me to deal with the business part of a health care practice. I wonder if it's possible to maintain *my* standards for quality care and still keep on practicing medicine."

Local Environment

The actual number of city residents had not changed appreciably since the early 1960s, although suburban areas had grown considerably. In the mid-1970s, a four-lane expressway, originally targeted for construction only one mile from the center of the downtown area, was put in place about eight miles farther away. Within five years, most of the stores followed the direction of that main highway artery and moved to a large mall situated about five miles from the original center of the city. Many of the former downtown shops then became empty. Government offices, banking and investment firms, insurance and real estate offices, and a university occupied some of this vacated space; it was used for quite different (primarily service-oriented) business activities.

Numerous residential apartments devoted to housing for the elderly and low-income families were built near the original, downtown shopping area. Several large office buildings (where much space was available for rent) and offices for a number of human services agencies relocated nearby.

As he headed across the street to lunch in the hospital dining room, Dr. Lou was again thinking about how things had changed. At first, he had been one of a few physicians in this area. Within the past ten years, however, many new physicians moved in.

Competition

Two large (500-bed) hospitals within easy access of the downtown area had been in operation for over 40 years. One was located immediately within the city limits on the north side of the city; the other was also just inside city limits on the opposite (south) side. They were approximately three miles apart and competed for a market share with City General, a 100-bed facility. This smaller hospital was only two blocks from the old business district; it was the only area hospital where Dr. Lou maintained staff privileges. Exhibit 8/7 contains a map showing the location of the hospitals and Dr. Lou's office.

Exhibit 8/7: Map of the Hospitals and Dr. Mickael's Medical Office

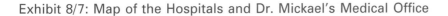

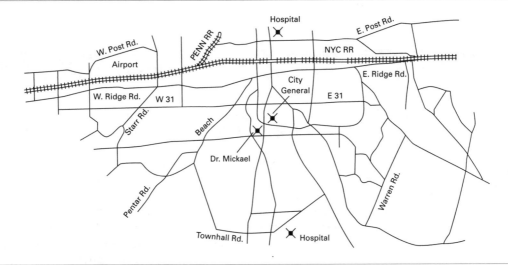

The two large hospitals had begun to actively compete for staff physicians (physicians in private practice who paid fees to a hospital for the privilege of bringing their patients there for treatment). In addition, these two health care institutions offered start-up help for newly certified physicians by providing low-cost office space and ensuring financial support for a certain period of time while they worked through the first months of practice.

City General recently began subsidizing physicians coming into the area by providing them with offices inside the hospital. Most of these physicians worked in specialty fields that had a strong market demand, and the hospital gave them a salary and special considerations, such as low rent for the first months of practice, to entice them to stay in the area.

These doctors served as consultants to hospital patients admitted by other staff physicians and could influence the length of time a patient remained in the hospital. This was an extremely important issue for the hospital, because under the new regulations a long length of stay could be costly to the facility. All third-party insurors reimbursed only a fixed amount to the hospital for patient care; the payment received was based on the diagnosis under which a patient was admitted. Should a patient develop complications, a specialist could validate the extension of reimbursable time to be added to the length of stay for that patient.

In the past few years, many services to patients provided by all these hospitals changed to care provided on an outpatient basis. Advancements in technology made it possible to complete in one day a number of services, including tests and some surgical procedures, which formerly required admission into the hospital and an overnight stay. Many such procedures could also be done by physicians in their offices, but insurance reimbursement was faster and easier if a patient had them done in a hospital. As an example of the degree of change involved, in the mid-1980s, outpatient gross revenue was only 18 percent of total gross revenue for City General. In 1992 this figure was projected to be approximately 30 percent.

January 8, 1994 (Lunchtime)

"May I join you?"

Dr. Lou looked up from his lunch to see Jane Duncan, City General's hospital administrator, standing across the table. "I'd like to talk with you about something."

Dr. Lou thought he knew what this was about. The hospital had been recruiting additional staff physicians (doctors who owned private practices in and around the city). A number of these individuals held family practice certification, a prerequisite for staff privileges in many hospitals. The recruitment program offered financial assistance to physicians who were family practice specialists wishing to move into the area, and also subsidized placement of younger physicians who had recently completed their residencies. In contrast to physicians designated as general practitioners, who had not received training beyond that received through medical school and a residency, "family practitioners" received additional training and passed state board exams written to specifically certify a physician in that field.

Last week after a hospital staff meeting, Duncan had caught him in the hall and wanted to know if Dr. Lou had thought about his retirement plans. "It's really not too soon," she had said. Dr. Lou knew that one of the methods used to bring in "new blood" was to provide financial backing to a physician wishing to ease out of practice, helping pay the salary of a partner (usually one with family practice certification) until the older physician retired.

"She wants to talk to me again about retirement and taking on a partner," he thought. "But I'm only in my late fifties. And I'm not ready to go to pasture yet! Besides, there's really no room to install a partner in my office."

January 8, 1994 (Afternoon)

After lunch Dr. Lou ran back to the office to take a look at Cathy's husband's arm before regular office hours started. This was a work-related case. As he treated the patient, he began thinking about industrial medicine as an alternative to full-time office practice. Right then the prospect seemed quite appealing. He had investigated the idea enough to know that there were only a few schools that provided this kind of training but one was within driving distance (Exhibit 8/8 contains information on industrial medicine).

As health costs rose over the past decade, manufacturing organizations began to feel the cost pinch of providing health care insurance to employees. Some larger companies in the area began to recognize the cost benefit of maintaining a private physician on staff who was trained in the treatment of health care needs for

Exhibit 8/8: Industrial Medicine as a New Career for Dr. Mickael

"Industrial Medicine" is an emerging physician specialty. Training in this new field entails postgraduate work and board certification.

As yet, only a few schools provide such training. One is located in Cincinnati, Ohio, which is geographically close enough to be feasible for Dr. Mickael. The time spent in actual attendance amounts to one two-week training period beginning in June of the year in which a physician is accepted for the training. Two additional training periods are each one week in duration: these take place in the months of October and March. After this, the physician was expected to individually study for and take the board certification exams, which were given only once per year; the exams were comprehensive and extended over a two-day period.

Training Program Costs: Industrial Medicine

University Residency:	
Three, on-site class sessions	$4,000.00
Per night cost for room	47.87
Books and supplies (total)	580.53
Transportation, Air:	
Three, round-trip fares	$1,650.00
Transportation, Ground:	
Car rental, per week with unlimited mileage	$125.45

industrial workers. Dr. Lou had been considering going back for postgraduate training in industrial medicine, and while wrapping the man's arm, he began to think about working for a large corporation.

"Work like that could have a lot of benefits; it would give me a chance to do something a little different, at least part time for now," he thought. "The income was almost comparable to what I net for the same time in the office, and some days I might even get home before 9:00 P.M.!"

End of the Day

As he was putting on his coat and getting ready to leave, Dr. Charles, the physician from across the hall, phoned to ask if Dr. Lou might be interested in buying him out. "I think you could use the space," he said, "and my practice is going down the tubes. I can't seem to get an upper hand with the finances. I've had to borrow every month to maintain the cash flow needed to pay *my* bills because patients can't keep up with theirs. City General has offered me a staff position, and I'm seriously considering it. I thought I'd give you first chance." After some minutes of other "office talk," Dr. Charles said good night.

"If I wanted to take on a new partner, that could work out well," thought Dr. Lou. "It might be interesting to check into this. I wonder what his asking price would be? It could not be too much more than the value of my practice; although his patients are a bit younger and some of his equipment is a little newer. The initial hospital proposal to buy me out indicated that my practice was worth about $175,000. So that means I should be able to negotiate with Dr. Charles for a little less than $200,000."

It was 9:30 P.M. when Dr. Lou finally left the office, and he still had hospital rounds to make. "This is another situation caused by these insurance regulations," he thought. "I feel as though I'm continuously updating patients' hospital records throughout the day, and more of my patients require hospitalization more often than they did when they were younger. All things being equal, I'm earning considerably less for doing the same things I did a decade ago, and in addition the paperwork has increased exponentially. There has to be a better way for me to deal with this business of practicing medicine."

CASE **9**

The New Office of Women's Health: Building Consensus to Establish a Strong Foundation

Patricia Clark, RN, MPH, newly appointed director of the Office of Women's Health at the State of Alabama Department of Public Health, sat quietly rereading Alabama Act 2002-141 (see Exhibit 9/1). The bill was unanimously passed by the Alabama Senate and overwhelmingly passed by the House (92 to 2, with 1 abstention). The legislation had been enacted during the last days of the administration of outgoing Alabama Governor, Don Siegelman. The Act created the Office of Women's Health, specified a steering committee to develop and recommend funding and program activities, and placed the Office within the Alabama Department of Public Health (ADPH).

The Mandate

Patricia's directive from Dr. John Thompson, State of Alabama Health Officer, had been to organize the office, work with the

This case was written by Julia Hughes of Tulane University and Peter M. Ginter and W. Jack Duncan of the University of Alabama at Birmingham. It is intended as a basis for classroom discussion rather than to illustrate either effective or ineffective handling of an administrative situation. Used with permission from the Alabama Department of Public Health.

Act 2002-141

Relating to the Alabama Department of Public Health; creating within the department an Office of Women's Health; specifying the purposes of the Office of Women's Health; providing staffing for the Office; and providing for an advisory committee for the office.

BE IT ENACTED BY THE LEGISLATURE OF ALABAMA:

Section 1. The Office of Women's Health is established within the Alabama Department of Public Health for the following purposes:

(1) To educate the public and be an advocate for women's health by requesting that the State Department of Public Health, either on its own or in partnership with other entities, establish appropriate forums, programs, or initiatives designed to educate the public regarding women's health, with an emphasis on preventive health and healthy life-style.

(2) To assist the State Health Officer in identifying, coordinating, and establishing priorities for programs, services, and resources the state should provide for women's health issues and concerns relating to the reproductive, menopausal, and postmenopausal phases of a woman's life, with an emphasis on postmenopausal health.

(3) To serve as a clearinghouse and resource for information regarding women's health data, strategies, services, and programs that address women's health issues, including, but not limited to, all of the following:
   a. Diseases that significantly impact women, including heart disease, cancer, hypertension, diabetes, and osteoporosis.
   b. Mental health.
   c. Substance abuse.
   d. Sexually transmitted diseases.
   e. Sexual assault and domestic violence.

(4) To collect, classify, and analyze relevant research information and data concerning women's health conducted or compiled by either of the following:
   a. The State Department of Public Health.
   b. Other entities in collaboration with the State Department of Public Health.

(5) To provide interested persons with information regarding the research results, except as prohibited by law.

(6) To develop and recommend funding and program activities for educating the public on women's health initiatives and information, including the following:
   a. Health needs throughout an Alabama woman's life.
   b. Diseases that significantly affect Alabama women, including heart disease, cancer, and osteoporosis.
   c. Access to health care for Alabama women.
   d. Poverty and women's health in Alabama.
   e. The leading causes of morbidity and mortality for Alabama women.
   f. Special health concerns of minority women.

(7) To seek funding from private or governmental entities to carry out the purposes of this Act.

(8) To prepare materials for publication and dissemination to the public on women's health.

(9) To conduct public educational forums in Alabama to raise public awareness and to educate citizens about women's health programs, issues, and services.

(10) To coordinate the activities and programs of the Office of Women's Health with other entities that focus on women's health or women's issues.

(11) To provide that the State Health Officer, within his or her annual report to the Governor and the Legislature, shall include information regarding the successes of the programs of the Office of Women's Health, priorities and services needed for women's health in Alabama, and areas for improvement.

(12) The Office of Women's Health will not advocate, promote, or otherwise advance abortion or abortifacients.

Section 2. The Alabama Department of Public Health may seek and accept financial contributions from corporations, limited liability corporations, partnerships, individuals, and other private entities for use by the Office of Women's Health.

Section 3. The State Health Officer shall appoint personnel to staff the Office of Women's Health including an individual who shall serve as the Director of the Office, in accordance with Departmental and State Personnel Department rules and regulations.

Section 4. (a) There shall be a steering committee called the Steering Committee on Women's Health that shall serve in an advisory capacity to the State Health Officer and the Director of the Office of Women's Health. The membership of the Committee shall include all of the following:

(1) Three physicians appointed by the Medical Association of the State of Alabama.
(2) Three nurses appointed by the Alabama State Nurses' Association.
(3) Three pharmacists appointed by the Alabama Pharmaceutical Association.
(4) Three employers appointed by the Business Council of Alabama.
(5) Three consumers, one appointed by the Governor, one appointed by the Lieutenant Governor, and one by the Speaker of the House.
(6) Three members to the Steering Committee of the Office of Women's Health appointed by the Alabama Hospital Association.
(7) Three registered dietitians appointed by the Alabama Dietetic Association.

The members of the Steering Committee shall serve two-year terms of office with the exception of the initial Committee on which one appointee from each group specified above shall serve a three-year term and one member from each group specified above will serve a one-year term. The Steering Committee shall be comprised of persons with an expertise in and knowledge of women's health issues in Alabama.

The Steering Committee shall reflect the racial, ethnic, gender, urban/rural, and economic diversity of the state.

(b) The State Health Officer Shall:

(1) Appoint a Chair for the Steering Committee from the Committee membership.
(2) Establish the policies and procedures under which the Steering Committee operates.
(3) Ensure that the Steering Committee will meet quarterly.

Section 5. The provisions of this Act shall be carried out to the extent that funds are available.

Section 6. The provisions of this Act are severable. If any part of this Act is declared invalid or unconstitutional, that declaration shall not affect the part which remains.

Section 7. This Act shall become effective immediately following its passage and approval by the Governor, or its otherwise becoming law.

Steering Committee, and begin developing programmatic and policy initiatives. Dr. Thompson had agreed to fund the Office until the legislature appropriated additional funds for its operation. Although the Office's current funding was quite limited, he suggested that establishing a "track record" could help when he went back to the legislature for funding and would aid in other fund-raising efforts for the Office as well.

The First Meeting of the Steering Committee

Patricia called the first meeting of the Steering Committee to order and introduced Dr. Thompson. "Welcome to the inaugural meeting of the Steering Committee," he said. "The new Office of Women's Health will be instrumental in identifying problem areas and resources needed to improve women's health in Alabama. I am delighted to be in attendance today and I look forward to working with each of you toward solving the issues facing women's health in Alabama."

Dr. Thompson introduced Alabama State House Representative Norma Jean Gordon, a key sponsor of the founding legislation, and thanked her for her support. Representative Gordon gave a brief history of Act 2002-141's passage, noting, "I was fortunate to have the Alabama State Nurses Association working with me on this legislation. Their support was instrumental to get the bill passed in the 2002 legislative session. Although funding for the Office of Women's Health is not included in this piece of legislation, I am prepared to help with future legislation to obtain funding. This initiative is long overdue for the women of Alabama. I want to express my appreciation to all of you on the Steering Committee for volunteering your valuable time. I also want to thank Dr. Thompson for agreeing to house the Office within the Alabama Department of Public Health."

Lynette Bush, president of the Alabama State Nurses Association (ASNA), commented, "ASNA is proud of its role as a creative impetus for the establishment of this new Office dedicated to women's health issues. We are prepared to work with you, the Steering Committee, and our state officials to assist the Office in promoting improvements in the health of the women of Alabama."

Next, Deborah Kirkland, with the Bureau of Family Health Services of ADPH, explained to the group, "The Bureau of Family Health Services provides services in five major areas: family planning, maternity, prenatal, smoking cessation, and unwed pregnancy. The main goal of the Bureau is to eliminate health disparities for women in Alabama."

Patricia then asked each Committee member to introduce him or herself (see Exhibit 9/2 for all the members' names and affiliations). As they were introducing themselves, Patricia noted the number of different viewpoints. General discussion ensued with various members representing the perspectives of their constituencies. Patricia hated to stop the great discussion but she wanted to have enough time for the group to hear the information to be presented by the guest speaker. Patricia introduced Dr. Elizabeth Wingerd, representing the Medical Association of the State of Alabama.

Exhibit 9/2: Alabama Department of Public Health, Office of Women's Health, Steering
        Committee Members

Name	Title and Organization	Representing
Richard Becker, MD	Department of Obstetrics/Gynecology, University of Alabama at Birmingham	Medical Association
Anne Magnus, MD	Internal Medicine, Simon-Williamson Clinic	Medical Association
Edith Reed, MD	Obstetrics/Gynecology, Miller Clinic	Medical Association
Karen Coplin, MSN, FNP	Retired Nurse Practitioner, faculty, University of South Alabama	Alabama State Nurses Association
Kristin Joplin, MSN, CRNP, MA	Program Director, Division of Neonatology, UAB Hospital	Alabama State Nurses Association
Erin Lawson, DSN, RN	Dean, College of Nursing & Health Sciences, Jacksonville State University	Alabama State Nurses Association
Susan Betts, RPh	St. Martin's in the Pines	Pharmaceutical Association
Violet Johanson, RPh, CDE	Jefferson County Department of Health	Pharmaceutical Association
Judith Skinner, Pharm.D.	Baptist Hospital	Pharmaceutical Association
Linda Bradley	Senior Governmental Affairs Manager, Pfizer, Inc.	Business Council of Alabama
Mary Francioni, RN	Medical Policy Analyst, Blue Cross Blue Shield of Alabama	Business Council of Alabama
Joel LeBlanc	Executive Director, Alabama Association of Health Plans	Business Council of Alabama
Tina Baker, JD	Attorney at Law	Consumer
Janise Jones-Hilton		Consumer
Vonnie Smith		Consumer
Terri Jeansomme	CEO, Jacksonville Medical Center	Alabama Hospital Association
Lois Stevenson	Associate Administrator/Chief Operating Officer, University of South Alabama Children's & Women's Hospital	Alabama Hospital Association
Victoria Williams	Director, Women's Center SE Alabama Medical Center	Alabama Hospital Association
Shanti Barnes, MPH, RD	Nutrition Director, Area I, Alabama Department of Public Health	Dietetic Association
Samantha Eggert, RD	St. Vincent Hospital	Dietetic Association
Antonia Joseph	Johnson City Nursing Home	Dietetic Association

Dr. Wingerd reported, "Alabama is ranked 49th in the nation for women's health issues. And a large portion of the health problems identified in Alabama and the South stem from poor diet and obesity." She continued, "We must educate the public and raise awareness about health issues. To address the most critical women's health threats of heart disease, cancer, hypertension, and diabetes, we must develop effective programs and find ways to fund them."

As Dr. Wingerd handed out copies of a summary of *Making the Grade on Women's Health: A National and State-by-State Report Card*, she recommended that the Steering Committee members read the introduction, executive summary, national statistics, and Alabama statistics sections in the full document. (Exhibit 9/3 contains a summary of the *Report Card*.) She continued, "The *Report Card*, developed by the National Women's Law Center, 'grades' 33 women's health status indicators and 32 policy indicators for each state as well as for the nation as a whole. Look at Alabama's grades on the heath status indicators." She summarized the results as follows:

- Alabama ranked 49th in overall women's health in the nation. Only two states – Mississippi (50th) and Louisiana (51st) – were worse than Alabama.
- Approximately 19 percent of Alabama women had no health insurance.
- The top three causes of death for Alabama women were heart disease, cancer, and stroke.
- Alabama's heart disease death rate for women ranked 49th in the nation.
- The prevalence of obesity was increasing for Alabama women. In 2000 Alabama ranked 42nd in percentage of overweight women; in 2003 Alabama ranked 49th in the nation.
- The increasing prevalence of obesity contributed to an increase in hypertension (Alabama ranked 50th), heart disease, and diabetes.
- Violence against women was a growing concern. According to the Alabama Criminal Justice Information Center, more than 20,000 cases of domestic violence were reported each year. The reported cases represented only 16 to 20 percent of these violent incidents. Most cases were never reported.
- The percentage of Alabama women who smoke had remained at 22 percent since 2000, but the Centers for Disease Control and Prevention (CDC) information cited an increase in smoking among youths.

Patricia thanked Dr. Wingerd for the thought provoking presentation. Glancing at her watch, she noted that they had run out of time. Patricia concluded with a recap of the meeting and reinforced to the committee, "The Office of Women's Health has no funding. However, we do have the opportunity to solicit funds from private agencies and we are the only office in the Department of Public Health that is authorized to do so." She closed the meeting with a reminder that the next Steering Committee meeting was to be held March 14, 2003.

What's Next?

"Dr. Wingerd did indeed present some disturbing facts for women in Alabama. She certainly reinforced my sense of urgency over the Office's strategic direction," thought Patricia.

"Today is December 13," she mused, "so I have just three months to establish the track record needed for funding. I simply have to get some focus and begin some policy or programmatic initiatives," she thought. "However, there are so

Exhibit 9/3: Summary of the Report Card for Alabama

Alabama		2001 Grade: U	Rank: 49
Status Indicators		2000 Grade: U	Rank: 49

Grading Key for Status Indicators	S Satisfactory	U Unsatisfactory	F Fail

I. Women's Access to Health Care Services

	White	White (Non-Hispanic)	Black	Black (Non-Hispanic)	Hispanic	American Indian, Alaskan Native	Asian/ Pacific Islander	18–44	45–64	2001 US Data	2000 State Overall Data	2000 State Grade	2000 State Rank	2001 State Overall Data	2001 State Grade	2001 State Rank
Women Without Health Insurance (%)		12.3		21.6	17.6			16.1	12.2	13.2	19.0	F	39	18.7	F	39
People in Medically Underserved Areas (%)										9.5	19.5	–	46	21.7	–	49
First Trimester Prenatal Care (%)	88.9	90.0	71.4	71.4	60.5					83.2	81.6	U	33	83.2	U	30
Women in County Without Abortion Provider (%)*										32	58	F	40	58	F	40

*This variable is graded against a state-specific benchmark.

II. Addressing Wellness and Prevention

	White (Non-Hispanic)	Black (Non-Hispanic)	Hispanic	American Indian, Alaskan Native	Asian/ Pacific Islander	18–44	45–64	50–64	65+	2001 US Data	2000 State Overall Data	2000 State Grade	2000 State Rank	2001 State Overall Data	2001 State Grade	2001 State Rank
Screening																
Pap Smears (%)	80.6	86.0	82.4	80.1	88.5	88.5	79.5		66.7	86.8	85.3	S	20	86.3	S	31
Mammograms (%)	72.4	67.8	60.4	54.2	85.8			77.1	72.9	78.8	76.1	S	24	76.7	S	41
Colorectal Cancer Screening (%)	41.8	36.0	44.3					36.7	45.4	41.3	41.0	S	16	41.0	S	31
Prevention																
No Leisure-Time Physical Activity (%)	29.2	44.7	38.9	29.7	17.0	29.2	33.9		44.0	28.6	33.5	F	36	35.9	F	47
Overweight (%)										33.3	34.0	F	42	37.7	F	49
Eating Five Fruits and Vegetables a Day (%)										26.9	24.3	F	39	22.8	F	47
Smoking (%)	25.4	14.1	15.7			25.6	21.9		11.6	21.2	22.3	F	36	22.0	F	32
Binge Drinking (%)	7.4	4.4				10.7	2.0			7.4	5.5	S	15	6.5	U	19
Annual Dental Visits (%)										70.5	62.1	F	45			

Exhibit 9/3: (cont'd)

III. Key Conditions	White	White (Non-Hispanic)	Black	Black (Non-Hispanic)	Hispanic	American Indian, Alaskan Native	Asian/Pacific Islander	18–44	45–64	65+	2001 US Data	2000 State Overall Data	2000 State Grade	2000 State Rank	2001 State Overall Data	2001 State Grade	2001 State Rank
Key Causes of Death for Women (per 100,000)																	
Heart Disease Death Rate	104.8	105.0	151.8	152.0	32.6	67.7					95.4	116.2	F	48	114.5	F	48
Stroke Death Rate	24.9	25.0	42.9	42.9							24.1	28.5	F	43	28.7	F	44
Lung Cancer Death Rate	27.4	27.5	20.3	20.4							26.9	25.3	S	17	25.8	S	17
Breast Cancer Death Rate	17.3	17.3	25.1	25.2							19.5	19.3	S	19	19.0	S	27
Chronic Conditions																	
High Blood Pressure (%)	28.8			42.7	27.3	29.5		16.6	42.7	58.1	24.7	32.5	F	50	33.4	F	50
Diabetes (%)	5.5			13.7				2.3	10.4	17.1	5.9	7.9	F	50	7.4	F	44
AIDS Rate (per 100,000)											8.7	5.5	S	31	5.8	S	33
Arthritis (%) (National Only)											21.8						
Osteoporosis (%) (National Only)											20.0						
Reproductive Health																	
Chlamydia (%)											5.5	10.8	F	49	10.0	F	48
Unintended Pregnancies (%) (National Only)											49.2						
Maternal Mortality Ratio (per 100,000)	6.7		21.1								7.7	11.7	F	46	11.7	F	46
Mental Health																	
Days Mental Health Was "Not Good" in Past 30 Days											3.8	4.3	–	47	4.1	–	38
Violence Against Women																	
Violence Experienced Over Lifetime (%) (National Only)											55.0						

IV. Living in a Healthy Community	White	White (Non-Hispanic)	Black	Black (Non-Hispanic)	Hispanic	American Indian, Alaskan Native	Asian/ Pacific Islander	Other Than White	18–44	45–64	65+	2001 US Data	2000 State Overall Data	2000 State Grade	2000 State Rank	2001 State Overall Data	2001 State Grade	2001 State Rank
Overall Health																		
Life Expectancy (years)	78.85		73.76					74.05				78.81	77.61	U	46	77.61	U	46
Days Activities Were Limited in Past 30 Days												3.5	5.1	–	45	4.4	–	45
Infant Mortality Rate (per 1,000)	7.8	7.7	14.7	14.7	8.4							7.2	9.8	F	48	10.0	F	49
Economic Security and Education																		
Poverty (%)	10.1		28.4		27.1		12.8		17.4	9.1	17.3	12.2	14.9	F	36	14.9	F	43
Wage Gap (%)												73.5	63.3	F	50	68.8	F	41
High School Completion	78.3		78.8		73.2		62.1					84.0	77.1	F	50	78.3	F	50

Source: National Women's Law Center website: http://www.nwlc.org/archive.cfm?section=archive, accessed on August 31, 2004.

many issues and they are all so critical to women in this state. What should be the focus of the Office? There are very capable people on this Committee and they have different expectations and priorities."

Patricia stared out the window, streaked with rain. "I am determined that the Office of Women's Health will make a difference," she reaffirmed to herself, "but how should the Office begin addressing women's health in Alabama?

"How can I develop consensus and focus with such a diverse and highly opinionated Steering Committee?" she wondered. Each member of the Steering Committee approached the issues a little differently and made excellent arguments as to what the Office should be doing.

Patricia knew the next three months would rush by with much of her time devoted to organizing the Office. She needed to figure out how the Steering Committee could set some priorities for the Office. The next meeting would be here before she knew it. No question but that the March meeting was critical!

The Rosemont Behavioral Health Center

During a flight from Los Angeles to Chicago, Charles Brown became involved in a conversation with Cates Lewis who happened to be sitting next to him. After five or ten minutes of the usual topics concerning the weather, promptness of the airline, and so forth, Cates asked Charles what he did for a living. With that, Charles and Cates entered into a conversation that would ultimately result in a long-term relationship.

Charles Brown was the CEO of a consulting firm called TM, Inc. His firm specialized in turning around failing companies and in some instances he bought out failed companies and resurrected them. Over the years TM was quite successful and Charles was in the enviable position of being able to choose his clients. TM was a virtual organization with a small core staff but with a network of associates that spanned numerous industries and disciplines. As a result, the company had been involved with organizations ranging from high-tech computer companies to low-tech manufacturing firms to health care organizations. Charles's background was health administration and he still gravitated toward projects that involved health care.

Cates Lewis was a successful publisher who owned a small firm that was very successful in a strong market niche. Several years ago Cates became the financial backer for a buyout of a behavioral health care center, The Rosemont. Cates's brother, Lloyd Lewis, spent over 20 years as a counselor for drug and alcohol abuse programs and in fact had worked for The Rosemont.

This case was written by Phil Rutsohn and Bob Forget, Marshall University. It is intended as a basis for classroom discussion rather than to illustrate either effective or ineffective handling of an administrative situation. Used with permission from Phil Rutsohn.

When he heardthat The Rosemont was on the market, he contacted his brother and asked if he would be interested in considering an acquisition. The arrangement would be that Cates would put up the seed money and Lloyd would be the CEO and manage The Rosemont.

The price was right and Lloyd was excited about the opportunity, so Cates put up $250,000 in cash and signed for a $750,000 note. At the time the $1 million commitment seemed to be a bargain. The buildings and equipment at Rosemont–Jackson and Rosemont–Bay Saint Louis were assessed at about $2.5 million with a small mortgage remaining on each. Admittedly the furniture and equipment at both locations were old and needed to be replaced but that could be phased in utilizing current earnings. The building in Jackson, which was configured with 50 two-bed rooms, was located in a rapidly deteriorating part of town but as Lloyd noted, "Wasn't that the plight of all urban health care facilities?" The buildings in Bay Saint Louis were located on a lovely piece of suburban property with older, nicely kept homes in the neighborhood. Although the outsides of the buildings were minimally presentable, the interiors would require a lot of work. Everything from new flooring to plumbing to electrical modifications would have to be undertaken if the institution was going to be able to establish itself as a premier health care delivery entity. Twenty-five rooms were available to handle 50 patients. However, if demand dictated and funds were available, the buildings could be modified to double patient load.

There were two satellite systems providing outpatient services (primarily to college students) in other parts of the state and there were corporate offices separate from both facilities. Because these functions were located in rental properties with no multi-year contracts, they were not seen as enhancing or inhibiting the value of the company. The only other asset that had any real value was accounts receivable. The A/R account was a mess and it was difficult to put a handle on how many accounts were actually collectable. However, Cates still felt pretty confident. If things didn't work out he could at least sell the fixed assets to a real estate developer and get his money back.

As was agreed, Lloyd assumed responsibility for managing the organization and Cates continued his concentration on publishing. Although Cates was a member of The Rosemont's board he readily admitted that he was "slack" concerning his board responsibilities. As long as Lloyd told him things were fine, Cates paid little attention to the details of running the center. Rather, he did not pay much attention until one of the board members, who was the CEO of the accounting firm handling The Rosemont financial statements, called him and told him The Rosemont was out of money. The accountant said to Cates, "Cash is so tight that payroll is not going to be met and suppliers are not going to be paid."

"Needless to say, I was a little upset," Cates reported. "I knew things were tight. The Rosemont didn't do very well under its past ownership but I thought things were turning around."

An emergency board meeting was called to see what could be done to improve the organization's financial position. Cates commented, "The problem was obvious. There just wasn't sufficient patient volume to generate the revenues necessary to cover expenses."

Lloyd insisted, "It's a temporary problem that will be rectified when the two new contracts are signed. One is with a local school system and one with the state."

As a result of Lloyd's confidence, Cates arranged for a $3 million line of credit with the local bank. He stated, "I wanted the line of credit to provide the organization with enough financial flexibility to get out of the woods!"

By the time Cates met Charles on the airplane things were bleak. Not only had patient volume continued to be insufficient to break even, The Rosemont had gone through most of the $3 million line of credit. The Rosemont was facing bankruptcy and needed help immediately. Cates asked Charles if he would be interested in consulting with The Rosemont and helping it get back on its feet. With the limited information provided by Cates, Charles was uncertain whether he could help but he agreed to make a two-day site consultation and report his findings to the board.

Charles Brown's Report to the Board

After two days of intensive investigation it was obvious to Charles that The Rosemont's problems would require two levels of intervention. First, a comprehensive crisis management program had to be installed to reduce costs and increase short-term revenues. Second, a long-term strategic plan had to be developed that would position the organization for successful penetration of future markets. In his presentation to the board, Charles laid out the following recommendations.

Crisis Management: The Rosemont would enter into a management contract with TM, Inc. for a nine-month period at a base rate of $25,000 a month. TM would be responsible only to the board, it would appoint a CEO for the length of the contract, and Charles would be appointed to the board.

Strategic Plan: At the conclusion of the nine-month contract, TM would provide the board with a five-year plan and strategic recommendations. At the end of the contract period, TM reserved the right to purchase 13 percent of The Rosemont stock at the fair market price on the day the contract was signed. Any future contracts with TM would be negotiated at the appropriate times.

Response from the Board

The response from the board was mixed. Some members felt that spending the additional $25,000 a month would just put the organization further in the hole. Others were unhappy with the stock option component of the contract. Lloyd was very unhappy about the TM-appointed CEO and the fact that the consultants would not be reporting to him. Although Cates was Lloyd's brother and the financial backer of the venture, he was the only "outsider." The remaining six board members included Lloyd and friends of Lloyd. Relationships ranged from "golfing buddy" to business partner in other ventures. One of the board's members was a retired judge whose participation on the board was not based on his legal expertise but rather his golf connections. He was a member of several local high-end country clubs and was viewed as "Mr. Network" among his peers. Two board members were partners in the accounting firm that audited The Rosemont's books, one board member owned several businesses that provided various nonmedical supplies to The Rosemont and one member was a recovering alcoholic whose only apparent qualification was that he was a product of The Rosemont program and played golf with Lloyd two days a week. Acquisition of 13 percent of outstanding stock would make TM the second largest stock holder and certainly shift the balance of power on the board.

Although there was a considerable amount of discussion over the merits of the proposal, the board realized that Cates had decided that he wanted TM. The bank was ready to call in its loans of approximately $4 million and the assessed market value of the organization was at best $2.5 million; therefore, liquidation was not a feasible alternative. The Rosemont had to be turned around!

TM's Challenge

With contract in hand, Charles began the process for turning The Rosemont around. His first task was to find a CEO with health care and crisis management experience. Matthew Ibrahim immediately came to mind. As a consultant Matthew had a limited amount of experience in managing a behavioral hospital, but he had a wealth of experience in managing group practices in financial distress. Matthew was currently available to take on the assignment and was immediately hired as the contract CEO.

After spending a week at The Rosemont, Matthew reported to Charles, "My time will be totally devoted to two tasks: one, improving the organization's efficiency to ensure a positive cash flow; and, two, improving employee morale." He continued, "Although improving the efficiency of The Rosemont is critical to the viability of the organization, I realize that the organization's long-run success will be determined by its ability to generate revenue. The Rosemont needs a marketing plan. We need a plan that will generate immediate revenues to bail the organization out of its current financial distress. Then we need to strategically position the organization for long-term success. I'd like to bring in DDN Marketing Systems. What do you think?"

DDN Marketing Systems was a database marketing group that had worked with TM on several previous projects and was highly regarded by Charles Brown. Charles readily agreed to subcontracting the marketing functions to DDN Marketing Systems.

All of the necessary expertise was now available to help The Rosemont. Given the precarious financial position the organization was in, Charles gave Matthew and DDN Marketing Systems a short lead time to recommend changes. Charles said, "I want a report identifying the major problems that have to be corrected and recommendations for correcting those problems within six weeks."

With this deadline in mind, Charles asked Lloyd to set up a board meeting in seven weeks. Charles thought to himself, "Although my company is empowered to make all of the operating decisions to immediately 'stop the bleeding' at The Rosemont, I think it's imperative that the board has a comprehensive analysis as soon as possible. The better informed the board is, the more willing it will be to bite the bullet when it's necessary."

The Rosemont's Organizational Structure

The Rosemont–Jackson had 100 beds and served mostly adult patients who primarily had problems with drug and alcohol abuse. Management staff at the Jackson facility included a chief operating officer (COO), a comptroller, a chief of nursing, a chief of patient support services, and an administrative coordinator. Support staff included patient care staff sufficient for the current patient population that fluctuated between 20 and 25 percent occupancy; and an administrative staff sufficient for full occupancy. Average reimbursement per patient day was $250. Approximately 95 percent of Rosemont–Jackson's revenues were generated by inpatients.

The Rosemont–Bay Saint Louis had 50 beds and served mostly adolescents who had problems primarily with drug and alcohol abuse. Its management staff included a COO, a chief of nursing, a chief of patient support services, and an administrative coordinator. Rosemont–Bay Saint Louis's support staff was short three nurses. However, the administrative staff was sufficient. Similar to Rosemont–Jackson, it had a reimbursement rate of about $250 per day and nearly 93 percent of its revenues were generated by inpatients.

At Bay Saint Louis there was leased office space for corporate staff including the executive offices. Corporate staff was responsible for overseeing corporate strategies and handling accounting and financial activities as well as corporate-level marketing. Management staff there included the chief financial officer, the chief executive officer, the marketing director, the accounting staff, and secretaries.

After several weeks' involvement with his management audit, Matthew faxed a memo to Charles (see Exhibit 10/1).

Within a day of receiving Matthew's communication, Charles received a fax from DDN Marketing Systems providing its analysis of The Rosemont (see Exhibit 10/2).

Decision Time at The Rosemont

With reports from Matthew and DDN in hand, Charles called a meeting of the board to decide what actions needed to be undertaken. Actually Charles knew what had to be done but he wanted the board's participation so that they would buy into the significant changes that were necessary. The organization was currently expending $60,000 a month more than it was bringing in and the bank was getting very concerned. Making all the necessary changes was not going to be accomplished in one session. In fact, Charles decided to hold a series of weekly meetings designed to incrementally move the board along to a desired end result. Of immediate concern was maintaining the organization as an ongoing entity – there was a list of short-term "action points" that had to be implemented immediately if the organization was going to stay afloat. If his change strategy worked correctly the board would "discover" these action points during the meetings.

Obviously the first step was to stop the bleeding and create a positive cash flow for The Rosemont. Unless the organization developed a long-term strategy that was responsive to the changing behavioral health market in the new millennium, the organization was doomed.

Exhibit 10/1: Memo to Charles Brown from Matthew Ibrahim

Date:	3/22/99
To:	Charles Brown
From:	Matthew Ibrahim
Re:	Audit Update

Charles, I have spent a considerable amount of time looking at the organizational structure of The Rosemont and believe that some basic restructuring could save the organization a significant amount of money. The Rosemont is divided into three interdependent but separate facilities. The Jackson and Bay Saint Louis facilities both see patients with similar medical problems, however the Bay Saint Louis facility predominantly attends to the needs of adolescents whereas the bulk of Jackson's patients are adult. In Bay Saint Louis there are executive offices and corporate staff that are housed independent of the treatment facility. The total cost of maintaining the executive offices and staff is approximately $40,000 to $60,000 per month which is about one-third of The Rosemont's total staffing budget. Jackson inputs all of its financial transactions, sends the source documents to the corporate offices to be reentered, and the corporate offices cut checks as appropriate. Essentially the same process holds true for the Bay Saint Louis facility. The Jackson and Bay Saint Louis computer systems are not compatible. As you know, both facilities are producing more expenses than revenues but in all fairness, you should know that the Jackson facility is being charged for all of the corporate expenses. The Jackson facility has a very competent comptroller.

All of the financial transactions for the Bay Saint Louis facility are being handled by the corporate staff. In fact, in an interview with the COO of Bay Saint Louis, I discovered that he has difficulty getting financial statements out of the corporate office. Most often he is merely told how far his facility is in the hole. The corporate offices house the CEO, marketing director, chief financial officer (the past CFO is still driving a Rosemont-leased vehicle and he's been gone for 12 months), two accounting staff, and two secretaries. Although marketing activities are approved at the corporate level, all "hands on marketing" is done by personnel at each facility. Financial information is housed at the corporate offices and is reluctantly shared with the management of the two patient care facilities. In fact, the administrators at both facilities do not have the required information on revenues or expenses that are necessary to effectively operate the facilities.

For an organization of this size, I feel that it is overkill to have corporate officers and operating officers. Do we need systems at both facilities and the corporate offices? Do we need a corporate finance and marketing position when we have people at both facilities handling these functions on a day-to-day basis?

Listed below are concerns that I have uncovered that require immediate action. Please do not assume that this list addresses all of the organization's problems, just the most immediate. Your recommendations and guidelines would be appreciated.

Concerns Requiring Immediate Action

1. Of immediate concern: telephone personnel are not closing the sale when prospective clients call either institution. Information is provided and personnel "suggest" that the caller come in for help but that is the extent of the effort!
2. Although commissioned referral agents have been effective in channeling patients to the Jackson facility, there are no contractual arrangements with commissioned referral agents at Bay Saint Louis.
3. Salary rates for Bay Saint Louis are below community norms.
4. Salaries for staff have been cut at both facilities and morale is low.
5. There is a general lack of financial information available to all of the management staff.
6. Because of a computer problem, Bay Saint Louis did not bill patients for a six-month period. At this point in time I estimate that less than 30 percent of total accounts receivable are collectable.
7. Managed care contracts are out of date for both facilities – many contracts have expired and fee schedules are old.
8. The recent Medicare Survey for the Bay Saint Louis facility suggests major changes have to be initiated. One building would not have passed inspection as a hospital. Luckily it was surveyed as business offices. We may not be that lucky next time. The other two buildings were only approved for the ground floor so the second floor cannot be used. Medicare indicated that in order to qualify for a contract we would need to spend in excess of $50,000 on renovations.
9. Patient furniture at the Bay Saint Louis facility is totally inadequate and most of the patient furniture at the Jackson facility will need to be replaced soon.
10. Checks and cash for services are being received in a multiple of locations.
11. The two facilities are using two different pre-certification and authorization forms.
12. Bill verification is not consistent between the two facilities.
13. At Bay Saint Louis patients are being carried on the census unless they have not been seen in 30 days – inflating its census significantly.
14. Bay Saint Louis is not validating the length of stay (LOS) with insurors to determine patient coverage.
15. Self-pay patients at Bay Saint Louis are really "no pay" patients.
16. No company-wide purchasing system or cost containment policy has been developed.
17. No uniform policy for petty cash between institutions has been established.
18. No uniform policy for accounts payable has been established.
19. No uniform policy for purchasing services has been established. This has resulted in significant price variances between the two facilities.
20. Medicaid contracts are far too slow in developing.
21. At least 25 percent of accounts payable are drastically in arrears.
22. Company-wide telephone services are too complicated and expensive. We have several different carriers and packages.
23. No criteria have been established concerning the need for cellular phones and personal calls are being paid for by the company.
24. Review of housekeeping costs for staffing, materials, and equipment suggests consideration of outsourcing this function.
25. Having clinical directors at both facilities seems redundant.
26. Having a director of nursing at both facilities seems redundant.
27. Jackson uses independent marketing contractors but Bay Saint Louis does not.
28. Although both facilities are part of the same organization, they operate as two separate entities with key management personnel failing to communicate.

Finally, I have to comment on the current and future financial position of the organization. With the limited, questionable, and poorly organized financial data available to me, I have determined a few expenses about which there is no question. We owe interest payments of $30,000 per month and insurance, payroll taxes, and automobile leases are $95,000 per month. It appears to me that well over one-half of our costs are fixed.

Exhibit 10/2: Memo from DDN Marketing to Charles Brown

Date: 3/23/99
To: Charles Brown
From: DDN Marketing Systems
Re: Marketing Audit

Charles, I have conducted a comprehensive audit of the marketing needs of The Rosemont. Attached is a report for your consideration. Please advise me as to where you would like to go from here.

Joshua

Marketing Background, Audit, and Strategy

Background

As a backdrop for repositioning the Company in the health care marketplace and to help establish the current trends, foibles, and reactions in the industry, a review of the big four in psychiatric centers was used to evaluate the market segment that the Company operates within. They are:

- Charter Medical
- National Medical Enterprises
- Community Psychiatric Centers
- Hospital Corporation of America

Although each has undergone various forms of reorganization, financial restructuring, etc. they seem to be surviving. It's also evident that they are not blowing away the market financially. Margins seem to be very tight. The only companies that appear to be making money in health care right now are the corporate acquisition oriented groups, which should be short lived.

There is little doubt that there has been a significant drop in demand for psychiatric services. The number of free-standing clinics is dropping at a rate of 6 percent a year. Profits are shrinking and ALOS is down virtually everywhere; also, many are experiencing public relations problems.

All of the large psychiatric chains are struggling financially because of managed care. Examples include:

- Community Psychiatric Centers, one of the big four, took a restructuring charge of $843,000 and a net operating loss of $1.3 million last year.
- Charter Medical Corp. emerged from bankruptcy in the early 1990s with $1.1 billion in debt.
- Last year four of the top five psychiatric chains experienced an 8 percent decline in patient days.
- A recent survey of 434 free-standing psychiatric hospitals found that patient revenues fell by 9.1 percent.
- Sandy Lutz, who writes extensively on psychiatric care for *Modern Health Care* contends that managed care is a far heavier influence on psychiatric hospitals than on acute care hospitals.
- About 70 percent of the largest companies in the United States offer employee assistance programs. General Motors has found that for every $1 spent on alcohol abuse treatment, it gains $3 in productivity.

A nationwide survey of mental health providers, insurors, employers, and others sought to find strategies that would work in this era of falling inpatient days, tighter cost controls, and greater demands

Exhibit 10/2: *(cont'd)*

for accountability. The survey found no clearly successful responses to the negative forces currently facing the industry. It did discover six common suggestions from the respondents:

- Aggressive inpatient utilization management: particular emphasis was placed on recognizing that the one paying the bills cannot be snubbed!
- Leverage strengths and tailor services to meet local markets.
- Market face-to-face with the true referral sources.
- Create a distinct organizational structure for outpatient services.
- Closely monitor program profitability.
- Implement responsive information systems.

Mac Crawford, president and CEO of Charter Medical Corporation, went one step further. Crawford stated that partnerships must be formed to survive and that Charter would initiate a major effort to form relationships with not-for-profit systems. In addition, Charter Medical Corporation initiated an aggressive vertical integration strategy by acquiring psychiatric group practices and other health professional practices.

McClean Hospital outside Boston demonstrates the changes and problems facing the industry. McClean is known nationally as an outstanding provider of inpatient treatment and has been the institution of choice for many well-known individuals. Because of managed care, it is now seeing much shorter lengths of stay. An average treatment unit historically would serve 90 patients a year. Now, in order to generate the same revenue, a unit is serving 500 patients a year.

To address these industry changes, McClean developed its Clinical Evaluation Center that is rapidly becoming a national model. The Clinical Evaluation Center is the entry point for patients in a continuum of care that emphasizes short-term stays and outpatient programs. Patients are evaluated by a team of medical specialists to determine the most appropriate treatment modality for them.

Intervention may range from outpatient services to residential services to inpatient services in a traditional hospital environment. Regardless of the modality selected it is obvious that the current trend is toward very short inpatient stays – as little as 24 hours for detoxification of the patient. Outpatient group and individual therapy sessions can range from 3 to 12 months depending on the individual and the type of addiction.

Although a 28-day inpatient stay was the norm for alcohol abuse up until the early 1990s it is now virtually impossible to get a 28-day inpatient stay funded. Although the numbers vary by institution, average length of stay for the typical behavioral health center has declined by 75 percent in the late 1990s and it appears that it will continue to decline in the new millennium.

Independent Audit

A marketing audit of Rosemont–Jackson and Rosemont–Bay Saint Louis was conducted on September 19th and 20th. The following analysis and recommendations are based on extensive interviews with key personnel at both facilities, an examination of marketing documents, and a general review of patient distribution at both facilities.

Although there is strong recognition of the need for extensive marketing at both facilities, most of the current marketing efforts are informal, appear to lack a strategic focus, and are reactive rather than proactive. The primary marketing tool utilized at both facilities involves networking. Although networking is a valid marketing strategy for all organizations (particularly small organizations) it should not be viewed as an exclusive strategy but, rather, incorporated into a planned mix of strategies. In addition, current networks may not be maximizing referrals, nor providing a patient mix that maximizes revenues.

Exhibit 10/2: (cont'd)

To maximize revenues there must be a mix of inpatient and outpatient services reimbursed by Medicare, Medicaid, and private pay insurors. Currently 90 percent of Rosemont–Jackson's patients are funded by Medicare and Medicaid. The remaining 10 percent of our patients are private pay or young people covered by contracts with local school systems. A major school system contract is up for renegotiation next month and I'm not sure if The Rosemont will win the award.

Our problem with low occupancy (20–25 percent) will be magnified but the trend is toward shorter stays in the coming years. In fact with the emphasis on shorter inpatient stays and more outpatient therapy sessions for both adults and adolescents, The Rosemont is going to have to increase its patient load threefold over the next two years.

Although the marketing audit did not focus on a financial analysis of the Company, it is difficult to evaluate the effectiveness of an organization's marketing efforts without evaluating the financial consequences of those efforts. A review of the financial information available suggests that there have been insufficient controls in place to allow one to compare revenue generation with marketing expenses.

One might infer from the patient mix that current marketing efforts have resulted in a skewed patient base weighted heavily toward beneficiaries of various social programs – particularly Medicaid. Obviously being a "Medicaid facility" does not produce the strongest revenue flow! Although there are a number of managed care contracts in place, patient distribution does not reflect a balanced demand schedule across payors. There is a loose leaf binder filled with managed care contracts and employer contracts, but the institution is currently not getting enough patients from these two sources to bother counting. It appears that somewhere along the line someone made an attempt to market The Rosemont to area employers and area managed care companies; however, there has been no follow-up, no effort to build referrals from physicians associated with these two sources, and in general a total lack of effort. One could not "guesstimate" the potential revenues from these contracts because they are out of date and it appears that the negotiated prices were based strictly on individual communication. The difference for an uncomplicated alcohol abuse treatment plan between managed care organizations ranges as much as 150 percent. Which pricing structure represents a careful analysis of actual costs is anyone's guess. Since managed care penetration has grown from 10 percent to 40 percent in the Jackson market over the past five years and Jackson is a leading industrial center in the state, these two sources of patients – managed care and business contracts – are critical to the organization's long-run success.

The physical facilities at both locations are not conducive to attracting insured and self-pay patients. One might argue that regardless of the marketing efforts of the company, its ability to penetrate nongovernment supported markets is going to be severely limited by its physical facilities. Because the Jackson facility represents a significant fixed asset for the organization, efforts should be undertaken to renovate it to accommodate the insured market or sell it and move to better facilities.

The treatment protocols for mental health and substance abuse are changing dramatically. Cost-driven decision-making is continuously pressuring health care providers to: (1) reduce average LOS; and, (2) shift more and more care to an outpatient basis. Interviews with key personnel at both facilities demonstrated keen insight into these changing trends but a lack of marketing focus to accommodate these trends is inhibiting the organization's ability to strategically position itself to target tomorrow's market. Although outsourcing marketing to independent marketing contractors has been quite beneficial for the Jackson location, it should be recognized that these referrals are primarily inpatient stays. Obviously, with a 100-bed facility, inpatient admissions are critical and there must be an ongoing effort to increase inpatient admissions; however, the future growth market in both mental health and substance abuse is in the outpatient arena.

Exhibit 10/2: (cont'd)

The Rosemont's Admissions

1. A physician may refer his or her patients. This accounts for about 20 percent of our patient population. The Medical Director of Rosemont–Jackson is well known and well respected, so this number should be considerably higher.
2. A patient learns of the facility from a friend, counselor, phone book, etc. and puts in a call for help. The patient is advised to come in, is evaluated by our Medical Director and admitted. This mechanism represents about another 20 to 25 percent of our patient admissions. A major problem here is that no one knows how many patients are lost; that is, they call but never come in.
3. Independent Marketing Contractors channel patients to the institution. There are numerous types of contractors and I will be happy to discuss them with you on a one-to-one basis but suffice it to say that at this time one independent marketing contractor accounts for over 20 percent of Rosemont's patient admissions and nearly all of them are funded by Medicare or Medicaid.
4. The remaining patients are mostly referred by state agencies, school counselors, and a sundry of other behavioral health care professionals.

Once again, very few of these patients are channeled from managed care organizations, individual employers, or other third-party payors.

The Company should immediately implement an ambulatory Detox care program. This strategy would accommodate two issues currently confronting the organization: (1) poor physical facilities, and (2) skewed patient mix. An ambulatory program should be initiated and targeted toward individuals requiring intervention but not inclined to stay at either of the Company's facilities and individuals who view the opportunity cost of an inpatient stay as exceeding the benefit. Interviews with key personnel suggest both the ability and interest in initiating an ambulatory care program. Although a competitive profile for both locations is in the development stage, it appears that the Company can develop a distinct competency that will allow it to differentiate itself from the competition should it choose to develop an ambulatory care program.

On-Site Evaluation

To evaluate the effectiveness of the Company's marketing efforts and identify areas for improvement, twelve specific questions were addressed. Each of these questions, along with our observations is provided.

Does the Organization Have a Marketing Department/Division?

Technically, the Company has a marketing department with several positions identified. The individuals filling these positions are responsible for virtually all of the marketing decisions for the organization. Although the efforts of the marketing group appear to be extensive, they are accomplished in a very loose structure and driven by informal communication among key personnel. There does not appear to be a clean division of responsibilities; for instance, an identified position responsible for mass media communication, direct mail, and telemarketing, and another designated for public relations, contract negotiations, etc. As a result, there appears to be some overlap of duties and responsibilities in some areas with voids in others. For example, Public Relations appears to be limited to participation in various groups, attendance at major functions, and one-on-one communication with key people in the community. However, organized efforts to ensure regular press releases, media coverage of innovative programs, etc. are nonexistent. The Jackson location recently solidified a relationship with a noted psychiatrist in the area to become its full-time Medical Director. There was no coverage in

Exhibit 10/2: (cont'd)

the local press. Efforts to stimulate demand through independent marketing contractors have been successful and should be continued. A recommendation for the continuation of this strategy is provided in the recommendations section.

Does the Organization Have Clear Marketing Goals?

Key personnel at neither facility were able to identify formal marketing goals for the Company. These goals may exist somewhere but they have not been communicated to those individuals who have the operational responsibility to implement them. Through interviews, it was evident that many individuals had informally identified a strategic direction for the Company, but there was no formal comprehensive focus directing the marketing efforts of the organization. Without some fundamental quantifiable goals it is very difficult for management to evaluate the efficacy of various marketing strategies or evaluate performance. For example, how does one evaluate the performance of the satellite programs without baseline criteria to measure against?

Does the Organization Have a Marketing Plan?

Market penetration and market development appears to be reactive, based on opportunity. Although opportunity should be a driving force in decision making, planned opportunity generally results in higher levels of success than spontaneous opportunity.

Does the Organization Have Clearly Defined Marketing Strategies?

In some areas marketing strategies are clearly defined although in others it appears that insufficient attention is paid to the relationship of specific strategies to specific outcomes. The strategy of utilizing independent marketing contractors to stimulate admissions is quantifiable and relatively easy to track. The Community Service Workshop Series is an excellent vehicle to build bridges with the referring community. However, it is difficult to measure the effectiveness of extensive networking with demand. Intuitively, one might logically argue that this strategy yields recognition for the Company throughout the community, but the current database system does not allow one to determine a cost/benefit relationship.

Is the Current Database System Market Oriented?

There is sufficient data being generated by both facilities concerning their captured market to generate effective marketing decisions. However, little information is being formally generated. There is no evidence of any formal market research being conducted which would provide the organization with the information necessary to develop strategies for capturing new markets or evaluating the attitudes/perceptions of the environment toward the company. All of the operating managers interviewed were universally unfamiliar with any financial information concerning the company. Although this is a problem of huge proportion, it is currently being rectified and managers will be provided with the financial information necessary to accomplish their jobs.

Does the Organization Maintain Clearly Defined Linkages with Potential Referring Physicians?

Efforts are made on an individual basis to keep physicians informed about patients and "thank you" notes are sent to referring physicians. However, no established policy is in place outlining a standardized procedure. Through networking, contacts are established with physicians but little emphasis is placed on sponsoring conferences, providing luncheons, distributing promotional items, and so forth.

Exhibit 10/2: (cont'd)

Does the Organization Maintain Clearly Defined Linkages with Social Agencies?

Many of the staff conduct seminars, provide lectures, and speak to various civic and professional groups. These activities appear to be done on a spontaneous basis reacting to requests from the community. There is no formal program outlining a strategy for developing linkages with the community.

Does the Organization Have Contractual Arrangements with Medicare and Medicaid?

A substantial portion of the revenues generated by the Company are through government programs. It appears that Bay Saint Louis will be eligible for Medicare in the very near future, providing increases in revenue for that facility. Although Medicare and Medicaid are excellent sources of patients for The Rosemont, caution should be used to ensure that patient distribution is not excessively skewed.

Does the Organization Have Managed Care Contracts?

The Company has a substantial number of managed care contracts, but many of them are out of date. A casual review of the pricing structure across contracts suggests significant variations in pricing. Although there are numerous contracts, the percentage of contract patients relative to total patient admissions is quite small. There must be constant interaction between the Company and local plan managers, MSOs, and managed care companies.

A plan must be developed to target mid- and small-size businesses, emphasizing personal contacts with operating managers within these organizations. Although it is the responsibility of corporate staff to negotiate contracts, the entire organization must speak from the same sheet of paper when talking with business and industry. Currently, the chaos in financial information makes it nearly impossible to determine the break-even point for specific patient services. There is no evidence that the Company is providing services under any contract at below the break-even point, but the potential certainly exists. Because of facility limitations at both locations (insured patients want a more pleasant looking facility), an ambulatory care program may be an excellent vehicle for increasing demand among businesses.

Does the Organization Have a Comprehensive Employee Assistance Program?

An employee assistance program (EAP) is in place but has not been operationalized. The demand for EAPs is growing rapidly and no longer provides an organization with an instant distinct competency. But, a comprehensive EAP can provide an organization with a competitive advantage if developed and marketed appropriately. The Company should consider developing an EAP that emphasizes a holistic approach to substance abuse and mental health – that is, counseling, education, and when necessary, treatment. Once again, emphasis should be placed on the mid- to small-size businesses. Many large organizations provide an in-house employee assistant program with full-time professionals employed by the company but it is rare to find an organization with 250 or fewer employees doing so. With some marketing efforts on The Rosemont's part, I see no reason why it cannot contract with multiple businesses in the area to provide these services.

Does the Organization Have a Distinct Competency That Differentiates It from Its Competitors?

When asked this question, employees consistently referred to quality as the company's distinct competency. Although quality may be the organization's distinct competency, the inadequacy of its physical facilities are contradictory to a quality image. For the Bay Saint Louis location, it appears that the company has a strong niche in adolescent care. Additional emphasis should be placed on

Exhibit 10/2: (cont'd)

capitalizing on this niche throughout the state and relationships should be developed with independent marketing contractors specializing in adolescent care.

Is the Organization Strategically Positioned to Respond to Increases in Outpatient and Decreases in Inpatient Services?

Programs and facilities must be developed to maximize on the trend toward outpatient care. It is not suggested that inpatient services be abandoned, but it is suggested that a balance must be obtained.

Assuming that quality is a distinct competency of the Company and recognizing the limitations of the physical facilities, one might make a strong argument that increases in outpatient services are a key to improving the *short-run* as well as the *long-run* financial health of the organization.

11

Riverview Regional Medical Center: An HMA Facility

Matt Hayes, executive director of Riverview Regional Medical Center (RRMC), reviewed the performance indicators for the 2004 fiscal year (see Exhibit 11/1). As he studied the numbers, he mentally reviewed key events and decisions over the past year that had contributed to some of the more dramatic changes in the annual profile. And, he considered what new challenges might confront him now that his chief competitor, Gadsden Regional Medical Center (GRMC), had a new executive director who would almost certainly attempt to alter the status quo in the local hospital market.

Health Care Providers

In 1993, Merrill Lynch predicted: "In the larger urban areas, HMOs would . . . continue to be the coordinator and provider of health care services. However, in nonurban markets, the hospital would be the cornerstone and coordinator of health care services for the health alliance purchasing cooperatives which would be formed under managed competition proposals."

At the individual provider level, some experts insisted that the financial power base was moving away from solo practices and independent small groups toward integrated, cost-competitive,

This case was written by Woodrow D. Richardson, Ball State University, and Donna J. Slovensky, The University of Alabama at Birmingham. It is intended to be used as a basis for class discussion rather than to illustrate either effective or ineffective handling of an administrative situation. Used with permission of Woody Richardson and Donna Slovensky.

Exhibit 11/1: RRMC Key Volume Indicators, FY 2002–FY 2004

Indicator	FY 2002	FY 2003	FY 2004
Open Heart	324	330	199
Cardiac Catheterization	7,661	9,704	6,548
Coronary Stents	942	1,420	795
Inpatient Endoscopy	1,300	1,360	1,227
Outpatient Endoscopy	2,354	2,263	2,283
Inpatient Surgery	2,922	2,873	2,068
Outpatient Surgery	3,047	2,806	3,301
Inpatient CT Scans	4,685	4,309	4,099
Outpatient CT Scans	6,087	5,753	6,440
Inpatient MRI	826	805	1,165
Outpatient MRI	2,915	2,534	2,434
Outpatient Visits	61,865	55,340	51,736
Births	887	433	0
Inpatient Admissions	10,530	9,710	8,482
Inpatient Admissions Via ER	5,527	5,253	5,011
ER Visits	25,452	24,764	24,347
Medicare Discharges	5,736	5,646	5,308
Medicare ALOS	6.28	6.33	6.2
Medicare Case Mix Index	1.53	1.62	1.46

comprehensive systems that produced a single patient bill including the charges of the physicians, the hospital, and the outpatient services. Integrated systems required a corporate structure to facilitate sharing of capitated risk. Throughout the 1990s, mergers and other types of strategic alliances between physicians' practices, and between hospitals and physicians' practices, had increased in an effort to reduce costs and become price competitive. Small group practices often lacked the administrative and management expertise as well as the material resources necessary to improve efficiency. They were advised to look for such capabilities when they sought potential partners.

Many physicians remained skeptical of mergers, partnerships, or alliances offering any competitive advantage. That skepticism occurred most often in areas where managed care was absent or limited. Exhibit 11/2 shows the penetration of managed care in selected southern states.

Rural and Nonurban Health Care Market

Forty-nine percent of the United States population resided in counties classified as rural or nonurban. Nonurban areas had 44 percent fewer doctors per 100,000 residents than urban-designated areas. Since 1981, more than 200 nonurban hospitals had closed. Many hospitals continued to underperform and were failing because of ineffective operations.[1]

Exhibit 11/2: HMO Penetration in Selected States

State	Percentage
Alabama	3.8
Florida	26.0
Georgia	13.4
Texas	12.8
California (reference point)	48.5

Source: InterStudy Staff, *The InterStudy Competitive Edge, Part II: Managed Care Industry Report* (St. Paul, MN: InterStudy, 2003). Data abstracted from: http://www.medicarehmo.com/mcmnu.htm, accessed September 20, 2004.

Rural and nonurban hospitals had become hot acquisition targets for investor-owned health care companies. For the nation's 2,400 rural hospitals – acute care facilities located outside of a metropolitan statistical area – the status quo was not acceptable.[2] Hospitals that chose to remain independent faced an uncertain environment where 60 percent to 75 percent of revenues were attributed to Medicare. Threatened by the prospect of declining federal reimbursement coupled with the lack of resources to invest in costly information systems, many local governments that owned rural and nonurban hospitals were looking for a way out.[3]

When it came to the inverted "field of dreams" logic used by small hospitals in the past, no other firm had been as successful as Health Management Associates, Inc., according to chairman of the board, William Schoen. "Whereas other hospitals [think], 'We are here and you will come,' we're in the customer service business," Schoen said.

Health Management Associates (HMA)

HMA was ahead of the growing throng of firms targeting rural and nonurban markets where the presence of managed care was less intense and where physicians perceived good opportunities. HMA generally employed a decentralized approach; operations were left to the executive directors of each hospital. Only financial controls were centralized. Founded in 1977, HMA acquired, improved, and operated hospitals in high-growth, nonurban areas in the Southeast and Southwest, where the growing population created a need for comprehensive health care services. HMA sought to turn around nonurban hospitals in growing communities with populations of 30,000 to 400,000 with a clear demographic need. The company looked for states with certificate of need (CON) regulations and an established physician base. Using a proven acquisition and management strategy, HMA consistently turned hospitals into efficient, state-of-the-art medical facilities that provided high-quality care. From 1991 to 2004, HMA acquired 38 hospitals, bringing its total count to 53 hospitals in 16 states. William Schoen, HMA chairman of the board, and Joseph Vumbacco, president and CEO, saw no shortage of acquisition prospects. Cost pressures coupled with inadequate coping resources would continue to affect many community hospitals adversely.

In 2003, HMA had a net income of $283.4 million on net patient service revenues of $2.56 billion. The company showed consistent growth from 1999, when net income was $150 million and revenues were $1.36 billion. Admissions rose 8.9 percent to more than 235,000 in 2003. Patient days and emergency room visits grew in 2003 to 1.1 million and to 914,000 respectively. Revenues of hospitals operated for at least 12 months grew by 7.9 percent over the year ended in 2003. Admissions for these hospitals were up 2.9 percent, and ER visits were up by 5.1 percent. Correspondingly, the hospitals' occupancy levels grew to 47.7 percent in 2003 versus 47.1 percent in 2002.

HMA had a small corporate overhead. The company employed about 100 people in its Naples, Florida, corporate office. Exhibit 11/3 provides information on the corporate officers' backgrounds.

Exhibit 11/3: HMA Board of Directors' Background Information

Name	Position	Year Elected
William J. Schoen	Chairman of the Board, Health Management Associates, Inc.	1983
Kent P. Dauten	President, Keystone Capital, Inc.	1981
Robert A. Knox	Senior Managing Director, Cornerstone Equity Investors, LLC	1985
Charles R. Lees	Director Emeritus, KPMG Peat Marwick LLP (retired)	1988
William E. Mayberry, MD	President and Chairman of the Board of Governors (retired), Mayo Clinic	1991
Randolph W. Westerfield, PhD	Dean, Marshall School of Business, University of Southern California	1982
Joseph V. Vumbacco	President and Chief Executive Officer, Health Management Associates, Inc.	1985
Donald E. Kiernan	Senior Executive Vice President and Chief Financial Officer (retired), SBC Communications, Inc.	1982
William C. Steere, Jr.	Chairman Emeritus of Pfizer, Inc.	1983

William J. Schoen served as Chairman of the Board since April 1986. He was first elected a director in February 1983, became President and Chief Operating Officer in December 1983, Co-Chief Executive Officer in December 1985, and Chief Executive Officer in April 1986. He served as President until April 1997 and Chief Executive Officer until January 2001. From 1982 to 1987, Mr. Schoen was Chairman of Commerce National Bank, Naples, Florida, and from 1973 to 1981 he was President, Chief Operating Officer, and Chief Executive Officer of The F&M Schaefer Corporation, a consumer products company. From 1971 to 1973, Mr. Schoen was President of the Pierce Glass subsidiary of Indian Head, Inc., a diversified company.

Kent P. Dauten served as a Director from March 1981 through May 1983, and from June 1985 through September 1988. He was again elected a Director in November 1988. Since February 1994, Mr. Dauten has been President of Keystone Capital, Inc., a private investment advisory firm he founded.

Exhibit 11/3: (cont'd)

Mr. Dauten was formerly a Senior Vice President of Madison Dearborn Partners, Inc., a private equity investment firm, and of First Chicago Investment Corporation and First Capital Corporation of Chicago, the venture capital subsidiaries of First Chicago Corporation, where he had been employed in various investment management positions since 1979.

Robert A. Knox became Senior Managing Director of Cornerstone Equity Investors, LLC, an investment advisory firm, in December 1996. From 1994 until December 1996, he was Chairman and Chief Executive Officer, and from 1984 to 1994 he was President, of Prudential Equity Investors, Inc., an investment capital firm. Prior to that, Mr. Knox was an investment executive of The Prudential Insurance Company of America. He served on HMA's Board of Directors since 1985.

Charles R. Lees was elected a Director in February 1989. Mr. Lees has been in the private practice of law, concentrating in tax matters, since May 1985. He was a Project Director for the Governor's Tax Reform Advisory Commission in California from August 1984 to September 1985. From 1979 to 1983 he was a visiting professor at the School of Accounting, University of Southern California. For more than 20 years prior to his retirement in 1979, Mr. Lees was a partner in the accounting firm of Peat, Marwick, Mitchell & Co., specializing in tax matters.

William E. Mayberry, MD was the retired President and Chief Executive Officer of the Mayo Foundation and the retired Chairman of the Board of Governors of the Mayo Clinic, Rochester, Minnesota, where he had been employed in various capacities from 1956 until his retirement in 1992.

Randolph W. Westerfield, PhD served as Dean, the Marshall School of Business, University of Southern California, Los Angeles, California, since 1993. For the previous 20 years he was a member of the finance faculty at the Wharton School of Business at the University of Pennsylvania. In addition, Dr. Westerfield served on the Board of Directors of William Lyon Homes and Nicolas Applegate Growth Equity Fund.

Joseph V. Vumbacco became Chief Executive Officer of the company in January 2001. Prior to that, and since April 1997, he was the Company's President, as well as serving as Chief Administrative Officer and Chief Operating Officer. He joined the company as an Executive Vice President in January 1996 after 14 years with The Turner Corporation (construction and real estate), most recently as an Executive Vice President. Prior to joining Turner, he served as the Senior Vice President and General Counsel for The F&M Schaefer Corporation, and previously was an attorney with the Manhattan law firm of Mudge, Rose, Guthrie & Alexander.

Donald E. Kiernan was the retired Senior Executive Vice President and Chief Financial Officer of SBC Communications Inc. (telecommunications), a position he held from October 1993 to August 2001. Prior to that, and since 1990, he served as Vice President of Finance for SBC Communications Inc. Mr. Kiernan was a Certified Public Accountant and former partner with Arthur Young & Company. Mr. Kiernan served on the Boards of Directors of Horace Mann Educators Corporation, LaBranche & Co Inc., Seagate Technology, and Viad Corp.

William C. Steere served as a director of the company since May 2003. He was the Chairman Emeritus of Pfizer Inc. since July 2001, a Director since 1987, and was Chairman of the Board from 1992 to April 2001 and Chief Executive Officer from February 1991 to December 2000. Mr. Steere served on the Board of Directors of Dow Jones & Company, Inc., MetLife, Inc., the New York University Medical Center, and The New York Botanical Garden, as well as on the Board of Overseers of Memorial Sloan-Kettering Cancer Center.

Source: Company documents.

Corporate Philosophy and Mission

HMA's Statement of Corporate Philosophy defined its goals and principles as a health care provider, employer, and publicly traded company. A cornerstone of HMA's philosophy was the conviction that all employees, at every hospital and at the corporate office, shared a common objective of providing quality service to the many different customers of its business. HMA's guiding objectives were as follows:

- To provide the highest quality of service to our patients, physicians, and the communities we serve.
- To provide employees with a satisfying and rewarding work environment.
- To provide an attractive return on investment to those who are investors in the Company.
- To function as a good corporate citizen in the communities we serve.
- To manage HMA in a manner that maintains uniform strength and identity while allowing individual hospitals the degree of independence necessary to maximize innovation and efficiency and meet the individual needs of the communities they serve.

Corporate Strategy

When originally established in 1977, HMA intended to compete as a national firm owning, leasing, and managing hospitals throughout the United States. In 1983, HMA redirected its focus to a niche of hospitals located in nonurban communities in the Southeast and Southwest with 30,000 to 400,000 in population. The officers believed the very nature and size of the facilities (generally 200 beds or fewer) located in nonurban communities precluded the individual, non-system-affiliated hospitals from attracting experienced and professional medical practitioners in each area of specialty. On the other hand, they believed that through system affiliation with HMA and its concomitant infusion of capital and management expertise, the same financially troubled hospitals could become profitable.

To penetrate the niche markets, HMA executives believed it was necessary to provide management expertise and medical technology in specific areas to reduce costs, attract physicians, and increase the scope and quality of service – all within a profitable framework that would halt the out-migration of patients to larger metropolitan areas for as many surgical procedures as possible. They believed that achieving these objectives allowed the communities HMA served to forge the viable and effective health care delivery facilities that they desperately needed.

Facilities

In August 2004, HMA operated 53 facilities (see Exhibit 11/4) consisting of just under 7,000 beds. HMA hospitals offered a broad range of inpatient and outpatient health services with an emphasis on primary care. Inpatient programs at all facilities included a wide variety of medical and surgical services, diagnostic

Exhibit 11/4: HMA Facilities in 2004

Location	Hospital	Facility Type	Licensed Beds
Alabama			
Anniston	Stringfellow Memorial Hospital	General Medical/Surgical	125
Gadsden	Riverview Regional Medical Center	General Medical/Surgical	281
Arkansas			
Little Rock	Southwest Regional Medical Center	General Medical/Surgical	125
Van Buren	Crawford Memorial	General Medical/Surgical	103
Florida			
Brooksville	Brooksville Regional Hospital	General Medical/Surgical	91
Crystal River	Seven Rivers Regional Medical Center	General Medical/Surgical	128
Dade City	Pasco Regional Medical Center	General Medical/Surgical	120
Greater Haines City	Heart of Florida Regional Medical Center	General Medical/Surgical	115
Key West	Lower Keys Medical Center	General Medical/Surgical	167
Lehigh Acres	Lehigh Regional Medical Center	General Medical/Surgical	88
Marathon	Fishermen's Hospital	General Medical/Surgical	58
Milton	Santa Rosa Medical Center	General Medical/Surgical	129
Orlando	University Behavioral Center	Psychiatric	80
Punta Gorda	Charlotte Regional Medical Center	General Medical/Surgical	156
Sebastian	Sebastian River Medical Center	General Medical/Surgical	52
Sebring	Highlands Regional Medical Center	General Medical/Surgical	129
Spring Hill	Spring Hill Regional Hospital	General Medical/Surgical	126
Tequesta	Sandy Pines	Psychiatric	75
Georgia			
Monroe	Walton Regional Medical Center	General Medical/Surgical	135
Statesboro	East Georgia Regional Medical Center	General Medical/Surgical	150
Kentucky			
Paintsville	Paul B. Hall Regional Medical Center	General Medical/Surgical	72
Mississippi			
Biloxi	Biloxi Regional Medical Center	General Medical/Surgical	153
Brandon	Rankin Medical Center	General Medical/Surgical	134
Canton	Madison Regional Medical Center	General Medical/Surgical	67
Clarksdale	Northwest Mississippi Regional Medical Center	General Medical/Surgical	195

Location	Hospital	Facility Type	Licensed Beds
Jackson	River Oaks Hospital	General Medical/Surgical	110
Jackson	Women's Hospital at River Oaks	General Medical/Surgical	111
Jackson	Central Mississippi Medical Center	General Medical/Surgical	473
Meridian	Riley Hospital	General Medical/Surgical	180
Natchez	Natchez Community Hospital	General Medical/Surgical	101
Missouri			
Kennett	Twin Rivers Regional Medical Center	General Medical/Surgical	116
Poplar Bluff	Poplar Bluff Regional Medical Center – North and South	General Medical/Surgical	423
North Carolina			
Hamlet	Sandhills Regional Medical Center	General Medical/Surgical	64
Louisburg	Franklin Regional Medical Center	General Medical/Surgical	85
Mooresville	Lake Normal Regional Medical Center	General Medical/Surgical	105
Statesville	Davis Regional Medical Center	General Medical/Surgical	149
Oklahoma			
Durant	Medical Center of Southeastern Oklahoma	General Medical/Surgical	120
Midwest City	Midwest City Regional Medical Center	General Medical/Surgical	247
Pennsylvania			
Carlisle	Carlisle Regional Medical Center	General Medical/Surgical	200
Lancaster	Community Hospital of Lancaster	General Medical/Surgical	154
Lancaster	Lancaster Regional Medical Center	General Medical/Surgical	261
South Carolina			
Gaffney	Upstate Carolina Medical Center	General Medical/Surgical	125
Hartsville	Carolina Pines Regional Medical Center	General Medical/Surgical	116
Tennessee			
Jamestown	Jamestown Regional Medical Center	General Medical/Surgical	85
Lebanon	University Medical Center	General Medical/Surgical	257
Tullahoma	Harton Regional Medical Center	General Medical/Surgical	137
Texas			
Mesquite	Medical Center of Mesquite	General Medical/Surgical	176
Mesquite	Mesquite Community Hospital	General Medical/Surgical	172
Virginia			
Pennington Gap	Lee Regional Medical Center	General Medical/Surgical	80
Washington			
Yakima	Yakima Regional Medical & Heart Center	General Medical/Surgical	226
Toppenish	Toppenish Community Hospital	General Medical/Surgical	63
West Virginia			
Williamson	Williamson Memorial Hospital	General Medical/Surgical	76

Source: Company documents.

services, intensive and cardiac care, plus emergency services that were staffed by physicians at all times. At various facilities, other specialty services, such as full-service obstetrics, oncology, and industrial medicine, were available. In addition, HMA operated two free-standing psychiatric hospitals.

Selected Financial Data and Operating Statistics

In 2004, HMA had a net income of $325 million on net patient service revenues of $3.2 billion and had shown consistent growth from 1999, when net income was $150 million and revenues were $1.36 billion. Total admissions rose 20.9 percent over fiscal year 2004, reflecting the admission contributions from hospitals acquired during the year. Patient days grew to 1.28 million in fiscal year 2004. Net patient revenues of hospitals that operated for at least 12 months increased by 3.7 percent during the fourth quarter of fiscal year 2004. Exhibit 11/5 shows the income statement and balance sheet for HMA.

Exhibit 11/5: Health Management Associates, Inc. Consolidated Statements of Income and Balance Sheets (in $ thousands, except per share data)

	Years ended September 30			
	2001	2002	2003	2004
Net Patient Service Revenue	1,879,801	2,262,601	2,560,576	3,205,885
Costs and Expenses:				
Salaries and Benefits	710,535	874,729	989,075	1,259,859
Supplies	535,926	650,852	741,487	956,891
Provision for Doubtful Accounts	143,923	172,430	186,826	240,074
Depreciation and Amortization	90,646	95,328	109,864	134,915
Rent Expense	40,850	47,048	50,401	65,766
Interest, Net	19,970	15,543	14,915	16,184
Write-off of Deferred Financing Costs	—	—	4,931	—
Noncash Charge for Retirement Benefits and Write-Down of Assets Held for Sale	17,000	—	—	—
Total Costs and Expenses	1,558,850	1,855,930	2,097,499	2,673,689
Income Before Minority Interests and Income Taxes	320,951	406,671	463,077	532,196
Minority Interests in Earnings of Consolidated Entities	—	1,009	4,341	5,716
Income Before Income Taxes	320,951	405,662	458,736	526,480
Provision for Income Taxes	125,973	159,226	175,312	201,381
Net Income	194,978	246,436	283,424	325,099
Net Income per Share:				
Basic	0.80	1.02	1.19	1.34
Diluted	0.76	0.97	1.13	1.32

Exhibit 11/5: *(cont'd)*

	2002	2003	2004
Assets			
Total Current Assets	695,786	1,093,336	941,594
Net Property, Plant, and Equipment	1,281,782	1,427,715	1,692,701
Funds Held By Trustee	1,450	15,924	55,942
Excess of Cost Over Acquired Net Assets, Net	342,113	397,825	748,156
Deferred Charges and Other Assets	43,186	75,726	68,895
	2,364,317	3,010,526	3,507,288
Liabilities and Stockholders' Equity			
Total Current Liabilities	273,743	267,613	320,131
Deferred Income Taxes	17,861	80,023	143,760
Other Long-Term Liabilities	42,793	63,752	96,803
Long-Term Debt	650,159	924,713	925,518
Minority Interests in Consolidated Entities	33,009	37,350	43,066
Stockholders' Equity:			
Preferred Stock	2,611	2,627	2,660
Additional Paid-in-Capital	373,214	399,782	445,270
Retained Earnings	1,271,583	1,535,322	1,830,736
	1,647,408	1,937,731	2,278,666
Less: Treasury Stock, 22,500 Shares at Both September 30, 2003 and 2002, Respectively	(300,656)	(300,656)	(300,656)
Total Stockholders' Equity	1,346,752	1,637,075	1,978,010
	2,364,317	3,010,526	3,507,288

Source: Health Management Associates, Inc. 2004 Annual Report.

Riverview Regional Medical Center

The 281-bed acute care facility was originally chartered as The Holy Name of Jesus Hospital, and was the first hospital built in Etowah County back in the early 1930s. Owned and operated by an order of Catholic nuns, it remained under their ownership and control until financial considerations persuaded them to sell the hospital to HMA in August 1991. At that time the name changed to Riverview Regional Medical Center. RRMC's mission statement was as follows:

> Riverview Regional Medical Center will provide services to the best of our ability, treating everyone with dignity and respect in a safe manner.

Local Demographics

RRMC was located in the city of Gadsden, Etowah County, in northeastern Alabama. Exhibit 11/6 shows the relationship and proximity of the cities of Etowah County as well as the county seat. Etowah County comprised 12 incorporated cities

Exhibit 11/6: Relationship and Proximity of Cities in Etowah County

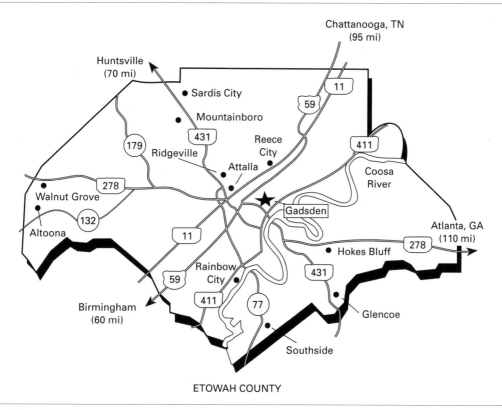

ETOWAH COUNTY

Source: *Birmingham News* (January 25, 1991), p. A12.

with a total population of 103,459 people in 2000.[4] Gadsden was the largest city (population 38,978) in Etowah County as well as the county seat (see Exhibit 11/7).

Gadsden was a transportation hub connecting many of the major metropolitan areas in the southeastern region of the country. It was located at the southern foothills of the Appalachian Mountains in an area 60 miles northeast of Birmingham, 70 miles southeast of Huntsville, 110 miles west of Atlanta, and 95 miles southwest of Chattanooga. Situated astride Lookout Mountain and the Coosa River, the city had grown from sparsely populated Indian country in the early 1800s to a city with a population that peaked at more than 58,000 residents in the early 1960s. Exhibit 11/8 shows the demographic makeup of Etowah County and Exhibit 11/9 shows the population of the surrounding counties.

Health Care Competition

Unlike many of the other facilities operated by HMA, RRMC was neither the sole community provider, nor even the dominant provider of health care in the

Exhibit 11/7: Population Trends, Etowah County/Gadsden 1960–2000

County/City	1960	1970	1980	1990	2000
Etowah County	92,980	96,980	103,057	99,840	103,459
Altoona	744	781	928	960	969
Attalla	8,257	7,510	7,737	6,859	6,952
Gadsden	58,088	53,928	47,565	42,523	38,978
Glencoe	2,592	2,901	4,648	4,670	5,143
Hokes Bluff	1,619	2,133	3,216	3,739	4,149
Mountainboro	–	311	266	261	338
Rainbow City	1,626	3,107	6,792	7,673	8,428
Reece City	470	496	718	657	634
Ridgeville	–	–	182	178	158
Sardis City	–	368	883	1,301	1,438
Southside	436	983	5,139	5,580	6,906
Walnut Grove	237	224	510	717	710

Source: http://www.census.gov/main/www/cen2000.html

Exhibit 11/8: Population Demographics

	1990	2000
Gadsden Population	42,523	38,978
County Population	99,840	103,459
Male	45.1%	46.0%
Female	54.9%	54.0%
White	70.5%	62.7%
Black	28.1%	34.0%
Under 5	6.3%	6.6%
65 or over	20.3%	2.1%
Median Household Income	$19,187	$24,823

Source: Gadsden Area Chamber of Commerce.

Exhibit 11/9: Population of Surrounding Counties

County	Area (sq. miles)	Population	County Seat	Workforce
Blount	643	51,024	Oneonta	23,896
Calhoun	611	112,249	Anniston	51,402
Cherokee	553	23,988	Centre	10,607
DeKalb	778	64,452	Fort Payne	30,903
Etowah	542	103,459	Gadsden	46,225
Jefferson	1,119	662,047	Birmingham	317,658
Marshall	567	82,231	Guntersville	38,900
St. Clair	646	64,742	Ashville	29,492

Source: http://censtats.census.gov/cgi-bin/pct/pctProfile.pl

market service area. Gadsden Regional Medical Center (GRMC), with 248 beds in service (346 licensed beds), offered considerable competition for RRMC. Both acute care hospitals were among the nine largest employers in Etowah County. Unlike the key GRMC medical staff members, who were housed in a hospital-owned professional office building, RRMC's key medical staff members and group practices maintained separate offices throughout the city. For the most part, the two hospitals had a common medical staff membership, with the exception of the Emergency Department and radiology physicians.

PRIMARY MARKET AREA

Although not owned by the Goodyear Tire and Rubber Company (Etowah county's largest employer and fourth largest taxpayer), GRMC was located on property adjacent to the Goodyear plant. The hospital, formerly known as Baptist Memorial Hospital, was sold to Quorum Health Group/Quorum Health Resources and renamed Gadsden Regional Medical Center in 1993. In April 2001, Triad acquired Quorum for $2.4 billion in cash and securities, creating the third largest investor-owned hospital chain in the United States.

Both RRMC and GRMC were accredited by the Joint Commission on Accreditation of Healthcare Organizations (JCAHO), certified for participation in the Health Insurance for the Aged (Medicare) Program by the DHHS, and contracted or participated in Blue Cross Plans as reported by the Blue Cross Association. However, only GRMC had a cancer program approved by the American College of Surgeons. In addition, GRMC offered neurosurgery, psychiatry, and obstetric services not offered by RRMC. For a comparison of the two facilities see Exhibit 11/10.

Another local provider of health care services was Mountain View Hospital, a psychiatric and chemical dependency facility for children, adolescents, and adults. Although by virtue of its target population Mountain View Hospital was not a

Exhibit 11/10: Facility Comparison

Category	RRMC[a]	GRMC[b]
Number of Beds	281	248
Number of Admissions	9,710	11,074
Census	129	135
Outpatient Visits	55,340	51,195
Births	*	1,163
Payroll (in thousands of dollars)	30,500	29,589
Personnel	850	939

*Obstetric services discontinued April 2003; 433 births between October 2002 and March 2003.

[a] **Source:** Riverview Regional Medical Center.

[b] **Source:** AHA Guide to the Health Care Field, 2003–04 edn (Chicago, IL: American Hospital Association, 2003).

direct competitor of RRMC, it nonetheless influenced the local market forces with respect to certain health care services.

Mountain View Hospital implemented professional and educational programs by recruiting national specialists in the field of mental health. Through a relationship with Northeast Alabama Psychiatric Services, neuropsychiatry was available as well as extensive outpatient services. In addition, the hospital specialized in treatment of attention deficit/hyperactivity disorders in children and adolescents. In June 1991, an adult psychiatric unit opened to treat depression, stress, anxiety, and panic disorders. An intensive care center for psychiatric care opened in January 1993. Other services provided by Mountain View Hospital included substance abuse treatment, a year-round academic program, a state licensed private school for inpatients, partial hospitalization, community education, and free 24-hour crisis evaluation. Physicians were being recruited from various nationally respected hospitals throughout the country with specialized areas of expertise in the field of mental health.

HealthSouth, one of the nation's largest providers of inpatient and outpatient services, operated rehabilitation and outpatient surgery facilities in Gadsden. In combination, these facilities offered a continuum of services, including acute medical care, inpatient rehabilitation, subacute care, day hospital, outpatient rehabilitation, home care, outpatient surgery, diagnostic imaging, and occupational medicine. In all, more than 30 medical specialties were available.[5] Many of the community physicians were part owners of the HealthSouth outpatient surgery facility; thus, they had a financial incentive to favor the facility over the hospital-based outpatient surgery units.

The HealthSouth Corporation was rocked by a multibillion dollar accounting scandal when it was accused of overstating its earnings in an effort to meet Wall Street expectations and bolster the stock price. Seventeen executives pleaded guilty to accounting fraud and violation of the Sarbanes-Oxley Act during the investigation.[6] The founder and CEO, Richard Scrushy, maintained his innocence but the board of directors forced him out of the company in March 2003. His trial on the 85-count indictment handed down in November 2003 began in March 2005.

RRMC increased its presence in nearby Anniston. In fact, one cardiologist had his primary care practice in Anniston, but sent his angioplasty patients to RRMC. With the military Base Realignment and Closure (BRAC) of Fort McClellan's Noble Army Base Hospital, RRMC was successful in obtaining the government contract for Tri-Care, thus bringing the area's military retirees to RRMC for service. HMA was present in Anniston through its ownership of Stringfellow Memorial Hospital, as well.

Out-migration to Birmingham

None of the hospitals in Gadsden could ignore the opportunity for residents to travel outside the local area for nonemergency care. Gadsden's proximity to the interstate network facilitated out-migration to urban areas boasting larger medical facilities. Although exact figures were unknown, the volume was estimated to be in excess of 25 percent. The Birmingham metropolitan area included approximately 20 hospitals, many of which offered specialty programs attractive to individuals who were predisposed to self-select health care services. Among those hospitals were HealthSouth, Baptist Medical Centers, St. Vincent's Hospital, Carraway Methodist Medical Center, Children's Hospital of Alabama, Brookwood Medical Center, the Eye Foundation Hospital, the Veterans' Administration Medical Center, and the University of Alabama at Birmingham (UAB) Medical Center.

The UAB Medical Center campus was located approximately one hour's drive from Gadsden via Interstate 59. It was a world-renowned patient care, education, and research complex, comprising: the Schools of Medicine, Dentistry, Nursing, Optometry, Health Related Professions and Public Health; the University of Alabama Hospital; and several of the specialty hospitals mentioned above. The University of Alabama Hospital, a 903-bed teaching facility with more than 50 clinical services, dominated the Medical Center. University Hospital encompassed the Alabama Heart Hospital, the Lurleen Wallace Complex for comprehensive cancer treatment, Spain Rehabilitation Center, and the Diabetes Hospital. More than 25 educational, instructional, and patient care "centers of excellence" and approximately 20 specialty units providing treatment, screening, and laboratory services were sponsored by the hospital. The UAB Hospital was consistently ranked as one of America's best hospitals by *U.S. News & World Report*.[7] In 2004, UAB ranked 6th in rheumatology, 13th in kidney disease, 17th in gynecology, and 19th in cancer. In all, *U.S. News & World Report* ranked 14 UAB programs in the top 50 for 2004. The medical staff (faculty for the UAB School of Medicine) practiced privately in the Kirklin Clinic, an ultramodern, high-technology facility that opened in 1992. The multispecialty Kirklin Clinic marketed aggressively throughout and beyond the Birmingham market area.

Operational Challenges at RRMC

HMA named Matt Hayes as executive director of RRMC in October 2003. From 2000 to 2003, Mr. Hayes served as executive director of Stringfellow Memorial Hospital, an HMA-leased facility in Anniston, Alabama. He was intimately familiar with RRMC, having served as its associate executive director from 1998 to 2000. He held a Master of Health Administration from the Medical University of South Carolina as well as an MBA from the University of Alabama at Birmingham.

Mr. Hayes faced many challenges in accepting the executive director's position at RRMC. First, his predecessor closed the Women's Pavilion in March 2003. Despite having a strong patient load, the unit was losing money because of its inability to capture the vast majority of births in the county and changes in reimbursement relating to disproportionate share monies. The decisions to close the Women's Pavilion and discontinue obstetrics created a perception in Gadsden that RRMC was in financial distress. Furthermore, the closing of the facility strained the relationship between management and the medical staff. Mr. Hayes established the Physicians' Leadership Group to improve communications with the medical staff. The group consisted of 25 core physicians that met quarterly. The goal was for this group to have more time to plan strategically, thereby minimizing implementation issues related to physician buy-in to changes at RRMC.

Physical Plant Changes at RRMC

The physical plant was originally constructed in 1931, with major additions in 1965 and in the 1970s. The acquisition of the hospital by HMA in 1991 ushered in more large-scale changes. By 1997, the facility had completed a $2 million renovation project that began with the hospital's entrance and included the emergency department (ED). The completely remodeled ED paralleled a level of medical sophistication usually observed only in larger urban hospitals. The ED was expanded to 18 patient treatment rooms with monitoring capabilities that included hardwire and telemetry electrocardiograms, noninvasive blood pressure measurement, noninvasive arterial blood gases, respiratory rate, and temperature. The ED was supported by a full-service, fully equipped 24-hour lab and state-of-the-art CT and ultrasound imaging units.

In 1994, HMA purchased the Medical Arts Building a few blocks from the hospital. Several of the older physician practices were located in this building and they had been reluctant to make technological and appearance upgrades. Thus, as tenants moved out, new tenants were hard to attract. HMA purchased the property, made some renovations, and leased the office space to physicians.

The hospital (when it was still Holy Name of Jesus) had an obstetrician with office space in the hospital. RRMC honored his lease until it expired in the mid-1990s, then turned the space into a separate entrance (rather than having outpatients enter through the ED, as was the old procedure). On his arrival, Mr. Hayes concluded, "Outpatient procedures aren't patient friendly. MRI and CT are on the first floor; outpatient registration is on the third floor; and the lab is on the second floor."

In August 2004, RRMC purchased the operations of a diagnostic center. The center was housed in a leased building one mile south of the hospital on the river. Mr. Hayes said, "Our goal is to have a full-blown diagnostic center with fast patient turnaround. The facility has an open MRI and a CAT scan scheduled to open by the end of the year. A PET scan will be available as a physician joint venture with the building landlord. Patients will perceive the PET as an HMA service since operations will be seamless, but the joint venture will hold the financial burden of the equipment."

Mr. Hayes commented, "The ED is the 'front door' for the facility because it accounts for nearly 60 percent of total admissions. We have initiated aesthetic renovations of the area over the past year and replaced the ED nurse manager to improve patient satisfaction." After renovating the ED in 1996, annual patient visits had increased from 23,000 to 26,000. In 2004, ED visits totaled over 24,000.

A Chest Pain Center was created across the hall from the ED, partially in response to the number of patients entering the ED complaining of chest pains

Exhibit 11/11: Top Ten "Chief Complaints" in Riverview's Emergency Department,
FY 2004

Chief Complaint	Number of Visits*
1. Chest Pain – Atraumatic	1,582
2. Abdominal Pain	1,509
3. Back Pain	1,131
4. Shortness of Breath	875
5. Fall	795
6. Nausea/Vomiting/Diarrhea	766
7. Headache – Frequent, with history	511
8. Knee Injury	353
9. Ankle Injury	346
10. Multiple Contusions	324

*Data from September 2004 not available.

(see Exhibit 11/11). There were ten beds in the Chest Pain Center; patients moved there after ED triage for tests and cardiac rule-out. Cardiac-diagnosed patients were transferred to the cardiac cath lab or admitted as inpatients. Evaluating ED patients with chest pain through the Center decreased the length of stay (LOS) in the ED to 3.25 hours. Although the national average for ED LOS is between four and five hours, the RRMC ED LOS is still above the HMA average of 2.0 hours, which is the ultimate goal.

The closing of the Women's Pavilion left a $3 million building vacant. Mr. Hayes stated, "I considered outpatient surgery, GI/endoscopy, and cardiac services as potential uses for the building. Ultimately, I decided to focus on what we do best." He continued, "The Heart and Vascular Center, a facility totally dedicated to cardiology, opened in October 2004. It has nine holding beds to serve the two cardiac catheterization labs and seven 23-hour beds. The building does have space for a third catheterization lab – if it's needed and we can get a CON. The old C-section suite is now the cardiac procedure room. If a patient needs immediate open heart surgery, the Center is connected to the open heart surgery suite by elevator."

In addition to these changes, all 180 patient rooms were converted to private occupancy, requiring major renovations to the 281 licensed-bed facility. This conversion occurred between April and August of 2004. Mr. Hayes contracted to have the exterior of the hospital painted to improve the community's "first impression" of RRMC.

Innovative Programs

In addition to the Heart and Vascular Center, RRMC opened the Heartburn Treatment Center. Hayes commented, "Do you realize that one out of every 14 Americans has severe, chronic heartburn? In fact, the American Gastroenterological

Association reports that heartburn affects more than 60 million people. Our Heartburn Treatment Center utilizes a nurse manager similar to the management model employed in the ED. One of our diagnostic procedures involves pH monitoring using the Bravo capsule.[8] If surgery is indicated, the 'lap Nissen' procedure[9] is performed at the hospital. Unfortunately, the manufacturer of the capsule has been unable to keep up with demand and the Center is only receiving two to four capsules per week. We could use twice as many each week."

Targeted at potential patients, the "Nurse First" program emphasized RRMC's commitment to patient care. The first person a patient saw in the ED was a nurse, not someone from the registration department. The ED utilized a computerized protocol system approved by an emergency department physician that aided in the triage of patients.

Targeted at physicians, the "One Call Scheduling" program attempted to simplify the admission process for physicians. The admitting physician called a dedicated number at RRMC, where staff could schedule appointments with any department at RRMC (preadmission testing, anesthesia, surgery scheduling, and so on).

Aimed at individuals and potential employers, the MedKey system employed computer technology to streamline patient registration and admission procedures with a plastic "smart card" containing a magnetic strip on which pertinent patient information was encoded and updated quickly and easily, as necessary. MedKey translated into increased operational efficiency and better service for patients by substantially decreasing the amount of time required to process an admission and record insurance coverage. HMA had over one million MedKey cards in use in 2004. All of the above programs portrayed a patient- and physician-oriented image.

Marketing

Subsequently, the MedKey system was a focused marketing strategy that used the patient database to promote RRMC facility utilization through membership incentives and rewards via discounts and extra services for MedKey "members." Marketing efforts were directed at recruiting potential individual members as well as employer-group memberships. As a marketing vehicle, Mr. Hayes viewed MedKey as more effective and cost efficient than mass advertising.

An in-house newsletter featuring new and existing programs and services as well as new benefits for MedKey members was developed and mailed on a regular basis. Promotional flyers were developed and mailed to inform members of upcoming events and activities.

The MedKey program created a win/win/win situation for area businesses, RRMC, and MedKey members. The hospital would win by improving its membership incentives through the discounts provided by the co-sponsoring enterprises. The companies would win by reaching a larger market through the hospital's direct-mailings to the ever-growing list of MedKey members to promote upcoming events, new services, and membership discounts. The members would win by receiving savings on services at RRMC as well as savings on the products and services of co-sponsoring enterprises.

A relatively new marketing tool for RRMC was the Internet. Its website made the hospital's programs and events easily accessible to current and prospective patients and staff. Of course, the competition offered websites as well.

As part of an ongoing image campaign, RRMC was filming a commercial. According to Mr. Hayes, "The basic message is that we've served the health care needs of the community since 1926 and will continue to do so for years to come." He continued, "The commercial combined with our campaigns on our new service lines and HealthGrade rankings should reflect positively on our image in the community. It also makes it easier to tell the RRMC story when I visit health fairs and speak to civic groups."

Operations

The hospital employed approximately 700 people, including nurses and housekeeping staff. The dietary department was contracted out. A local rather than a national vendor provided the laundry service. This decision allowed for a perceived luxury amenity in that the hospital had monogrammed towels as opposed to those with the stamped-on hospital logo available from national vendors.

In an effort to achieve a quality-driven level of patient-focused care, the patients' room telephones provided direct lines to the nurse manager, housekeeping, and food service (in the event of an error in dietary restriction meals). This allowed for direct contact to the service provider rather than waiting for information to pass through a chain of command.

Future Challenges for RRMC

Ongoing reimbursement issues presented a constant challenge for all health care administrators. Medicare reimbursement for Alabama was the lowest rate in the nation. Over 65 percent of Alabama hospitals were operating "in the red." The rumor among state health care leaders was that the Alabama Medicaid program would decrease beneficiary coverage from 16 inpatient days per year to 12 per year because of funding issues. Eighty percent of RRMC's patients were Medicare or Blue Cross. In addition to the fixed pricing constraints inherent in Medicare, Blue Cross's monopoly prevented negotiations to achieve better rates for those patients.

Mr. Hayes knew that the Heartburn Center and Diagnostic Center were important steps in generating outpatient revenues. These centers, along with initiating the nurse manager positions, helped improve patient satisfaction. The opening of the Heart and Vascular Center in October 2004 was expected to bolster RRMC's reputation in the community. In fact, HealthGrades.com's fall 2004 ratings listed RRMC as the no. 1 cardiovascular surgery hospital in Alabama. HealthGrades recognized the hospital's orthopedics and stroke programs as well.

Despite the strong gains made in operational efficiencies and improved service lines, Mr. Hayes knew closing the Women's Pavilion was an unpopular decision with the community citizens and with the medical staff. Improving relations with these groups would have to be his focus in the immediate future. However, the corporate goal to improve further the efficiency of the ED "front door" and gaining market share for the newly opened Heart and Vascular Center needed his attention as well.

NOTES

1. Ernst and Young, *Health Management Associates, Inc., 1995 Annual Report.*
2. B. Japsen, "Investor-owned Chains Seek Rich Rural Harvest," *Modern Healthcare* 26, no. 27 (July 1, 1996), pp. 32–37.
3. Ibid.
4. "State of Alabama – 2000 Census" available at: http://www.ador.state.al.us/licenses/census.html, accessed September 11, 2004.
5. See http://www.healthsouth.com.
6. "Scrushy Accused of Plane Misuse," *Toronto Star* (July 3, 2004), p. D20.
7. "Best Hospitals 2004," *U.S. News & World Report*, http://www.usnews.com/usnews/health/hosptl/tophosp.htm, accessed September 13, 2004.
8. The Bravo capsule (microchip) was inserted in the esophagus via the throat to monitor and record acid reflux. After the data were retrieved from the monitor, the chip sloughed off and passed through the digestive tract. This technique was much more comfortable for the patient than the commonly used procedure of passing a probe through the nostril into the esophagus, and leaving the probe physically attached to an external monitor for 24 hours.
9. The "lap Nissen" procedure, or fundoplication, was used to control acid reflux by wrapping the upper portion of the stomach (the fundus) around the bottom of the esophagus. The procedure was performed laparoscopically through five small incisions instead of one large abdominal incision. Surgical trauma was lessened and recovery time shortened with laparoscopic procedures.

CASE **12**

AIDSCAP Nepal

Background

It was September 1996 and Ravin Lama, Managing Director of
Stimulus Advertizers, one of Nepal's larger advertising agencies,
looked out of his Kathmandu office window pondering his
future course of action. (See Appendix A for an overview of Nepal.)
He had just received a copy of a qualitative, quickly conducted,
small sample study that had been developed by a research
agency in order to assess the impact of *The AIDS Awareness and
Condom Promotion Multimedia Campaign* which his agency had
helped develop and implement since mid-1995. The main focus
of this campaign was to increase people's access to condoms,
promote their correct and consistent use (particularly when engaging in high-risk behaviors), and communicate HIV/AIDS
awareness messages. He had an upcoming meeting with Joy
Pollock, Resident Advisor to the AIDS-CAP (AIDS Control and
Prevention) project, at which they had to both evaluate the
impact of the current campaign, which was to conclude in April
1997, and develop a strategy for Phase II of their communication
program. AIDSCAP was the primary sponsor of the campaign.

Launched in July 1995, the campaign to reduce the rate of
sexually transmitted HIV infection in AIDSCAP's project area –
the Terai/Central region of the country – had been ongoing for
over a year. Lama was preparing for a meeting where he had
to present a thorough evaluation of the progress made thus far in
this phase, recommend any necessary changes, and develop his

agency's plans for Phase II, which was to address issues of fear in the general public regarding people living with AIDS. Specifically, his task was to determine whether the results of the small sample study were sufficient to assess the effectiveness of the present campaign and, if not, to design an appropriate assessment tool. Phase II, the fear issue, had become important because the media were reporting that a large number of HIV-positive Nepalese commercial sex workers (CSWs) were returning home from brothels in India. Once Lama was satisfied that the current phase's objectives were being met, he had to set specific objectives for Phase II and design the promotion campaign.

Many Nepalese women worked as prostitutes in several large Indian cities such as Mumbai (formerly called Bombay) and Delhi. Mostly from rural areas where economic prospects were poor, they were often part of an elaborate network where they were recruited, ostensibly for legitimate employment, and once in India were either coerced into or drifted into prostitution. Often abused and abandoned by their husbands and in-laws and having no means of financial support, many became CSWs. Although prostitution had not always been legal, attempts by Indian authorities to regulate it were sporadic and half-hearted. Once infected with HIV, the women were usually thrown out of the brothels, the only real "family" many of them had so far away from home. They generally returned home to Nepal in anticipation of receiving better care from their families than they would get in India. However, fear and rejection from society, frequently based on ignorance of the disease and how it spread, meant that they were often shunned.

AIDS: A Historical Perspective

Although AIDS was first recognized internationally in 1981, it was identified in Nepal in 1988. Data presented at a conference in Kathmandu in the mid-1990s indicated that although the HIV/AIDS epidemic in Nepal was at a relatively early stage compared to other countries, the incidence of AIDS was increasing. The total number of HIV/AIDS cases reported in the country was in the hundreds according to the National Centre for AIDS and STD Control (NCASC), but NCASC projected HIV cases at 15,000 in 2000. His Majesty's Government of Nepal and national and international nongovernment organizations were actively participating in an attempt to control its spread. The NCASC chief stated that "the situation offers, therefore, a unique opportunity to support and undertake preventive activities before the disease reaches an epidemic stage in the country."

The evidence in the mid-1990s was that:

- Extensive or epidemic spread of HIV had not been documented in Nepal;
- A large proportion of HIV infections had been and would be acquired outside the country – Nepal had a long, open border with India and many Nepalese worked in India;
- An estimated 15,000 HIV cases and 1,000 AIDS cases and deaths would occur annually by the year 2000;
- HIV/AIDS surveillance needed to be strengthened and behavioral surveillance started as soon as possible – that is, more extensive screening and testing for

infection and more detailed assessment of the extent of high-risk behaviors such as unprotected sex with CSWs was needed; and

- STD services, condom distribution and promotion, and behavior change communications to high-risk groups needed to be strengthened.

Additionally, epidemiological evidence indicated that the primary modes of transmission of HIV/AIDS in Nepal were through heterosexual contact with CSWs followed by intravenous drug use. Some of the identified high-risk behaviors were pre-marital and extramarital sexual practices, wide availability of CSWs, and low condom use. Much of the pre- and extramarital sexual activity was with CSWs, given the taboos and social norms against such activity among "respectable" people, particularly for women. CSWs were a major medium of the spread of HIV/AIDS because once a client became infected, he could become the core transmitter of the virus as he traveled through Nepal and infected other CSWs, who in turn infected their other clients, if condoms were not used.

Despite the AIDS threat not being very immediate in Nepal, the issue was complicated by the close contacts between Nepal and India. A significant portion of Nepal's male population worked in India, and if they acquired the infection there it could rapidly spread in Nepal when they had sexual contacts during their visits home. In addition, many Nepalese CSWs worked in brothels in large Indian cities such as New Delhi and Mumbai. Data from India indicated that the HIV infection rate among CSWs in Mumbai had increased from 0.5 percent in 1986 to 69 percent in 1995. Mumbai had an estimated 70,000 CSWs. India had almost 2.5 million CSWs out of a total population of over 900 million.

Several studies had been conducted to measure awareness, attitudes towards and usage of condoms, oral and injectable contraceptives, brand awareness and image, and general views about HIV/AIDS in Nepal. One such study was conducted in 1994 among CSWs and their clients along the highway route in AIDSCAP's project area and from similar groups in a control area where AIDSCAP did not have a campaign. This study interviewed 100 CSWs and 209 of their clients in the project area and 62 CSWs and 103 clients in the control area. This study's key findings from the project and control areas are presented in Exhibits 12/1 to 12/5. This study reported on the general awareness of AIDS, condom use and purchase patterns, and also identified the main sources of information about AIDS and perceptions regarding means of prevention.

AIDSCAP

AIDSCAP, part of Family Health International, had its activities funded by the US Agency for International Development (USAID). Futures Group International was appointed as the consultant for the project. For the initial phase, the activities of both Stimulus, which handled the communication program, and Contraceptive Retail Sales Company, which handled condom distribution, were managed by the Futures Group. For Phase II of the project, Stimulus would deal directly with AIDSCAP.

Exhibit 12/1: Socio-demographics of CSWs and Clients: 1994 Baseline Study

	CSWs		Clients	
	Project Area **(n = 100)**	**Control Area** **(n = 62)**	**Project Area** **(n = 209)**	**Control Area** **(n = 103)**
Variable	%	%	%	%
Age (In Years)				
0–19	13.0	24.2	54.5 (15–24)	41.7
20–29	63.0	45.2	37.3 (25–34)	50.5
30–39	18.0	27.4	8.1 (35–44)	7.8
40+	6.0	3.2	0.0 (45+)	0.0
Mean Age	26	26	24.9	25.8
Education				
Literate	44.0	40.3	90.5	93.2
Illiterate	56.0	59.7	10.5	6.8
Marital Status				
Married	93.0	83.9	56.5	66.0
Unmarried	7.0	16.1	43.5	34.0
Presently Living With **Husband/Wife**	(n = 93)	(n = 52)	(n = 118)	(n = 68)
Yes	43.0	42.3	83.9	83.8
No	57.0	57.7	16.1	16.2
Children	(n = 93)	(n = 52)		
Yes	68.8	19.4	Not	Not
No	31.2	80.6	Available	Available

Note: The age ranges used for categorizing CSWs and their clients were different.

Given all the available evidence, AIDSCAP decided that its goal was to reduce the rate of sexually transmitted HIV infection in the Terai/Central region through the implementation of three major prevention and control strategies:

• Reduce sexually transmitted diseases.
• Increase the use of condoms among the risk populations.
• Reduce risk behaviors through communications and outreach activities to targeted populations.

It was decided to focus on the Terai/Central region because of the relatively high concentrations of CSWs working in these areas, the presence of major highways, and the movement of large numbers of people (including CSWs and their clients) across the border with India. Several studies had noted the pattern of Nepalese women working as CSWs in India, Indian clients crossing the border to patronize sex workers in Nepal, and Nepalese migrant workers returning

Exhibit 12/2: CSW's Condom Use and Purchase Behavior, 1994 Baseline Study

Condom Use/Purchase Behavior	Project Area (%)	Control Area (%)
Ever Bought Condoms for Clients	(n = 100)	(n = 62)
Yes	26.0	24.2
No	74.0	75.8
Price of Condom	(n = 26)	(n = 15)
Expensive	15.4	26.7
Reasonable	55.7	60.0
Cheap	26.9	13.3
Most Convenient Location to Buy/Get	(n = 96)	(n = 57)
Pharmacy	59.4	61.4
Retail Store	50.0	66.7
Health Worker/Volunteer	29.2	0.0
Health Post/Center/Hospital	25.0	1.8
Hotel/Lodge	16.7	15.8
Public Place	9.4	0.0
NGOs	0.0	14.0
Others	8.3	5.3
Clients Using Condoms	(n = 100)	(n = 62)
All of Them	13.0	14.5
Most of Them	16.0	29.0
Half of Them	14.0	14.5
A Few of Them	13.0	19.4
None of Them	44.0	22.6
Use by Last Client	(n = 100)	(n = 62)
Yes	35.0	48.4
No	65.0	51.6
Decision Maker	(n = 35)	(n = 30)
Last Client	42.9	50.0
CSW	57.1	50.0
Condom Bought By	(n = 35)	(n = 30)
Client	57.1	56.7
CSW	42.9	43.3
Ever Requested Client to Use Condom	(n = 100)	(n = 62)
Yes	30.0	33.9
No	70.0	66.1
Any of Those Clients Refused	(n = 30)	(n = 21)
Yes	60.0	47.6
No	40.0	52.4

Exhibit 12/3: Clients' Condom Use and Purchase Behavior, 1994 Baseline Study

Condom Use/Purchase Behavior	Project Area (%)	Control Area (%)
Ever Used	(n = 209)	(n = 103)
Yes	52.6	55.3
No	47.4	44.7
Price of Condom	(n = 108)	(n = 57)
Expensive	11.1	24.6
Reasonable	60.2	47.4
Cheap/Inexpensive	28.7	28.1
Most Convenient Location to Buy/Get	(n = 209)	(n = 102)
Pharmacy	66.5	68.6
Retail Store	49.8	40.2
Health Worker/Volunteer	7.7	10.2
Health Post/Center/Hospital	17.2	9.8
Hotel/Lodge	16.3	3.9
Public Place	3.8	0.0
NGOs	8.1	4.9
Others/Don't Know	6.3	15.7
Frequency of Condom Use with CSWs	(n = 209)	(n = 103)
Always	22.0	6.8
Mostly	16.7	16.5
Sometimes	5.3	15.5
Rarely	5.7	14.6
Never	50.2	46.6
Reasons for Not Using Condoms	(n = 63)	(n = 48)
Unavailability/No Time	60.3	52.1
Complexity	34.9	12.5
Sexual Dissatisfaction	27.0	64.6
Unreliability/Others	6.3	22.9
Person Who First Mentioned Condom	(n = 71)	(n = 22)
Myself	95.8	100.0
CSW	4.2	0.0

occasionally from India to visit their families. The targets of the campaign were the individuals at highest risk: CSWs and their clients (who included transport workers, migrant laborers, military, and police). Transport workers – truck drivers and their helpers – were seen by AIDSCAP as a high-risk group because they tended to be away from home for long periods of time. In addition, because they traveled, once infected they could easily spread the disease to the other CSWs they frequented along the highway. Military and police were targeted because the lower ranks usually were not provided family accommodations when posted

Exhibit 12/4: Knowledge of AIDS: 1994 Baseline Study

	CSWs		Clients	
Knowledge of AIDS	**Project Area (n = 100)** %	**Control Area (n = 62)** %	**Project Area (n = 209)** %	**Control Area (n = 103)** %
Ever Heard of AIDS				
Yes	82.0	59.7	90.4	91.3
No	18.0	40.3	9.6	8.7
AIDS is				
A Disease	79.0	54.8	88.5	70.9
Others	3.0	4.8	3.8	20.4
Not Heard of AIDS	18.0	40.3	9.6	8.7
Is AIDS Transmitted				
Yes	53.0	38.7	75.1	80.6
No	47.0	61.3	15.3	10.7
Don't Know	0.0	0.0	9.6	8.7
Modes of AIDS Transmission				
Sex Without Condom	23.0	21.0	29.2	44.7
Multiple Sex Partners	29.0	24.2	51.2	47.6
Sexual Intercourse	22.0	27.4	23.0	35.9
By Blood	5.0	3.2	9.6	20.4
By Syringe	1.0	3.2	5.3	7.8
Sex with AIDS-Infected People	0.0	1.6	1.4	8.7
Sex with CSW	0.0	0.0	4.8	5.8
Other	1.0	1.6	0.5	1.0
Don't Know	47.0	61.3	0.0	0.0
Consequences of AIDS				
Death	66.0	40.3	72.7	61.2
Remain Sick for Long	9.0	14.5	12.0	22.3
Others	4.0	3.2	4.8	5.8
Don't Know	21.0	41.9	10.5	15.5
Preventive Measures				
Use Condom	34.0	27.4	54.5	51.5
Stop Sex with Multiple Partners	25.0	22.6	30.1	45.6
Stop Going to CSW	2.0	1.6	23.9	27.2
Use Disposable Syringe	1.0	0.0	1.9	2.9
Use Tested Blood	1.0	0.0	0.0	0.0
Don't Use Others' Shaving Material	0.0	0.0	2.4	2.9
Don't Know	54.0	62.9	0.0	0.0
Knowledge of AIDS Among Those Exposed to Condom Advertising				
Yes	50.0	44.4	79.4	85.4
No	50.0	55.6	20.6	14.6

Exhibit 12/5: Sources of Knowledge about HIV/AIDS: 1994 Baseline Study

	CSWs		Clients	
	Project Area (n = 82)	Control Area (n = 37)	Project Area (n = 189)	Control Area (n = 94)
Source	%	%	%	%
Friends/Neighbors	68.3	54.1	52.4	42.6
Radio	40.2	70.3	60.3	72.3
Health Post/Hospital	22.2	0.0	9.0	13.8
Newspapers/Posters/Magazines	13.4	18.9	43.9	46.8
Television	12.2	24.3	29.1	28.7
Health Workers/Volunteers	9.8	0.0	3.7	2.1
Pharmacy	7.3	16.2	16.4	9.6
Billboards	6.1	18.9	30.7	29.8
Clients	3.7	0.0	–	–
Street Drama/Theater	2.4	0.0	2.1	0.0
NGOs	1.2	18.9	5.3	7.4
Hotel/Shop	0.0	0.0	2.1	0.0
Others/Don't Know	4.9	2.7	3.7	6.4

away from home. They generally were housed in barracks while their families stayed behind in their home villages. This forced separation, along with peer pressure, made them high risks for HIV transmission. AIDSCAP felt that migrant workers were a high-risk group because they left their homes in search of construction jobs (such as road and bridge building) that were easier to find along the highway routes. Again, living away from home for long periods made them more likely to patronize CSWs.

Phase I

Condom Distribution

AIDSCAP recognized that in order for AIDS preventive communication strategies to work, increased accessibility of condoms was a vital element. To this end it subcontracted with Futures Group International to conduct condom promotion and distribution activities in the target area. The issue was complicated by the fact that condom promotion in Nepal had traditionally focused primarily on its benefit as a family planning method, not so much as a means of disease prevention. In addition, AIDSCAP had to keep in mind that Nepalese society was very traditional and frowned on pre-marital and extramarital sexual activity. Any attempt to promote condom use for other than family planning activity had to be sensitive to this.

Futures Group worked with Contraceptive Retail Sales Company to improve condom accessibility and availability through retail and nontraditional outlets in the AIDSCAP target region. A rapid assessment study conducted by AIDSCAP indicated that clients of CSWs wanted condoms to be easily available at all hours through nontraditional distribution outlets such as tea shops, *paan pasals* (small shops selling cigarettes and other frequently purchased consumer products), hotels, and truck stops. Distribution efforts were therefore put into these outlets, especially along major truck routes, so as to make access easy for the primary target market of the effort – clients of CSWs. Two brands of condoms, Panther and *Dhaal* ("shield" in Nepali), donated by USAID were marketed in Nepal. Panther was targeted primarily at the upper social class and *Dhaal* at the middle and lower classes.

Condom Promotion

The other major element in AIDSCAP's strategy was the communication program. This was where Lama's organization, Stimulus, entered the picture. The responsibility for communicating the goals of the project rested with him and his agency.

OBJECTIVES

Based on AIDSCAP's overall goals, three specific communication goals for the campaign were established:

- To increase the existing levels of awareness among the target audience that sexual transmission was the primary mode of acquiring HIV infection and AIDS.
- To increase perception of individual risk of acquiring HIV/AIDS.
- To promote consistent and correct condom use as a method of protection from HIV/AIDS.

These goals were expected to be achieved sequentially, following the traditional communication hierarchy of effects model, which suggested that consumer responses moved from the least serious or involved through the most serious or complex. One classic approach, the AIDA model, proposed that a message's impact began with *attention*, moves to *interest*, then *desire*, and finally *action*. First, AIDSCAP wanted to develop awareness among the target audience about HIV/AIDS and its modes of transmission, heighten attention and interest by communicating its risks, and finally motivate action to take preventive measures.

TARGET AUDIENCES

AIDSCAP identified clients of CSWs as the project's primary target audience. In order to reach the clients, the media selected should match the target – defined as sexually active men aged 15–35 who engaged in commercial sex. CSWs were made the secondary target because of the difficulty in reaching them via mass media vehicles given their generally low levels of literacy, high mobility along the transportation routes, and limited reach of media away from the major cities. Thus interpersonal counseling, peer counseling, and other such efforts conducted by AIDSCAP would be used to reach CSWs in addition to the efforts of this communication campaign.

CREATIVE

The first creative task for Stimulus was to develop a logo that would serve as the HIV/AIDS awareness campaign ID to be used in all communication and training material for the entire project. This logo was intended to communicate protection from HIV/AIDS and symbolize positive behavior change (namely, use of condoms). Other considerations were that it represent positive feelings (no fear), represent positive outcomes of condom use, symbolize strength, and be easily understood. After initial focus groups and in-depth interviews with target group members, four logos were developed based on "structured brainstorming" (where participants were asked to suggest how best to visually communicate strength, lack of fear, and so on) by a group of AIDSCAP implementing partners. Subsequently, a survey was conducted in early 1995 among the target group (bus/truck drivers and conductors) to test these logos. Based on this study, a logo showing an animated condom (named *Dhale Dai*) holding a shield and kicking the AIDS virus (see Exhibit 12/6) was selected as the one with the highest ranking in terms of overall liking; conveying the impression of strength, confidence, attractiveness, protection against AIDS; and encouraging the use of condoms. This character was used in a message (*Dhale and Dhaal Bahadur*) to communicate correct and consistent condom use.

To develop a slogan for the campaign, several condom benefit statements were tested. These revealed that protection and freedom from worry were the most strongly received concepts. As a result, the slogan *Condom lagaon . . . AIDS bhagaon* (use a condom – drive away AIDS) was selected.

The creative strategy was developed around four primary ideas: (1) dispel myths regarding how HIV/AIDS was/was not transmitted (such as via dirty glasses and food, mosquitoes); (2) build awareness that anyone could become infected with AIDS even with one sexual contact in the same way as sexually transmitted diseases (epidemiological studies suggest that the possibility of AIDS transmission per exposure increased substantially when the presence of STDs was high in a population); (3) create general awareness about HIV/AIDS and the dangers of casual, unprotected sex; and (4) communicate the widespread availability of condoms and the lack of a need to feel fear or embarrassment about using them.

MEDIA

A combination of media was used to communicate the key creative messages of the campaign. Billboards featuring the condom character *Dhale* along with the

Exhibit 12/6: *Dhale Dai*

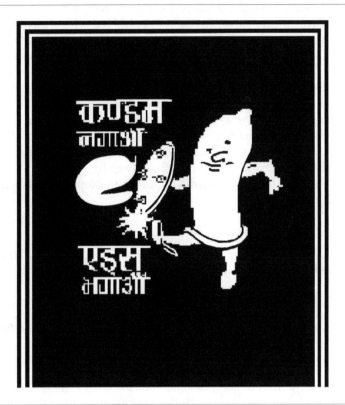

slogan "Use a Condom . . . Drive away AIDS" were placed at several points along the main highways in the project area. For radio, four 60-second spots and a jingle were developed. FM Radio was used in Kathmandu; Radio Nepal, which has widespread reach across most of the country, was also used. The state-owned TV channel, Nepal TV, was used to telecast a 60-second animated spot of *Dhale* in Nepali.

The van that Contraceptive Retail Sales used for its condom distribution activity was equipped with a video screen that was used to show a 45-minute soap opera-style film that was developed by Stimulus in mid-1996. This film's primary characters were a truck driver (named *Guruji*) and his assistant (*Antare*) and the main ideas – how to protect from AIDS and other STDs, their means of transmission, the value of correct condom use, dangers of unprotected sex and other risk behaviors – were communicated in a conversational setting between these two characters. In addition, a film version of the TV spot and a shortened (19-minute) version of the *Guruji and Antare* video were screened at movie theaters in five towns in the target area. The *Guruji and Antare* story was also developed in the form of a comic book. Because of high visual content, comic books were seen as more interesting than text-heavy material. Given Nepal's high levels of illiteracy, particularly among truck drivers and laborers, comic books were an effective way to deliver the message. AIDSCAP contracted with a traveling group of street performers who enacted the contents of the film at several villages along the highway. At these live performances and the video showings, copies of the comic book were distributed. A few days before these activities were scheduled for an area, project workers would put up posters and make public announcements to alert the residents about the upcoming arrival of the video van or the live performers. On these occasions as well, the project workers would distribute comic books. Other printed material, in Nepali, included brochures, stickers, and condom wallets. Metal signs, posters, and calendars were distributed to shops, pharmacies, health centers, and community buildings for display.

Details of the major media available in Nepal are presented in Exhibits 12/7 and 12/8.

Exhibit 12/7: Media Data: Broadcast

Medium	Broadcast Time	Content	General Rate* (30 sec.)	Sponsorship* Rate (30 sec.)
1. Radio				
FM				
Hits FM	7:15 a.m.–3 p.m.	Nepali, English, Hindi Songs	Rs. 300–800	Rs. 325–900
Image Plus	4 p.m.–5 p.m.	Nepali, English, Hindi Songs	Rs. 600	
Classic FM	6 p.m.–7 p.m.	Songs, Phone-ins, Business Briefs	Rs. 300	Rs. 3,300 (30 min.)
Kantipur FM	7 p.m.–10 p.m.	Songs, Phone-ins, Comedy	Rs. 275	
Good Nite FM	10 p.m.–12 midnight	Music	Rs. 200–250	
Medium Wave				
Radio Nepal	7:45 a.m.–10:55 p.m.	News, Music, Educational, Agriculture, Health, Sports, Environment, etc.	Rs. 500–800	Rs. 6,700–9,000 (30 min.)
2. TV				
Nepal TV	7 a.m.–7:40 a.m. daily 6 p.m.–10:15 p.m. daily 12 p.m.–5 p.m. (Sat.)	News, English and Nepali Educational and Entertainment, Indian and Pakistani Music and Serials	Rs. 2,750–6,500	

* Rs. = rupees. In 1996, US$1 = Rs. 56.75.

Notes: 1. Radio: 2,000,000 sets, 5 listeners/set, FM coverage in Kathmandu Valley only, MW coverage national and parts of neighboring countries.   2. TV: 250,000 sets, 6 viewers/set, coverage over most of the country. 3. A 60-sec. spot costs twice as much as a 30-sec. spot.

Exhibit 12/8: Media Data: Print

Publication	Language and Frequency	Content	Circulation	Cost* Black and White	Color
Newspapers				col/cm	col/cm
Kantipur	Nepali, Daily	All Newspapers – Daily and	45,000–50,000	Rs. 90	Rs. 250
Gorkhapatra	Nepali, Daily	Weekly – Contain: domestic	40,000	Rs. 90	
Aajo Samacharpatra	Nepali, Daily	and International News,	10,000	Rs. 75	
Himalaya Times	Nepali, Daily	Business Reports, Sports, etc.	10,000	Rs. 59	
Sagarmatha	Nepali, Daily		5,000	Rs. 75	Rs. 250
Kathmandu Post	English, Daily		12,000	Rs. 90	
Rising Nepal	English, Daily		8,000	Rs. 90	
Independent	English, Weekly		5,000		Rs. 55 (1 color) Rs. 69 (2 colors)
Saptahik	Nepali, Weekly			Rs. 40	Rs. 200
Magazines				**Full Page (B&W)**	**Full Page (Color)**
Kamana	Nepali, Monthly	Movie News	30,000	Rs. 4,000	Rs. 11,000
Sadhana	Nepali, Monthly	General Interest, Family	25,000–35,000	Rs. 3,000	Rs. 6,500
Asmita	Nepali, Monthly	Women's Issues	15,000	Rs. 4,000	Rs. 15–20,000 (cover)
Yuva Manch	Nepali, Monthly	Children and Youth, 8–21	15,000		
Wave	English, Monthly	Youth, 12–22		Rs. 4,000	
Spotlight	English, Monthly	Political, News, Sports, Business, Leisure South Asian focus, Tourism	5,000		
Himal	English and Nepali, Monthly		10,000	US$ 1,000	US$ 1,200

* Rs. = rupees. In 1996, US$1 = Rs. 56.75.

Note: Average number of readers per copy: 5.

Exhibit 12/9: Phase I Media Schedule: 1995–97

Medium	Period	Number of Spots, Performances, Shows	Cost*
1. Radio			
Radio Nepal	July 1995–April 1997	1,096	Rs. 1,982,700
FM	Nov. 1995–Feb. 1996	151	Rs. 121,400
	May 1996	8	Rs. 5,040
	Sep. 1996–April 1997	80	Rs. 53,700
2. NTV	Feb. 1996–April 1997	128	Rs. 902,840
3. Cinema	Feb. 1996–Aug. 1996	3,125	Rs. 17,005
(in 5 towns)	Oct. 1996–April 1997	3,155	Rs. 19,058
4. Street Drama	Aug. 1995–July 1996	60	Rs. 300,000
	Oct. 1996–April 1997	64	Rs. 355,840
5. Video Van	Sep. 1996–March 1997	61	Rs. 500,000
Total Media Cost			Rs. 4,257,583

* Rs. = rupees. In 1996, US$1 = Rs. 56.75.

BUDGET

Because of uncertain funding levels, Lama was not given a budget at the start of the Phase I campaign. He had to make periodic funding requests, which, if approved after review, determined how much he had available to spend on different aspects of the campaign. Details of the media budget and schedule for Phase I are provided in Exhibit 12/9.

The Assessment

In May 1996, the AIDSCAP commissioned a market research agency to conduct a quick, small sample assessment of the impact of the program on behavior change among CSWs (with "CSW" defined as a woman who was involved in multiple sexual encounters for financial benefit) and their clients (with "client" defined as a person who had sexual contact with at least one CSW within three months from the date of the interview). A convenience sample of 25 CSWs and 25 clients from the AIDSCAP intervention area transportation routes was surveyed using personal interviews. The target sample was identified based on information supplied by hotels and teashops, bars, pimps, local people, as well as through the CSWs and their clients themselves. The respondents were compensated for their participation in the interviews. The specific goals of this study were to:

• assess target groups' awareness and understanding of HIV/AIDS,
• assess target groups' awareness of AIDSCAP communication messages,

Exhibit 12/10: Socio-demographics of CSWs and Clients: 1996 Study

Variable	CSWs (n = 25)	Clients (n = 25)
Age		
0–20	16.0	20.0
21–25	40.0	28.0
26–30	16.0	16.0
Over 30	24.0	36.0
Not Known	4.0	–
Education		
Literate	48.0	96.0
Illiterate	52.0	4.0
Marital Status		
Ever Been Married	88.0	72.0
Unmarried	12.0	28.0
Children		
Yes	36.0	44.0
No	64.0	56.0

- assess target groups' self-risk perception, and
- collect information of target groups' recent condom use.

The study concluded that the awareness of the campaign slogan (*condom lagaon ... AIDS bhagaon*) was high, with most respondents having been exposed to it via radio or through billboards. A sizable number had heard some of the other campaign messages as well. It appeared that the AIDSCAP promotional campaign did have a positive impact on AIDS awareness levels; however, perceptions of risk from AIDS were low. Details of the study are provided in Exhibits 12/10 through 12/13.

The Future

As Lama contemplated his upcoming meeting with Pollock, two sets of issues confronted him. The first, and more immediate, was to determine whether the results of the small sample study gave him sufficient information with which to evaluate the impact of the communication campaign thus far. His initial reaction was that since these results were based on a limited sample of CSWs and their clients, perhaps a more detailed follow-up was necessary, using a larger sample from the intervention area along with a sample from the control area. This was especially significant because a successful execution of this phase's communications goals was essential before Phase II could be launched; without successful execution, the effectiveness of Phase II would be limited. Specifically, Lama had to determine, if he decided to initiate a detailed assessment, the methodology he

Exhibit 12/11: Condom Use Behavior: 1996 Study

Condom Usage	CSWs (n = 25)	Clients (n = 25)
Ever Use Condom		
Yes	76.0	68.0
No	24.0	32.0
Used Condom With Last CSW/Client		
Yes	60.0	44.0
No	16.0	24.0
Not Applicable	24.0	32.0
First to Initiate Use of Condom		
CSW	28.0	20.0
Client	32.0	24.0
Not Applicable	40.0	56.0
Condom Provided By		
CSW	24.0	16.0
Client	36.0	28.0
Not Applicable	40.0	56.0
Always Use Condoms With CSWs	Not Applicable	
Yes		28.0
No		16.0
Not Applicable		56.0
Condoms Used By		Not Applicable
All the Clients	12.0	
Most of the Clients	48.0	
Few of the Clients	16.0	
None of the Clients	24.0	

should employ (research design, measures, data collection) to evaluate the current phase. Was the methodology used in the small sample study adequate, or were more comprehensive data necessary?

The second issue was to start thinking about Phase II, due to be launched in mid-1997. His task was to address issues of fear in the general public regarding people living with AIDS. This was of particular concern in Nepal given the large number of HIV-positive women who had returned from brothels in Mumbai and elsewhere in India and the resulting fear among many sections of the Nepalese population. Lama wondered whether launching Phase II was the correct decision at this point in time. Was it timely to move ahead with these new issues, or should he focus on strengthening the current prevention campaign? If he decided to tackle the fear issue, Lama had to design the entire communications strategy for Phase II of the campaign. He had to develop specific objectives, generate the creative and media strategies, and identify appropriate measures to assess the communications effectiveness of this phase of the AIDS-CAP project.

Exhibit 12/12: Knowledge of AIDS: 1996 Study

Knowledge of AIDS	CSWs (n = 25)	Clients (n = 25)
Ever Heard of AIDS		
Yes	96.0	100.0
No	4.0	0.0
AIDS is		
A Disease	88.0	100.0
A Fatal Disease	8.0	0.0
Not Heard of AIDS	4.0	0.0
Is AIDS Transmitted		
Yes	76.0	96.0
No	20.0	4.0
Don't Know	4.0	0.0
Modes of AIDS Transmission		
Sex Without Condom	52.0	44.0
Multiple Sex Partners	36.0	56.0
Sexual Intercourse	32.0	24.0
By Blood	–	20.0
By Syringe	–	16.0
Other	4.0	4.0
Don't Know	24.0	–
Consequences of AIDS		
Death	60.0	76.0
Remain Sick for Long	20.0	28.0
Don't Know	20.0	8.0
Preventive Measures		
Use Condom	64.0	84.0
Stop Sex with Multiple Partners	44.0	64.0
Stop Going to CSW	–	4.0
Use Disposable Syringe	–	8.0
Avoid Blood Transfusion from AIDS patient	–	8.0
Don't Know	24.0	4.0

Exhibit 12/13: Awareness of AIDSCAP Messages: 1996 Study

	Heard/Seen Condom Ad In Past 3 Months		Heard/Seen Condom Lagaon AIDS Bhagaon		Heard/Seen Dhale and Dhaal Bahadur		Heard/Seen Guruji and Antare	
	CSWs (n = 25)	Clients (n = 25)	CSWs (n = 25)	Clients (n = 25)	CSWs (n = 25)	Clients (n = 25)	CSWs (n = 25)	Clients (n = 25)
Radio	18	18	16	19	5	10	1	0
Billboards	15	12	13	8	1	3	0	1
Pharmacy	8	9	8	4	1	2	0	0
Cinema Hall	8	6	8	4	1	2	7	6
Outreach Workers	8	5	8	7	4	5	0	0
Print Material	7	8	6	11	5	9	3	8
Video Van Film	3	4	2	5	0	5	3	6
TV	2	4	3	2	2	0	2	0
Street Drama	2	1	2	1	0	1	0	2
Friends	–	1	2	8	1	7	0	0
Health Centers	–	2	1	3	0	1	0	0
Not Seen/Heard	0	3	2	2	18	11	14	9

Appendix A: Nepal – A Brief Overview

Topography and Climate

Nepal is a landlocked country with a total land area of 147,181 sq. km. It is roughly rectangular in shape and extends approximately 885 km east–west and between 145 km and 241 km north–south. It is bordered on the north by China, and by India in the south, east, and west. The topography ranges from the mountainous high Himalayas in the north to the mid-Himalayas in the middle, with their terraced slopes and fertile valleys, to the flat, subtropical Terai region along the country's southern border with India. Many of the world's tallest peaks, including Mount Everest, lie within Nepal.

The climate varies from the subtropical in the Terai to the alpine in the mountains. Kathmandu, the capital, is located in a valley and has a pleasant climate, with none of the extremes of the north or the south. The southwest monsoon brings rainfall during the period June to August, mostly in the Kathmandu valley and the east. The western portion of the country gets most of its rainfall in the winter.

History and Political System

Nepal, which has never been under foreign domination, consisted of several small autonomous kingdoms that were unified by King Prithvi Narayan Shah in 1769.

The powerful Rana line of hereditary prime ministers ruled the country from the early nineteenth century until their overthrow in 1951 after a popular revolution led by King Tribhuvan. In 1959, the country held its first election and a parliamentary government ran the country for a brief period. This experiment with democracy ended in 1960 and from then until 1990, when a people's movement ushered in democracy again, the country was governed by the monarchy with the assistance of a *Rashtriya Panchayat* (National Parliament). The members of this parliament were not affiliated with any party and were initially indirectly elected. Later, from the early '80s, the people directly elected parliamentary representatives but it was still a partyless system. In 1990, the country adopted a new constitution with a parliamentary system of government based on multiparty democracy with a constitutional monarchy.

Social and Cultural Environment

Nepal is a highly diverse country ethnically, linguistically, and culturally. The people are mostly of either Indo-Aryan or Tibeto-Burmese stock. While almost 90 percent of the population is Hindu, there are significant numbers of Buddhists and a small number of Muslims and Christians as well. Nepali is the *lingua franca* of the country, although several other languages are spoken as well, such as Newari, Tamang, Gurung, Maithili, Magar, and so on. English is spoken and understood by the educated people and in most urban centers.

The country is very rich culturally and this finds its expression in art, music, dance, and in the exquisite and intricate wood, stone, and bronze images found in the many temples, pagodas, and palaces.

Economic

Nepal is classified as a least developed country on the basis of several macro-economic indicators. Per capita income is around $200 annually and the country is primarily agrarian with less than 10 percent of GDP coming from the manufacturing sector. The population is close to 19 million with a growth rate of a little over 2 percent annually. As is usually the case in many developing countries, the birth rate and infant mortality rates are very high and average life expectancy is only 56.5 years. While the overall literacy rate is almost 40 percent, it is 54 percent for males and only 25 percent for females.

The country's major trading partners are India, USA, Japan, and Germany. The bulk of industrial, consumer, and durable products are imported from India, a country on which Nepal is very reliant. The country has been running a trade deficit and had 1994 exports of $363 million and $1,176 million in imports. Its primary exports are carpets and garments and it imports petroleum products, raw wool, manufactured products, and so on. The currency is the rupee (Rs.) with an exchange rate in 1996 of $1 = Rs. 56.75.

13 *CASE*

Emanuel Medical Center: Crisis in the Health Care Industry

The Haley Eckman Story

On Friday, four-year-old Haley Eckman stayed home from school because of a slight fever. She complained that she was feeling very tired. That night, Haley's temperature increased to 104°F. At 3:15 A.M., Mr. and Mrs. Eckman took Haley to the emergency department (ED) of Emanuel Medical Center (EMC) in Turlock, California. They registered at the admissions desk and waited for someone to see them. After what seemed like forever to the Eckmans, a triage nurse came out to evaluate Haley. He asked several questions, but failed to take her temperature – a routine procedure in that situation. He then disappeared, leaving the Eckmans to wait yet again.

While they waited, Haley vomited. She said she felt very weak. The family asked if Haley could lie down in a bed while they waited to see a doctor. A staff member told them that there were no available beds, and that they would have to wait. The Eckmans saw several empty beds across the hall from where they sat as the staff member said this.

At 4:35 A.M., the Eckmans were led to a room where a nurse took Haley's temperature and the physician on duty examined her. The physician assessed Haley's condition and ordered medicine that

This case study was prepared by Randall Harris, Kevin Vogt, and Armand Gilinsky as a basis for class discussion rather than to illustrate either effective or ineffective handling of an administrative situation. © 2004 by Randall Harris, Kevin Vogt, and Armand Gilinsky. Used with permission from Randy Harris.

Haley could not keep down. Finally, the physician told the Eckmans that Haley had the stomach flu and that they should take her home to rest.

The following night, Haley's temperature hit 106°F. This time the family drove to Memorial Medical Center in Modesto, California, where she was diagnosed with a urinary tract infection and was treated with the appropriate antibiotics.

Mrs. Eckman was so upset about Haley's treatment at EMC that she contacted the California Department of Health Services and registered a complaint. She then contacted the local newspaper about the incident. The Department of Health Services came to EMC, conducted an investigation, and concluded that standard ED procedures were not followed and that the staff did not act in a considerate and respectful manner.

More Problems Than the ED

Mr. Robert Moen, EMC president and CEO, was experiencing a number of challenges in 2002. First, there had been significant negative attention for Emanuel Medical Center following the newspaper accounts and a state investigation of the Haley Eckman incident. The emergency department at EMC was experiencing greater pressure to deliver services in an increasingly difficult health care environment, particularly in light of federal EMTALA (Emergency Medical Treatment and Active Labor Act) legislation that required access to emergency medical care for all, regardless of ability to pay. Bernadette Khanania, EMC's ED Director, said, "I think when the EMTALA rules changed, it had an impact. The trend is sicker patients in the ED. It has to do with managed care, full practices, and older patients. It's not just our ED; every ED is seeing these changes."

The cost of operating the emergency department had risen precipitously and patient flows vastly exceeded the capacity for which the ED had been designed. Moen commented, "We don't get paid enough for the emergency department patients that we see. Not being paid adequately means that we can't build for the future."

An ED nurse agreed: "The patients are much sicker when they come in because they wait longer, so the pace is faster."

In addition, reimbursements for services from health maintenance organizations (HMOs) and government programs had been drastically reduced, at the same time that paperwork and other regulatory burdens had increased. EMC was beginning to experience labor shortages, particularly of nurses, that were driving up EMC's cost of operations. And, for-profit managed care facilities were making significant incursions into EMC's service area. According to Moen, "Kaiser Permanente has announced plans to build a facility in our area."

The net effect of all of these factors was increasing pressure on the profitability of EMC. EMC's operating margins had been negative for some time, contributing to increased pressures on cash flow. Moen said, "I am beginning to think that the pressures placed on us by our stakeholders potentially threaten the hospital's survival. I don't know whether we should merge the hospital with a competing organization or one of the HMOs, try to sell the hospital, close the ED, close the hospital outright, or work harder to alter operations and turn it around."

US Health Care Industry

US national health expenditures totaled $1.553 trillion in 2002. This amount represented 14.9 percent of US gross domestic product (GDP) according to the US Centers for Medicare and Medicaid Services.[1] By way of contrast, US national health expenditures in 1980 were $245.8 billion and 8.8 percent of US GDP. Growth in national health expenditures began to outpace growth in US GDP in 1999 and this trend was forecasted to continue well into the twenty-first century.

Growth in spending on hospitals, physicians, and pharmaceuticals rose rapidly during this time period. National spending on hospital services rose from $378.5 billion in 1998 to $486.5 billion in 2002, an increase of 28.5 percent. Spending on physician and clinical services rose 32.2 percent, from $256.8 billion to $339.5 billion, during this same time period. The largest increase, however, was spending on pharmaceuticals. US consumers spent $162.4 billion on pharmaceuticals in 2002, an increase of 87.3 percent from 1996. From 1994 to 2002, annual US spending on pharmaceuticals almost tripled, according to the US Centers for Medicare and Medicaid Services.[2] Exhibit 13/1 contains key statistics of the US health care industry.

The precipitous rise in health care expenditures was accompanied by a rapid consolidation of health care facilities. The total number of hospitals in the United States actually decreased from 1996 to 2002 as consolidation and

Exhibit 13/1: US Health Care Industry Key Statistics: 1998 to 2002

	Year				
	1998	**1999**	**2000**	**2001**	**2002**
National Health Expenditures ($ billions)	1,150.3	1,222.6	1,309.4	1,420.7	1,553.0
Annual Percent Growth Rate in Expenditures	5.3	6.3	7.1	8.5	9.3
US GDP ($ billions)	8,782	9,274	9,825	10,082	10,446
Annual Percent Growth Rate in GDP	5.6	5.6	5.9	2.6	3.6
National Health Expenditures as a Percent of GDP	13.1	13.2	13.3	14.1	14.9
US Medicare Expenditures ($ billions)	204.0	206.2	217.5	239.2	259.1
US Medicaid Expenditures ($ billions)	93.2	100.9	109.8	122.5	137.0
US Hospital Facilities					
Number of Hospitals	5,015	4,956	4,915	4,908	4,927
Not-for-Profit Hospitals	3,026	3,012	3,003	2,998	3,025
State/Local Government Hospitals	1,218	1,197	1,163	1,156	1,136
For-Profit Hospitals	771	747	749	754	766

Source: Centers for Medicare and Medicaid Services; American Hospital Association.

closures occurred. In 1996, there were 5,134 community hospitals, but that number decreased to 4,927 by 2002. Fully 61 percent of US hospitals were operated as not-for-profit entities. In 2002, state and local governments operated 1,136 hospitals, 14.6 percent less than in 1996. Corporate, for-profit hospitals were actually the smallest group, numbering 766 hospitals in the US in 2000, according to the American Hospital Association.[3]

Regardless of the ownership status or size, all hospitals were subject to the same cumbersome governmental regulations. From the workplace safeguards of the Occupational Safety and Health Administration (OSHA) to the patient safety mandates of Title XXII of the Federal Health and Safety Code, regulation played a large role in health care. It was rumored in the industry that if a person were to gather together all of the documents that related to federal billing regulations for Medicare, it would fill a 40-ft tractor-trailer. At the federal level, the Office of the Inspector General (OIG) was mandated to oversee regulatory compliance in the health care industry.

EMTALA

A significant change in the regulatory environment occurred in 1986. The Emergency Medical Treatment and Active Labor Act (EMTALA) was made federal law that year. The legislation was passed after a gang member died in the parking lot of a hospital in plain view of emergency department staff. In passing this law, the federal government mandated access to emergency medical care for all people, regardless of their ability to pay, once they were present on the grounds of a hospital. It was designed to address emergency facilities' refusal to treat patients with serious conditions who were not able to pay for the services. Although the legislation was passed in 1986, it was not until the late 1990s that it began to be actively enforced. Investigations of EMTALA violations increased markedly at that time and fines up to $50,000 per incident were levied on both hospitals and physicians.[4]

With rapid growth in the number of underinsured and uninsured US citizens during the same period, the EMTALA legislation posed a significant challenge for hospitals and their emergency departments. Although it made perfect sense to care for those who were in critical condition before asking any financial questions, the EMTALA regulations had turned the most expensive department in a hospital into a free clinic for underinsured and uninsured patients that were largely in need of routine primary – not emergency – medical care. It was rapidly bankrupting many hospitals in the process.

The Role of Government

All of this regulation came with a direct cost to consumers, and consumers were increasingly concerned. "Health care ranks as the voters' top concern; recent spurts in costs have provoked more pressure – from employers and consumers

– for changes than at any time since the failure of the Clinton national health-insurance initiative in 1994," according to J. Cummings in the *Wall Street Journal*.[5] The federal government, through the Balanced Budget Act of 1997, contributed to cost pressures in the industry by decreasing reimbursements for Medicare.

Staffing Shortages

Hospitals were dealing with chronic staff shortages. Demand for health care services was increasing rapidly at the same time that the labor pool for nurses, in particular, was leveling off. The increasing average age of active nurses was further exacerbating this problem.[6] (See Exhibit 13/2 for estimated imbalance between nurse supply and demand in the United States through 2020.)

Consequently, salaries paid to nurses were rising rapidly. Health care employers were attempting to increase the attractiveness of nursing jobs for qualified professionals. Employers had become increasingly willing to offer

Exhibit 13/2: Registered Nurses, Estimated Supply and Demand from 2000 to 2020

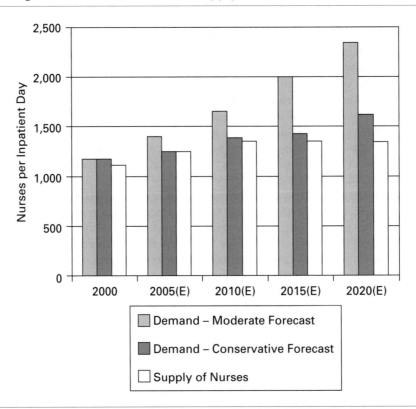

Source: Health Care Advisory Board, 2000.

flextime and other nontraditional staffing arrangements to accommodate an increasingly stretched labor pool. These trends were expected to continue nationally for at least the next 20 years.

California Health Care Industry

In January 2001, the California Medical Association (CMA) produced its report, *California's Emergency Services: A System in Crisis*. The CMA president, Dr. Frank E. Staggers, commented on the report: "Because our emergency and trauma system is woefully underfunded, it may not be able to fully respond when we need it the most. This report shows we have much to do if we want to preserve an emergency medical system that's always available and truly protects the public." He continued, "California's health care system is struggling to adjust to serious underfunding of all services and provide care to more than 7 million uninsured Californians. The 'safety net' – that part of the system that serves as the first line of defense – has begun to unravel."[7]

Health care in California has been described as the "perfect storm." Declining reimbursements combined with increasingly onerous regulation and a shortage of nurses had led to negative operating margins for over half of California hospitals. From 1996 to 2000, 7 percent of the hospitals in California closed.[8] That left fewer emergency departments to care for the immediate needs of more patients and fewer beds to care for the chronically ill. These factors, combined with an aging population that increasingly demanded quality health care, produced a sharp increase in demand at exactly the time that the health care system had a reduced capacity to handle the patient load.

Of the hospital closures in California, the largest reduction had been in state and local government-owned facilities. Since 1996, 17 percent of state and county hospitals in California had closed. At the same time, the number of for-profit facilities decreased by 11 percent. The only sector resisting this trend was the not-for-profits. The not-for-profit sector closed less than 2 percent of its facilities during the 1996–2000 time period, placing intense pressure on the not-for-profit sector to handle the increasing demands of the health care system.[9]

On the expense side of the equation, California's hospitals confronted a challenging climate relative to other hospitals in the nation. They had higher patient costs than the national average (because of the impact of managed care on patient treatment patterns), higher wages for hospital employees, a significant nursing shortage, and the third-largest uninsured population in the nation.

Managed Care

Managed care exploded in California in the early 1990s because cost pressures on insurance premiums caused employers to look for ways to manage rising health care costs. Although HMO premiums held constant or decreased during this time period, the real pressure was on health care providers. Managed care shifted the risk of providing services from insurors to hospitals and physicians. These arrangements made the provider responsible for a person's health care, regardless of how much health care was consumed or how much it cost.

The new HMO payment arrangements created a need to manage the entire health care process, not just hospital care or medical care. This change gave rise to contractual and ownership interests in horizontal and vertical health care networks. "Vertical integration was seen by many as the solution to the problem that capitation posed for providers because it theoretically allowed a system to control the whole delivery system and therefore manage costs and utilization. During the past five years, empires have been built and have fallen," according to the Standard & Poor's industry survey.[10] Unfortunately, the tremendous costs associated with these networks forced some HMOs out of business and many health care networks and systems simply abandoned the experiment. Fortunately for the rest of the country, California tried it first.

Medi-Cal

Medi-Cal was the California state health insurance program for low-income families. In 2001, a total of 5.5 million persons per month in California were eligible for Medi-Cal (an increase of 8.2 percent over 2000). A total of $1.3 billion in nondental medical service fees were reimbursed by the State of California through Medi-Cal in 2001, representing a 14.0 percent increase over 2000, according to the California Department of Health Services.[11] During this time, California ranked 42nd out of 50 states in the level of per capita payments for health care.[12]

In 2001, the California Hospital Association litigated successfully to increase reimbursements, arguing that the state had failed to pay California hospitals at a reasonable rate. The settlement required the state to increase rates by 30 percent (an effective 2 percent increase per year) as well as paying a lump sum of $350 million to be split by all of the hospitals in the state.[13] Even with these increases, physicians and hospitals were reluctant to serve a high percentage of Medi-Cal patients because of the low reimbursements. According to an ED nurse at EMC, "The patients who are mostly on Medi-Cal . . . They come here to our ED at EMC." Dr. Robert Craig, an ED physician added, "Hospitals are having trouble dealing with the volume of patients that they treat."

Medicare

Beginning in 1983, Medicare (the federal program for the elderly) had reimbursed inpatient care at preestablished rates (the prospective payment system or PPS), but had paid for outpatient services at provider costs. In August 2000, however, a new policy was established to pay a fixed fee for all outpatient services as well. It decreased overall payments by 5 percent and greatly increased the paperwork associated with reimbursements. The new payment policy reduced out-of-pocket expenses to Medicare beneficiaries by lowering co-payments and standardized patient co-payments across facilities in the United States so that patients would pay the same co-payment for services they received no matter where the care was provided. Prior to this change, Medicare patients paid 20 percent of their bills. Since charges varied widely across facilities throughout the country, a patient could end up paying ten times as much in out-of-pocket expenses at one hospital compared with another. For most hospitals in California, the mandated co-payment rate resulted in significantly lower reimbursements from Medicare.

HMOs

Health maintenance organizations routinely negotiated reduced fees with hospitals in exchange for sending their patients to the contracting hospital's facilities. In California, this arrangement had been around for over 20 years, but in the past 10 years the payment scheme had shifted to capitation. HMOs began to match Medicare reimbursements, routinely underfunding the expenses that hospitals incurred, making it unaffordable for the hospitals to provide patient treatment. By 2001, a large percentage of hospitals in California had exited from HMO capitation contracts; hospitals returned to adversarial negotiation, as had been done previously.

The result of this new, more adversarial relationship was to once again shift the rising cost of health care to HMOs and the employers that paid them. Hospitals, squeezed by underfunded and inadequate payments from government-sponsored programs and faced with rising costs (such as EMTALA mandated emergency care), began extracting higher payments from commercial payors. Cost shifting drove commercial payments higher for the first time in several years. As the shifting continued, employers began to see dramatic increases in health care costs for their employees. Employers, as a consequence, then began to pass these costs on to their employees or to reduce the benefits provided. Employees, both directly or indirectly, began to pay more for their health care and became increasingly underinsured.

Physician Concerns

Physicians began seeing their incomes fall as managed care programs began to decrease reimbursements for medical services as well as hospital and other services. In the central valley of northern California, in particular, the high mix of Medi-Cal patients among all patients lowered the overall compensation of physicians, particularly those in specialty practices. In addition, managed care programs, and in particular Medi-Cal, had taken a great deal of autonomy away from physicians. Physicians complained that they were second-guessed by medical directors at HMOs as well as administrators at Medi-Cal. Physicians began being required to obtain administrative authorizations from managed care programs before proceeding with treatment and were increasingly denied these authorizations if adequate documentation was not presented. Physicians found dealing with the process to be time consuming and increasingly frustrating. Service delivery and patient/customer satisfaction were seriously affected. In addition, a growing number of physicians simply refused to treat Medi-Cal patients because the cost of providing care to these patients exceeded what the State of California would reimburse.

Emanuel Medical Center

Emanuel Medical Center (EMC) of Turlock, California, was founded in 1917. Turlock was located approximately 100 miles east of San Francisco (see Exhibit 13/3 for a map). The hospital was established to serve the medical needs of all people in the local community, regardless of social, ethnic, or religious background. Founded by two pastors of the Swedish Mission Church, EMC operated on behalf of the Board of Benevolence of the Evangelical Covenant Church.

Mission, Vision, and Values

An early motto attributed to its founders described the mission of EMC as a "Christian service institution." In 2002, the mission of Emanuel Medical Center was to "create a healthier community." EMC's vision was to be "a caring community, caring for our community." The culture of EMC was built on a set of core values and beliefs that included: the affirmation of *life*, the pursuit of *justice* in the treatment of all individuals, *stewardship* of the lives entrusted to it, *integrity* in all of their actions, *collaboration* with individuals and the community to achieve their shared goals, and *excellence* in a commitment to exceed all expectations for their institution.

Emanuel Medical Center dedicated itself to implementing performance improvement measures for all critical hospital functions, providing excellent customer service, and continuously improving patient satisfaction. EMC identified three organizational goals around which it based its operating strategies and resource decisions. These three organizational goals were: caring for their customers and each other; providing clinical, operational, and service excellence; and growing revenue, facilities, and people.

Major Products and Divisions

Emanuel Medical Center was organized into three units: the acute-care 150-bed hospital, a 145-bed skilled-nursing facility, and a 49-bed assisted living facility. The central hospital facility handled acute inpatient services, including intensive care, monitored care, and general medical and surgical services. The site housed a comprehensive emergency department that never closed. Although there were 150 licensed beds, the occupancy rate of the hospital was typically little more than

Exhibit 13/3: Map of Turlock and Northern California

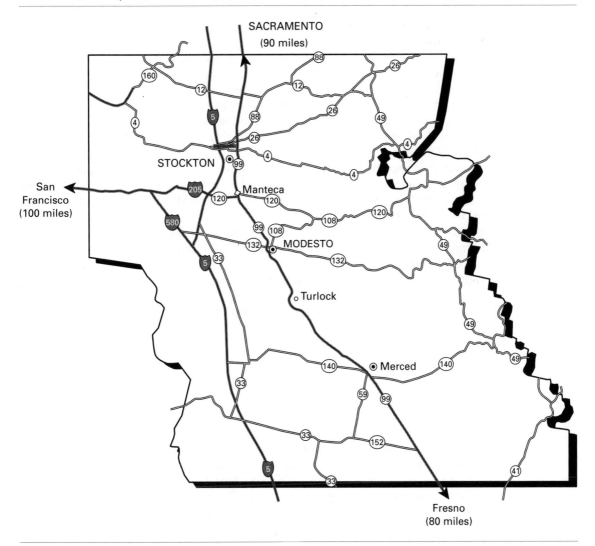

50 percent. Many of the rooms were semiprivate (two patients per room) and that tended to reduce patient satisfaction. However, one patient often received the exclusive use of a semiprivate room, if space allowed; that was typically the case with occupancy at 50 percent.

EMC's emergency department, on the other hand, was running well beyond full capacity. Built in the 1970s, the ED was designed for 16,000 visits per year. Over 45,000 patient visits were made to the ED during 2001. In addition, at any given time, over half of the patients admitted to the hospital for an extended stay came through the ED. This had increased the financial pressure on EMC, because patients admitted through the ED were often the least able to pay or reimburse the hospital for services provided. Patients admitted to the hospital through a physician referral were much more likely to have comprehensive health insurance.

A full complement of outpatient services was available at the hospital site, including radiology, a clinical laboratory, and outpatient surgery. In addition, a separate diagnostic and rehabilitation center was housed on the hospital campus. This center enabled patients to have routine radiology exams, mammograms, and speech and occupational therapy on an outpatient basis.

Brandel Manor, the 145-bed skilled-nursing facility, rendered nursing and physical therapy services to patients needing around-the-clock care following surgery or a prolonged illness. Brandel Manor offered services for patients who could no longer live at home and required care because of the loss of mobility or some mental impairment. Brandel Manor maintained an average occupancy rate of better than 90 percent each year.

Finally, EMC owned and operated Cypress of Emanuel, a 49-bed assisted living facility. Cypress was an apartment-like setting for patients who had full mobility, but preferred the communal aspects of living. Residents received oversight for medication administration and group dining experiences to stay socially active. Occupancy was close to 100 percent. A constant waiting list existed for Cypress of Emanuel because it was an affordable alternative to other facilities in the area.

EMC's Service Area

EMC's primary service area consisted of the city of Turlock and eight smaller surrounding towns. Eighty percent of EMC's patients were residents of this primary service area; nearly 64 percent of patients were residents of Turlock. The secondary service area consisted of the additional 12 small towns that were geographically between 5 and 15 miles from EMC. Fourteen percent of EMC's patients were residents of the secondary service area. The remaining six percent of EMC's patients were from outside both these service areas.

CUSTOMER DEMOGRAPHICS

EMC's customer base was growing, aging, and becoming more culturally diverse. EMC's primary service area had a population of approximately 200,000 in 2002, up from approximately 168,000 in 1998 (an increase of 19 percent). Baby boomers made up a fast growing proportion of the rapidly aging EMC patient population. In 1999, 40.1 percent of hospital patients at EMC were 65 years of age or older, 33.2 percent of patients were aged 15 to 44, and 10.2 percent were 14 years old or younger. EMC's service area had an estimated Hispanic population of approximately 65,000 (32.5 percent). By 1999, Hispanic patients were the fastest growing segment of ED admissions at EMC.

EMC Hospital Operations

Emanuel Medical Center was an organization with long-term employees working in a close-knit environment. They liked to project a caring, friendly feeling to those that visited their medical center. Many larger hospitals had multiple layers of management, high turnover rates, and little connection between employees. EMC had largely been able to maintain a small-town atmosphere at the hospital. They took complaints, such as the one made by the Eckmans, personally.

EMC had ranked in the 90th percentile for the past three Press Ganey Corporation surveys in total patient satisfaction. The initiative to improve these scores from beginning marks in the 70th percentile had involved the entire facility in an effort to deliver high-touch, friendly patient care.

One of the many benefits from EMC's intense focus on the patient was a reduction in costs. EMC had been benchmarked as a low-cost provider of services against statewide measures within its comparison group. Surveys through the Solutient Corporation against a national database showed that EMC was a benchmark hospital for salary cost per admission, supply cost per admission, and overall cost per admission.

Being a small-town hospital had some drawbacks, however. Larger hospitals tended to acquire new technology first. Although the hospital constantly updated equipment, EMC was sometimes perceived as low-tech because of a lack of some specialties, such as specialized cardiology services. Heart catheterization and surgery were not offered at EMC, but were available at hospitals in Modesto. This lack of specialization in some areas affected the bottom line of the hospital, because these high-tech specialties tended to be quite profitable.

The emergency department was a growing area of concern. The department was built for patient volumes that existed over 25 years ago. An additional ED waiting room was built in the 1980s, but it had been outgrown. Many days the waiting room was full, the beds in the department were all full, and more patients and family members were becoming increasingly frustrated. Moen summed it up: "There are probably other things, but fundamental to the whole crisis is the lack of reimbursement. It squeezes us. We cannot finance out of operations the major expansions that we see we really need to do."

Top Management Team

The senior management team at EMC consisted of the president/chief executive officer and six vice presidents. These vice presidents led the divisions of finance, professional services, support services, patient care services, human resources, and development.

Robert Moen, president and CEO since 1986, had been at EMC for over 30 years. He had seen many changes as the facility grew through the late 1960s and early 1970s, but one of his biggest challenges was the emergency department. Moen believed that the problems experienced by patients such as Haley Eckman in

Exhibit 13/4: Percentage of EMC Emergency Department Visits by Insurance Status, Fiscal Years 2000 to 2002

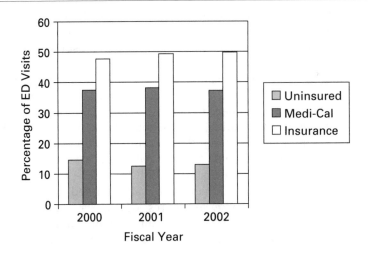

Source: EMC Company Documents.

the ED were partly systemic. He said, "In much of the past 20 years, we were able to get by . . . In many cases it was because we were creative, careful, and selective in what we did. To ensure the future profitability of the hospital and our ability to provide services, we were able to build facilities when we needed to. However, we are in a place right now that, due to drastic cuts in reimbursements, we can barely stay up from an operational standpoint, let alone try to put money aside to build for the future."

Moen continued, "I'm concerned that over half of all emergency department patients admitted to EMC are either underinsured through programs like Medi-Cal or uninsured. From 2000 to 2002, our ED admissions increased 9.77 percent. During that time period, however, no more than 49 percent of ED admits had full health insurance coverage." Exhibit 13/4 shows a breakdown of payment types for EMC emergency department admissions.

Strategic Goals and Current Issues

EMC's top management team had set several strategic priorities for fiscal year 2003 (FY03) to FY06 to enhance EMC's position as a hospital of choice for both patients and the workforce:

- *Physician Development:* Recruit and retain the finest physicians, both general practice and specialists.
- *Product Mix:* Optimize product and service offerings to create growth and increase market share.

- *Facilities and Technology:* Create a "techno-edge" by wisely acquiring new technologies, as well as providing appropriate facilities for operations.
- *Contract Management:* Manage contracts with HMOs and governmental organizations for maximum reimbursement, keeping EMC a provider where financial conditions were favorable.
- *Quality Workforce:* Assure a quality workforce through offering competitive wages and benefits, as well as actively recruiting and retaining the best employees.

Moen had several operational issues on his mind. He said, "I'm concerned about shortages of critical care monitor beds and a lack of staff. Staffing is a statewide issue, but it affects all of us and causes management diversion from other operational concerns. On the physician backup side, we are struggling right now with recruiting and retaining a number of physician specialties and subspecialties. We don't always have adequate numbers of physicians with the right specializations locally to properly back up the demand in the emergency department."

He continued, "Another looming issue is the rising influence of managed care organizations. Since the 1990s, a number of health care facilities have been assimilated into managed care networks. For example, Memorial Hospital in Modesto was acquired by the Sutter network in 1996. In addition, Kaiser Permanente has made significant inroads." In 1998, Kaiser had 10,000 people insured in EMC's service area; at the end of 2001, that number had grown to 60,000. As of 2002, EMC no longer contracted to provide health care services to Kaiser's clients because Moen was unable to agree with Kaiser on reimbursement rates for services.

Moen constantly felt the pressure from government regulations and declining reimbursement rates. Changes in mandatory staffing levels for nurses, for example, had reduced the number of beds that EMC could offer for acute care at any given time. Moen stated, "I'm unclear about the future impact of other pending government legislation. Federal and state reimbursement rates are inadequate to meet hospital costs; yet state and federal budgets are strained, making any increases in reimbursement rates unlikely. I am certain that these outside forces will continue to exert tremendous downward pressure on EMC's bottom line."

Competitive Environment

Because of closures and consolidations, EMC was facing an increasingly hostile external environment. Four major health systems competed for business in EMC's service area: Sutter Health, Catholic Healthcare West, Tenet Healthcare Corporation, and Kaiser Permanente (see Exhibit 13/5).

Sutter Health

Sutter Medical Centers treated more inpatients than any other network in Northern California. Sutter Health was one of the nation's leading not-for-profit networks of community health care services, serving more than 20 Northern California

Exhibit 13/5: Competitors in EMC's Service Area

Company	Facility	Location	Number of Beds
Sutter Health	Memorial Medical Center	Modesto	300
Catholic Healthcare West	Mercy Hospital	Merced	115
	St. Joseph's Hospital	Stockton	294
Tenet Healthcare Corporation	Doctors Medical Center	Modesto	397
Kaiser Permanente	Doctors Hospital	Manteca	73
	Memorial Medical Center (under contract)	Modesto	300
	Dameron Hospital (under contract)	Stockton	192
Independent Hospital	Emanuel Medical Center	Turlock	150

Source: American Hospital Association, California Office of Statewide Health Planning and Development.

counties, from the Oregon border to the San Joaquin Valley, and from the Pacific coast to the Sierra foothills. In EMC's service area, Sutter owned Memorial Medical Center, a 300-bed full-service hospital. Memorial was located in Modesto, 20 miles north of Turlock. In 2001, Memorial Medical Center had 57,191 ED visits and had an average occupancy rate of 82.2 percent.[14] Memorial specialized in cardiac care, cancer services, and outpatient surgery and offered a family birthing center.

Catholic Healthcare West

Catholic Healthcare West, a not-for-profit health care provider, spanned a service area that encompassed parts of Arizona, Nevada, and most of California. It was the largest not-for-profit health care provider in California and the largest Catholic hospital system in the western part of the United States. Mercy Hospital of Merced, located in Merced, California, approximately 30 miles south of EMC, joined Catholic Healthcare West in 1996. Mercy was a 115-bed acute care hospital that specialized in maternity care, surgical services, critical care, emergency medicine, laboratory, radiology, and respiratory services and boasted an accredited sleep disorder lab. In 2001, Mercy had 45,561 ED visits and had an average occupancy rate of 42.1 percent.[15] In addition, Catholic Healthcare West owned St. Joseph's Hospital in Stockton, approximately 50 miles north of EMC. St. Joseph's had 294 beds and specialized in sports medicine, cancer, and cardiac care and offered an outpatient surgical center.

Tenet Healthcare Corporation

Tenet Healthcare Corporation, a nationwide for-profit provider of health care services, owned or operated 116 acute care hospitals and related businesses serving communities in 17 states. The company, headquartered in Santa Barbara, California, employed approximately 113,000 people nationwide. In EMC's service area, Tenet operated Doctors Medical Center of Modesto and Doctors Hospital of Manteca.

Doctors Medical Center of Modesto began as a small 56-bed facility, but grew to become a full-care hospital, licensed for 397 beds. Located 20 miles north of Turlock, DMC Modesto held the contract to service the Yosemite National Forest, covering emergency evacuations and injury treatment. In 2001, Doctors had 52,487 ED visits and had an average occupancy rate of 60.7 percent.[16] It specialized in cancer treatment, neurosurgery, cardiac care, and pediatrics.

Doctors Hospital of Manteca was a much smaller facility. Located 35 miles north of Turlock, the Manteca facility had 73 beds with an average occupancy rate of 42.4 percent. In 2001, Doctors Hospital of Manteca had 14,145 ED visits, and specialized in occupational medicine.[17]

Kaiser Permanente

Kaiser, though a relative newcomer, was becoming a major player in local health care, with 60,000+ people insured in Stanislaus County. In EMC's secondary service area, Kaiser operated under contract through Dameron Hospital in Stockton, about 50 miles north of Turlock. Dameron had 192 beds, a 62.2 percent average occupancy rate, and 31,125 ED visits in 2001.[18]

Kaiser patients in Stanislaus County (EMC's primary service area) were treated at Memorial Hospital in Modesto, a Sutter affiliate. The partnership agreement between Kaiser and Memorial Hospital was to expire in February 2003. In November 2001, Kaiser announced plans to spend $1 billion in the Central Valley of California on medical facilities in or around Sacramento, Stockton, and Modesto. Thus, Kaiser's plans included a new hospital in EMC's service area. Kaiser had been aggressive in its marketing and promotion in Stanislaus County. Moen and the board anticipated that Kaiser would continue to push for greater coverage in EMC's primary service area.

Independent Hospitals

Of the four independent hospitals that were operational in EMC's primary service area in 1995, only EMC Medical Center remained open. The other independent hospitals, Bloss Memorial Hospital, Stanislaus Medical Center (the Stanislaus County-run facility), and Del Puerto Hospital, had all closed during the late 1990s. These closures mirrored the nationwide trend of hospital closures that occurred during the same time period.

Financial Status of EMC

With the dramatic growth in managed care in the late 1990s, EMC was under pressure to accept capitation or risk having no patients. Under the capitation payment system, an HMO would pay a set amount per member per month (PMPM) to EMC to cover patient care costs for their covered members. PMPM was actually a prepayment, because fees were paid to EMC each month for each HMO member enrolled in its program, rather than paid out to EMC after services were rendered. Capitation reduced accounts receivable for EMC and improved EMC's cash flow on the front end. On the back end, however, the HMO payment rates and the relative risk that EMC faced were not aligned. Fully allocated costs for patient treatments regularly exceeded HMO payments to EMC and EMC began to experience significant losses from HMO-covered patient care.

The financial trends for EMC closely matched the HMO capitation experiment experienced by many hospitals in California. Although EMC saw the move into capitation in 1997 as a defensive strategy to retain HMO patients, the effect on EMC's bottom line became increasingly negative. As the contracts began to expire, EMC exited the HMO-sponsored capitation arrangements, restoring the hospital to marginal profitability.

EMC Revenues

EMC posted total income of $4.7 million in 2001, which was a net margin of 6.3 percent. During the same year, however, EMC lost $4.1 million on operations – a direct result of the rising costs of employee salaries and wages, as well as the growing losses from HMO capitation programs. Over the five-year period of capitation for EMC, all but the first year resulted in operating losses. Exhibits 13/6 and 13/7 present income statements and balance sheets for EMC from 1997 to 2002.

EMC's primary source of revenue was from operations, related to caring for patients, either inpatient (with an overnight stay) or outpatient. The more common types of outpatient care were same-day surgery, emergency department visits, and routine radiology procedures.

Over the past five years, EMC had developed significant revenues from nonoperating related sources. The primary source was income on investments that were made in the mid-1990s. During that time, the board of directors had adopted a capital structure that favored liquidity on EMC's balance sheet. By borrowing funds for expansion and investing unspent funds allocated for capital expenditures, EMC increased its capital reserves from $4 million to $23 million within three years. With strong returns from the stock market in the late 1990s, this reserve ballooned to over $50 million by the end of the decade. In the early years of the twenty-first century, this base provided a source of income that was sorely needed to shore up operating losses.

The second significant nonoperating source of income was fund raising. EMC was a not-for-profit charity and donors were given a tax advantage for their contributions. Over the history of EMC, the community had supported facility expansions and the ongoing activities of the development office. In 2001, EMC implemented an aggressive program to involve the community in building for the future. With a matching grant from the Mary Stuart Rogers Foundation, the

Exhibit 13/6: Emanuel Medical Center Income Statements, Fiscal Years 1997 to 2002 (in $ thousands)

	1997	1998	1999	2000	2001	2002
Net Patient Revenue	53,787	46,654	46,329	46,700	47,457	65,653
Other Revenue	720	821	939	1,084	1,022	1,192
Premium Revenue	1,265	7,115	7,198	8,187	7,666	1,715
Total Operating Revenue	**55,772**	**54,590**	**54,466**	**55,971**	**56,145**	**68,560**
Operating Expenses:						
Salaries and Wages	21,516	22,336	22,339	23,640	25,274	27,506
Employee Benefits	7,405	8,486	8,336	7,883	7,887	9,073
Professional Fees	2,749	2,590	1,783	2,271	2,368	4,643
Supplies	8,879	8,981	8,487	8,750	9,093	10,081
Purchased Services	3,603	2,981	2,749	2,897	3,195	3,774
Depreciation	3,563	3,627	3,774	3,768	3,623	3,533
Utilities	681	727	668	689	667	677
Insurance	826	920	591	405	393	527
Interest Expense	1,552	1,777	1,765	1,584	1,303	475
Bad Debt	1,389	1,978	2,627	2,938	4,357	6,155
Other	1,424	1,381	1,682	1,877	2,124	2,248
Total Expenses	**53,587**	**55,784**	**54,801**	**56,702**	**60,284**	**68,692**
Operating Income	**2,185**	**(1,194)**	**(335)**	**(731)**	**(4,139)**	**(132)**
Nonoperating Revenue						
Interest and Dividend Income	968	1,217	1,284	1,465	2,620	2,084
Realized Gains (Losses) on Investments	1,005	2,733	3,578	7,885	5,707	(2,160)
Contributions	390	299	268	415	489	688
Total Nonoperating Revenue	**2,363**	**4,249**	**5,130**	**9,765**	**8,816**	**612**
Net Income	**4,548**	**3,055**	**4,795**	**9,034**	**4,677**	**480**
Unrealized Gains on Investments	1,792	(1,055)	2,394	2,848	(8,357)	(2,676)
Increase in Net Assets	6,340	2,000	7,189	11,882	(3,680)	(2,196)
Acute and ICU Patient Days (Actual)	26,048	25,342	23,895	25,330	25,051	27,006
ED Visits (Actual)	36,214	34,363	32,071	37,485	38,931	41,145

Source: California Office of Statewide Health Planning and Development.

community took part in a fund drive to expand the birthing center at EMC. During a five-week kick-off campaign, volunteers and employees raised over $1.4 million toward the $4 million project.

EMC Expenses

Expenses over the past three years had grown at a rate of 7.7 percent per year, with salaries and wages combined with benefits accounting for 4.1 percent. In addition, during 2002, EMC had to raise salaries for beginning nurses by as much as

Exhibit 13/7: Emanuel Medical Center Balance Sheets, Fiscal Years 1997 to 2002 (in $ thousands)

	1997	1998	1999	2000	2001	2002
Current Assets						
Cash and Cash Equivalents	2,108	1,572	2,076	4,315	650	484
Trustee Held Funds	505	766	685	599	574	524
Accounts Receivable	7,693	8,967	8,722	7,708	9,650	10,987
Other Receivables	589	877	1,867	1,434	1,423	2,806
Inventory	925	952	977	1,054	1,073	1,043
Prepaid Expenses	288	22	44	15	246	365
Total	12,108	13,156	14,371	15,125	13,616	16,209
Investments						
Board Designated Investments	30,944	33,956	41,803	54,781	52,689	47,589
Trustee Held Funds	2,223	2,122	2,135	2,033	2,300	2,228
Total	33,167	36,078	43,938	56,814	54,989	49,817
Property and Equipment						
Land	1,509	1,509	1,509	1,509	1,509	1,509
Buildings and Improvements	39,811	39,932	40,935	41,206	43,152	44,099
Equipment	19,610	21,194	23,070	23,942	25,593	27,130
Construction in Progress	1,369	897	753	1,551	596	833
Property and Equipment (at cost)	62,299	63,532	66,267	68,208	70,850	73,571
Less Accumulated Depreciation	26,262	29,814	33,524	36,956	40,264	43,744
Property and Equipment, Net	36,037	33,718	32,743	31,252	30,586	29,827
Other Assets	658	603	902	1,784	1,316	1,165
Total Assets	81,970	83,555	91,954	104,975	100,507	97,018
Current Liabilities						
Accounts Payable	2,032	1,194	1,281	1,238	1,929	1,617
Payroll and Related Liabilities	2,055	2,314	2,440	2,692	3,088	2,171
Interest Payable	435	446	428	430	423	415
Other Current Liabilities	936	1,726	2,856	2,672	2,268	2,056
Current Portion of Long-Term Debt	627	685	804	964	630	615
IBNR Liability	545	450	1,085	1,273	1,582	288
Estimated Third-Party Settlements	1,537	1,515	1,373	3,047	2,184	2,272
Total Current Liabilities	8,167	8,330	10,267	12,316	12,104	9,434
Long-Term Debt	27,216	26,638	25,911	25,022	24,426	24,114
Total Liabilities	35,383	34,968	36,178	37,338	36,530	33,548
Total Net Assets	46,587	48,587	55,776	67,657	63,977	63,470
Total Liabilities and Net Assets	81,970	83,555	91,954	104,975	100,507	97,018

Source: California Office of Statewide Health Planning and Development.

27 percent to be competitive. The nursing shortage in California had increased the use of temporary nurses – that added significantly to labor costs.

EMC entered capitation in 1997 with a relatively low number of patients as HMO members. More important to EMC than the absolute dollars paid out for treatment of HMO patients under capitation payments was the percentage of this premium revenue that was given to other health care providers for services rendered. In 1997, 34 percent of HMO premium revenue received by EMC was paid out to other providers for health care services (such as cardiac surgery) that EMC was not equipped to provide for its members. In 2001, 54 percent of the HMO revenue EMC received went to other health care providers. This substantially increased EMC's losses on HMO capitation programs and contributed to EMC's eventual exit from this payment mechanism in 2002.

By 1998, however, EMC had 17,000 patients per year under this arrangement. This number of HMO-contracted patients remained fairly constant through the next four years. Capitation expenses had grown during the five-year period from $655,000 in 1997 to $8.9 million in 2001.

EMC management observed a significant increase in uncollectable debts payable to EMC after the county medical facility in Modesto closed in 1997.

Bottom Line

The EMC board of directors' decision to invest assets in stocks and bonds in the mid-1990s had a dramatic impact on EMC's financial health. Moen concluded, "If the board had not made these investments beginning in 1993, the financial viability of EMC would be in jeopardy."

Mr. Bruce Metcalf, chairman of EMC's board of directors, stated, "Given the size of our reserves, we are at least hopeful that we can weather the ups and downs of the current market environment as well as continue to plan for the future."

The Future of Emanuel Medical Center

Moen stated, "I have seen a number of significant changes in the health care industry, but nothing like I'm seeing now. I am concerned about EMC's ability to survive and prosper in this radically altered health care environment."

"Yes, we're at risk if we continue to get influxes of patients who are not financially solvent. I mean, at some point somebody could decide this is costing us more money than it's worth. That's why EDs close," Dr. Robert Craig, an ED physician, agreed.

Moen continued, "We have a number of challenges, including a new landscape of state and federal regulation, unfunded mandates from government programs, and a growing financial misalignment between health care providers, facilities, and patients. These issues are most serious in our emergency department. Open access to the emergency department has become the fail-safe mechanism for what I regard as an increasingly broken health care system." He acknowledged,

"Just about everybody is unhappy with the emergency department. Haley Eckman's treatment seems to personify the current dilemma of our ED. Service standards are declining, morale is slipping, and staffing is challenging as we try to handle patients arriving at our ED for care." Moen concluded, "Emergency departments across the state are becoming inundated with people seeking primary medical care because they have little or no access to a physician. Unfortunately, this is the most expensive form of health care delivery, and it is increasingly impacting the bottom line at EMC. Although we are a not-for-profit, the situation is grave."

Half jokingly, Moen suggested to an influential EMC donor, "Maybe we should consider closing the hospital."

"Closing the hospital is not an option," the individual growled back.

Moen replied, "Support for the hospital is very strong in the community. Closing the ED doesn't really seem an option either. Half of EMC's hospital admissions come through the ED. Medical inpatient care and general surgery are the hospital's most profitable areas and they are closely aligned with ED admits."

Moen worried: "We are the last independent hospital in this area. All of the other independent hospitals in our primary service area have closed. How long can we resist the incursion of managed for-profit health care facilities? Kaiser Permanente, in particular, has achieved significant growth in this region during the past four years." He continued, "Depending on the course of future events, EMC could come under significant pressure to either contract with or be acquired by Kaiser or another major for-profit provider. Kaiser is poised to make significant inroads into our service area in the next 18 months. The outcome of Kaiser's actions could change this market dramatically.

"We are addressing operational issues affecting EMC," Moen went on. "Physicians are in short supply, as well as other health care professionals. Nurses, in particular, are really difficult to retain. When we have nursing shortages, we can hire temporary nurses, but it is very expensive. And, it's difficult to integrate temporary nurses into the EMC community. The staffing situation has become critical enough sometimes to affect emergency department operations."

Moen continued, "We've looked at the problem of the medically underinsured and uninsured that the ED is experiencing. I've thought about becoming a federally funded clinic to cope with these pressures. And we – the medical staff, the board, and me – have discussed the need to expand the ED facility. Either option, however, requires capital that is in short supply. We need to improve the overall patient mix for the hospital. We need to attract and retain patients with a greater ability to pay full fees, including elective surgeries.

"Margins at EMC are under pressure. I'm thankful for the board's investments in the late 1990s: that cushioned the blow, but for how long? The rising salaries have caused operating margins to remain negative. Our withdrawal from HMO capitation programs helped increase revenues but the increases are not enough to offset the underfunded government programs. We have to restore the hospital to profitability," he concluded. Moen paused and thought for a moment about little Haley Eckman, scared and sick in the emergency department of Emanuel Medical Center. "We have to do better."

NOTES

1. Centers for Medicare and Medicaid Services at http://www.cms.hhs.gov/statistics/nhe/historical/
2. Ibid.
3. American Hospital Association, *Hospital Statistics 2002* (New York: Health Forum, 2002).
4. American College of Emergency Physicians, *EMTALA*. Retrieved April 16, 2002, from http://www.acep.org/3,393,0.html
5. J. Cummings, "New Budget Blueprint Mandates Austerity from Agencies Unrelated to Terror Fight," *Wall Street Journal* (January 10, 2002). Retrieved January 1, 2002, from http://www.wsj.com/
6. A. M. Joseph and J. R. Melick, *Public Finance: Health Care Staffing Shortage* (New York: Fitch, June 27, 2001).
7. California Medical Association, *California's Emergency Services: A System in Crisis* (California: 2001). Retrieved April 16, 2002, from http://www.cmanet.org/upload/ERWhitePaper.pdf
8. R. Kagan, L. Simonson Maiuro, J. Schmittdiel, and Y. Wil, *California's Closed Hospitals, 1995–2000*. Unpublished manuscript, University of California, Berkeley, 2001.
9. Ibid.
10. Standard & Poors, *Healthcare Facilities Industry Survey* (New York: Standard & Poors, 2002).
11. G. Heihle and M. Cline, *California's Medical Assistance Program, Annual Statistical Report, Calendar Year 2001* (Sacramento, CA: California Department of Health Services, 2002).
12. "Medi-Cal Ranks 42nd Nationwide in Pay Rates for Medicaid Treatment," *AHA News Now* (July 15, 2001). Retrieved April 16, 2002, from http://www.healthforum.com/HFPubs/asp/Archive.asp
13. K. A. Smith, "State OKs Hospital's Fix-it Plan," *The Modesto Bee* (Modesto, CA: November 27, 1998). Retrieved April 16, 2002, from http://www.Modbee.com
14. Sutter Health, *About Sutter Health*. Retrieved April 16, 2002, http://www.sutterhealth.org/about/
15. Catholic Healthcare West, *About Us*. Retrieved April 16, 2002, from http://www.chwhealth.org/
16. Tenet Healthcare Corporation, *About Us*. Retrieved April 16, 2002, from http://www.tenethealth.com/TenetHealth/OurCompany
17. Ibid.
18. Kaiser Permanente, http://newsmedia.kaiserpermanente.org/kpweb/facdir

14 CASE

Cooper Green Hospital and the Community Care Plan

An Overworked CEO

There are certain days when life seems unbearable. For Max Michael, MD, it had been one of those days. He had the difficult responsibility of balancing costs with access to care, of rationing procedures with policy, and of juggling personnel with budgets, performance, and demand. Dr. Michael, a former chief of staff at the hospital and now its chief executive officer (CEO), had spent the better part of his day fighting a losing battle in an understaffed, understocked, overflowing outpatient clinic. It was there, on the front lines, where he had first encountered the nature of the health care problem and developed his vision for its solution. As Dr. Michael left the clinic that evening, he mulled over a looming decision he was going to have to make. It was his last patient that reminded him of the importance of that decision.

Martha James Spent Her Day at Cooper Green Hospital

It was the second day in a row that Martha James missed work because she was running a fever and ached all over. She dared not miss another day for fear of losing the job she had with a small local business that paid above minimum wage but offered no health

This case was written by Alice Adams and Peter M. Ginter, University of Alabama at Birmingham, and Linda E. Swayne, The University of North Carolina at Charlotte. It is intended as a basis for classroom discussion rather than to illustrate either effective or ineffective handling of an administrative situation. Used with permission from Alice Adams.

insurance. Her husband also was employed full time but did not receive any insurance benefits. Money was very tight for the couple and their two children, yet, based on federal guidelines, they were not eligible for financial assistance from the Aid to Families and Dependent Children (AFDC) welfare program; nor were they eligible for state Medicaid benefits. With no money to spare, the cost of a visit to a physician's office was a luxury Martha felt she could not afford. She did the only thing she knew to do: she headed for the emergency room at Cooper Green Hospital.

It was nearly 9:00 A.M. when Martha arrived after a 45-minute bus ride. She waited for more than two hours before her name was finally called. The nurse asked her about her symptoms. Barely even looking up, the nurse said Martha would have to be seen over at the Outpatient Clinic because her case was not truly an "emergency." She was told to sign in at the Clinic desk and they would try to "work her in."

After more than four hours of sitting in the overcrowded waiting room, Martha finally heard her name called again. The doctor who took her case was a silver-haired man with sharp eyes and a concerned demeanor. Dr. Michael quickly determined the problem: a respiratory tract infection that had been "going around" for weeks. When asked, she admitted she had been coughing for more than a week, but had hoped the severe cough would go away on its own. "Besides," she said, "I can't afford to take a day off work to go to the doctor for just a cold."

"The problem," Dr. Michael explained, "is the infection is now affecting your lungs, which requires more intensive treatment than if you had come for help a week ago."

Glancing at her chart, he realized she lived near Lawson State College, the location of one of the hospital's Community Care Plan (CCP) clinics. He asked, "Martha, are you aware of the Community Care Plan clinics and the services they offer? They have medical office visits with much shorter waiting times."

She replied, "I have heard something about them, but don't really know what it is about or how it could help me."

Martha still had to stop by the hospital pharmacy to pick up two medications and it was nearly 5:30 P.M. She knew she could get them much faster at a local drug store, but they would be several times as expensive. Instead, she settled in for another wait. By the time she headed back to the bus stop – some nine hours after she left home – Dr. Michael was wrapping up his afternoon in the clinic.

Dr. Michael Wraps up His Day

As Dr. Michael entered his office, Martha James was still on his mind. It had been nearly four years since he launched the Community Care Plan, but in many ways it was still struggling. In his heart, he still believed it was a good model to provide access to preventive and routine medical services to the population traditionally served by Cooper Green Hospital: the poor and uninsured of Jefferson County. It placed small outpatient clinics within local neighborhoods. They were staffed by physician assistants or nurse practitioners, who were supervised by a physician. For a quarterly fee, members could receive routine medical care at the CCP clinics. When needed, they also received care from specialists, and even inpatient hospital care at Cooper Green. To Dr. Michael it made perfect sense; the CCP offered better access to services, less waiting time, less travel time, and a better atmosphere.

But the numbers did not agree. Although some of the CCP clinics established a reasonably sized patient base, others were struggling to attract members. If Martha James had been a CCP member, she could have been seen and received treatment before the infection had migrated to her lungs and she would not have had such a long waiting time. "For her, and thousands more like her," Dr. Michael thought, "it's important to keep the CCP running – if at all possible." But few people knew about the CCP and even fewer had joined.

The five-year funding that enabled the hospital to launch the CCP was about to run out. Dr. Michael knew he was facing a critical decision: should he push forward with expansion plans for the CCP, maintain the clinics that existed, or fold the program altogether?

Cooper Green Hospital

In 1998, Cooper Green Hospital (CGH) was the current incarnation of Mercy Hospital. Built in 1972 with Alabama State and Hill-Burton funding, Mercy Hospital served the vision of the Alabama legislature to provide care for the indigent population of Jefferson County. Despite numerous organizational, structure, and name changes, the mission of the facility remained essentially the same: to provide quality medical care to the residents of Jefferson County, regardless of their ability to pay.

Mercy Hospital opened with 319 inpatient beds – a number based on an epidemiological study using the number of indigent cases reported in county hospitals during the mid-1960s. The study projected that the hospital would operate near 80 percent capacity. Occupancy never reached the initial projections. The highest average census for the hospital was 186.3 in fiscal year 1974. The numbers of inpatient admissions, discharges, and length of stay for 1998 are shown in Exhibit 14/1.

The role CGH played in the community faced constant scrutiny from a county commission with increasing budget pressures. Media and public challenges

Exhibit 14/1: Inpatient Statistics for Cooper Green Hospital, Fiscal Year 1998

Location	Admissions	Discharges	Average Length of Stay
4 West	1,464	1,518	4.1
7 West	1,742	2,197	4.6
MSICU	673	145	3.8
5 East	303	1,827	2.3
Labor And Delivery	1,596	75	1.0
Nursery	1,444	1,441	2.1
Total	7,222	7,203	3.0

about the quality of care provided by CGH limited its ability to attract patients with private insurance. For the first two decades of the hospital's operations, cost overruns were common, as the county's indigent population grew and medical costs soared. Facing increasing costs, Dr. Michael and the administrative staff initiated a stringent budget-cutting program that included personnel lay-offs, taking beds out of service, postponing most capital improvements, and eliminating some services. The hospital's financial statements for the fiscal years 1993–1998 are included in Exhibits 14/2 and 14/3.

Early in his tenure as CEO, Dr. Michael initiated a strategic planning program for the hospital. Mission, vision, and value statements were developed (see Exhibit 14/4), strategic goals were outlined, and plans for meeting them were created. Each year, the strategic goals for the upcoming fiscal year were developed by the "management group" (consisting of the CEO, COO, CFO, Medical Chief of Staff, and Nursing Administrator) and distributed to all departmental supervisors.

As a result of ongoing strategic planning, Dr. Michael took the initial steps to transform Cooper Green Hospital into the Jefferson Health System (JHS) in 1998. JHS consisted of CGH (the inpatient facility) and Jefferson Outpatient Care (comprised of the outpatient clinics located in the hospital and six satellite clinics of CCP). JHS provided services to patients through two plans: HealthFirst, a traditional fee-for-service plan, and the Community Care Plan (CCP), a pre-paid membership plan.

Part of the motive for the transformation and expansion of CGH was to enhance its ability to generate external revenue, including attracting patients with private insurance. If CGH could attract paying patients on the basis of quality and satisfaction, it could mold itself from a provider of last resort into a true competitor in the market.

HealthFirst

Charges for services under the HealthFirst plan were determined by a sliding-fee scale that was based on federal poverty guidelines. Depending on the number of

Exhibit 14/2: Cooper Green Hospital/Jefferson Health System Sources of Revenue

	1994	1995	1996	1997	1998
Indigent Care Fund	$13,126,249	$23,168,333	$31,638,294	$34,824,238	$36,199,381
Disproportionate Share Fund	$4,419,644	$8,854,308	$3,329,871	$3,596,076	$3,238,323
Medicare (total payments)	$10,566,183	$9,566,505	$9,974,860	$10,033,547	$7,056,823
Medicaid	$7,107,137	$11,442,428	$8,934,432	$7,900,835	$15,604,803
Blue Cross	$449,653	$262,415	$258,808	$296,152	$264,792
Commercial Insurance	$350,978	$307,604	$925,646	$458,266	$362,785
Self-Pay (payments from patients)	$915,047	$914,589	$1,129,513	$1,067,686	$1,015,164

Exhibit 14/3: Cooper Green Hospital/Jefferson Health System Statements of Revenue
           and Expense

Operating Revenue	1994	1995	1996	1997	1998
Inpatient Revenue	$37,288,811	$34,529,493	$33,248,117	$32,217,566	$35,830,206
Outpatient Revenue	$12,097,455	$13,791,112	$14,568,700	$15,197,207	$16,470,205
Total Patient Revenue	$49,386,266	$48,320,605	$47,816,817	$47,414,773	$52,300,411
Deductions from Revenue	$28,956,540	$25,313,448	$26,224,910	$28,682,168	$33,024,781
(Bad debt, subsidized care)					
Net Patient Revenue	$20,429,726	$23,007,157	$21,591,907	$18,732,605	$19,275,630
Other Operating Revenue	$2,256,812	$2,719,377	$3,111,157	$2,845,788	$3,792,735
Total Operating Revenue	$22,686,538	$25,726,534	$24,703,064	$21,578,393	$23,068,365
Operating Expenses					
Salaries & Wages	$19,390,676	$20,547,467	$20,976,332	$21,275,798	$23,017,889
Fringe Benefits	$4,681,390	$4,680,937	$4,607,439	$4,731,080	$4,976,824
Contract Services	$1,690,145	$1,833,616	$1,443,654	$1,558,705	$2,416,836
Utilities	$986,035	$921,191	$866,758	$844,867	$911,943
Outside Services	$1,489,785	$1,132,401	$826,958	$975,837	$1,229,699
Services from Other Hospitals	$2,567,655	$2,447,907	$1,881,087	$2,129,683	$1,915,322
Jefferson County Dept. of Health	$2,003,193	$1,861,591	$1,933,874	$2,040,062	$1,800,396
Physician Services	$9,843,577	$10,068,571	$10,200,031	$10,681,650	$11,370,273
County Maintenance	$1,059,678	$1,094,720	$1,045,600	$1,032,207	$1,619,744
Indirect County Appropriation	$3,693,500	$1,281,983	$1,281,983	$1,278,006	$1,558,907
All Other	$10,134,544	$11,095,892	$12,248,708	$11,399,367	$11,378,434
Total Operating Expense	$57,540,178	$56,966,276	$57,312,424	$57,947,262	$62,196,267
Gain/(Loss) from Operations	$(34,853,640)	$(31,239,742)	$(32,609,360)	$(36,368,869)	$(39,127,902)
Non-Operating Revenue					
Indigent Care Fund	$13,126,249	$23,168,333	$31,638,294	$34,824,238	$36,199,381
Disproportionate Share Fund	$4,419,644	$8,854,308	$3,501,061	$3,565,485	$3,238,323
County Appropriation	$19,581,071				
Transfer from County General Fund	$579,179				
Interest and Other Income	$70,244	$124,406	$117,249	$90,577	$144,192
Total Non-Operating Revenue	$37,776,387	$32,147,047	$35,256,604	$38,480,300	$39,581,896
Gain/(Loss) before Depreciation	$2,922,747	$907,305	$2,647,244	$2,111,431	$453,994
Depreciation	$1,581,901	$1,615,024	$2,098,569	$1,833,237	$2,040,682
Net Gain/(Loss)	$1,340,846	$(707,719)	$548,675	$278,194	$(1,586,688)

people in the family and the family's income, patients were assigned to one of
eight financial support categories. At the lowest level, patients paid as little as
$2 for an office visit. At the highest level, patients paid full price for services
(approximately $50 for an office visit). The HealthFirst financial support cat-
egories are shown in Exhibit 14/5. Initially, HealthFirst patients could only
be seen at the outpatient clinic located at the hospital. However, in 1998 these

Exhibit 14/4: Mission, Vision, and Value Statements of Cooper Green Hospital

Mission Statement

Cooper Green Hospital is committed to serve Jefferson County residents with quality health care regardless of ability to pay. We strive to attract and maintain a dedicated and compassionate staff of professionals who believe in the worth of our services. We seek to continuously improve our services and adapt to meet the changing health needs of the communities we serve.

Vision Statement

Cooper Green Hospital is the leader to an equitable and just health care system through excellence, quality, compassion, and trust.

Values Statements

We are committed to health and well-being of those we serve.
We expect from ourselves the highest levels of excellence.
We know the vital importance of advocacy for those we serve.
We are committed to our staff having opportunities for personal and professional growth.
We expect for ourselves the highest ethical standards.
We understand that creativity and innovation are essential.
We recognize the importance of working with the patient and the community.
We are dedicated to all levels of education for health professionals.

Exhibit 14/5: HealthFirst Membership Categories

Family Plan

Total Family income per year	Membership fee per year	Co-payment per visit	Co-payment per prescription or refill
Up to $1,850	$35	$2	$0.50
$1,851 to $3,700	$65	$2	$0.50
$3,701 to $5,500	$95	$2	$1
$5,501 to $7,400	$130	$2	$1
$7,401 to $11,000	$195	$2	$2
$11,001 to $14,800	$260	$2	$2

Individual Plan

Total individual income per year	Membership fee per year	Co-payment per visit	Co-payment per prescription or refill
Up to $920	$15	$2	$0.50
$921 to $1,840	$25	$2	$0.50
$1,841 to $2,760	$40	$2	$1
$2,761 to $3,680	$65	$2	$1
$3,681 to $5,520	$100	$2	$2
$5,521 to $7,360	$150	$2	$2

regulations were relaxed, allowing HealthFirst patients to be seen at any of the satellite (CCP) clinics.

Community Care Plan

An important part of Dr. Michael's vision for JHS was the CCP. His initial approach to developing the plan was best described as a "Field of Dreams" strategy: if you build it, they will come. "I envisioned offices filled with patients who were appreciative of the opportunity to receive quality medical care for a fair and affordable price – with less time waiting," Dr. Michael remembered.

CCP was developed around the ideas that catastrophic care was more expensive, patients waited until their conditions worsened, and they were treated in the more costly CGH Emergency Department. Dr. Michael asked himself, "Why not avoid these unanticipated high health care costs by allowing patients to pay a low monthly premium for unlimited services?" This would require that CGH, as well as the patients, change the way they thought about health care. Further, for the system to survive, Dr. Michael and his executive staff would have to understand and respond to the rapidly changing health care environment.

The Health Care Environment

Change in the US health care system was occurring dramatically and pervasively. Managed care was altering how providers interacted with patients, funding for care was being restricted, and many health care systems were using non-physician providers to cut costs.

The Changing US Health Care System

Because of its mission to provide medical care to the poor and uninsured, Cooper Green Hospital was considered one of the "safety net providers" across the United States. Safety net providers had large Medicaid and indigent care caseloads relative to other providers and were willing to provide services regardless of a person's ability to pay. Although safety net providers were the primary source of care for the poor and uninsured, they also provided critical access to health services in areas where health care was difficult to obtain.

Safety net providers faced many challenges in covering the cost of uncompensated care because they relied on Medicaid and fee-for-service reimbursement from other patients as major sources of revenue. Because of increased interest in Medicaid patients by for-profit Medicaid managed care programs, there was a decrease in the number of Medicaid patients using safety net providers, resulting in a financial drain and necessitating cuts in service levels.

Experts agreed that because of health care reform and cutbacks in funding, increased demand for uncompensated care and decreased capacity of the health care delivery system to meet this need would continue. This forced safety net providers to focus on improving operational efficiency as well as utilizing financial and staffing resources more effectively. Flexibility in the rapidly changing health care environment was essential to future survival; however, many safety net pro_____ ____ _nable to adapt quickly to changing market conditions, in part be_____ _____ ___ ____l regulati__ _s, labor relations, and depend__

MANAGED CARE

Health_____ _e mid-1980s to the mid-
1990s,_____ 14 percent of the United
States_____ : century, the health care
indus_____ percent of GDP. Health
care_____ l individuals) were seeking v_____ y turned to managed care
as a_____ an workers were insured
by h_____ ed provider organizations
(PP_____ ly 27 percent in 1987. By
199_____ ce in the United States and
enr_____

T_____ e attempt to control health
car_____ ices through utilization re-
vie_____ nts, and case management.
_____ were regulated in the state
of_____ ealth under Title 27 Chapter
21_____ njunction with the Alabama
D_____)s operating within the state.

MEDICARE AND

_____ l Security Act. The Medicare
_____ l coverage for the aged and
_____ ed to encompass other popu-
_____ ccurity or Railroad Retirement
_____ th end-stage renal disease who
_____ nother provision allowed non-

_____ : programs: Part A – Hospital
Insurance and Part B – _____ _____ surance. Medicare Part A provided coverage for medical expenses incurred from hospital admissions, skilled-nursing facilities, home health services, and hospice care. Part A was free of charge for qualified Medicare beneficiaries. Medicare Part B, a supplemental coverage purchased by the Medicare beneficiary at a monthly fee, covered ancillary medical expenses such as noninpatient lab fees, physician fees, outpatient services, and medical equipment and supplies. In 1997, Medicare as a whole covered 38 million people. Utilization of Part A, Part B, or both, was 87 percent of enrollees.

Exhibit 14/6: Medicare Enrollment Statistics, 1995

Category	National	Alabama
Aged (Part A and/or B)	27.4 million	541,225
Disabled (Part A and/or B)	3.3 million	101,123
Total Enrolled (Part A and/or B)	30.7 million	642,398

Exhibit 14/7: Population and Medicaid Eligibles

Year	Population	Eligibles	Percent
1996	4,127,562	635,568	15.4%
1997	4,141,341	632,472	15.3%
1998	4,155,080	637,489	15.3%

Medicare enrollment statistics for 1995 for the United States and Alabama are shown in Exhibit 14/6.

In 1996, Medicare was the largest health coverage program in the nation. Benefits were estimated to be $191 billion that year; 6,273 hospitals nationwide were Medicare Certified. The Health Care Financing Administration (HCFA), a federal agency under the Department of Health and Human Services, was responsible for formulating Medicare policies and managing the Medicare program.

Title XIX of the Social Security Act of 1965 gave rise to Medicaid as part of the federal-state welfare structure to aid America's poor population. Title XIX allowed federal funding for state-run programs. To receive funding, the state programs were required to make provisions for basic health services, including hospital inpatient care, outpatient services, laboratory and X-ray services, and physician services, among others. If funding allowed, states could offer additional services, including medicine, eyeglasses, and dental care.

Providers of services for Medicaid recipients received payment directly from the State Medicaid Agency. Providers were required to accept the Medicaid reimbursement as payment in full. Medicaid agencies could require cost sharing by the recipient in the form of co-payments, but the recipient's inability to meet the co-pay could not be used to deny services.

In 1998, the Alabama Medicaid program provided some benefits for a variety of populations, but the majority of expenses were for indigent women and children, indigent elderly persons in nursing homes, and the disabled. Exhibit 14/7 shows the percent of Alabama residents who were eligible for the Medicaid program from 1996 through 1998. In fiscal year 1998, 15.3 percent of Alabama's population was eligible for Medicaid services, up nearly 5 percentage points from FY 1990 (10.4 percent). Medicaid expansion to cover more populations (particularly children) and the increase in the elderly population increased the budget.

The population actually enrolled in the Medicaid program averaged 267,258 recipients per month in FY 1998. Of the 637,489 individual Medicaid eligibles in FY 1998, approximately 83 percent actually utilized services.

BALANCED BUDGET ACT

The Balanced Budget Act of 1997 was labeled the most significant change to the Medicare and Medicaid programs since their inception. A significant change for Alabama hospitals was the CHIP (Children's Health Insurance Program) initiative that infused an additional $23 million into Alabama's health care reimbursement for children under the age of 19. Phase I of the Alabama plan was a Medicaid expansion that funded Medicaid coverage to children from age 16 through 18 whose family income was less than 100 percent of the poverty level. Phase II, known as the ALLKIDS program, provided payments for insurance coverage of Alabama children through age 18 if the family income was under 200 percent of the poverty level and the child was not eligible for any other Medicaid program. The ALLKIDS program was a little different in coverage because a third-party payor was responsible for provider reimbursement, not Medicaid. ALLKIDS was not an entitlement program like Medicaid or the CHIPs Medicaid expansion; coverage was on a first come, first served basis. Therefore, if funding ran out to pay the insurance premiums for the ALLKIDS program, applicants were put on a waiting list.

NONPHYSICIAN PROVIDERS

Nonphysician providers (NPPs) such as physician assistants, nurse practitioners, certified nurse midwives, nurse anesthetists, and clinical nurse specialists, were health care professionals licensed to practice medicine with physician supervision. Nurse practitioners were registered nurses who received additional education and clinical training in the "nursing model." Physician assistants were trained by physicians in the "medical model." Physician assistant programs were structured similar to – but were shorter in duration than – medical school programs.

Although the scope of services that they could legally perform varied by state, most NPPs provided primary care services such as well-care physical examinations, tests, diagnosis and treatment for acute illnesses, as well as diagnosis, treatment, and monitoring of chronic conditions (such as diabetes and hypertension). In addition, in most states they were licensed to write prescriptions (with some limitations that varied by state). For more complex tasks and cases, NPPs sought consultation from their supervising physician or referred patients to a specialist.

Nurse practitioners and physician assistants were often viewed as more appropriate for primary care services because these professionals tended to take a more holistic view of patient care, focused on health care prevention and education, and spent more time with their patients than most physicians. It was estimated that NPPs could perform 60 to 80 percent of services traditionally done by physicians in family practice settings. In addition, NPPs were viewed as good economic alternatives for primary care physicians because their salaries were usually 50 to 65 percent of those earned by physicians. Although they were required to be "supervised" by a physician, one physician could supervise three to four NPPs. Thus, NPPs were often referred to as "physician extenders." In 1998, there were estimated to be over 48,000 nurse practitioners and over 34,000 physician assistants in clinical practice in the United States.

The Local Environment

Once known as a center of the steel-making industry, Jefferson County, Alabama, boasted a diversified economy by the 1990s. Biotechnology, health care, research, engineering, and a vast array of financial and service industries had supplanted much of the industrial core that had built the city in the early part of the twentieth century. As of 1998, the Birmingham metropolitan statistical area (MSA) population was approximately 875,000; Jefferson County population was approximately 652,000.

According to a 1993 survey conducted by CGH's Center for Community Care, more than one-third of Jefferson County residents were uninsured. Many poor residents delayed getting necessary medical care because they had no health insurance; an estimated 48,000 residents had been denied care within the past 12 months because they lacked health insurance. When asked what issues were most important to their community, low-income residents overwhelmingly listed crime, violence, housing, and drugs as the highest-priority issues. On average, health care was listed as the sixth most important issue, despite the fact that more than 64,000 residents reported their health status as fair or poor.

Exhibit 14/8 provides additional demographic and socioeconomic data for Jefferson County.

Exhibit 14/8: Selected Jefferson County Statistics

Total Population	1997	659,524
Births	1997	9,352
Deaths	1997	7,096
Urban and Rural	Urban	581,973
	Rural	69,552
Sex	Male	303,713
	Female	347,812
Race	White	417,881
	Black	228,187
	American Indian	1,242
	Asian	3,643
	Other	572
Household Income	Less than $5k	22,749
	5k–10k	27,477
	10k–15k	24,802
	15k–20k	24,294
	20k–30k	42,879
	30k–40k	34,373
	40k–50k	25,108
	50k–60k	17,124
	$60k+	32,488
Median Household Income		$32,632
Per Capita Income		$21,915
People of all ages in poverty		105,779
Under 18 in poverty		40,006
Medicare Beneficiaries	Aged	93,443
	Disabled	32,503

Other Health Care Providers in Birmingham, Jefferson County

Twelve acute care hospitals were located in Birmingham, the largest city in Jefferson County. In 1998, 8 of the 12 hospitals reported a decline in admissions; inpatient capacity in the area exceeded demand. As a result many Jefferson County hospitals were scrambling to earn a share of the rapidly developing outpatient market. In their efforts to reposition themselves to respond to these and other changes in the health care environment, several hospitals had entered into alliances. For instance, Brookwood Medical Center, Medical Center East, and Lloyd Noland Hospital formed an alliance in 1995.

Exhibit 14/9 provides a brief description of each of the other acute care hospitals in Jefferson County. Exhibit 14/10 contains selected operating statistics for

Exhibit 14/9: Descriptions of Other Jefferson County Hospitals

Princeton Baptist Medical Center
As part of the Baptist Health System (http://www.BHSALA.com), Princeton Baptist served primarily those citizens located on the west side of the Birmingham MSA.

Montclair Baptist Medical Center
As one of 13 tertiary care and acute care hospitals in the Baptist Health System, Montclair served those residing on the east side of the Birmingham MSA.

Brookwood
The medical center (http://www.brookwood-medical.com) was part of the Tenet Healthcare System (http://www.tenethealth.com) and had a staff of more than 300 physicians, representing every major specialty. Brookwood also had a Women's Medical Center, specializing in OB/GYN and other health services for women.

Carraway Methodist
As the flagship of the Carraway system (http://carraway.org), Carraway Methodist placed special emphasis on emergency medicine, laser surgery, cardiology and cardiac surgery, cancer treatment, diabetes care, hyperbaric medicine, and other high-tech services.

Children's Hospital
Children's Hospital (http://www.chsys.org) was the leading provider of comprehensive pediatric services in Alabama.

HEALTHSOUTH Medical Center
Home of the corporate headquarters, HEALTHSOUTH (http://www.healthsouth.com) was the nation's leading provider of comprehensive outpatient and rehabilitative health care services.

Lloyd Noland Hospital
Affiliated with Tenet Health System, this hospital became the South's first industrial medical experiment. As one of the state's first teaching hospitals, Lloyd Noland (http://www.tenethealth.com/LloydNoland) continued to provide excellent disease control and health care maintenance.

Exhibit 14/9: (cont'd)

Medical Center East
This hospital was Birmingham's most modern medical center. As the flagship of Eastern Health System (http://www.ehs-inc.org), there were more than 300 physicians on staff, representing nearly 70 medical specialties.

Saint Vincent's Hospital
As a member of the Daughters of Charity National Health System, St. Vincent's (http://www.stv.org) was dedicated to providing quality health care to the public by offering patient-centered, economical services, with a special emphasis on the sick and poor. They focused on cardiology, maternal and pediatric, neurological, oncology, and occupational health services.

University Hospital of Alabama
As a major teaching and research institution, University Hospital (http://www.health.uab.edu) provided patients with the most advanced health care available. University Hospital offered a comprehensive range of primary care and specialty services.

Bessemer Carraway Medical Center
As part of the Carraway Medical System, Carraway Bessemer was the principal provider of tertiary care services to the residents of the city of Bessemer (in Jefferson County).

Exhibit 14/10: Selected Operating Statistics for Jefferson County Hospitals

Hospital	No. beds	Admissions in 1996	Discharges to SHPDA in 1997	Status
Baptist Medical Center – Princeton	499	14,103	1,143	Not-for-Profit Church Affiliated
Baptist Medical Center – Montclair	534	19,650	1,510	Not-for-Profit Church Affiliated
Brookwood Medical Center	586	20,651	1,586	For-Profit
Carraway Methodist Medical Center	617	13,449	1,174	Not-for-Profit Church Affiliated
The Children's Hospital of Alabama	225	10,727	950	Not-for-Profit
Cooper Green Hospital	319	5,938	451	Not-for-Profit County Owned
HEALTHSOUTH Medical Center	219	6,615	494	For-Profit
Lloyd Noland Hospital	319	5,095	411	For-Profit
Medical Center East	282	11,467	1,172	Not-for-Profit
Saint Vincent's Hospital	338	14,540	1,281	Not-for-Profit Church Affiliated
University Hospital	908	37,226	3,176	Not-for-Profit State Owned
Bessemer Carraway Medical Center	300	6,452	564	Not-for-Profit

Source: Compiled from SMG Marketing Group, Inc. data for 1998.

Exhibit 14/11: Jefferson County Managed Care Organizations

MCO	Commercial Enrollment*	Ownership
UnitedHealthcare of Alabama	82,485	UnitedHealthcare, Inc.
Health Partners of Alabama	80,386	Baptist Health System
CACH HMO	36,562	Children's Hospital
Viva Health	25,610	University of Alabama at Birmingham
Apex Healthcare	5,855	DirectCare, Inc.

*Commercial enrollment includes self-insured covered lives under HMO-style medical management by region. The Birmingham region includes Blount, Calhoun, Etowah, Jefferson, Shelby, St. Clair, and Tuscaloosa Counties.

Source: Compiled using data from Harkey Associates, *Health Maintenance Organizations* (Managed Care Research and Publishing, March 1999).

each of them. Exhibit 14/11 provides enrollment and ownership information for each of the managed care organizations that were operating in Jefferson County in 1998.

Jefferson County Department of Health

CGH and the Jefferson County Department of Health (JCDH) established a working alliance to improve continuity of care for the county's indigent patients. JCDH physicians were accorded staff privileges at CGH and JCDH agreed to refer to CGH its patients who needed diagnostic testing or acute care. CGH and JCDH maintained a close working relationship, at times partnering on individual projects. They also explored the idea of a more comprehensive alliance, but no such plans had come to fruition by 1999.

JCDH operated an extensive health care network, providing pediatric and adult health care services to approximately 80,000 people every year. The JCDH network consisted of 8 community-based health centers and 19 school health programs. Health care services were available to any resident of Jefferson County, with the cost of services based on the patient's ability to pay. Services available at the centers included maternity care; family planning; well- and sick-child care; adult primary care; the Women, Infants, and Children (WIC) nutritional program; social services; dental care; pharmacy; and sexually transmitted disease testing and treatment. In addition, health centers sponsored seminars on disease prevention and health promotion topics. The locations of the JCDH clinics are shown on the map in Exhibit 14/12.

County Government/Authority for CGH

The Alabama State legislature granted county governments the authority to develop, own, and operate hospitals and other health care facilities for the benefit

Exhibit 14/12: Jefferson County Department of Health Primary Care Center Locations

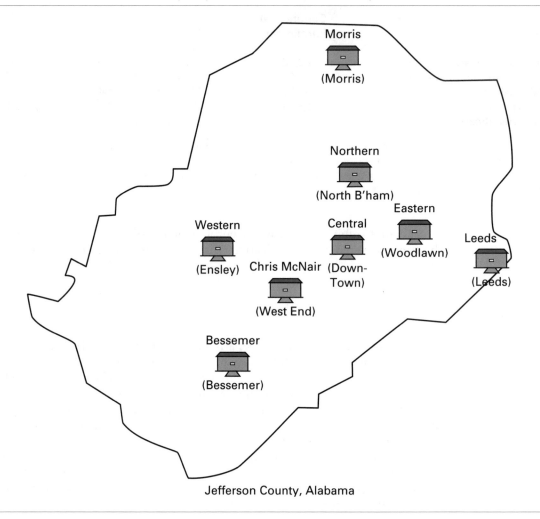

Jefferson County, Alabama

of county residents. Jefferson County was governed by a five-member county commission that was elected for four-year terms. The Commission was responsible for administering finances, collecting taxes, allocating resources, and providing for the delivery of services such as law enforcement, sewer services, and health care.

In 1998, the Commission oversaw the reorganization of Cooper Green Hospital into the Jefferson Health System (JHS). County Commissioner Jeff Germany assumed responsibility for governmental oversight of JHS as its Commissioner of Health and Human Services, a position he had held for Cooper Green Hospital during the past 12 years.

Whereas some county hospitals operated as independent organizations or under the auspices of independent "health authorities," JHS was an operational department of the county government. Although Dr. Michael, as the CEO, had operational and administrative control over the hospital, it remained very closely tied to the county government system. The most restrictive aspects of this were regulations that mandated the hospital's use of the county's personnel system as well as its financial services system.

Hospital Operations

Prior to the 1998 reorganization, the hospital was broadly divided into out-patient and inpatient divisions. All department managers reported to then-COO, Antoinette Smith-Epps. The 1998 reorganization into the JHS structure created distinct inpatient and outpatient divisions. Ms. Smith-Epps was named Hospital Administrator and remained in charge of inpatient services and most of the support and administrative services. Responsibility for outpatient services was assigned to Jerome Calhoun, who was named Administrator of Jefferson Out-patient Care. The organizational chart for the JHS (reflecting changes made in the 1998 restructuring) is shown in Exhibit 14/13.

Throughout the 1990s the number of outpatient visits continued to increase at CGH. This followed the national trend, in which there was an increasing emphasis on outpatient care driven by the need to reduce costs, coupled with new technology that enabled more types of care to be delivered on an outpatient basis. Exhibit 14/14 contains outpatient visits, by specialty, for fiscal years 1993 to 1998.

According to Ms. Smith-Epps, JHS faced several problems. The first was one that most health care providers confronted in the late 1990s: the problem of tight revenue. The Balanced Budget Act of 1997 had reduced the revenue of most providers and had affected CGH significantly because CGH served the indigent population and had few sources of revenue. Fortunately, during the late 1990s losses had been somewhat offset by an increase in the county's indigent care fund (ICF). Funded by county tax revenues split among several organizations, including CGH, Children's Hospital, and JCDH, ICF revenues were distributed on a straight percentage basis, so when the economy was good (and therefore tax revenues high), the hospital received more income.

A second issue was the lack of resources to invest in capital projects such as upgrades and enhancements to the information system, new medical equipment, or renovations to improve patient flow and access. Because the facilities were con-structed in the late 1960s, when the focus was on inpatient services, the physical layout of the hospital and the outpatient clinics was not conducive to providing outpatient services efficiently. The shortage of examination rooms, work space for nurses and clerks, and waiting room space was particularly acute in the out-patient clinics. This resulted in very long waiting times to get an appointment as well as very long waiting times to be seen by a health care provider on the day of the appointment.

Exhibit 14/13: Organizational Chart

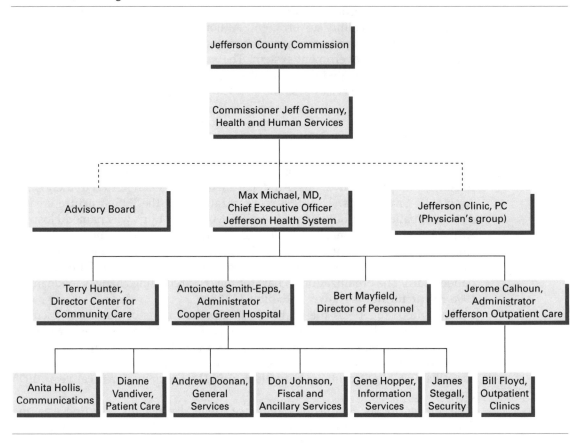

The frustration experienced by the patients was sometimes compounded by discourteous staff members. JHS employed over 600 staff, all part of the "civil service" structure of the county personnel system. Compared to other health care providers, staff turnover at JHS was low. There were many very dedicated, talented staff members who could have easily worked elsewhere, in better working conditions and for more money. They chose to work at JHS because they believed in its mission and enjoyed serving those in need. However, the hospital had its share of employees who were primarily attracted by the job security of the civil service system. Some of these employees tended to perform at minimally acceptable levels and display negative attitudes to patients and others. The administration had made several efforts to improve the morale and customer service orientation of the staff, although with limited success. Annual employee satisfaction surveys indicated there had been a slight improvement from 1993 to 1998, but there seemed to remain a core of "negative" individuals whose attitudes demoralized other staff members and angered patients.

Exhibit 14/14: Outpatient Visits for Cooper Green Hospital

	FY 1993	FY 1994	FY 1995	FY 1996	FY 1997	FY 1998
Cardiac	1,164	603	795	846	670	0
Medicine	21,723	23,361	25,340	24,690	23,903	22,873
Neurology	1,239	1,300	1,488	1,260	1,182	1,273
Pulmonary	828	1,081	1,242	1,221	1,155	1,033
Renal	431	443	593	659	861	907
Rheumatology	1,183	1,160	1,286	1,295	1,206	1,415
Dermatology	1,713	1,791	1,677	1,666	1,562	1,678
Ear, Nose, Throat	2,991	2,760	2,726	2,469	2,402	2,474
Ophthalmology	5,812	5,368	6,120	7,148	7,110	6,561
Coagulation	422	581	669	820	831	683
Gynecology	6,472	6,756	8,015	9,453	9,965	10,128
Chemotherapy	361	279	353	518	558	867
St. George (AIDS Clinic)	1,332	1,331	1,904	2,124	2,566	2,505
Genitourinary	1,495	1,563	1,764	1,616	1,414	1,558
Hematology / Oncology	1,453	1,508	1,828	2,048	2,425	2,364
Surgery	9,193	8,999	8,716	8,017	8,609	8,196
Orthopedics	4,932	4,748	4,706	4,207	3,813	4,108
Teens First	0	0	0	28	28	15
Total Clinics	62,744	63,632	69,222	70,085	70,260	68,638
Emergency	39,262	37,982	36,959	33,736	34,124	34,671
Labor & Delivery	3,420	3,997	3,169	2,903	3,018	3,228
Same Day Surgery	2,147	2,106	2,199	2,045	2,169	2,195
Referred Testing (from JCDH)	14,103	14,680	17,994	14,155	13,745	15,127
Physical Therapy	0	0	0	3,914	3,968	5,251
Community Care Clinics	0	0	0	1,706	3,025	4,997
Total Non-Clinics	58,932	58,765	60,321	58,459	60,049	65,469
Grand Total	121,676	122,397	129,543	128,544	130,309	134,107

Patients at Jefferson Health System had widely varying views about the service and quality of care received. Overall patient satisfaction with JHS, as measured by patient surveys, averaged about 90 percent. Patients recorded the most satisfaction with aspects related to the health care providers; they recorded the least satisfaction with issues related to making appointments, waiting times, and the facility. On the surveys, many patients expressed gratitude for the care they received at the hospital and had high praise for various staff members. They often remarked that without JHS, they would have no way of obtaining health care. One of the most common phrases seen on the written responses was "God Bless Cooper Green Hospital."

Some patients, however, expressed frustration over long waiting times and poor customer service. Some complained about specific staff members, often citing a lack of respect or a lack of caring about patients. Other complaints involved poor coordination between departments that sometimes resulted in patients experiencing long waits in two or three different departments and difficulty in scheduling appointments in a timely manner. Many patients had to wait three weeks to see a doctor, and when they arrived at the hospital on the appointment date they experienced long waits before being seen. Patients also cited the small, uncomfortable waiting rooms and the overall layout of the hospital as sources of frustration.

The Community Care Plan

When Dr. Michael assumed the position of CEO of Cooper Green Hospital in 1992, managed care was growing nationwide. Through coordinating health care and creating an organized system for receiving medical care, "managing care" was supposed to reduce costs. Managed care reached into every sector of health care – investor-owned health plans, not-for-profit organizations, Medicare plans, and state-run Medicaid projects.

It was within that context that Dr. Michael began to formulate his idea for a means of providing affordable, quality care to the poor, underserved residents of Jefferson County. Just as other managed care plans were using primary care physicians as gatekeepers to monitor the health of their patients on a long-term basis, the local CCP clinics would serve as the members' first stop for receiving health care and preventive services. Specialists at Cooper Green Hospital would serve their needs for services that extended beyond the capacity of the clinics. Dr. Michael envisioned this concept as a coordinated hub-and-spoke configuration for the provision of more effective and efficient health care.

Funding

Given the financial pressures facing the hospital, Dr. Michael had known that funding CCP would be a challenge. With pledges of $250,000 from funding partners, including local businesses, foundations, and government agencies, CGH was awarded a matching grant from the Robert Wood Johnson Foundation (RWJF) for $500,000 for the development of six clinics over the four-year project period.

In 1995, the first CCP clinic opened. It was located in the public housing community of Cooper Green Homes (neither affiliated with nor located next to the hospital). The second clinic opened shortly thereafter in Pratt City (approximately 10 miles southwest of the hospital). The Cooper Green Homes site was chosen for the first clinic for three reasons: (1) as a public housing community its residents clearly had a need for affordable health care; (2) the housing community's Resident Advisory board was very active and supported the placement of the CCP clinic; and (3) the Birmingham Housing Authority had pledged to provide and renovate space for the clinic. The third and fourth clinics, Southtown (2 miles northeast of the hospital) and Bessemer (15 miles southwest

Exhibit 14/15: Community Care Plan Membership Fees and Co-payments

Family Plan

Total income per year	Membership fee per year	Co-pay per visit	Co-pay per prescription or refill
Up to $1,850	$35	$2	$0.50
$1,851 to $3,700	$65	$2	$0.50
$3,701 to $5,500	$95	$2	$1
$5,501 to $7,400	$130	$2	$1
$7,401 to $11,000	$195	$2	$2
$11,001 to $14,800	$260	$2	$2

Individual Plan

Total income per year	Membership fee per year	Co-pay per visit	Co-pay per prescription or refill
Up to $920	$15	$2	$0.50
$921 to $1,840	$25	$2	$0.50
$1,841 to $2,760	$40	$2	$1
$2,761 to $3,680	$65	$2	$1
$3,681 to $5,520	$100	$2	$2
$5,521 to $7,360	$150	$2	$2

of the hospital), were opened in the fourth quarter of 1997. In early 1998, the Cooper Green Homes clinic was closed because of continuing problems with vandalism, gang violence, and low enrollment; it was relocated to the Lawson area.

CCP Member Services

To receive services, patients were required to enroll in the CCP. Only residents of Jefferson County were eligible for membership. Members paid an enrollment fee that was due at the beginning of each year or could be paid in four installments. Co-payments were required to receive services (see Exhibit 14/15). Similar to the HealthFirst program, co-payments and membership fees were based on a sliding scale determined by family income. Those covered by Medicaid, Medicare, or certain qualified insurance plans did not have to pay a membership fee.

Membership began with a complete physical (at no extra charge) that served as a health assessment. In addition, the CCP wellness program, HealthPoints, was an incentive plan to keep members healthy. It provided participants with discounts on their co-payments and membership fees. The program's motto was *With HealthPoints, it pays to improve your health*. To participate in the HealthPoints program, members set quarterly goals and visited their health care provider every three months to monitor progress. Members received "points" for met goals.

Examples of HealthPoints goals included getting regular check-ups, obtaining referrals before visiting the ER, exercising 20 minutes three times per week, eating a balanced diet, following the "well baby" schedule, quitting smoking, and losing weight.

CCP membership included both outpatient and inpatient services. Satellite health clinics provided primary care outpatient services such as immediate treatment of illnesses and minor injuries; lab tests; care for chronic illnesses (diabetes, arthritis, high blood pressure); yearly check-ups; immunizations; family planning services; special health classes; and prescription drugs from the JHS pharmacy (located at the hospital). Members were referred to specialists when necessary. With a written referral, members were also eligible to receive home care services, hearing tests, eye exams, and glaucoma screenings. Additionally, social services and other programs were provided through JHS, JCDH, and other local agencies.

Staffing

Each clinic had at least three full-time staff members: a nurse practitioner or a physician assistant, a registered nurse, and a receptionist/licensed practical nurse. The RN and LPN were employed by the county and reported directly to Bill Floyd, manager of Outpatient Services at JHS. The nurse practitioners and physician assistants were employed by Jefferson Clinic (the physician practice group affiliated with CGH through a contract with the Jefferson County Commission), and reported to Mark Wilson, MD, Medical Director of Outpatient Services (Jefferson Clinic). As medical director and supervisor for the non-physician providers, Dr. Wilson rotated throughout all of the clinics.

Turnover rate for employees at each of the outpatient clinics was extremely low and morale was generally high. Staff members at the clinics tended to be satisfied with their work and remained employed at the CCP for extended periods. When new positions opened up at a CCP site, many employees from JHS applied to work there.

For the first three years, the CCP did not have any full-time administrative staff; administrative duties were handled by a team of JHS staff and interns who each devoted part of their time to the CCP. As manager of the JHS Outpatient Clinic and the CCP clinics, Bill Floyd spent approximately 25 percent of his time on CCP matters. In mid-1997, Jerome Calhoun was hired to oversee all outpatient operations and could devote approximately 30 percent of his time to CCP.

Costs

Each CCP site required approximately $225,000 for start-up and general operating expenses during its first year. The estimated ongoing operating costs for one clinic with 1,000 patients were $170,000. During the initial years of CCP, approximately 30 percent of costs was provided through the RWJF grant. The remaining

70 percent was provided through local matching funds (30 percent), in-kind support from JHS (34 percent), and operating revenues (6 percent). The program was designed so that as individual sites increased enrollments, a greater percentage of operating expenses would be covered by operating revenue. The break-even point for a given clinic was estimated to be 1,000 members, although that number was somewhat low because the calculation did not include in-kind support or subsidies from JHS in the form of administrative resources and specialist physician services. It was expected that each clinic would reach the break-even point by its third year of operation; however, by mid-1999, none of the Community Care Plan Clinics had done so.

Enrollment and Utilization

Enrollment for the CCP generally fell below expectations, although the experiences of the clinics were varied. The first clinic, initially located in a public housing community, experienced the slowest growth. Although somewhat expected because of its "pioneering" role, this clinic's growth continued to be slow even after other clinics opened. The clinic and administrative staff felt that growth at that site had been limited by the problems with gang violence and vandalism. The other clinic located within a public housing community, Southtown, experienced somewhat slower growth as well. The clinics in Pratt City and Bessemer appeared to be on track to reach 1,000 members by their fourth year of operation. Enrollment for each of the clinics as of March 1999 is shown in Exhibit 14/16.

According to Bill Floyd, members tended to readily use the services available to them. As of March 1999, the average patient load per day at Lawson was 15 patients, at Pratt City 20 patients, at Southtown 10 patients, and at Bessemer 13 patients. One nurse practitioner or one physician assistant was located at each site and could handle seeing between 22 and 25 patients per day. Mr. Floyd expected patient loads to increase as HealthFirst members became aware of the option to receive services at the CCP clinics.

Exhibit 14/16: CCP Enrollment

SITE (opening date)	Oct. 1995	Oct. 1996	Oct. 1997	Oct. 1998	As of March 1999
Lawson (4/95)	143	262	323	560	700
Pratt City (10/95)	N/A	242	498	728	852
Southtown (9/97)	N/A	N/A	N/A	219	350
Bessemer (9/97)	N/A	N/A	N/A	355	424
TOTAL	**143**	**504**	**821**	**1,862**	**2,326**

Marketing and Market Research

Marketing for the CCP was still largely a work-in-progress. In an effort to publicize the first clinic, a health fair was scheduled at the site approximately two months before opening. However, because of construction delays, the clinic did not open for several months after the fair, nullifying the impact of the publicity efforts. The primary approaches to marketing during the first two years were appearances by Dr. Michael, Mr. Floyd, and staff members at community organizations, church groups, and schools along with promotional materials placed within the hospital.

A more formal marketing effort began in 1997. The intention was to educate the staff of Cooper Green Hospital, neighboring communities, county health departments, Social Services, uninsured populations, small businesses, and other hospitals in the area regarding CCP and how to access the services. Clinic staff members, interns, and administrative staff made appearances at schools, churches, neighborhoods, and local shelters, and held or attended 12 to 15 health fairs each year. Additionally, promotional materials were placed more prominently at Cooper Green Hospital in hopes of raising awareness among patients. Printed materials were often used because they could be printed at low cost, but CCP staff members realized they were beyond the reading level of many of the patients and potential patients. Word-of-mouth had proven to be the most promising and reliable avenue of enrolling and retaining patients.

Because of limited administrative staff, no one person was responsible for coordinating the marketing effort. Although Bill Floyd, as manager, set the tone for the marketing activities, specific duties were handled by a number of different people. Radio spots were placed sporadically with stations serving a predominantly African-American audience. In late 1995, eight billboards were placed on the western side of town, in the general vicinity of the first two clinics; they remained for approximately two months. Later, in conjunction with St. Vincent's Hospital, a television advertisement was developed that aired once a week for eight weeks. According to Mr. Floyd such promotions generated a great deal of interest, but it was not clear how effective they were in recruiting members.

Prior to opening the first clinic, focus groups were used to assess the printed membership information packet, but there were no surveys to assess patient awareness, attitudes, or understanding about CGH or CCP specifically, or about prepaid health plans generally. Additionally, although some information from the 1993 HealthWatch needs assessment survey was available to guide placement of CCP clinics, that process was driven more by long-standing political promises and community lobbying than systematic data analysis.

Coordination Efforts between CCP and CGH

Coordination efforts between the CCP and CGH developed slowly. The first challenge was staff education and training for all hospital employees regarding the purpose and function of CCP. Although progress was slow during the initial years of CCP, Antoinette Smith-Epps felt that by 1999, most hospital employees were aware of CCP and had a basic understanding of its purpose.

A second challenge involved coordinating the administrative functions of CCP with those of CGH. For example, billing functions were carried out both at CCP and in the business office of CGH, resulting in overlapping systems and confusion about patients' accounts. As CCP grew, communication of employee concerns, issues, and suggestions became more complex. Whereas the staff members of the first clinic had been part of a tightly knit team that included both clinical and administrative staff members from CGH and CCP, each new clinic presented the challenge of developing effective channels of communication.

The CCP experienced "growing pains" in the area of information services. It outgrew current hardware capacities and enhanced software was needed to link the clinics and CGH. Because CGH and CCP shared the same computer and medical records system, this modernization was vital to the success of the project. Another complication was the need for compatibility with the information system of Jefferson County.

HMO License

Alabama state law required any organization operating a health maintenance organization (HMO) or similar health plan to have an HMO license. The CCP development team did not consider the plan to be a true HMO or insurance product because it was essentially just a different way of offering the same health services to the same population for which the county had always provided services. Nonetheless, preferring to err on the side of caution and prior to opening the first CCP clinic, Dr. Michael inquired with the appropriate agency. Because of the uniqueness of the CCP model in a public hospital, the agency was not able to immediately determine whether the CCP would be required to obtain an HMO license, and essentially "tabled" the matter indefinitely. The first CCP clinic opened shortly thereafter.

Following favorable press coverage of the first CCP clinic, the state agency received a complaint from a Birmingham health plan alleging that Cooper Green Hospital was operating an HMO without a license. Although the agency had previously declined to make a ruling on whether a license was required, following the complaint it informed CGH that CCP would be required to obtain an HMO license or shut down within 90 days. Unable to complete the complex and expensive application process within the allotted time frame, Dr. Michael instead entered into an agreement with United Healthcare of Alabama to operate CCP under its HMO license. JHS paid United Healthcare approximately $20,000 each year to operate the plan under its HMO license, but JHS retained all operational control over the plan. The affiliation with United was not marketed, so members were not aware of any affiliation. Although United Healthcare underwent several leadership changes that created some administrative delays in processing renewal applications for CCP, Dr. Michael described the situation as "a good working relationship and a bargain for JHS. If we tried to obtain our own HMO license, I estimate that it would cost JHS between $750,000 and $1,000,000."

Issues for the Future

As Dr. Michael left his office that evening, he glanced at his calendar – May 1999. He thought, "In less than a year, the RWJF funding will run out and the CCP clinics will have to make it on their own. There isn't enough excess in the JHS budget to subsidize their operations to any greater extent. Yet, I believe that CCP represents the system's best chance to improve the delivery of care for the underserved population, as well as ease the strain of overcrowded waiting rooms at CGH."

The original plan, as funded by RWJF and the local funding partners, had called for six clinics to be opened within five years. "We only have four now," he mused. "Should we forge ahead with expansion plans to try to achieve a critical mass, hold steady until we work out the 'growing pains,' or give up on the plan altogether?"

As he pulled out of the parking lot, he noticed the crowd from the ER waiting room had spilled out onto the sidewalk . . .

US HealthSolutions

Don Hernandez, CEO of US HealthSolutions (USHS), no longer saw or heard the television set as he sat staring at it. His mind was back at the office. He had a meeting with Jim Keister, Vice President of Marketing for USHS, the next morning and Jim was pushing for a decision regarding a new product launch. Jim was sure this was a winner if employers could be made aware of the financial savings. Don thought, "It all sounded good but was it? Lots of legal and technological issues to consider – profitability ones, too. Yet . . ." He was brought back to the television set by a beeping sound and a weather warning appearing at the bottom of the screen. It would be a stormy night in Charlotte.

It had already started raining. Don turned off the television, settled back in his favorite over-stuffed leather chair, and began reviewing the proposal for the next day's meeting one more time.

The Company

USHS was a privately held venture that was considering whether to offer a service that was not available elsewhere from a single company. Fast and secure access to significant electronic medical records, advance health care directives, Universal Data Forms, plus Internet links to insurance forms needed to file workers' compensation claims were the combination of services that USHS had developed as a package to offer large organizations. The electronic medical record was to include specific information that would be useful in an emergency, rather than individual total medical history. An advance directive allowed a person to make decisions about end-of-life care when they were

This case was written by Linda E. Swayne, The University of North Carolina at Charlotte. It is intended as a basis for classroom discussion rather than to illustrate either effective or ineffective handling of an administrative situation. Used with permission.

conscious and competent to do so. Use of "heroic means," life support equipment, do-not-resuscitate orders, and so on could be specified. Universal data forms allowed for one generic form for insurance claims regardless of the carrier.

The service had evolved over time through the efforts of an experienced emergency and acute care physician, an attorney with a vast amount of experience in end-of-life decisions, a retired insurance industry CEO, and an information technology (IT) company that specialized in health care and security issues. The documents could be accessed via the Internet or faxed to any medical facility, anywhere in the world, with the individual's approval.

USHS contracted with two separate business entities to provide its unique service. Healthcare Planning Services (HPS) would provide all legal counsel and educational training for USHS's customers, and Firstline Consulting Services (FCS) would provide the creation and technical support needed to manage the USHS's software and web-based products.

Through its service offering, USHS developed three significant organizational goals:

- To add value to the health care system by connecting the physician and the patient via Internet-based data, providing faster physician access to medical records.
- To add value to the corporate human resources programs by introducing electronic medical records, electronic Universal Data Forms, Internet links to workers' compensation, and advance health care directives.
- To add value to the individual employees of the client companies through faster access to electronically controlled medical records (that needed to be initiated for first time use and then simply updated), online worker's compensation forms to expedite the claim process, and quicker access to advance health directives to ensure that the patient had the ultimate control over resuscitative measures.

End-of-Life Care

A significant portion of the population (approximately 43 percent) had not been exposed to discussions with a health care provider concerning end-of-life care. Discussions regarding end-of-life care, by those who actually had discussions, prompted low numbers of people to take action. Only 18 percent completed a living will and 11 percent completed a durable power of attorney for health care (DPAHC) after a discussion concerning end-of-life care. Social and demographic differences affected interest and perceived need for advance directives. Factors for not engaging in end-of-life planning conversations or establishing advance directives included age, level of education, marital status, and residence location. Older, better educated, married, nonrural individuals were most likely to have executed an advance directive.[1]

Slightly more than 70 percent of the population encountered an end-of-life crisis during their lifetime, either a death or nonlethal significant medical event of a family member or friend. Approximately one-third of persons under age 55 had a DPAHC or living will. One-third of DPAHCs and 35 percent of living wills were completed within the last week before death. People tended to be reactive rather than proactive regarding end-of-life care. The majority of conversations were prompted by some significant medical event that might occur too late for individuals to execute advance directives. Only one-third of living wills completed by seriously ill patients were actually included in their medical charts by the time of discharge or death.[2] Therefore, despite advance directives being executed, there was no guarantee that the patient's wishes concerning end-of-life care would be made known to health care providers.

Additional Details about the Proposed Service

USHS's core service was face-to-face education associated with its comprehensive package, but especially the advance directive component. The service offered unlimited logistical access to legally executed advance directives, providing confidence to employees that their wishes would be made known to caregivers. Periodic reminders to employees would keep medical records information up to date. Qualified clinicians were employed to glean only significant and necessary client medical record information; the employee was relieved of the responsibility to determine the information that should or should not be included.

Companies that purchased the USHS service were provided management reports allowing them to monitor the effectiveness of the advance directive program both in terms of employee participation and cost savings. The cost savings could be significant given recent accounting changes. Under SFAS 106, an accounting standard guideline, organizations that provided health insurance for retired employees were required to place cash into reserve accounts equal to a percentage of that future health care cost – effectively removing it from operations (see Exhibit 15/1 for more detail on SFAS 106). USHS could save corporations with large numbers of employees (and large numbers of retired employees) huge sums of money.

The comprehensive service included:

- *Electronic medical record storage*: A person's medical records were stored in a summarized format. Critical care information concerning surgeries, allergies, current prescriptions, or other significant information was stored and maintained. USHS employed an emergency medicine physician specialist to edit the patient's electronic medical record into a document that would be useful to other physicians in an emergency. None of the competing companies offered an edited version of a medical record.
- *Advance health care directives*: An employee's end-of-life directive was stored and maintained on the web-based system. At any time, this form could be retrieved by a medical facility wherever the need arose.
- *Universal Data Forms*: Forms for patient demographic, insurance, and financial information required for general admission into a hospital or by a physician

Retirement benefits are appropriately viewed as a form of deferred compensation, the cost of which the employer logically recognizes during the period of active employment of the individual who will receive benefits or whose beneficiaries or dependents will receive benefits.

The *expected postretirement benefit obligation* for an employer is the actuarial present value as of a particular date of the postretirement benefits expected to be paid to the employee, the employee's beneficiaries, and any covered dependents. The *accumulated postretirement benefit obligation* is the present value of all future benefits attributed to an employee's service rendered to the date of the evaluation.

Net postretirement benefit cost, the name assigned the periodic expense associated with providing retirement benefits other than pensions, is made up of five diverse and offsetting components summarized as follows:

Cost Component

Service Cost
The portion of the expected postretirement benefit obligation attributed to employee services during that period.

Interest Cost
The increase in the accumulated postretirement benefit obligation to recognize the effects of the passage of time.

Return on Plan Assets
The change in the value of the plan assets, adjusted for contributions and benefit payments.

Prior Service Cost
The effects of plan amendments which increase or reduce benefits to employees.

   If benefits are increased
   If benefits are reduced

Gains and Losses
Changes in the amount of the accumulated postretirement benefit obligation or plan assets resulting from experience different from that assumed or from changes in assumptions.

   If loss is recognized
   If gain is recognized

In the past, most companies accounted for postretirement benefits other than pensions on a cash basis. That is, they expensed benefits as they were paid rather than as they were earned by employees, provided no funding in advance of the time benefits were paid, and recognized no obligation of the provision of benefits.

The second section of the note explains the company's postretirement health care and life insurance benefits. The disclosure is similar to that for pensions, with the components of net periodic postretirement benefit cost presented first, followed by the accrued postretirement benefit cost. Following that disclosure is a discussion of the assumed health care cost trend rate that was used in determining the information that is presented, including the impact of a 1% increase in that rate. This is a disclosure required by SFAS No. 106 and is intended to alert financial statement readers to the impact this important estimate has on the amounts in the financial statements and notes.

In fact, these important employee benefit plans often represent some of the most significant obligations and expenses recognized by companies, and the uncertainties surrounding their measurement require an even higher level of professional judgment than many of the other areas of financial reporting.

would be stored and made accessible through the website. Employees needed to fill out the original data only once and it could be transferred to any new health care provider with the employee's authorization.

- *Insurance link to worker's compensation forms*: A direct link to the forms required to process workers' compensation claims for a state could be accessed through the website. This feature offered an early reporting system for employees with potential workers' compensation claims and notified employees of the importance of reporting incidents in a timely manner.

USHS's service was to deliver these features to an organization's employees through educational seminars tested by qualified professionals from the medical and legal communities. USHS's contracted legal representatives were responsible for providing the specifics behind the advance directives as well as providing assistance during the official registration of forms pertaining to the end-of-life directive. By carefully explaining the benefits and responding to employee concerns, all employees could make informed and intelligent decisions concerning their end-of-life directives. Over 90 percent of a pre-market test group that attended a USHS seminar had executed advance directives. Research had indicated that typically only 57 percent of the population that had discussions concerning end-of-life care could be expected to commit to the advance directive.[3]

USHS provided three facilitators to staff each seminar – at least one was a physician and at least one was an attorney. Seminar sizes were limited to a maximum of 125 employees per three-hour seminar. Time was used to present an overview of the various products and sufficient time was provided to enable each person to have some individual time with an expert if desired. Exhibit 15/2 illustrates client capacity for USHS. Because employer cost savings could be maximized through execution of advance directives, the main objectives in the informational seminars would be:

- Education of employees regarding living wills and advance directives;
- Distribution of approved forms for completion by interested employees; and
- Giving information on the edited medical record and how to keep it updated through training to use the website.

Employees could leave the seminar with legal documents at no cost to themselves.

Competition

There were several other companies providing products and services that incorporated varying degrees of medical records storage and advance directive information. Most competitors were marketing their product/services through the Internet directly to end users.

Companies that offered at least one product that competed with USHS were HealthCare Decisions (advance directive forms, consultation, and storage and retrieval of executed advance directives), VitalWorks (patient medical records online

Exhibit 15/2: Annual Capacity and Class Size

1. A classroom size ranging from 20 to 45 students per instructor was appropriate for an interactive training session requiring a three-hour time period.* Interactive was defined as a highly involved session between student and instructor. Role-play, scenario development, and in-class written assignments constituted a class high in student/instructor interaction.
2. Class Timeframe:

   • One work shift – approximately eight hours.
   • One lunch shift – approximately one hour.
   • Approximately seven hours of the work shift would be open for teacher/instructor interaction.

   Three facilitators were necessary to instruct each class. Professionals from the medical and legal community would attend each seminar to instruct, answer questions, and aid in completing all documents. The workshop was expected to require approximately three hours, based on pre-market tests performed in South Carolina.

*Anne Monnin, *Team Training Strategies for the 90s*, Scott Aviation Team Training Manual, 1998.

for physician practices), and Legal Health Documents (advance directives documents and do-it-yourself kits). In addition, local hospitals and clinics sometimes provided electronic patient records storage and retrieval.

Another competitor, McKessonHBOC (McKHBOC) enjoyed name recognition and relationships with 25,000 drugstores, 6,500 physicians, 5,000 hospitals, and 10,000 nursing homes. McKHBOC announced the launch of its online health care unit, iMcKesson on June 12, 2000. It handled two million prescriptions online from the 6,500 physicians that the company was serving and maintained good referral relationships. iMcKesson announced its plans to include and maintain electronic medical records in the near future.

Healtheon/WebMD offered storage and transmission of medical records in an electronic format. The consumer registered and managed the medical information and updated the information themselves. This service was free to consumers after they registered with WebMD. Healtheon/WebMD's goal was to be the medical portal for consumers, physicians, and other health care companies to health care information and products.

The Customer

USHS's target customers were large employers. Companies must have a minimum of 1,500 employees to provide a situation where an advance directive would have the potential to impact health care expenses. In the city of Charlotte, where Jim Keister lived, there were 23 organizations that had more than 1,500 employees (see Exhibit 15/3). Further, each employee carried an average of two additional dependants on the company's medical plan. Providing educational programs for dependants increased the customer base. Company benefits managers, CEOs, vice presidents of human resources, in companies that had more than 1,500 employees, represented potential *primary* customers for the USHS venture. Self-insured large

Exhibit 15/3: Charlotte Area Employers with more than 1,500 Employees

Company	Number of Employees
First Union	15,000
Charlotte-Mecklenburg Schools	12,383
Carolinas Healthcare System	11,566
Bank of America	11,495
Duke Energy Corporation	7,161
Presbyterian Healthcare/NovantHealth	6,700
USAirways	6,000
North Carolina State Government	5,777
City of Charlotte	4,745
US Government	4,662
Mecklenburg County	4,500
Ruddick/Harris-Teeter, Inc.	3,254
US Postal Service	3,124
BellSouth Telecommunications	3,000
Solectron Technology, Inc.	3,000
Winn-Dixie	3,000
Food Lion	2,250
IBM	2,000
Continental General Tire, Inc.	1,950
UNC-Charlotte	1,895
Wal-Mart Stores/Sam's Club	1,883
Family Dollar Stores	1,527
Metrolina Restaurant Group, LLC. (Wendy's)	1,500

companies were most likely to benefit from USHS's service. The employees of the companies and their spouses and other family members would be *secondary* customers for USHS. The degree of penetration of this secondary market would be instrumental for USHS to demonstrate savings in medical expenses.

When health care expenses for retired employees could be documented, SFAS 106 benefits emerged for companies. SFAS 106 (adopted in 1998) required companies to set aside cash reserves to cover health benefits for retired employees. With advance directives, costs could be reduced by, on average, $65,000 per employee or retiree who did in fact die without extended life support, and so on. Once the health care cost savings were documented, cash reserves could be maintained at a much lower level providing additional cash to the organization.

Pricing

USHS had first-year enrollee break-even costs of between $69 and $119 per employee (primarily from the costs of producing the seminars and developing/ updating the medical record), depending on the number of employees participating

Exhibit 15/4: 100 Employee/Day Unit Volume and Sales Figures (2001–2003)

Year	New Employees (Units)*	Retained Employees (Units)	New Employee Revenue	Retained Employee Revenue	Total Revenue
2001	14,079	N/A	$1,210,794	N/A	$1,210,794
2002	14,079	12,671	$1,210,794	$1,089,706	$2,300,500
2003	14,079	24,075	$1,210,794	$2,070,450	$3,281,244

- Based on training 100 employees per day at a break-even cost of $86 per employee, reference Exhibit 15/7.
- In 2001, 14,079 units will be sold, generating sales revenue of $1,210,794. New members will comprise 100 percent of sales.
- In 2002, 14,079 units will be sold, generating new employee sales revenue of $1,210,794. Retained employees from the previous year were expected to decrease by 10 percent due to employee turnover. Sales generated from retained employees were projected to be $1,089,706. Total sales equated to $2,300,500.
- In 2003, 14,079 units will be sold, generating new employee sales revenue of $1,210,794. Retained employees from the previous two years were each projected to decrease by 10 percent per year, respectively, due to employee turnover. Sales generated from retained employees were projected to be $2,070,450. Total sales equated to $3,281,244.

*Values based on Burg's 57 percent prediction.

in the sessions and the strategy that USHS decided on for entering the market. The break-even cost for the second and subsequent years would be from $7 to $8 per employee per year.

If an organization had 5,000 employees, approximately 49 percent (2,450) could be expected to execute an advance directive. Among the 2,450 with executed advance directives, risk tables indicate that 13 would die during one year. At savings (on average) of $65,000, the organization would reduce its annual medical expenses by $633,750 as well as reducing its required reserve under SFAS 106.

Jim's calculations using a cooperative agreement with a managed care organization showed slightly over $1 million in revenue for the first year of operation, increasing to over $3 million in the third year. If they could present to 100 employees per day, Jim had calculated the break-even cost to be $86 per employee; however, if they could train 125 employees per day the break-even cost fell to $69 (see Exhibits 15/4 and 15/5). If USHS chose to sell to large companies directly through their own sales force, the numbers were higher. USHS expected to convert at least 14,000 of the prospective clients into customers, generating sales revenue of approximately $1,200,000 during the first fiscal year.

The Company planned to sell 1.1 million shares of stock in order to raise $1.1 million in capital, resulting in outside ownership of 11 percent of the company's common stock. USHS planned to pass break even and achieve profitability by the third year, with a minimum gross profit of $1,025,194 by 2003 (a 31 percent gross margin).

Exhibit 15/5: 125 Employee/Day Unit Volume and Sales Figures (2001–2003)

Year	New Employees (Units)*	Retained Employees (Units)	New Employee Revenue	Retained Employee Revenue	Total Revenue
2001	17,598	N/A	$1,214,262	N/A	$1,214,262
2002	17,598	15,838	$1,214,262	$1,092,822	$2,307,084
2003	17,598	30,092	$1,214,262	$2,076,361	$3,290,623

- Based on training 125 employees per day at a break-even cost of $69 per employee, reference Exhibit 15/7.
- In 2001, 17,598 units will be sold, generating sales revenue of $1,214,262. New members will comprise 100 percent of sales.
- In 2002, 17,598 units will be sold, generating new employee sales revenue of $1,214,262. Retained employees from the previous year were expected to decrease by 10 percent due to employee turnover. Sales generated from retained employees were projected to be $1,092,822. Total sales equated to $2,307,084.
- In 2003, 17,598 units will be sold, generating new employee sales revenue of $1,214,262. Retained employees from the previous two years were each projected to decrease by 10 percent per year, respectively, due to employee turnover. Sales generated from retained employees were projected to be $2,076,361. Total sales equated to $3,290,623.

*Values based on Burg's 57 percent prediction.

Challenges

USHS's major challenge was that it was difficult to demonstrate savings to companies and managed care organizations (MCOs). Theoretically it was understandable, logical, and made good business sense but there was no *evidence* concerning the cost savings. Further, revenues were generated through promotion of the dying process, something that Americans did not discuss freely. In addition, USHS did not have proven infrastructure for delivering the product – getting information to hospitals and other health care providers – and maintaining information in a web-accessible format. The staff was not in place to provide services to employees; nor were the software/systems in place.

USHS products could remain as an employee benefit even if a company changed insurance carriers; therefore USHS's product offered MCOs a benefit in landing a large company's business but it was not sustainable for the MCO. Would it be sustainable for USHS if the large company switched plans? The first year was the most expensive and least profitable for USHS.

Advance directives education and storage were provided free of charge by hospitals and other health care organizations, although typically there was still need for legal guidance. Most conversations regarding end-of-life care were with family members and attorneys; therefore, these conversations were largely viewed as personal and legal matters. Insurance companies could independently develop a product line and, given their large size and marketing ability, take the market from USHS.

Delivery Strategy: Sales Force or Alliance?

Don realized from his reading that a major strategic issue was whether USHS should offer the service on its own through a corporate sales force to sell to major employers or attempt an alliance with a managed care organization. There were two distinct markets to which USHS could target its product and service offering – large employers and managed care organizations that would market the product to large employers.

Hire a Sales Force

USHS would have to hire and train a sales force to call on vice presidents of human resources and CEOs to recruit and retain clients. In addition, USHS needed a call-center available as a 24/7 operation for customer support. Without having historical data to demonstrate actual health care savings, sales of the product to human resource managers and CEOs might be difficult.

Once a major employer was sold, product delivery was fairly easy to determine. Based on presentations to a minimum of 100 new employees per day, equal to a maximum annual capacity of 24,700 new employees, USHS has a break-even cost of $86 per new employee per year (see Exhibit 15/6).

Partner with a Managed Care Organization

USHS could utilize an MCO client to charge a per-employee, per-month price that would cover the break-even cost for each new employee. The break-even cost for an MCO-related customer was lower because of the reduced marketing costs (see Exhibit 15/7). In year two the new employees became retained employees, which equated to a break-even cost of $8 per employee per year because of the reduction in resources required to maintain and store the records of retained employees. The MCO continued to charge a premium for each employee based on the $86 per employee per year break-even cost which equated to a $78 gross profit per retained employee per year.

There were three main reasons why the MCO market should be the targeted customer base for USHS:

- USHS was going to "partner" with the MCO to market its product offering to subscribers of the MCO's health plans. USHS's product would be packaged with the MCO's health plans. The partnership would prove to be beneficial to USHS as it allowed the company to quickly reach a large secondary market with a minimal amount of marketing expenditures.
- The partnership between USHS and the MCO would allow USHS to obtain actual cost savings data rather than being forced to rely on actuarial data. Actual data would enable USHS to entice other MCOs to include the USHS product with their health plans.

Exhibit 15/6: Break-Even Analysis Using a Direct Sales Force

The initial annual expense budget, based on selling direct to companies with a minimum of 1,500 employees, was projected to be $2,940,500 less accounts receivable (see Exhibit 15/11). The break-even costs for new employees and retained employees were expected to be:

	Costs for New Employees	Cost of Retained Employees
Personnel	$334,500	$33,750
Cost of Sales	$525,300	N/A
Operations		
(Less Accounts Receivable)	$1,700,450	$82,000
Web		
(Hardware and Software)	$380,250	N/A
Total Costs:	**$2,940,500**	**$115,750**

Analysis

Costs are based on the minimum training capacity of 24,700 new employees. Based on the results from Burg et al.'s studies, only 57 percent of this population is expected to commit to the advance directive,[a] although in a market pre-test in South Carolina, USHS achieved nearly 90 percent partipation in advance directives by employees.

Based on 100 employees per eight-hour work shift:
Cost Per New Employee = $2,940,500/24,700 employees = $119 per new employee.
Cost Per Retained Employee = $115,750/14,079 employees = $8 per retained employee.

Based on 125 employees per eight-hour work shift:
Costs Per New Employee = $2,940,500/30,875 employees = $95 per new employee.
Cost Per Retained Employee = $115,750/17,598 employees = $7 per retained employee.

[a] M. A. Burg, C. McCarty, W. L. Allen, and D. Denslow, *Advance Directives: Population Prevalence.*

- USHS would be able to ride the coattails of the MCO with which it formed a partnership, allowing USHS to achieve a significant brand awareness for its product offering. Although USHS's product would be marketed in conjunction with the MCO's health plans, the USHS brand would be at the forefront throughout the educational seminars and contact for product maintenance (updating of medical records).

The primary benefit for the MCO would be a reduction in its medical loss ratio (MLR). Because USHS did not have actual cost-savings data, it could partner with a North Carolina managed care organization in an alliance or joint venture to gain statistical data that validates the cost savings of USHS products. Three MCOs in North Carolina could be targets for such an arrangement: Partners National Health Plan, Coventry Health Care, and United HealthCare. These three would be attractive because:

- All three were aggressively trying to increase their North Carolina market share.

Exhibit 15/7: Break-Even Analysis Using the Managed Care Organization Strategy

If an affiliation with an MCO can be accomplished, cost reductions could be realized in the following areas (reference Exhibit 15/11):

- Eliminate costs associated with a sales force.
- Eliminate sales commissions.
- Eliminate costs associated with marketing brochures.
- Eliminate advertising costs.
- Eliminate seminar site costs.
- Eliminate costs associated with company car leases.
- Reduce costs associated with employee benefits.
- Reduce costs associated with employee insurance.
- Reduce costs associated with payroll taxes.

Utilizing the MCO strategy, the annual expense budget was projected to be $2,140,300 (less accounts receivable), as illustrated in Exhibit 15/11. The costs associated with an alliance with an MCO as the customer for both new employees and retained employees are:

	Cost of New Employees	Cost of Retained Employees
Personnel	$322,500	$33,750
Cost of Sales	$28,050	N/A
Operations	$1,409,500	$82,000
(Less Accounts Receivable)		
Web	$380,250	N/A
(Hardware and Software)		
Total Costs:	**$2,140,300**	**$115,750**

Analysis
Based on 100 employees per eight-hour work shift:
Cost Per New Employee = $2,140,300/24,700 employees = $86 per new employee.
Cost Per Retained Employee = $115,750/14,079 employees = $8 per retained employee.

Based on 125 employees per eight-hour work shift:
Costs Per New Employee = $2,140,300/30,875 employees = $69 per new employee.
Cost Per Retained Employee = $115,750/17,598 employees = $7 per retained employee.

Assumptions
- There are 247 workdays per calendar year.
- 24,700 employees can be trained over a 247 workday period based on 100 employees per day. Based on the Burg et al. studies, approximately 57 percent of the population is expected to exercise their end-of-life option.
- 30,875 employees can be trained over a 247 workday period based on 125 employees per day. Based on the Burg et al. studies, approximately 57 percent of the population is expected to exercise their end of life option.[a]

---

[a] M. A. Burg, C. McCarty, W. L. Allen, and D. Denslow, *Advance Directives: Population Prevalence.*

- Expansion strategies for these MCOs in North Carolina were similar to USHS's plan – Charlotte first and then on to the Triangle area (Raleigh, Durham, Chapel Hill).
- Each of these MCOs already had business relationships with several businesses that USHS would want to target.
- USHS's innovative cost-saving strategy might help the MCO partner to take market share from Blue Cross/Blue Shield and Aetna (two other major carriers in Charlotte and North Carolina).

These markets could include other MCOs that have a significant presence in other areas; agencies such as AAA and AARP, which serve huge target markets; and agencies such as Humana that sell Medicare supplements. In addition to these entities, USHS could market its products and services to large companies that were self-insured.

Exhibit 15/8: Savings Example for a Managed Care Company

Given:

1. Medical Loss Ratio (MLR) = Total Medical Expenses pmpm/Total Revenues from Premiums[a]
2. Target MLR = 85 percent[b]
3. $65,000 saved in medical expenses when advance directive indicates lack of desire for futile medical care at end of life (Chambers et al., 1994 – note 4)
4. 1997 NC age adjusted death rate: 518.1 deaths/100,000 population (National Vital Statistics Report, vol. 47, no. 25). *Please note deaths represented are all deaths and would include some deaths where advance directives would be irrelevant such as homicide, suicide, accidents, etc.*

Assume premium of $135 pmpm for managed care company (MCO)
For MLR = 85 percent: medical expenses = 85 percent × $135 pmpm = $114.75 pmpm
For MCO with 100,000 members: medical expenses/yr. = $114.75 × 100,000 × 12 = $137,000,000
Deaths/yr. for 100,000 members = 518 deaths/yr.
Medical Savings for 100 percent advance directive participation = $33,670,000
Medical Savings for 10 percent advance directive participation = $3,367,000
Medical Savings for 50 percent advance directive participation with 75 percent adherence = $12,675,000
Adjusted annual medical expenses after 10 percent advance directive savings = $133,633,000
Medical expense as pmpm = $133,633,000/100,000/12 = $111.36
Adjusted MLR with 10 percent advance directive savings = $111.36/$135 × 100 = 82 percent
Therefore if only 10 percent of the members predicted to die have advance directives that restrict end-of-life care, the MCO could anticipate a 3 percent decrease in MLR.
Adjusted annual medical expenses after 50 percent advance directive and 75 percent adherence: savings = $124,325,000
Medical expense as pmpm = $124,325,000/100,000/12 = $103.60
Adjusted MLR with 50 percent advance directive and 75 percent adherence savings = $103.60/$135 × 100 = 77 percent
Therefore using reasonable predictions of members executing advance directives and probability ADs will be adhered to, the MLR could be anticipated to decrease 8 percent to 77 percent.

[a] pmpm = per member per month.
[b] statements 1 and 2 are accepted industry standards corroborated by two separate managed care companies.

Exhibit 15/8 illustrates a sample MLR calculation as well as potential savings for an MCO.[4,5,6] Of the three companies previously mentioned, Partners National Health Plans might be the easiest one to reach a joint venture agreement with since the entire company was based in North Carolina. The others, Coventry and United, have North Carolina regional operations, but corporate leadership is elsewhere. Another advantage to Partners was that it was a subsidiary of NovantHealth, the parent company of Presbyterian HealthCare. Reaching a joint venture agreement with Partners would allow USHS access to Presbyterian's 6,700 employees. These employees should be easier to sell on the idea of executing advance directives given their medical backgrounds. Exhibit 15/9 illustrates estimated cost savings using sales to Presbyterian HealthCare as a model. Obtaining 6,700 customers instantly would be nearly 50 percent of USHS's first-year client recruitment goal. Exhibit 15/10 provides cost savings for other sized organizations.

Exhibit 15/9: Cost Savings Example for Potential MCO Customer (Presbyterian HealthCare/NovantHealth)

Given:

1. $65,000 saved in medical expenses when advance directive indicates lack of desire for futile medical care at end of life (Chambers et al., 1994)
2. 1997 NC age adjusted death rate: 518.1 deaths/100,000 population (National Vital Statistics Report, vol. 47, no. 25). *Please note deaths represented are all deaths and would include some deaths where advance directives would be irrelevant, such as homicide, suicide, accidents, and so on.*
3. Number of Presbyterian employees in Charlotte is 6,700 (Charlotte Chamber of Commerce)
4. 49–57 percent of population predicted to exercise advance directive with education and time (McKinley et al., 1996; Burg et al., 1995)
5. Advance directives will be adhered to 75 percent of time (Danis et al., 1991)

Optimistic Number of Presbyterian Employees Predicted to Execute AD = 6,700 × 57% = 3,819
Pessimistic Number of Presbyterian Employees Predicted to Execute AD = 6,700 × 49% = 3,283
Number of Anticipated Deaths Among Employees with AD = 3,283 × 0.52% to 3,819 × 0.52% = 17 to 20
Adherence to AD in Employees at Risk for Death = 17 × 75% to 20 × 75% = 13 to 15
Predicted Annual Medical Expense Savings with AD = 13 × $65,000 to 15 × $65,000 = $845,000 to $975,000

Exhibit 15/10: Annual Medical Expense Savings for Other Company Sizes

Number of Employees	Predicted Number of Executed AD (49%)	Predicted Deaths Among Executed AD (0.52%)	Annual Medical Expense Savings (with 75% adherence)
20,000	9,800	51	$2,486,250
10,000	4,900	25	$1,218,750
5,000	2,450	13	$633,750

Exhibit 15/11: US Healthcare Solutions – Expense Budget (July, 2000–June, 2001): *Initial Budget*

	July	August	Sept	Oct	Nov	Dec	Jan	Feb	March	April	May	June	Total
PERSONNEL													
Don Hernandez	10,000	10,000	10,000	10,000	10,000	10,000	10,000	10,000	10,000	10,000	10,000	10,000	$120,000
Bob Miller	0	0	0	0	0	0	0	0	0	0	0	0	$0
Sales Director Jim Kiester	4,000	4,000	4,000	4,000	4,000	4,000	4,000	4,000	4,000	4,000	4,000	4,000	$48,000
Receptionist/Accounting	0	0	2,500	2,500	2,500	2,500	2,500	2,500	3,000	3,000	3,000	3,000	$27,000
Telephone&Data Entry	0	0	0	4,500	4,500	4,500	4,500	4,500	4,500	4,500	4,500	4,500	$40,500
Telephone&Data Entry	0	0	0	0	0	0	4,500	4,500	4,500	4,500	4,500	4,500	$27,000
Medical Director	5,000	5,000	5,000	5,000	5,000	5,000	5,000	5,000	5,000	5,000	5,000	5,000	$60,000
Salesperson #1	0	0	0	0	0	0	2,000	2,000	2,000	2,000	2,000	2,000	$12,000
Salesperson #2	0	0	0	0	0	0	0	0	0	0	0	0	$0
Salesperson #3	0	0	0	0	0	0	0	0	0	0	0	0	$0
TOTAL	19,000	19,000	21,500	26,000	26,000	26,000	32,500	32,500	33,000	33,000	33,000	33,000	$334,500
COST of SALES													
HPS Royalty	0	0	0	14,025	0	14,025	0	0	0	0	0	0	$28,050
Commissions	0	0	0	87,750	0	0	87,750	0	87,750	0	234,000	0	$497,250
TOTAL	0	0	0	101,775	0	14,025	87,750	0	87,750	0	234,000	0	$525,300
OPERATING													
Advertising	0	5,000	5,000	5,000	5,000	5,000	15,000	15,000	15,000	15,000	15,000	15,000	$115,000
Marketing Consulting	10,000	10,000	5,000	5,000	5,000	5,000	2,500	2,500	2,500	2,500	2,500	2,500	$55,000
Marketing Brochures, etc.	15,000	10,000	5,000	2,000	2,000	2,000	2,000	2,000	2,000	2,000	2,000	2,000	$48,000
Accounts Receivable	0	0	0	268,125	0	0	268,125	0	268,125	0	715,000	0	$1,519,375
Seminar Site Cost	0	0	0	7,500	0	0	7,500	0	7,500	0	20,000	0	$42,500
Seminar Doctor Fees	0	0	0	37,500	0	0	37,500	0	37,500	0	100,000	0	$212,500
Seminar Attorney Fees	0	0	0	30,000	0	0	30,000	0	30,000	0	80,000	0	$170,000
Seminar Supplies & Handouts	0	0	0	30,000	0	0	30,000	0	30,000	0	80,000	0	$170,000
Document Scanning	0	0	0	15,000	0	0	15,000	0	15,000	0	40,000	0	$85,000
Depreciation	0	0	0	0	0	0	0	0	0	0	0	0	$0
Dues and Subscriptions	1,000	1,000	1,000	1,000	1,000	1,000	1,000	1,000	1,000	1,000	1,000	1,000	$12,000
Employee Benefits	4,750	4,750	5,375	6,500	6,500	6,500	7,625	7,625	7,750	7,750	7,750	7,750	$80,625
Employee Insurance	1,900	1,900	2,150	2,600	2,600	2,600	3,050	3,050	3,100	3,100	3,100	3,100	$32,250
Payroll Taxes (SS, etc.)	1,900	1,900	2,150	2,600	2,600	2,600	3,050	3,050	3,100	3,100	3,100	3,100	$32,250
Company Car (Lease)	1,500	1,500	1,500	1,500	1,500	1,500	1,500	1,500	1,500	1,500	1,500	1,500	$18,000
Interest	0	0	0	0	0	0	0	0	0	0	0	0	$0
Legal and Accounting	10,000	6,000	6,000	6,000	6,000	6,000	6,000	6,000	6,000	6,000	6,000	6,000	$76,000
E&O and other Insurance	7,500	7,500	7,500	7,500	7,500	7,500	7,500	7,500	7,500	7,500	7,500	7,500	$90,000
Office Supplies & Postage	2,000	2,000	2,000	2,000	2,000	2,000	2,000	2,000	2,000	2,000	2,000	2,000	$24,000
Rent	2,500	2,500	2,500	2,500	2,500	2,500	2,500	2,500	2,500	2,500	2,500	2,500	$30,000
Property Taxes	200	200	200	200	200	200	200	200	200	200	200	200	$2,400
Telephone	2,000	2,300	2,645	3,042	3,498	4,023	4,626	5,320	6,118	7,036	8,091	9,305	$58,003
T & E	5,000	5,500	6,050	6,655	7,321	8,053	8,858	9,744	10,718	11,790	12,969	14,266	$106,921
Other	20,000	20,000	20,000	20,000	20,000	20,000	20,000	20,000	20,000	20,000	20,000	20,000	$240,000
TOTAL	85,250	82,050	74,070	462,222	75,219	76,475	475,534	88,989	479,111	92,975	1,130,210	97,720	$3,219,825
WEB													
Server Equipment	25,000	6,250	2,500	2,500	2,500	2,500	2,500	2,500	2,500	2,500	2,500	2,500	$56,250
Colocation Cost	4,000	4,000	4,000	4,000	4,000	4,000	4,000	4,000	4,000	4,000	4,000	4,000	$48,000
Telecomm Cost	3,000	3,500	3,500	4,000	4,000	5,000	5,000	5,000	5,000	5,000	5,000	0	$48,000
Employee Equipment	4,000	4,000	6,000	8,000	8,000	8,000	10,000	10,000	10,000	10,000	10,000	10,000	$98,000
Software Development	20,000	10,000	10,000	10,000	10,000	10,000	10,000	10,000	10,000	10,000	10,000	10,000	$130,000
TOTAL	56,000	27,750	26,000	28,500	28,500	29,500	31,500	31,500	31,500	31,500	31,500	26,500	$380,250
TOTAL	160,250	128,800	121,570	618,497	129,719	146,000	627,284	152,989	631,361	157,475	1,428,710	157,220	$4,459,875

Exhibit 15/12: US Healthcare Solutions – Expense Budget (July, 2000–June, 2001): *MCO Budget*

	July	August	Sept	Oct	Nov	Dec	Jan	Feb	March	April	May	June	Total
PERSONNEL													
Don Hernandez	10,000	10,000	10,000	10,000	10,000	10,000	10,000	10,000	10,000	10,000	10,000	10,000	$120,000
Bob Miller													$0
Sales Director Jim Kiester	4,000	4,000	4,000	4,000	4,000	4,000	4,000	4,000	4,000	4,000	4,000	4,000	$48,000
Receptionist/Accounting			2,500	2,500	2,500	2,500	2,500	2,500	3,000	3,000	3,000	3,000	$27,000
Telephone&Data Entry				4,500	4,500	4,500	4,500	4,500	4,500	4,500	4,500	4,500	$40,500
Telephone&Data Entry							4,500	4,500	4,500	4,500	4,500	4,500	$27,000
Medical Director	5,000	5,000	5,000	5,000	5,000	5,000	5,000	5,000	5,000	5,000	5,000	5,000	$60,000
TOTAL	19,000	19,000	21,500	26,000	26,000	26,000	30,500	30,500	31,000	31,000	31,000	31,000	$322,500
COST of SALES													
HPS Royalty	0	0	0	14,025	0	14,025	0	0	0	0	0	0	$28,050
TOTAL	0	0	0	14,025	0	14,025	0	0	0	0	0	0	$28,050
OPERATING													
Accounts Receivable	0	0	0	268,125	0	0	268,125	0	268,125	0	715,000	0	$1,519,375
Seminar Doctor Fees	0	0	0	37,500	0	0	37,500	0	37,500	0	100,000	0	$212,500
Seminar Attorney Fees	0	0	0	30,000	0	0	30,000	0	30,000	0	80,000	0	$170,000
Seminar Supplies & Handouts	0	0	0	30,000	0	0	30,000	0	30,000	0	80,000	0	$170,000
Document Scanning	0	0	0	15,000	0	0	15,000	0	15,000	0	40,000	0	$85,000
Depreciation	0	0	0	0	0	0	0	0	0	0	0	0	$0
Dues and Subscriptions	1,000	1,000	1,000	1,000	1,000	1,000	1,000	1,000	1,000	1,000	1,000	1,000	$12,000
Employee Benefits	3,750	3,750	4,375	5,500	5,500	5,500	6,625	6,625	6,900	7,750	7,750	7,750	$71,775
Employee Insurance	1,900	1,900	1,900	1,900	1,900	1,900	2,050	3,000	3,000	3,000	3,100	3,100	$28,650
Payroll Taxes (SS, etc.)	1,900	1,900	2,150	2,600	2,600	2,600	3,050	3,050	3,100	3,100	3,100	3,100	$32,250
Interest	0	0	0	0	0	0	0	0	0	0	0	0	$0
Legal and Accounting	10,000	6,000	6,000	6,000	6,000	6,000	6,000	6,000	6,000	6,000	6,000	6,000	$76,000
E&O and other Insurance	7,500	7,500	7,500	7,500	7,500	7,500	7,500	7,500	7,500	7,500	7,500	7,500	$90,000
Office Supplies & Postage	2,000	2,000	2,000	2,000	2,000	2,000	2,000	2,000	2,000	2,000	2,000	2,000	$24,000
Rent	2,500	2,500	2,500	2,500	2,500	2,500	2,500	2,500	2,500	2,500	2,500	2,500	$30,000
Property Taxes	200	200	200	200	200	200	200	200	200	200	200	200	$2,400
Telephone	2,000	2,300	2,645	3,042	3,498	4,023	4,626	5,320	6,118	7,036	8,091	9,305	$58,003
T & E	5,000	5,500	6,050	6,655	7,321	8,053	8,858	9,744	10,718	11,790	12,969	14,266	$106,921
Other	20,000	20,000	20,000	20,000	20,000	20,000	20,000	20,000	20,000	20,000	20,000	20,000	$240,000
TOTAL	57,750	54,550	56,320	439,522	60,019	61,275	445,034	66,939	449,661	71,875	1,089,210	76,720	$2,928,875
WEB													
Server Equipment	25,000	6,250	2,500	2,500	2,500	2,500	2,500	2,500	2,500	2,500	2,500	2,500	$56,250
Colocation Cost	4,000	4,000	4,000	4,000	4,000	4,000	4,000	4,000	4,000	4,000	4,000	4,000	$48,000
Telecomm Cost	3,000	3,500	3,500	4,000	4,000	5,000	5,000	5,000	5,000	5,000	5,000		$48,000
Employee Equipment	4,000	4,000	6,000	8,000	8,000	8,000	10,000	10,000	10,000	10,000	10,000	10,000	$98,000
Software Development	20,000	10,000	10,000	10,000	10,000	10,000	10,000	10,000	10,000	10,000	10,000	10,000	$130,000
TOTAL	56,000	27,750	26,000	28,500	28,500	29,500	31,500	31,500	31,500	31,500	31,500	26,500	$380,250
TOTAL	132,750	101,300	103,820	508,047	114,519	130,800	507,034	128,939	512,161	134,375	1,151,710	134,220	$3,659,675

After customers have been successfully recruited, retention of these customers would be critical for USHS to be profitable. USHS should concentrate on providing excellent customer service at its call center and through its website. This would likely require substantial investment in personnel.

Expansion into the North Carolina Triangle area would be a logical next step. Again, a large number of firms with more than 1,500 employees was available. If the joint venture idea were pursued, expansion into the Raleigh area dovetails into both Partners' and Coventry's growth strategy, making the joint venture idea a win–win for both companies. If USHS were successful, expansion could proceed with the same model into South Carolina and Virginia.

Financials Project Profit

Jim's projections for either the sales force or MCO alternative looked good (see Exhibits 15/11 and 15/12). Dan did have a few questions about some of the assumptions he had used.

The Meeting

The lights flickered after a deafening crack of thunder. The television weather warning had not been wrong. As the rain and wind rattled the panes of his study bay window, Don began setting the agenda for the next day's meeting. "If we reach slightly over 14,000 employees in the first year, things should work out. We should certainly discuss compatibility with our company goals. What about the changing technology? The competition? Do we have to be first to market to succeed? How should we reach the market? Wow, there was a lot to discuss, but we will have to accomplish more than just talk. By the end of the meeting we will have to have a decision and implementation plan. What activities will be required to pull this off successfully?" Don knew there were many questions. Did they have the right answers?

NOTES

1. Foundation for Healthy Communities, End-of-Life Planning in New Hampshire: A Statewide Survey (May 2000).
2. E. J. Mundell, *Medical Charts Often Lack Advance Directives*, www.lougehrigsdisease.net (January 8, 1999).
3. M. A. Burg, C. McCarty, W. L. Allen, D. Denslow, *Advance Directives: Population Prevalence*; C. V. Chambers, J. J. Diamond, R. L. Perkel, and L. A. Lasch, "Relationship of Advance Directives to and Demand in Florida," *Journal of the Florida Medical Association* 82 (1995), pp. 811–814.
4. C. V. Chambers, J. J. Diamond, R. L. Perkel, and L. A. Lasch, "Relationship of Advance Directives to Hospital Charges in a Medicare Population," *Archives of Internal Medicire* 154 (1994), pp. 541–547.
5. E. D. McKinley, J. M. Garrett, A. T. Evans, and M. Danis, "Differences in End-of-Life Decision Making Among Black and White Ambulatory Cancer Patients," *Journal of General Internal Medicine* 11 (1996), pp. 651–656.
6. M. Danis et al., "A Prospective Study of Advanced Directives for Life Sustaining Care," *New England Journal of Medicine* 324 (1991), pp. 882–888.

16 CASE

C. W. Williams Health Center: A Community Asset

The Metrolina Health Center was started by Dr. Charles Warren "C. W." Williams and several medical colleagues with a $25,000 grant from the Department of Health and Human Services. Concerned about the health needs of the poor and wanting to make the world a better place for those less fortunate, Dr. Williams, Charlotte's first African American to serve on the surgical staff of Charlotte Memorial Hospital (Charlotte's largest hospital), enlisted the aid of Dr. John Murphy, a local dentist; Peggy Beckwith, director of the Sickle Cell Association; and health planner Bob Ellis to create a health facility for the unserved and underserved population of Mecklenburg County, North Carolina. The health facility received its corporate status in 1980. Dr. Williams died in 1982 when the health facility was still in its infancy. Thereafter, the Metrolina Comprehensive Health Center was renamed the C. W. Williams Health Center.

"We're celebrating our fifteenth year of operation at C. W. Williams, and I'm celebrating my first full year as CEO," commented Michelle Marrs. "I'm feeling really good about a lot of things – we are fully staffed for the first time in two years, and we are a significant player in a pilot program by North Carolina to manage the health care of Medicaid patients in Mecklenburg County (Charlotte area) through private HMOs. We're the only organization that's approved to serve Medicaid recipients that's

This case was written by Linda E. Swayne, The University of North Carolina at Charlotte, and Peter M. Ginter, University of Alabama at Birmingham. It is intended as a basis for classroom discussion rather than to illustrate either effective or ineffective handling of an administrative situation. Used with permission from Linda Swayne.

Exhibit 16/1: C. W. Williams Health Center Mission, Vision, and Values Statements

Mission

To promote a healthier future for our community by consistently providing excellent, accessible health care with pride, compassion, and respect.

Values

- Respect each individual, patient, and staff member as well as our community as a valued entity that must be treasured.
- Consistently provide the highest quality patient care with pride and compassion.
- Partner with other organizations to respond to the social, health, and economic development needs of our community.
- Operate in an efficient, well-staffed, comfortable environment as an autonomous and financially sound organization.

Vision

Committed to the pioneering vision of Dr. Charles Warren Williams, Charlotte's first Black surgeon, we will move into the twenty-first century promoting a healthier and brighter future for our community. This means:
- C. W. Williams Health Center will offer personal, high-quality, affordable, comprehensive health services that improve the quality of life for all.
- C. W. Williams Health Center, while partnering with other health care organizations, will expand its high-quality health services into areas of need. No longer will patients be required to travel long distances to receive the medical care they deserve. C. W. Williams Health Center will come to them!
- C. W. Williams Health Center will be well managed using state-of-the-art technology, accelerating into the twenty-first century as a leading provider of comprehensive community-based health services.
- C. W. Williams Health Center will be viewed as Mecklenburg County's premier community health agency, providing care with RESPECT:
Reliable health care
Efficient operations
Supportive staff
Personal care
Effective systems
Clean environments
Timely services

not an HMO. We have a contract for primary care case management. We're used to providing care for the Medicaid population and we're used to providing health education. It's part of our original mission (see Exhibit 16/1) and has been since the beginning of C. W. Williams."

Michelle continued, "I've been in health care for quite a while but things are really changing rapidly now. The center might be forced to align with one of the two hospitals because of managed care changes. Although we don't want to take

Exhibit 16/2: Michelle Marrs, Chief Executive Officer of C. W. Williams Health Center

Michelle Marrs had over 20 years' experience working in a variety of health care settings and delivery systems. On earning her BS degree, she began her career as a community health educator working in the prevention of alcoholism and substance abuse among youth and women. In 1976 she pursued graduate education at the Harvard School of Public Health and the Graduate School of Education, earning a masters of education with a concentration in administration, planning, and social policy. She worked for the US Public Health Service, Division of Health Services Delivery; the University of Massachusetts Medical Center as director of the Patient Care Studies Department and administrator of the Radiation Oncology Department; the Mattapan Community Health Center (a comprehensive community-based primary care health facility in Boston) as director; and as medical office administrator for Kaiser Permanente. Marrs was appointed chief executive officer of the C. W. Williams Health Center in November 1994.

away the patient's choice, it might happen. In order for me to do all that I should be doing externally, I need more help internally. I believe we should have a director of finance. We have a great opportunity to buy another location so that we can serve more patients, but this is a relatively unstable time in health care. Buying another facility would be a stretch financially, but the location would be perfect. The asking price does seem high, though. . . ." (Exhibit 16/2 contains a biographical sketch of Ms. Marrs.)

Community Health Centers[1]

When the nation's resources were mobilized during the early 1960s to fight the War on Poverty, it was discovered that poor health and lack of basic medical care were major obstacles to the educational and job training progress of the poor. A system of preventive and comprehensive medical care was necessary to battle poverty. A new health care model for poor communities was started in 1963 through the vision and efforts of two New England physicians – Count Geiger and Jack Gibson of the Tufts Medical School – to open the first two neighborhood health centers in Mound Bayou, in rural Mississippi, and in a Boston housing project.

In 1966, an amendment to the Economic Opportunity Act formally established the Comprehensive Health Center Program. By 1971, a total of 150 health centers had been established. By 1990, more than 540 community and migrant health centers at 1,400 service sites had received federal grants totaling $547 million to supplement their budgets of $1.3 billion. By 1996, the numbers had increased to 700 centers at 2,400 delivery sites providing service to over 9 million people.

Community health centers had a public health perspective; however, they were similar to private practices staffed by physicians, nurses, and allied health professionals. They differed from the typical medical office in that they offered a broader range of services, such as social services and health education. Health centers removed the financial and nonfinancial barriers to health care. In

Exhibit 16/3: Ethnicity of Urban and Rural Health Center Patients

Urban Health Center Patients		Rural Health Center Patients	
African American/Black	37.0%	African American/Black	19.6%
White/Non-Hispanic	29.9%	White/Non-Hispanic	49.3%
Native American	0.8%	Native American	1.1%
Asian/Pacific Islander	3.2%	Asian/Pacific Islander	2.9%
Hispanic/Latino	27.2%	Hispanic/Latino	26.5%
Other	1.9%	Other	0.6%

addition, health centers were owned by the community and operated by a local volunteer governing board. Federally funded health centers were required to have patients as a majority of the governing board. The use of patients to govern was a major factor in keeping the centers responsive to patients and generating acceptance by them. Because of the increasing complexity of health care delivery, many board members were taking advantage of training opportunities through their state and national associations to better manage the facility.

Community Health Centers Provide Care for the Medically Underserved

Federally subsidized health centers must, by law, serve populations that are identified by the Public Health Service as medically underserved. Half of the medically underserved population lived in rural areas where there were few medical resources. The other half were located in economically depressed inner-city communities where individuals lived in poverty, lacked health insurance, or had special needs such as homelessness, AIDS, or substance abuse. Approximately 60 percent of health center patients were minorities in urban areas whereas 50 percent were white/non-Hispanics in rural areas (see Exhibit 16/3).

Typically, 50 percent of health center patients did not have private health insurance; nor did they qualify for public health insurance (Medicaid or Medicare). That compared to 13.4 percent of the US population that was uninsured (see Exhibit 16/4). Over 80 percent of health center patients had incomes below the

Exhibit 16/4: Insurance Status of US Health Center Patients, C. W. Williams Health Center Patients, the US Population, and North Carolina Population

	Health Center Patients	US Population	North Carolina Population	C. W. Williams Health Center Patients
Uninsured	42.7%	13.4%	14%	21%
Private Insurance	13.9%	63.2%	64%	10%
Public Insurance	42.9%	23.4%	22%	69%

federal poverty level ($28,700 for a family of four in 1994). Most of the remaining 20 percent were between 100 percent and 200 percent of the federal poverty level.

Community Health Centers Are Cost Effective

Numerous national studies have indicated that the kind of ongoing primary care management provided by community health centers resulted in significantly lowered costs for inpatient hospital care and specialty care. Because illnesses were diagnosed and treated at an earlier stage, more expensive care interventions were often not needed. Hospital admission rates were 22 to 67 percent lower for health center patients than for community residents. A study of six New York city and state health centers found that Medicaid beneficiaries were 22 to 30 percent less costly to treat than those not served by health centers.[2] A Washington state study found that the average cost to Medicaid per hospital bill was $49 for health center patients versus $74 for commercial sector patients.[3] Health center indigent patients were less likely to make emergency room visits – a reduction of 13 percent overall and 38 percent for pediatric care. In addition, defensive medicine (the practice of ordering every and all diagnostic tests to avoid malpractice claims) was less frequently used. Community health center physicians had some of the lowest medical malpractice loss ratios in the nation.

Not only were community health centers cost efficient, patients were highly satisfied with the care received. A total of 96 percent were satisfied or very satisfied with the care they received, and 97 percent indicated they would recommend the health center to their friends and families.[4] Only 4 percent were not so satisfied, and only 3 percent would not recommend their health center to others.

Movement to Managed Care

In 1990, a little over 2 million Medicaid beneficiaries were enrolled in managed care plans; in 1993 the number had increased to 8 million; and in 1995 over 11 million Medicaid beneficiaries were enrolled. Medicaid beneficiaries and other low-income Americans had higher rates of illness and disability than others, and thus accumulated significantly higher costs of medical care.[5]

C. W. Williams Health Center

C. W. Williams was beginning to recognize the impact of managed care. Like much of the South, the Carolinas had been slow to accept managed care. The major reasons seemed to be the rural nature of many Southern states, markets that were not as attractive to major managed care organizations, dominant insurers that continued to provide fee-for-service ensuring choice of physicians and hospitals, and medical inflation that accelerated more slowly than in other areas.

Major changes began to occur, however, beginning in 1993; by 1996 managed care was being implemented in many areas at an accelerated pace.

Challenges for C. W. Williams

Michelle reported, "One of my greatest challenges has been how to handle the changes imposed by the shift from a primarily fee-for-service to a managed care environment. Local physicians who in the past had the flexibility, loyalty, and availability to assist C. W. Williams by providing part-time assistance or volunteer efforts during the physician shortage are now employed by managed care organizations or involved in contractual relationships that prohibit them from working with us. The few remaining primary care solo or small group practices are struggling for survival themselves and seldom are available to provide patient sessions or assist with our hospital call-rotation schedule. The rigorous call-rotation schedule of a small primary care facility like C. W. Williams is frequently unattractive to available physicians seeking opportunities, even when a market competitive compensation package is offered. Many of these physician recruitment and retention issues are being driven by the rapid changes brought on by the impact of managed care in the local community. It is a real challenge to recruit physicians to provide the necessary access to medical care for our patients."

She continued, "My next greatest challenge is investment in technology to facilitate this transition to managed care. Technology is expensive, yet I know it is crucial to our survival and success. We also need more space, but I don't know if this is a good time for expansion."

She concluded, "One of the pressing and perhaps most difficult efforts has been the careful and strategic consideration of the need to affiliate to some degree with one of the two area hospitals in order to more fully integrate and broaden the range of services to patients of our center. Although a decision has not been made at this juncture, the organization has made significant strides to comprehend the needs of this community, consider the pros and cons of either choice, and continue providing the best care possible under some very difficult circumstances."

Hospital Affiliation

Traditionally, the patients of C. W. Williams Health Center that needed hospitalization were admitted to Charlotte Memorial Hospital, a large regional hospital that was designated at the Trauma I level – one of five designated by the state of North Carolina to handle major trauma cases 24 hours a day, 7 days per week (full staffing) as well as perform research in the area of trauma. Uncompensated inpatient care was financed by the county. Charlotte Memorial became Carolinas Medical Center (CMC) in 1984 when it began a program to develop a totally integrated system. In 1995, C. W. Williams provided Carolinas Medical Center with more than 3,000 patient bed days; however, the patients were usually seen by their regular C. W. Williams physicians. As Carolinas Medical Center purchased physician practices (over 300 doctors were employed by the system) and purchased or managed many of the surrounding community hospitals, some C. W. Williams patients became concerned that CMC would take over C. W. Williams and that their community health center would no longer exist.

"My preference is that our patients have a choice of where they would prefer to go for hospitalization. Our older patients expect to go to Carolinas Medical, but many of our middle-aged patients have expressed a preference for Presbyterian. Both hospitals have indicated an interest in our patients," according to Michelle. She continued, "We may not really have a choice, however. We recently received information that reported the 12 largest hospitals in the state, including the teaching hospitals – Duke, University of North Carolina at Chapel Hill, Carolinas Medical Center, and East Carolina – have formed a consortium and will contract with the state to pay for Medicaid patients. At the same time all 20 of the health centers in the state – including us at C. W. Williams – are cooperating to develop a health maintenance organization. We expect to gain approval for the HMO by July 1997. Since 60 percent of our patients are Medicaid, if the state contracts with the new consortium, then we will be required to send our patients to Carolinas Medical Center."

Services

C. W. Williams Health Center provides primary and preventive health services including: medical, radiology, laboratory, pharmacy, subspecialty, and inpatient managed care; health education/promotion; community outreach; and transportation to care (Exhibit 16/5 lists all services). The center was strongly linked to the Charlotte community, and it worked with other public and private health services to coordinate resources for effective patient care. No one was denied care because of an inability to pay. A little over 20 percent of the patients at C. W. Williams were uninsured.

The full-time staff included five physicians, two physician assistants (PAs), two nurses, one X-ray technician, one pharmacist, and a staff of 28. Of the five physicians, one was an internist, two were in family practice, and two were pediatricians. The PAs "floated" to work wherever help was most needed. With the help of one assistant, the pharmacist filled more than 20,000 prescriptions annually.

Patients at C. W. Williams

All first-time patients at C. W. Williams were asked what type of insurance they had. If they had some type of insurance – private, Medicare, Medicaid – an appointment was immediately scheduled. If the new patient had no insurance, he or she was asked if they would be interested in applying for the C. W. Williams discount program (the discount could amount to as much as 100 percent, but every

Exhibit 16/5: C. W. Williams Health Center Services

Primary Care and Preventive Services
Diagnostic Laboratory
Diagnostic X-ray (basic)
Pharmacy
EMS (crash cart and CPR-trained staff)
Family Planning
Immunizations (MD-directed as well as open clinic – no relationship required)
Prenatal Care and Gynecology
Health Education
Parenting Education
Translation Services
Substance Abuse and Counseling
Nutrition Counseling
Diagnostic Testing
  HIV
  Mammogram
  Pap Smears
  TB Testing
  Vision/Hearing Testing
  Lead Testing
  Pregnancy Test
  Drug Screening

person was asked to pay something). The discount was based on income and the number of people in the household. If the response was "no," the caller was informed that payment was expected at the time services were rendered. Visa, Mastercard, cash, and personal check (with two forms of identification) were accepted. At C. W. Williams, all health care was made affordable.

C. W. Williams made reminder calls to the patient's home (or neighbor's or relative's telephone) several days prior to the appointment. When patients arrived at the center, they provided their name to the nurse at the front reception desk and then took a seat in a large waiting room. The pharmacy window was near the front door for the convenience of patients who were simply picking up a prescription. The reception desk, pharmacy, and waiting room occupied the first floor.

When the patient's name was called, he or she was taken by elevator to the second floor where there were ten examination rooms. After seeing the physician, physician assistant, or nurse, the patient was escorted back down the elevator to the pharmacy if a prescription was needed and then to the reception desk to pay. Pharmaceuticals were discounted and a special program by Pfizer Pharmaceuticals provided over $60,000 worth of drugs in 1995 for medically indigent patients.

The center's patient population was 64 percent female between the ages of 15 and 44 (see Exhibit 16/6). Nearly 80 percent of patients were African Americans, 18 percent were white, and 2 percent were other minorities. Patients

Exhibit 16/6: C. W. Williams Health Center Patients by Age and Sex

Females	1991	1992	1993	1994	1995
<1	343	408	263	198	101
1–4	434	552	692	647	417
5–11	322	572	494	641	658
12–14	376	197	150	148	124
15–17	361	168	146	121	92
18–19	264	152	85	82	67
20–34	749	1,250	967	964	712
35–44	869	617	479	532	467
45–64	583	567	617	658	658
65+	400	488	531	527	524
	4,701	4,971	4,424	4,518	3,820
Males					
<1	367	471	328	199	119
1–4	439	516	707	625	410
5–11	440	644	598	846	738
12–14	171	175	128	120	104
15–17	180	133	79	76	155
18–19	126	67	28	23	69
20–34	296	389	219	187	126
35–44	313	296	182	205	132
45–64	229	316	273	294	235
65+	151	248	190	190	181
	2,712	3,255	2,732	2,765	2,269
Total	7,413	8,226	7,156	7,283	6,089

Exhibit 16/7: Patient Satisfaction Study

Rank	Selected Service Indicators	Mean Score
1	Helpfulness/attitudes of medical staff	3.82
2	Clean/comfortable/convenient facility	3.65
3	Relationship with physician/nurse	3.58
4	Quality of health services	3.28
5	Ability to satisfy all medical needs	3.20
6	Helpfulness/attitudes of nonmedical staff	2.72

were quite satisfied with the services provided as indicated in patient surveys conducted by the center. Paralleling national studies, 97 percent of C. W. Williams patients would recommend the center to family or friends. Selected service indicators by rank from the patient satisfaction study are included as Exhibit 16/7.

C. W. Williams Organization

The center was managed by a board of directors, responsible for developing policy and hiring the CEO.

Board of Directors

The federal government required that all community health centers have a board of directors that was made up of at least 51 percent patients or citizens who lived in the community. The board chairman of C. W. Williams, Mr. Daniel Dooley, was a center patient. C. W. Williams had a board of 15, all of whom were African Americans and four of whom were patients and out of the workforce. Two members of the board were managers/directors from the Public Health Department (which was under the management of CMC). There were two other health professionals – a nurse and a physician. Other board members included a CPA, a financial planner, an insurance agent, a vice president for human resources, an executive in a search firm, and a former professor of economics. A majority of the board had not had a great deal of exposure to the changes occurring in the health care industry (aside from their own personal situations); nor were they trained in strategic management.

The Staff

The center was operated by Michelle Marrs as CEO, who had an operations officer and medical director reporting to her (see Exhibit 16/8 for an organization chart).

Eventually the director of finance, who had worked at the center for over ten years, resigned. "She was offered another position within C. W. Williams," said Michelle, "but she declined to take it. Frankly, I have to have someone with greater expertise in finance. With capitation on the horizon, we need to do some very critical planning to better manage our finances and make sure we are receiving as much reimbursement from Washington as we are entitled."

There were some disagreements between the board and Ms. Marrs over responsibilities. Employees frequently appealed to the chairman and other members of the board when they felt that they had not been treated fairly. Ms. Marrs would prefer the board to be more involved in setting strategic direction for C. W. Williams. "A two-year strategic plan was developed late in 1995 that has not been moved along, embraced, and further developed. Committees have not met on a regular basis to actualize stated objectives."

C. W. Williams Was Financially Strong

The center received an increasing amount of federal grant money for the first ten years of its operation as the number of patients grew, but leveled off as most government allocations were reduced (see Exhibit 16/9). Although the amount collected from Medicare was increasing, the amount collected compared with the

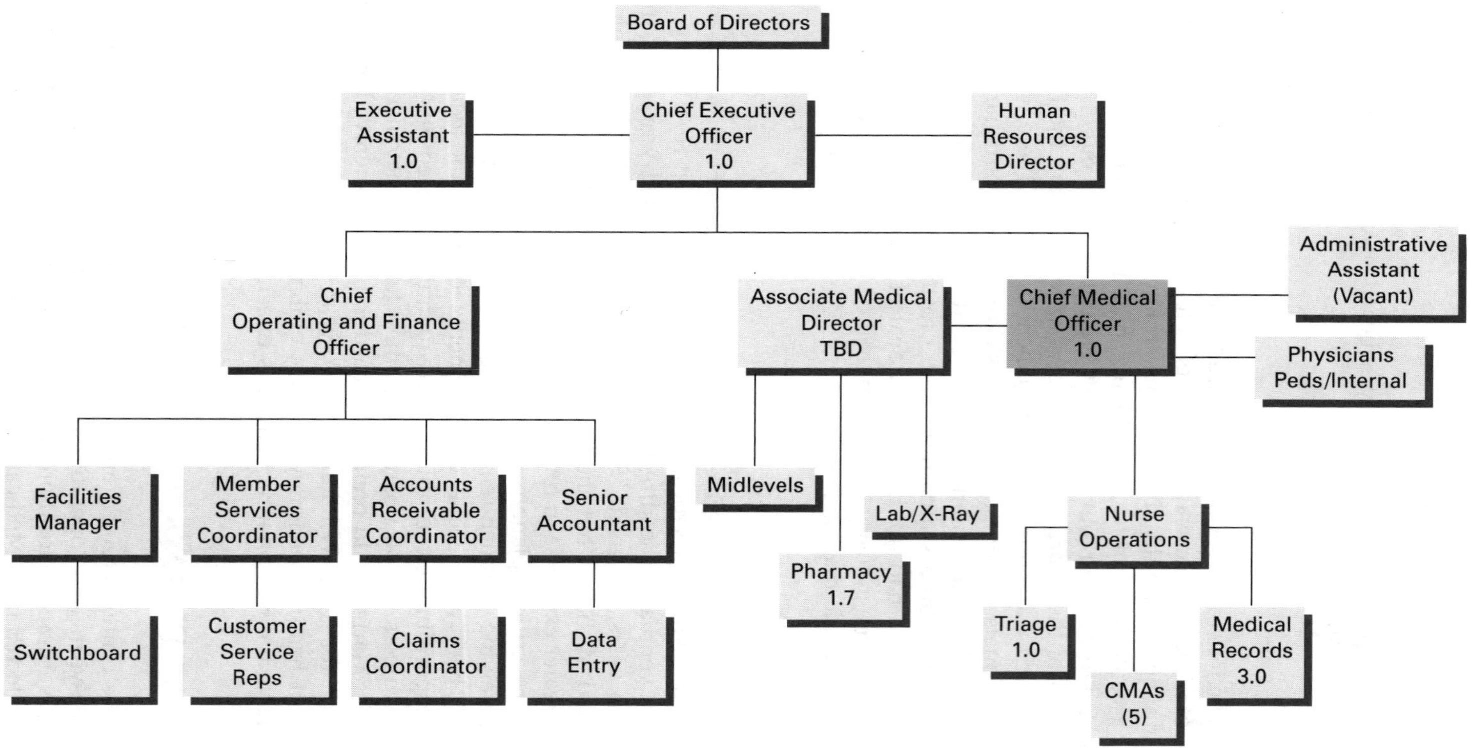

Exhibit 16/8: Metrolina Comprehensive Health Center, Inc. dba C. W. Williams Health Center

full charge was decreasing (see Exhibit 16/10). Exhibits 16/11 to 16/14 provide details of the financial situation.

Carolina ACCESS – A Pilot Program

In fiscal year 1994 (July 1, 1994 to June 30, 1995), North Carolina served more than 950,000 Medicaid recipients at a cost of over $3.5 billion. The aged, blind, and disabled accounted for 26 percent of the eligibles and 65 percent of the expenditures. Families and children accounted for 74 percent of the eligibles and 35 percent of the expenditures. Services were heavily concentrated in two areas: inpatient hospital – accounting for 20 percent of expenses – and nursing-facility/intermediate care/mentally retarded services – accounting for 34 percent of expenses. Mecklenburg County had the highest number of eligibles within the state at 50,849 people, representing 7 percent of the Medicaid population.

What started out in 1986 as a contract with Kaiser Permanente to provide medical services for recipients of Aid to Families with Dependent Children in four counties became a complex mixture of three models of managed care. Carolina ACCESS was North Carolina Medicaid's primary care case management model of managed care. It began a pilot program named "Health Care Connections" in Mecklenburg County on June 1, 1996.

Exhibit 16/9: C. W. Williams Funding Sources

Funding Source	1991	1992	1993	1994	1995
Grant (Federal)	740,000	666,524	689,361	720,584	720,584
Medicare	152,042	157,891	258,104	260,389	301,444
Medicaid	381,109	453,712	641,069	562,380	456,043
Third-Party Pay	25,673	14,128	84,347	90,253	51,799
Uninsured Self-Pay	300,748	441,508	174,992	262,817	338,272
Grant (Miscellaneous)	0	0	0	11,500	48,000
Total	1,599,572	1,733,763	1,847,873	1,907,923	1,916,142

Exhibit 16/10: Funding Accounts Receivable

	1994		1995	
	Full Charge	Amount Collected	Full Charge	Amount Collected
Medicare	436,853	260,389	369,306	301,444
Medicaid	914,212	562,380	725,175	456,043
Insured	99,202	90,253	61,021	51,799
Patient Fees	899,055	262,817	754,864	338,272

Exhibit 16/11: C. W. Williams Health Center Balance Sheets

	1992–1993	1993–1994	1994–1995	1995–1996
Assets				
Current Assets				
Cash	280,550	335,258	339,459	132,925
Certificates of Deposit	23,413	24,496	25,446	529,826
Accounts Receivable (net)	213,815	285,934	202,865	160,230
Accounts Receivable (other)	5,661	4,721	2,936	10,069
Security Deposits	1,847	97	-0-	-0-
Notes Receivable	-0-	-0-	29,825	10,403
Inventory	26,191	23,777	30,217	26,844
Prepaid Loans	12,087	21,605	9,722	11,159
Investments	269	269	269	51,628
Total Current Assets	563,833	696,157	640,739	933,084
Property and Equipment				
Land	10,000	10,000	10,000	10,000
Building	311,039	311,039	311,039	311,039
Building Renovations	904,434	904,434	909,754	915,949
Equipment	282,333	312,892	328,063	387,178
Less Depreciation	(393,392)	(452,432)	(523,384)	(597,275)
Total Property and Equipment	1,114,414	1,085,933	1,035,472	1,026,891
Total Assets	1,678,247	1,782,090	1,676,211	1,959,975
Liabilities and Net Assets				
Liabilities				
Accounts Payable	11,066	31,582	13,136	34,039
Vacation Expense Accounts	36,694	42,857	19,457	28,144
Deferred Revenue	42,641	37,910	43,400	59,433
Total Liabilities	90,401	112,349	75,993	121,616
Net Assets				
Unrestricted				1,838,350
Temporary Restricted	-0-	-0-	-0-	-0-
Total Net Assets	1,587,846	1,669,741	1,600,218	1,838,350
Total Liabilities and Net Assets	1,678,247	1,782,090	1,676,211	1,959,976

Health Care Connections

The state of North Carolina wanted to move 42,000 Mecklenburg County Medicaid recipients into managed care. The state contracted with six health plans and C. W. Williams, as a federally qualified health center, to serve the Mecklenburg County Medicaid population. Because one organization was dropped from the program, Medicaid recipients were to choose one of the following plans to provide their health care:

- Atlantic Health Plans (*type*: HMO; *hospital affiliation*: Carolinas Medical Center, University Hospital, Mercy Hospital, Mercy South, Union Regional Medical, Kings Mountain Hospital).
- Kaiser Permanente (*type*: HMO; *hospital affiliation*: Presbyterian Hospital, Presbyterian Hospital – Matthews, Presbyterian Orthopedic, Presbyterian Specialty Hospital).
- Maxicare North Carolina, Inc. (*type*: HMO; *hospital affiliation*: Presbyterian Hospital, Presbyterian Hospital – Matthews, Presbyterian Orthopedic, Presbyterian Specialty Hospital).
- Optimum Choice/Mid-Atlantic Medical (*type*: HMO; *hospital affiliation*: Presbyterian Hospital, Presbyterian Hospital – Matthews, Presbyterian Orthopedic, Presbyterian Specialty Hospital).
- The Wellness Plan of NC, Inc. (*type*: HMO; *hospital affiliation*: Carolinas Medical Center, University Hospital, Mercy Hospital, Mercy South, Union Regional Medical, Kings Mountain Hospital).
- C. W. Williams Health Center (*type*: partially federally funded, community health center; *hospital affiliation*: Carolinas Medical Center, University Hospital, Mercy Hospital, Mercy South, Union Regional Medical, Kings Mountain Hospital or Presbyterian Hospital, Presbyterian Hospital – Matthews, Presbyterian Orthopedic, Presbyterian Specialty Hospital).

Exhibit 16/12: Statement of Support, Revenue, Expenses, and Change in Fund Balances

	1992–1993	1993–1994	1994–1995	1995–1996
Contributed Support and Revenue				
Contributed	720,712	720,584	732,584	768,584
Earned Revenue				
Patient Fees	1,213,919	1,186,497	1,183,904	1,129,030
Medicare				465,248
Contributions				5,676
Interest Income	7,228	9,666	12,567	14,115
Dividend Income				2,387
Rental Income				1,980
Miscellaneous Income	5,962	5,941	4,772	11,055
Total Earned	1,227,109	1,202,104	1,201,243	1,629,491
Total Contributed Support and Revenue	1,947,821	1,922,688	1,933,827	2,398,075
Expenses				
Program	1,782,312	1,840,447	2,002,633	2,157,768
Other	442	349	217	2,166
Total Expenses	1,782,754	1,840,796	2,002,850	2,159,934
Increase (decrease) in Net Assets	165,062	81,892	(69,523)	238,141
Net Assets (beginning of year)	1,310,155	1,587,849	1,669,741	1,600,218
Adjustment	112,629*	-0-	-0-	-0-
Net Assets (end of year)	1,587,846	1,669,741	1,600,218	1,838,359

*Federal grant funds earned but not drawn down in prior years were not recognized as revenue. The error had no effect on net income for fiscal year ended March 31, 1992.

Exhibit 16/13: Statement of Functional Expenditures, Fiscal Year Ended March 31

	1992–1993	1993–1994	1994–1995	1995–1996
Personnel				
Salaries	937,119	1,016,194	1,102,373	1,181,639
Benefits	190,300	210,228	210,674	211,705
Total	1,127,419	1,226,422	1,313,047	1,393,344
Other				
Accounting	5,250	5,985	6,397	7,200
Bank Charges	840	300	213	1,001
Building Maintenance	38,842	54,132	49,586	53,828
Consultants	26,674	2,733	39,565	44,923[a]
Contract MDs	-0-	-0-	-0-	87,159
Dues/Publications/Conferences	17,371	21,655	22,066	24,258
Equipment Maintenance	28,732	27,365	30,402	27,352
Insurance	15,182	3,146	3,215	3,292
Legal Fees	688	2,774	3,652	3,582
Marketing	6,358	1,958	5,734	15,730
Patient Services	28,959	28,222	35,397	43,815
Pharmacy	271,542	237,761	225,762	188,061
Physician Recruiting	14,171	32,929	56,173	21,395
Postage	8,435	11,622	10,019	14,182
Printing	729	963	2,405	9,696
Supplies	73,020	62,828	72,977	84,064
Telephone	16,755	17,967	20,914	25,002
Travel – Board	2,713	1,202	4,977	3,476
Travel – Staff	13,889	14,576	12,631	15,978
Utilities	15,782	18,305	16,548	16,536
Total Other	585,932	546,423	618,633	690,530
Total Personnel and Other	1,713,351	1,772,845	1,931,680	2,083,874
Depreciation	(68,966)	(67,604)	(70,952)	(73,891)
Total Expenses	1,782,317	1,840,449	2,002,632	2,157,765

[a] Includes contracted medical director.

An integral part of the selection process was the use of a health benefits advisor to assist families in choosing the appropriate plan. By law, none of the organizations was permitted to promote its plan to Medicaid recipients. Rather, the Public Consulting Group of Charlotte was awarded the contract to be an independent enrollment counselor to assist Medicaid recipients in their choices of health care options.

"More than 33,000 of the Medicaid recipients were women and children. Sixty percent of the group had no medical relationship. Slightly over 50 percent of C. W. Williams's patients are Medicaid recipients," said Michelle Marrs. See Exhibit 16/15 for C. W. Williams users by pay source.

Exhibit 16/14: C. W. Williams Health Center Statement of Cash Flows, Fiscal Year Ended March 31

Net Cash Flow from Operations	1992–1993	1993–1994	1994–1995	1995–1996
Increase in Net Assets	165,062	81,892	(69,523)	238,141
Noncash Income Expense Depreciation	68,966	67,604	70,952	73,891
Increase in Deposits	(1,750)	1,750	-0-	-0-
Decrease in Receivables	(86,620)	(71,179)	55,028	65,328
(Increase) in Prepaid Expenses	(2,277)	(9,518)	11,980	(1,437)
(Increase) Decrease in Inventory	(4,105)	2,414	(6,440)	3,373
Increase in Payables	14,094	20,516	(18,445)	20,903
Increase (Decrease) in Vacation Expense Accrual	(8,583)	6,163	(23,400)	8,688
(Increase) in Notes Receivable	-0-	-0-	-0-	(10,403)
Increase in Deferred Revenue	(2,992)	(4,731)	5,490	16,032
Net Cash Flow from Operations	141,795	94,911	25,642	414,516
Cash Flow from Investing in Fixed Assets	(52,547)	(39,120)	(20,491)	(65,311)
Purchase Marketable Securities	-0-	-0-	-0-	(51,359)
Net Cash Used by Investments	(52,547)	(39,120)	(20,491)	(116,670)
Net Cash from Financing Activities	112,629	-0-	-0-	-0-
Increase in Cash	201,877	55,791	5,151	297,846
Cash + Cash Equivalents				
Beginning of Year April 1	130,274	332,151	387,942	393,093
End of Year March 31	332,151	387,942	393,093	690,939

"We have about 8,000 patients coming to us for about 30,000 visits," according to Michelle (see Exhibit 16/16). "So there are approximately 4,000 people who currently come to us for health care that are now required to choose a health plan. The state decided that an independent agency had to sign people up so that there would be no 'bounty' hunting for enrollees. In the first month, about 2,300 Medicaid recipients enrolled in the pilot program. Almost half of the people who signed up chose Kaiser Foundation Health Plan. It has a history of serving Medicaid patients. We received the next highest number of enrollees, because we too have a history of serving this market. We had 402 enrollees during that first month. Of those, only 38 were previous patients. What we don't know yet is whether we have lost any patients to other programs. The lack of up-to-date information is frustrating. We need a better information system."

Michelle continued, "We decided that we could provide care for up to 8,000 Medicaid patients at C. W. Williams. I embrace managed care for a number of reasons: patients must choose a primary care provider, patients will be encouraged to take an active role in their health care, and there will be less duplication of medical services and costs. In the past, some doctors have shied away from Medicaid patients because they didn't want to be bothered with the paperwork, the medical services weren't fully compensated, and Medicaid patients tended to have numerous health problems.

Exhibit 16/15: Users by Pay Source

Source	Percent of Users	Number of Users	Income to C. W. Williams	Number of Encounters
1994–1995				
Medicare	13%	791	301,444	2,392
Medicaid	56%	3,410	456,043	10,305
Full Pay	10%	609	318,424	1,840
Uninsured	21%	1,279	42,421	3,865
		6,089	1,118,332	18,402
1993–1994				
Medicare	12%	1,037	195,352	2,880
Medicaid	53%	4,579	585,446	12,720
Full Pay	11%	950	178,525	2,640
Uninsured	24%	2,074	101,569	5,760
		8,640	1,060,892	24,000
1992–1993				
Medicare	10%	853	189,927	2,304
Medicaid	36%	3,072	401,355	8,294
Full Pay	10%	853	158,473	2,304
Uninsured	44%	3,755	186,708	10,138
		8,533	936,463	23,040
1991–1992				
Medicare	20%	1,614	162,980	4,032
Medicaid	30%	2,419	312,680	6,048
Full Pay	10%	806	157,101	2,016
Uninsured	40%	3,225	159,855	8,064
		8,064	792,616	20,160

Exhibit 16/16: C. W. Williams Health Center Patient Visits

Primary Care Visits

Internal Medicine	8,248
Family Practice	4,573
Pediatrics	2,643
Gynecology	236
Midlevel Practitioners	3,609
Total	19,309

Subspecialty/Ancillary Service Visits

Podiatry	82
Mammography	101
Immunizations	1,766
Perinatal	429
X-ray	1,152
Dental	17
Pharmacy Prescriptions	20,868
Hospital	1,762
Laboratory	13,103
Health Education	412
Other Medical Specialists	1,032
Total	40,724

"There are seven different companies that applied and were given authority to provide health care for Medicaid recipients in Mecklenburg County. Although I understand one had to withdraw, we are the only one that is not an HMO. Although we don't provide hospitalization, we do provide for patients' care whether they need an office visit or to be hospitalized. Our physicians provide care while the patient is in the hospital."

She continued, "Medicaid beneficiaries have to be recertified every six months. We are three months into the sign-up process or approximately halfway. Kaiser has enrolled the highest number, about one-third of the beneficiaries (see Exhibit 16/17). We have enrolled over 12 percent. The independent enrollment counselor is responsible for helping Medicaid recipients enroll during the initial 12 months. I expect the numbers to dwindle for the last six months of that time period. Changes will primarily come from new patients to the area and patients who are unhappy with their initial choice."

Medicaid patients were going to be a challenge for managed care. Because many of them were used to going to the emergency room for care, they were not in the habit of making or keeping appointments. Some facilities overbooked appointments to try to utilize medical staff efficiently; however, the practice caused very long waits at times. Other complicating factors included lack of telephones for contacting patients for reminder calls or physician follow-ups, lack of transportation, the number of high-risk patients as a result of poverty or lifestyle factors, and patients that did not follow doctors' orders.

Health Connection Enrollment

Medicaid recipients were required to be recertified every six months in the state of North Carolina. During this process, a time was allocated for the Public Consulting Group of Charlotte to make a presentation about the managed care choices available. The presentation included a discussion of:

- managed care and HMOs and how they were similar to and different from previous Medicaid practices;
- benefits of Health Care Connections such as having a medical home, a 24-hour, seven-day-a-week hotline to ask questions about medical care, physician choice, and plan choice; and

Exhibit 16/17: ACCESS Enrollment Data for the Week Ended September 6, 1996

	Atlantic	Kaiser Permanente	Maxi-care	Optimum Choice	Wellness Plan	C. W. Williams	Total
Week Totals	229	347	66	114	189	124	1,069
Month-to-date	229	347	66	114	189	124	1,069
Year-to-date	3,708	5,384	1,164	1,507	2,238	2,016	16,017
Project-to-date	3,708	5,384	1,164	1,507	2,238	2,016	16,017

- methods to choose a plan based on wanting to use a doctor that the patient has used before, hospital choice (some plans were associated with a specific hospital), and location (for easy access).

If Medicaid recipients did not choose a plan that day, they had ten working days to call in on the hotline to choose a plan. If they had not done so by that deadline, they were randomly assigned to a plan. Public Consulting Group's health benefits advisors (HBAs) made the presentations and then assisted each individual in determining what choice he or she would like to make and filling out the paperwork. More than 80 percent of the Medicaid recipients who went through the recertification process and heard the presentation decided on site. Most others called back on the hotline after more carefully studying the information. About 3 percent were randomly assigned because they did not select a plan.

New Medicaid recipients were provided individualized presentations because they tended to be new to the community, had recently developed a health problem, or were pregnant. Because they might have less information than those who had been "in the system" for some time, it took a more detailed explanation from the HBA.

HBAs presented the information in a fair, factual, and useful manner for session attendees. For the first several months they attempted to thoroughly explain the difference between an HMO and a "partially federally funded community health center," but the HBAs decided it was too confusing to the audience and did not really make a difference in their health care. For the past month they explained "managed care" more carefully and touched lightly on HMOs. C. W. Williams was presented as one of the choices, although some of the HBAs mentioned that it was the only choice that had evening and weekend hours for appointments.

Strategic Plan for C. W. Williams

With the help of Michelle Marrs, the C. W. Williams Board of Directors was beginning to develop a strategic plan. Exhibit 16/18 provides the SWOT analysis that was developed. "Part of our strategic plan was to go to the people – make it easier for our patients to visit C. W. Williams by establishing satellite clinics. We recently became aware of a building that is for sale that would meet our needs. The owner would like to sell to us. He's older and likes the idea that the building will 'do some good for people,' but he's asking $479,000. The location is near a large number of Medicaid beneficiaries plus a middle-class area of minority patients that could add to our insured population. I just don't know if we should take the risk to buy the building. We own our current building and have no debt. We are running out of space at C. W. Williams. We have two examination rooms for each physician and all patients have to wait on the first floor and then be called to the second floor when a room becomes free. I know that ideally for the greatest efficiency we should have three exam rooms for each doctor."

Exhibit 16/18: C. W. Williams Health Center SWOT Analysis

Strengths	Weaknesses
Community-based business	Need for deputy director
Primary care provider with walk-in component	Lack of RN/triage director
Large patient base	Staffing and staffing pattern
Fast, discounted pharmacy	Managed care readiness
Cash reserve	Number of providers
Laboratory/X-ray	Recruitment and retention
Clean facility in good location	Limited referrals
Satellites	Limited services
Good reputation with community and funders	No social worker/nutritionist/health educator
Resources for disabled patients	No on-site Medicaid eligibility
Strong leadership/management	Weak relationship with community MDs
Growth potential	Limited hours of operation
Property owned with good parking	Transportation
Excellent quality of care	Organizational structure
Culturally sensitive staff	Management information systems
Nice environment	Market share at risk of erosion
Dedicated board and staff	Staff orientation to managed care

Opportunities	Threats
Many in the community are uninsured and have multiple medical care needs	Uncertain financial future of health care in general
A number of universities are located in the Charlotte area	Health care reform
Health care reform	Competition from other health care providers for the medically underserved
Oversupply of physicians means that many will not set up private practices or be able to join just any practice	Loss of patients as they choose HMOs rather than C. W. Williams
Managed care	Managed care
Charlotte market	Reimbursement restructuring
	Shortage of health care professionals

"We have had an architect look at the proposed facility. He estimated that it would take about $500,000 for remodeling. According to the tax records, the building and land are worth about $250,000. Since we don't yet know how many patients we will actually receive from Health Care Connection or how many of our patients will choose an HMO, it's hard to decide if we should take the risk."

What to Do

"At the end of the week I sometimes wonder what I've accomplished," Michelle stated. "I seem to spend a lot of time putting out fires when I should be concentrating on developing a strategic plan and writing more grants."

NOTES

1. This section is adapted from Mickey Goodson, *A Quick History* (National Association of Community Health Centers Publication, undated).

2. *Utilization and Costs to Medicaid of AFDC Recipients in New York Served and Not Served by Community Health Centers* (Columbia, MD: Center for Health Policy Studies, June 1994).

3. *Using Medicaid Fee-for-Service Data to Develop Community Health Center Policy* (Seattle, WA: Washington Association of Community Health Centers and Group Health Cooperative of Puget Sound, 1994).

4. *Key Points: A National Survey of Patient Experiences in Community and Migrant Health Centers* (New York: Commonwealth Fund, 1994).

5. *Health Insurance of Minorities in the US* (Report by the Agency for Health Care Policy and Research, US Department of Health and Human Services, 1992) and *Green Book, Overview of Entitlement Programs Under the Jurisdiction of the Ways and Means Committee* (US House of Representatives, 1994).

Regional Memorial's Institutional Ethics Committee: Work To Do

"And learn to play the game fair, no self-deception, no shrinking from the truth; mercy and consideration for the other man, but none for yourself, upon whom you have to keep an incessant watch."

Sir William Osler
Physician and Educator (1849–1919)

Prologue

Mr. Blackwell decided to consult the Institutional Ethics Committee (IEC) of Regional Memorial Hospital. Blackwell was the CEO of this large, public health facility that had over 900 beds and serviced a countywide population of over 1.2 million. His concerns centered around several cases that plagued his medical and administrative staffs for months. The questions just did not go away. The cases of Baby Boy-X and Annie O. were not typical, and neither were the free baby formula case and the vendor ethics case, but they all raised ethical issues that were troublesome, fairly common, and not easily managed.

This case was written by John M. Lincourt, The University of North Carolina at Charlotte. The first two situations come from *Ethics Without a Net, a Case Workbook in Bioethics* by John M. Lincourt (Dubuque, IA: Kendall/Hunt Publishing Company, 1991). Reproduction of the cases is by permission of the publisher. The prologue, background sections, and latter two cases were written especially for *Strategic Management of Health Care Organizations*, 5th edn. Used with permission from John Lincourt.

Even with a combined expenditure of over $0.5 million, questions about the nature, duration, and efficacy of care provided remained in the cases of Baby Boy-X and Annie O. As CEO, Blackwell sought the advice of the hospital's IEC on the appropriateness of the care given and special help on what would constitute a fair level of care in these medical cases.

Because of perceived conflicts of interest in the other two cases, Blackwell sought the advice of the hospital's IEC on the fair course of action. In his book, W. H. Shaw explained the problems associated with the free baby formula and the vendor ethics clearly when he wrote that "a conflict of interest arises when employees at any level have a private interest in a transaction substantial enough that it does or reasonably might affect their independent judgment."[1] Patients had the right and hospitals had the responsibility to expect those who made decisions to be as free as possible from conflicts of interest.

Background

R. E. Cranford and A. E. Doudera's description of hospital ethics committees was useful: "Institutional ethics committees are interdisciplinary groups within health care institutions that advise about pressing ethical problems that arise in clinical care."[2] IECs were founded on the primary assumption that cooperative, reasoned reflection was likely to assist decision makers to reach better conclusions. These committees provided information and education to staff and the surrounding communities about ethical questions, proposed policies related to ethically difficult issues, and reviewed patient care situations (prospectively and retrospectively) in which ethical questions were at stake. Assets provided by IECs were that: (1) they served as a locus for discussion, clarification, dialogue, and advice (not decisions); (2) they supplied protection and support for health care providers making difficult decisions; and (3) they increased awareness of and sensitivity to ethical dimensions of clinical cases.

IECs were not without their critics. Some claimed such advisory groups threatened to undermine the traditional doctor–patient relationship and imposed new and untested regulatory burdens on patients, families, physicians, and hospitals. Labeling an issue as "ethical" removed it from the category of those that were strictly medical or managerial and declared that relevant considerations were not just technical in nature. Many health care providers were unaccustomed to working in this area of ethical values, and some insisted their training and experience provided scant preparation for it. Conversely, others claimed that ethical values were woven into the very fabric of medical practice and management, thereby rendering them eminently suitable, if not the most suitable, as the basis for making such decisions. These individuals tended to view IECs as "God Squads" – that is, generally lacking in moral authority and ill-equipped to handle the ethical challenges of vexing and sometimes urgent hospital decisions. Such attitudes still persisted in some quarters.[3]

The operation of IECs was similar to other hospital committees, but there were some important differences. These included the interdisciplinary composition, sliding orientation period, and varied utilization pattern. IECs tended to be large committees having between 10 and 20 members. Membership included: nurses and physicians (frequently from oncology and pediatrics); administrators, including an outside attorney; members of the clergy and social services; a citizen or two; plus an ethicist (if available). Orientation for a new committee or new members ranged from a week or two up to a full year. Typically this period was devoted to a careful review of institutional and community standards of care, and introduction to the bioethical literature (which was becoming vast), and, most importantly, practice sessions involving ethics cases. Such reviews were usually retrospective in nature and came from that institution, one of similar status, or the literature.

Committee utilization patterns varied as well. The IEC might be convened on a case requiring immediate action, the careful review of past cases that were known to include ethical misjudgment, and cases that after review were not considered to be ethical issues at all but rather some other problem or issue (legal or procedural, for instance). Finally, the Patient Self-Determination Act, passed by Congress as part of the Omnibus Reconciliation Act of 1990 (effective December 1, 1991), helped to legitimize IECs and to socialize them more completely into hospital medical practice.

Increasingly, the arenas of business ethics and biomedical ethics intersected in important ways. No longer was the assertion heard that health care was not a business but rather a profession that somehow stood above the adversarial and competitive features of typical business practices. Hospitals were businesses and health care was an industry. In fact, the business aspects of health care were now the object of much discussion, concern, debate, and study.

The Case of Baby Boy-X

Baby Boy-X was born to a 37-year-old woman at 36 weeks' gestation. The birth was a spontaneous vaginal delivery and the patient's medical history gave no clue to the future difficulties associated with the birth of this child. The first indications of fetal risk were revealed when the Apgar scores were computed. This child had scores of 2 at one minute and 1 at five minutes. These scores were used to assess the general conditions of the neonate, by rating the child's status using the following criteria: color, pulse, respiration, reflex response, and muscle tone. A total score of 10 denoted a newborn in the best condition. Neonatal mortality rose rapidly as the total Apgar score approached 0. For example, scores of 1 and 2 predicted a 12 to 15 percent survival rate. Baby Boy-X's score was cause for serious concern for the medical staff at Regional Memorial.

The patient's clinical, physical, and social histories supported the Apgar assessment. These included:

- Deformed right leg;
- Hydrocephalus;
- Nonfunctioning GI track;

- Irregular cessation of breathing that required a ventilator;
- Chronic anemia, requiring transfusions and nutritional supplements;
- Repeated grand mal seizures during the first two months;
- Probable blindness;
- Lowered and malformed ears;
- Severe contraction of the limbs, including fingers and toes;
- Cerebral shrinkage and degeneration caused by lack of oxygen to the brain;
- Little brain activity except during seizures; and
- Gastrostomy, colostomy, and ileostomy tubes inserted surgically for proper nutrition and excretion.

Baby Boy-X was kept in the neonatal intensive care unit (NICU) for four months. He was on a ventilator and given drugs for his seizure disorder. The consensus among the NICU personnel was the prognosis was poor, and they expected the patient to die from massive infection or following violent seizure activity. The cost at four months was $182,265. The mother and father were separated and the family was on welfare. The father had not visited the child.

On numerous occasions, members of the medical and administrative staffs initiated discussions with the mother about her son's grim prognosis and poor quality of life. These conversations were started in the hopes she would realize the futility of all the heroic measures being employed and allow her son to die naturally and soon. Staff members stated privately that scarce and costly medical resources were being wasted. This patient would never leave the hospital alive and his life in the hospital was severely compromised and painful. Some administrators asked pointed questions about rethinking the "medical full-court press" for this patient. Resources expended here could be redirected to clients whose chances for survival and normal lifestyles were markedly better.

In the face of all these remarks, the mother remained adamant. The following text was taken from the NICU nursing notes and poignantly reflected the mother's attitude at the same time. "She [the mother] does not identify her child as a person with serious health problems. She does not understand the nature and extent of his high-risk problems plus his levels of pain and discomfort. She feels the baby is alright and she seems quite unrealistic about treatment outcomes. Because of car problems, she visits only once each week and usually for about one hour. She holds the baby briefly and combs his hair. The child's father has yet to visit the patient. She continually insists that everything medically possible should be done for her child."

The Case of Annie O.

This case ranged over three years, cost the taxpayers in excess of $310,000, and could be considered "a classic worst-case scenario" in allocation. The initial encounter with the patient occurred in the emergency room of Regional Memorial Hospital. A description of some of the medical and nonmedical facts that shaped the case and led to the ethical dilemma follows.

The patient was a 41-year-old white female who was hospitalized 41 times over a period of three years. The hospitalizations ranged from 4 to 21 days, and on several occasions the patient signed herself out of the hospital against medical advice. She was a wheelchair-bound paraplegic subsequent to a gunshot wound to the spine. Her former husband was tried and convicted of the assault and was in prison. The patient's only child was placed in a foster home because the court deemed the patient "an unfit mother."

The patient presented to the emergency room with the following problems and history:

- Fever >103°F;
- Insulin dependent diabetic;
- Chronic urinary track infection;
- Recurrent depression;
- Allergies to most antibiotics;
- Recurrent vaginal infection and pelvic rash;
- Intermittent alcohol and substance abuse;
- Multiple fractures due to osteoporosis (hollowing of bones);
- Poor nutrition and overweight (5'4" and 197 pounds); and
- Deep and pitting ulcers on both buttocks caused by poor hygiene/sanitation.

The social history was relevant. The patient lived in an abandoned garage owned by a local farmer. There was no electricity or running water, and the garage had a dirt floor. Water and electricity were supplied by way of a garden hose and extension cord from the farmer's house. There were no toilet facilities. The patient was well known to the local medical community for her consistent non-compliance. Over the years, many adjectives were used by health care providers and others to describe her behavior. These included: "rude," "hostile," "obstinate," "uncooperative," "cunning," "mean," and "blatantly self-destructive." One physician described Annie as "a bitch on wheels." Although Annie had many serious medical problems, her uncooperative attitude and risky lifestyle made her case extremely difficult to manage. On her most recent admission, she spiked a fever of >103°F, had a raging urinary tract infection, and one of her ulcers had become reinfected. This combination of medical problems, though serious, was fairly typical for this patient. However, a new problem surfaced on this visit to the hospital. Annie O. was also pregnant.

Free Baby Formula

The business–health care overlap was highlighted in the way three hospitals dealt with the issue of breast-feeding. At question was a curious phenomenon. Health professionals were virtually unanimous in the belief that breast milk was best for infants. Evidence was overwhelming that breast milk reduced a baby's susceptibility to illnesses, such as ear infections and stomach flu, and played a positive role in many other ways, such as mental and hormonal development.

Why, then, did so many mothers who gave birth in hospitals choose synthetic baby formula? The reasons were many and varied, including opposition to breast-feeding from family and friends, lack of good information, unsympathetic work settings, and trends of custom and fashion. However, in addition, many health professionals believed hospitals undermined breast-feeding by the widespread practice of giving new mothers free formula supplied by formula manufacturers. Research indicated the practice did make a difference. One study at Boston City Hospital, cited in the *Wall Street Journal*, found that 343 low-income women, who received free formula from the hospital, breast-fed their infants for a median duration of 42 days, compared with 60 days for those who received no free formula – a difference of 30 percent. The article concluded with the observation that breast-feeding rates were not much higher than they were ten years ago.

At a joint meeting of the IECs of the three local hospitals, this issue of conflict of interest between formula manufacturers who supplied the free formula and the three hospitals was raised. At the time, all three hospitals accepted free baby formula. One breast-feeding proponent candidly described her suspicion of the close ties between hospitals and formula companies hoping to promote their product. Discussion of the issue by IEC members at this joint meeting resulted in four main options for dealing with the issue: (1) accept no free formula at all despite its availability; (2) give no free formula to those who breast-feed; (3) charge patients a nominal fee for the free formula, so families considered the cost of formula when making the breast-feeding decision; and (4) continue to issue free formula but also distribute information about the benefits of breast-feeding. The four options were not prioritized.

At Mr. Blackwell's request, the IEC of Regional Memorial Hospital was to advise him on a morally justifiable course of action relative to the hospital's free baby formula practice.

Vendor Ethics

Hospitals were not self-sustaining, independent entities. They depended on the goods and services provided by others. These ranged from the rare to the commonplace and included such items as radioactive material, laboratory testing, security apparatus, laundry services, waste removal, and a vast array of drugs, medicines, and surgical instruments. A current label among health care managers to describe this operation was "outsourcing." All of these goods and services were outsourced by hospitals to vendors. Conflicts of interest involving vendors occurred when the self-interest of employees of the hospital led them to carry out their duties in ways that might not be in the best interest of the patients, health care providers, or the hospital itself.

A leading cause of conflict of interest between hospitals and vendors was the perk. Promotional perks were marketing incentives provided by vendors to influence the decisions of hospital purchasing agents. So overzealous were some of these marketing practices that the distinction between persuasion and bribery was often blurred.

Vendors offered a wide range of incentives. These included dinners and concerts, trips to resorts, tickets to sporting events, frequent flier miles, use of company planes, free drug samples, and other expensive inducements such as computers, fax machines, and cellular phones. Inexpensive gratuities such as pens, doughnuts, and tee-shirts were standard practice. Employees who defended the practice argued that because health care was an industry, it was unrealistic, if not foolish, to think standard business practices would not come into play. They rejected the argument that perks jeopardized their objectivity and independent judgment. They claimed further that if a conflict did arise, it was invariably transparent and easily managed, so as not to compromise the trust the employee held by virtue of his or her office.

Conversely, the practice of offering gratuities to employees who were responsible for vendor access and sales raised important ethical concerns for hospital administrators. They worried about the real or perceived conflict of interest between the employee working for the overall welfare of the institution and the distracting effect gifts from vendors had on such purchasing decisions. One caveat deserved mentioning. This was the mutual need to establish reliable and trustworthy relationships between hospitals and vendors. Hospitals needed to believe that goods ordered from vendors would be delivered on time, in the right way, to the appointed location, and at the agreed price; vendors needed to believe that unreasonable demands would not be made, invoices would be paid on time, and company representatives would not be abused, but treated in a professional and respectful manner.

The specific issue that Mr. Blackwell brought to the IEC was a rumor he heard and later confirmed. It involved a purchasing agent employed by the hospital. She was responsible for overseeing a fairly extensive landscaping project. The work cost over $100,000 and took a full year to complete. One part of the project involved the purchase and installation of 24 Japanese cherry trees. These were ornamental hybrids – *Prunus serrulata* – with a minimum height of 20 ft. The going price for the trees was reported by the agent to be $600 per tree.

On visiting the purchasing agent's home, Blackwell saw three 20-ft Japanese cherry trees in the front yard. Somewhat embarrassed by the surprise visit, the agent explained to her CEO that when the nursery learned the agent was relandscaping her property they provided the trees. "It was merely a gesture of goodwill. That's all," the agent explained. Asked if she felt the free trees influenced her choice of nursery for the hospital, she replied: "Absolutely not, I would have chosen Green Thumb Nursery even if they had not given me the trees. I decided objectively. Mr. Blackwell, I know my job and I am always impartial."

Mr. Blackwell's first thoughts were "precedent setting." He knew that his decisions regarding such matters would be the subject of much discussion by a variety of people and indeed set precedent. The purchasing agent had been an excellent employee. He referred this case to the IEC for a full, open hearing.

The Meeting

At Mr. Blackwell's request, the IEC of Regional Memorial Hospital was to meet to advise him on a morally justifiable course of action relative to the hospital's free baby formula practice and handling of the employee who received "free" trees as well as to offer advice on what to do about Baby Boy-X and Annie O. It would be a full agenda.

NOTES

1. W. H. Shaw, *Business Ethics* (Belmont, CA: Wadsworth Publishing Co., 1991), p. 258.
2. R. E. Cranford and A. E. Doudera, "The Emergence of Institutional Ethics Committees," *Proceeding of the American Society of Law and Medicine* (April 1983), p. 13.
3. M. Siegler, "Ethics Committees: Decision by Bureaucracy," *Hastings Center Report* 16 (June/July 1986), pp. 3, 22.

CASE **18**

The *Premier* Health Care Alliance Emerges

"Significant changes have been occurring for health care alliances," said Ben Latimer, president and CEO of SunHealth Alliance until November 1995. "Consolidation, integration, and growth and acquisitions by investor-owned health care organizations are all impacting alliances. Take for example, what happened in St. Louis. Barnes Hospital, Jewish Hospital, and Christian Health Services merged to form BJC Health System. Each one of them belonged to a different health care alliance – Barnes was associated with Voluntary Hospitals of America (VHA), Jewish was allied with Premier, and Christian was a member of American Healthcare Systems. After the merger, BJC extensively studied the three different alliances and chose one – VHA."

In 1995, there were over 700 hospitals involved with mergers or acquisitions and 1996 would probably have more, based on the number that occurred in the first half of the year. Latimer continued, "Although consolidation has occurred somewhat more slowly in the South, we are observing more and more of it. SunHealth had the largest market share in our 15-state area, but we had little room to grow. Consolidation meant that SunHealth was going to gain some partners and lose some others. It was a real challenge to grow in that kind of environment."

"In addition, investor-owned health care organizations were acquiring hospitals. Many of those that they purchased were for-profits, but increasingly they were not-for-profits in need of cash. The Columbia/HCAs and Tenets were ready to buy these hospitals and in some instances, after purchasing them, closed them.

This case was written by Linda E. Swayne, The University of North Carolina at Charlotte, and Peter M. Ginter, University of Alabama at Birmingham. It is intended as a basis for classroom discussion rather than to illustrate either effective or ineffective handling of an administrative situation. Used with permission from Linda Swayne.

"The investor-owned organizations tout their ability to buy at lower prices. They promote this idea to combat the profit-making image and to induce communities to sell the local hospital to them. Because they own the hospital, they can mandate compliance. They also require that all their units buy from a single source in order to obtain those lower prices.

"Integrated networks or health care systems have been formed in many areas of the country. This organizational alternative, if it is of sufficient size, was able to compete with SunHealth if we didn't continue to grow. We wanted to grow, but not at the cost of sacrificing quality.

"One way we could get larger was to require our partners to belong only to SunHealth Alliance and set a specific amount of purchasing that was required. But then we would have to decide if we would require partners to disassociate if they didn't meet these requirements and whether we would pay them a 'market value' for their shares and how we would determine that market value.

"Another way to grow would have been to acquire another regional alliance in New England or the West, but our partners' goal was to be a 'premier' alliance. They wanted to be part of a strong alliance with a great deal of market power as well as prestige. So we began thinking about becoming much larger and the way to do that was through a merger.

"We began talking with VHA in February 1995 about a possible merger. I signed a nondisclosure and confidentiality agreement but it was not limiting – meaning that I was not prohibited from talking with others. Consultants were hired to determine the interest and compatibility of the two organizations. The consultants and lawyers had been talking for nine months when Robert O'Leary of AmHS contacted me at the American Hospital Association annual meeting with a proposal that SunHealth merge with the very new AmHS/Premier. Those two alliances had merged in August. I owed it to the SunHealth partners to talk with O'Leary.

"We quickly realized that AmHS/Premier had a good geographic fit with SunHealth and there was a good fit with services. We had some overlap with VHA. In addition, there was a difference in the organization of SunHealth and VHA. VHA was organized by regions. SunHealth and AmHS/Premier had similar organizations.

"One month after the contact with O'Leary, our Board approved a merger of equals with AmHS/Premier. We think it was the right choice for us. SunHealth partners liked Rob O'Leary's vision and the 'fit' between the organizations. In the final analysis, the 'fit' was the most important variable."

History of SunHealth Alliance

In 1969, SunHealth was founded as Carolinas Hospital and Health Services, Inc. (CHHS), by the state hospital associations of North Carolina and South Carolina as a free-standing, not-for-profit, shared services corporation. The South Carolina Hospital Association (SCHA) had contacted the Duke Endowment, a major foundation, to determine whether it had any interest in helping SCHA set up something similar to a California program – the Commission for Administrative Services to Hospitals (CASH). In the mid-1960s, hospitals cooperated more than they competed, and CASH and other similar organizations were emerging to assist with planning and applying industrial and management engineering techniques to hospitals for increased efficiencies.

Although receptive, the Duke Endowment leadership was concerned that the 20 or so hospitals in South Carolina were too few to be able to develop such a program. In addition, they knew that a similar group was under way in North Carolina. The Duke Endowment proposed one organization with a board of directors comprising hospital CEOs from both states. The two Carolinas had many commonalities, including culture, social structure, and economy. The hospital communities were similar in philosophy and maintained close ties. In addition, the Duke Endowment was chartered to improve higher education and health care in both North Carolina and South Carolina and saw an opportunity to leverage its grants to benefit more hospitals in the two states.

The two state hospital association CEOs developed the plan and bylaws for the organization. Dr. John Canada, a professor at North Carolina State University, put together a proposal for introducing management engineering and management education for the hospitals. Canada took the responsibility for finding the first staff. According to Latimer, "He considered a number of folks, I understand, but he had some contact with Dr. Harold Smalley at Georgia Tech who suggested that I be considered. I met with the eight-member board and was fortunate to be selected by that group."

Ben Latimer Assumes Leadership of CHHS

Ben W. Latimer earned a BME degree from Georgia Tech University in 1962 and then worked for somewhat over a year at Procter & Gamble in the Department of Industrial Engineering as a management trainee. He returned to Georgia Tech and studied under Dr. Harold Smalley, one of the pioneers in applying industrial engineering and quantitative analysis techniques to health care. (The term *management engineering* was more acceptable to hospital administrators and physicians and thus was used in health care.) Just before he completed the master of science degree in industrial engineering, Latimer was recommended by Smalley for a position with Methodist Hospital in Memphis, Tennessee. There Latimer worked on improving staffing and scheduling, particularly in the area of nursing. He realized early on that management techniques would be interwoven with the newly developing computer technology and management information systems. Although satisfied with the progress he was making in introducing management engineering at Methodist Hospital, he was intrigued by the opportunity at CHHS.

"Though independent of direct hospital association control or ownership, CHHS did serve *in effect* as the associations' operational arm for some services developed or wanted by them for hospital members," wrote Ben Latimer and Pat Poston in a 1976 *Topics in Health Care Financing* article. As an example, they cited group purchasing that was researched and developed by the South Carolina Hospital Association but operationalized by CHHS. Latimer stated, "However, CHHS was never limited to implementing only those activities assigned it by the associations. In fact, CHHS operated as an expansion-minded company and would assess user needs and organize services to meet those needs.

"This organizational model was especially applicable to states in which size, density, and health care patterns precluded the existence of enough mid-sized hospitals to support shared services economically," commented Ben. "In addition, the separate but 'associated' corporation provided additional benefits – services could cross state lines, we had to be cost effective in order to survive, we had greater flexibility to recruit and pay employees differently than the associations, we could provide some services that associations were not able to provide, and members did not pay 'dues' but rather membership fees plus fees for the services that they selected. . . .

"The first service provided was management engineering known originally as the Carolinas Hospital Improvement Program or CHIP. It was designed to move hospital administration toward developing strategies for quality improvement and cost containment. It included such things as work and cleaning schedules and management education because most hospital administrators were educated in various health professions and had to learn management skills 'on the job.' For the CHIP program, all the development support came from the Duke Endowment. But as that was followed by other programs in the biomedical engineering and clinical engineering areas, the W. K. Kellogg Foundation supported our efforts as did the Kate B. Reynolds Health Care Trust.

"We used foundation support for development funds to establish new programs. However, each service we added was designed to be self-supporting. If the service was not good enough and the member hospitals weren't willing to pay for it, then it was not continued."

The Growing Alliance Expanded Beyond the Carolinas

When CHHS was originally developed, the support from the Duke Endowment and the composition of the governing board dictated that it was a service organization for the two Carolinas. "It never crossed our mind to serve anyone other than North and South Carolina," Latimer said. "In the mid-1970s, the question was first raised about offering services beyond our two states. The board decided that it would not harm the current partners and would allow for a larger staff that would have the opportunity to gain more from a broader representation of health organizations, and there would be broader forums for development and expansion.

"Up until the mid-1970s, CHHS served all sizes of hospitals in the Carolinas. Because of our location and the mix of hospitals in the area, most people probably thought we only served small and medium-sized hospitals. Some of the large hospitals – those with 400-plus beds – thought they had more in common with other large-sized hospitals across a broader region. So we formed the Sun

Alliance, which corresponded loosely with the geographic area of the Southeastern Hospital Conference. We [CHHS] provided services for Sun Alliance."

CHHS Becomes SunHealth Alliance

"Eventually we determined that having two separate organizations was not beneficial. On the advice of Dr. Howard Zuckerman, a consultant from the University of Michigan, we merged the two organizations into SunHealth Corporation in 1985," Latimer stated. The planning consultants laid out the concept of a regional health services network and encouraged the development of a network organization that in effect mirrored the composition of the hospital industry in the region – small community hospitals, large hospital systems, university hospitals, public hospitals, and so on. Given that the purpose of SunHealth was to provide health services to a large share of the population in the region, the consultants encouraged alignment of hospitals corresponding to actual patient flow patterns among facilities and physicians.

The board and management of SunHealth did not want the organization to be thought of as an "investment vehicle designed to return earnings," but rather as a service organization to help partners fulfill their missions. *Partner* was consciously selected to be used when referring to shareholder hospitals to constantly remind all involved parties that SunHealth was a shared alliance where partners worked together to share risk and improve health care.

Requirements for SunHealth Membership

SunHealth Alliance offered membership to hospitals that met the following criteria:

1. A candidate must be a tax-exempt organization engaged principally in the operation, directly or through an affiliated entity, of a not-for-profit hospital with total assets of $5 million or more.
2. It must not be contract managed by an entity other than one that is controlled by or under common control with the member.
3. It must have approval in accordance with board policies and procedures.

In terms of recruiting for new partners in the Alliance, priority was given to (1) hospital organizations in population areas not served by existing partners, (2) those readily able to hold equity interest, (3) those demonstrating interest in existing alliance activities, and (4) those having commitment to improve region-wide health care delivery.

A new partner was evaluated on the basis of the characteristics it conveyed in its management team, relationships with other providers (competing and cooperative), recommendations from existing members, and the candidate's objectives in seeking network membership. SunHealth used the term *multihospital system* to refer to partners who operated multiple hospital facilities in different service areas. The term *emerging integrated health care system* was used to refer to those partners that operated acute care hospitals but had related (diversified and nondiversified) hospital services.

Because of its regional orientation, the SunHealth Alliance (more so than other major alliances in the country) was composed of diverse segments of membership, including public, general, denominational, rural, community, not-for-profit, and regional referral hospitals, plus academic medical centers that served patients from throughout the world. Some of the implications of this diversity among members were reflected in the establishment of membership criteria and requirements. Although members shared some objectives in networking, their local strategies were typically diverse. Some members, constrained by law, organizational relationships, or philosophy, could not make certain types of institutional commitments. For example, public general hospitals and tax-district hospitals were subject to public bidding. Denominational, university, and foundation operated hospitals were subject to systems or organizational investment requirements for purchasing.

A partner's rights might be terminated if that shareholder failed to continue to meet the technical eligibility requirements, such as loss of its tax exemption, being no longer engaged in the operation of a not-for-profit hospital, being acquired or contract managed by a nonrelated organization, or failure to pay its approved assessment.

SunHealth's Goals and Benefits for Partners

SunHealth's overarching goal was supporting partners to achieve their goals. "I think that our support is one of the things that distinguishes SunHealth from other multihospital organizations and arrangements," said Latimer. "We are so committed to helping our partners reach their goals. We do that through a variety of means:

- collecting and sharing information and experience;
- creating new and better ways through research, development, and testing; and
- supporting the installation and implementation of new and better ways at alliance hospitals."

Services Provided for Partner Hospitals

The impact of the prospective payment system (implemented in 1983) on hospitals caused considerably more concern with improving efficiency. Because hospitals were reimbursed at a predetermined level for each diagnosis related group, those hospitals that could provide the service at a cost below the reimbursement rate had greater revenues over costs and thus greater flexibility. The hospital could choose to spend the money on expansion, development of new services, new technology, and so on. Therefore, CHHS served the hospital members by helping them to increase efficiency.

After CHIP, Carolinas Hospital Engineering Support Services (CHESS) was established to assess and provide feedback on the rapidly emerging new health care technologies. CHIP and CHESS were followed shortly by group purchasing developed in the mid-1970s to offset inflation, the money crunch, and cost-justification requirements. SunHealth did not actually purchase or warehouse items that partners needed. Rather it negotiated terms and conditions to ensure the quality of goods and services, plus sought value-added arrangements.

To provide the best in quality and price, SunHealth developed "corporate partnerships" in the mid-1980s with a small number of selected companies. SunHealth Alliance partners purchased approximately $2 billion annually, encouraging vendors to provide an array of value-added offerings as well as an excellent price. Purchasing included medical and surgical supplies, dietary products, pharmaceuticals, medical imaging products, capital equipment, and laboratory supplies. According to Latimer, "We go beyond trading volume for price. With our corporate partners we want to work closely together for our mutual benefit. Some of our corporate partners are Johnson & Johnson, Abbott Labs, DuPont, Juran, and General Medical."

Consulting and Other Services

SunHealth's consulting unit had been in operation for more than 20 years. A variety of consulting services allowed hospitals to increase their efficiency in both administrative and clinical areas. Consulting expertise included nursing management, financial management, cost management, decision support, quality management, telecommunications, materials management, facilities management, human resources management, productivity management, health care planning (both strategic and operational), managed care issues, information systems, and medical staff services.

"Each consulting service provided partners with new techniques or new services not previously employed to maximum benefit in typical hospitals in the region," Latimer said. As SunHealth was better able than individual hospitals to locate, recruit, and compensate scarce technical and professional personnel, these programs made staff expertise available economically on a shared basis.

Partner hospitals were able to obtain support services that assisted in the planning, development, operation, and management of integrated managed-care programs, including contract evaluation and negotiation. The SunHealth staff provided assistance to hospitals in strategic consulting and health care planning services designed to strengthen alliance members as market leaders and improve interactions among hospitals, physicians, patients, and payors.

SunHealth joined with a variety of outside organizations to assist in the planning, development, and management of more specialized areas such as malpractice, general liability and workers' compensation insurance services, mental health, addictive disease and rehabilitation service, financial management consulting, human resources consulting, executive and physician search, medical claims collection, housekeeping, dietary plan operations and laundry management, electronic claims processing, employee health benefits, and utilization review services.

"Our services offered to partners must be of sufficient value to be used by the hospitals without resorting to mandates or dues. In essence, we had to be self-sufficient, including generating some surplus so that we could develop new programs or improve existing programs that were of benefit for our partners."

Partners were charged for the consulting and clinical technology services they used in three different ways. One was the per diem rate, or a fixed amount per "expert day." Another was a per project charge: "We quote a charge to carry out the project and if the quote is off we have to absorb the loss, or if it comes in under the quote, it is to our advantage," Latimer explained. The third way was a continuing service arrangement. "We place a full-time industrial engineer in the hospital to manage a department. The hospital reimburses us for the compensation of the individual.

"We use incentives to encourage purchasing from SunHealth vendors," Latimer stated. "Financial incentives are offered in those situations that are likely to produce financial results. For example, volume purchasing achieves greater savings for the alliance; the savings are returned to partners through rebating of the service fees. Other services, such as consulting, are offered purely on a fee basis as volume usage does not generate discounts."

SunHealth in 1995

Approximately 650 employees at SunHealth provided services to its 151 partners. The partners provided nearly $25 billion worth of health services annually through 350 hospitals that accounted for over 72,000 licensed beds. Located primarily in 15 southeastern and south central states, hospital bed-size of partners varied as illustrated in Exhibit 18/1. SunHealth had clearly stated its mission and vision (see Exhibit 18/2).

SunHealth was extremely successful in serving its partners' needs and remaining financially strong, as evidenced by its key indicators and comparisons of its hospitals with other hospitals nationally and regionally (see Exhibit 18/3). Purchasing volume was $1.5 billion for fiscal year 1992 or $28,253 per adjusted occupied bed.[1] Purchasing incentives of $1.9 billion and $16.6 million in vendor dividends were credited to partner organizations in fiscal year 1992.

Exhibit 18/1: SunHealth's Partners by Bed Size

Number of Adjusted Occupied Beds	Percent of Partners
1–199	34.2
200–299	32.2
300–399	10.7
400–499	12.2
Over 500	10.7

Exhibit 18/2: SunHealth Mission and Vision

Vision
Together, we improve the health status of people in our communities.

Purpose and Mission
The SunHealth Alliance is a working partnership committed to improving the health status of people in our communities. The alliance exists to help partners and their allies succeed in carrying out this commitment by:

- Providing sustained leadership for the positive transformation of health services organization and delivery;
- Transferring knowledge and experience relating to health services delivery, and developing new methods and knowledge;
- Supporting the linkage of efforts and integration of services in networks, so as to serve communities better; and
- Providing cost-effective resources for the improvement of health status.

History of AmHS[2]

American Healthcare Systems (AmHS), located in San Diego, California, restricted its membership to hospital systems. AmHS was founded in 1984 by merging two previous alliances, Associated Health Systems headquartered in Phoenix, Arizona, representing 11 systems, and United Health Care Systems, located in Kansas City, Missouri, with 14 systems. By 1995, its board was comprised of 40 CEOs of the shareholder systems that owned, leased, or operated 397 hospitals and had affiliation agreements with 528 other hospitals. AmHS shareholders and affiliates were located in 46 states and the District of Columbia.

Since its founding in 1984, the organization had three different leaders. First was Charles Ewell who left in 1986 to become president of the Governance Institute in La Jolla, California. From 1986 to 1995, Monroe Trout, MD, was president, chief executive officer, and chairman. Robert O'Leary assumed the position in 1995.

In January 1987, AmHS adopted a strategic plan that called for eliminating programs that directly involved the alliance in health care delivery and expanded services that could best be offered on a national scale.[3] The plan had the following objectives:

- AmHS will develop profit-making ventures that offer high-quality products and services to AmHS shareholders and other health care providers. These ventures will complement rather than compete with AmHS shareholders.
- AmHS will broaden its shareholder base to achieve maximum geographic coverage. This will permit AmHS to take full advantage of economies of scale and mass purchasing, as well as to provide a wide base for distribution of its products.

- AmHS will remain financially self-sufficient by sustaining a variety of revenue sources.
- AmHS will strengthen its key core services, including marketing and the AmHS Institute's representational and educational endeavors.

AmHS developed a number of ventures to benefit shareholders. AmHS Insurance Management Services (IMS) was designed to improve AmHS shareholders' access to cost-effective liability insurance coverage. It created two insurance companies (AEP and ADRL) to share risk, exerting a measure of stability and control over the market in areas such as excess liability insurance. IMS group purchased insurance from major insurors at substantial discounts, often with profit-sharing provisions.

AmHS Capital Corporation was a financial services company that provided customized programs such as a taxable medium-term rate program (when tax-exempt financing was an issue), a consolidated credit card program to serve hospitals and nonacute care sites such as doctors' offices, and a capital asset protection program to better manage and control capital equipment servicing expenses.

The AmHS Business Group focused on initiating new programs. As an extension of the strategic partnering concept, AmHS Business Group attempted to add value for shareholders by reducing operating costs while maintaining or improving medical efficacy. It purchased equity positions in various manufacturers in exchange for achieving market-share objectives, assessed products and services of health care suppliers (such as those that provided high-technology equipment for potential investment by AmHS), and coordinated two venture capital funds in which AmHS was a special limited partner. By 1995, more than $45 million had been invested in emerging medical companies.

The AmHS Institute, located in Washington, DC, was the organization's public policy center. The Institute served three functions: advocacy, education, and communication. New initiatives were in the areas of managed care, physician integration, information systems, and alternative care purchasing for nonacute care facilities.

These ventures, and AmHS's corporate partnerships in the purchasing area, were structured to generate capital for the corporation and the systems. AmHS prided itself on its small, highly professional management staff. With a total roster of less than one hundred employees, fewer than any other similar-sized alliance, AmHS made the best possible use of shareholders' assets – maximizing benefits while minimizing overhead expenses. AmHS was able to maintain this staffing level by relying on the talents of its multihospital system shareholders.

In the summer of 1989, AmHS initiated a program to improve member compliance in some group purchasing programs.[4] The compliance improvement program encouraged members to participate at specified levels. Shareholders were rewarded for total compliance in the program with up to 10 percent of annual dividends. Shareholders falling below specified levels were penalized. The eventual goal was 100 percent compliance, which would result in higher returns on investments for members. In 1995, AmHS had accomplished better than

Exhibit 18/3: SunHealth Key Financial Indicators

Key Indicator	FY 1991	FY 1992	FY 1993	FY 1994
Current ratio	2.4	2.2	1.9	1.6
Total assets	$14.2 million	$16.2 million	$18.3 million	$20.8 million
Total shareholder equity	$8.8 million	$9.5 million	$9.8 million	$10.0 million
Book value per share	$123.98	$130.68	$131.00	$132.00
Enrollment of alliance	141	145	149	155

Comparisons of SunHealth Hospitals with Other Health Care Institutions

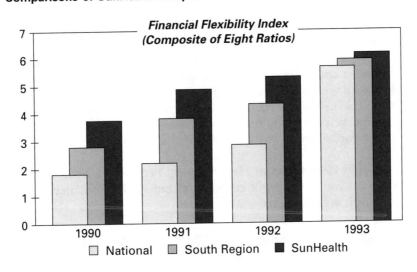

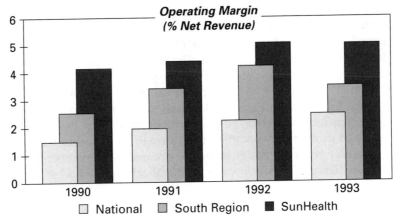

Source: HFMA Reports and Company Records.

90 percent compliance. If a purchasing group cannot guarantee commitment from its members, it had no bargaining leverage. It was not only the number but the commitment that vendors desired.

AmHS was a shareholder-driven national alliance of 40 distinguished multi-hospital systems working together to improve their competitive positions, realize the economic advantages of size, and create innovative solutions addressing common needs. Its statement of mission is included as Exhibit 18/4.

To be considered as a shareholder in AmHS, an applicant should:

- be a not-for-profit health care corporation;
- be a high-quality prestigious health care organization;
- have a mission consistent with that of AmHS;
- complement the operations of existing shareholders;
- have a sizable market share within its major markets;
- have a strong financial position and be large enough to participate fully;
- have a well-respected management team;
- be able to fulfill certain AmHS program commitments, such as a requirement to participate in the AmHS purchasing program; and
- not participate in any other national alliance.

In July 1995, Quorum Health Group became a corporate affiliate of AmHS. Quorum was a for-profit corporation but its 105 affiliated hospitals were not-for-profit organizations.

History of Premier Health Alliance[5]

Based in Westchester, Illinois, Premier Health Alliance began in 1983 as a consortium of 16 Jewish hospitals that agreed to develop a formal arrangement to handle common concerns. Originally the organization limited its membership to community teaching hospitals. The leadership did not plan for growth because of its focus on community teaching hospitals.

Alan Weinstein became the first president. Two years later the organization changed its name to Premier Hospitals Alliance to reflect the admission of non-Jewish members. It changed names again in 1993 to Premier Health Alliance as many of its members became health care systems rather than single hospitals.

Premier offered a wider range of services to its members than other broader-based alliances. This was because its member hospitals had similar needs and wants

Exhibit 18/4: AmHS Mission

AmHS mission is to ensure the availability of high-quality health care services to patients at a reasonable and affordable cost. AmHS supports this mission by linking outstanding multihospital systems that share this goal and recognize the benefit of leveraging their resources through collaboration. It is through the strengthening of its shareholders that the success of AmHS can be measured.

Exhibit 18/5: Premier Health Alliance Mission

Premier Health Alliance is a national alliance owned by preeminent hospitals, systems, and provider networks that are responsible for improving the health of the people who live in their communities. Premier provides hospitals, systems, and provider networks strategic advantages to improve health – through collaborating with other organizations, sharing meaningful information, pursuing economies of scale, and preserving community resources. Premier provides member hospitals, systems and provider networks the strategies and services they need to sustain a leadership role in healthcare excellence, community service, education, and research.

and the group was small enough so that the staff maintained personal contact with each hospital. Premier services fell into three areas: services that saved hospitals money directly, such as group purchasing and investment programs; services that enhanced the member's market share, such as home care, imaging, and physician bonding; and information sharing services.[6] Premier had 70 programs that were evaluated continuously. A program that did not meet its expectations was marked and studied to see if it should be dropped. Between 7 and 12 programs were dropped in a year, but at least that many were added. Premier was expanding its managed care consulting and management services for its members.[7]

In 1995, 55 hospitals and health systems owned Premier, representing 280 hospitals. Together the hospitals accounted for nearly $2 billion in purchasing. Premier developed a committed buying program that was designed to reward the hospitals that bought more of their products and services from vendors that Premier had under contract. Hospitals that agreed to buy 80 percent of applicable products under five national contracts earned 12 percent lower prices, on average, than other Premier contracts.

According to Weinstein, president of Premier Health Alliance, "Our commitment to being a member-driven organization is the cornerstone to our success. No alliance offers more to its members in program depth and breadth, quality, or service. We have high expectations of those we work with and serve. Premier boasts a proud heritage that will carry us well into the future, side by side with our membership." Premier's mission statement is included as Exhibit 18/5.

Premier's operating philosophy incorporated the following:

- Premier provides programs and services that support members as they pursue cost savings, management efficiencies, medical excellence, and the integration of health services in their communities.
- Premier delivers meaningful, strategic solutions to the management, clinical, and operating issues facing members during an era of unprecedented health reform.
- Premier programs are tailored to serve members in their individual environments and foster collaboration with other local health organizations. Programs must provide immediate financial value, long-term strategic value, or both.
- Premier is governed by its owners, yet is responsive to the needs of its member organizations.

- While voluntary in nature, Premier strives to build compliance in and, thereby, increase the success of its programs.
- Premier members' staffs participate in Premier projects at every step, lending their expertise and ensuring relevance and appropriateness. Premier's own employees are an equally valuable asset, and the alliance is committed to their ongoing training, development, and recognition.
- All Premier relationships – with owners, members, business partners, and employees – are characterized by personal service, mutual respect, integrity, and the highest ethical standards.

AmHS and Premier Merge

In July 1995, AmHS and Premier agreed to merge. In August, the organization formally became AmHS/Premier – the largest hospital alliance representing over one-quarter of all community hospitals in the United States and $8 billion in purchasing. Robert O'Leary, CEO of AmHS, became CEO of the new organization, and Alan Weinstein, president of Premier, became president and chief operating officer. AmHS brought shareholders experience in systems and competing in managed care environments. Premier had developed expertise in technology assessment, information systems, and quality measurement.

AmHS/Premier had 95 shareholders operating 400 facilities representing 1,400 hospitals with 240,000 licensed beds in 49 states. They operated in most major metropolitan areas providing the potential for the development of regional networks. The new company was less well represented in the Southeast and the Rocky Mountain areas. It represented $45 billion in revenues making it three times larger than Columbia/HCA and 30 percent larger than the next largest alliance, VHA.

A 13-member board was to govern the organization – 4 members from AmHS, 4 from Premier, 3 outside members, and O'Leary and Weinstein. Joint committees were expected to draft new policies for the merged organization; a high level of compliance was a priority. AmHS required that 90 percent of eligible goods be bought under its corporate contracts, and Premier guaranteed 80 percent compliance under selected contracts.

AmHS/Premier and SunHealth Agree to Merge

Four months later in November 1995, the recently merged AmHS/Premier formally merged with SunHealth. The new alliance had 240 shareholders with 650 facilities and 1,700 hospitals in 50 states. It represented over 30 percent of the community hospitals in the United States and was five times larger than Columbia/HCA in terms of members and purchasing volume. Annual purchases would be $10 billion, making it a formidable customer and competitor. SunHealth provided geographic coverage in the Southeast, added buying clout, and enhanced services including technology assessment, benchmarking, and physician integration. Exhibit 18/6 provides a map of the location of the new organization's hospitals.

Exhibit 18/6: Geographic Location of AmHS/Premier/SunHealth Hospitals

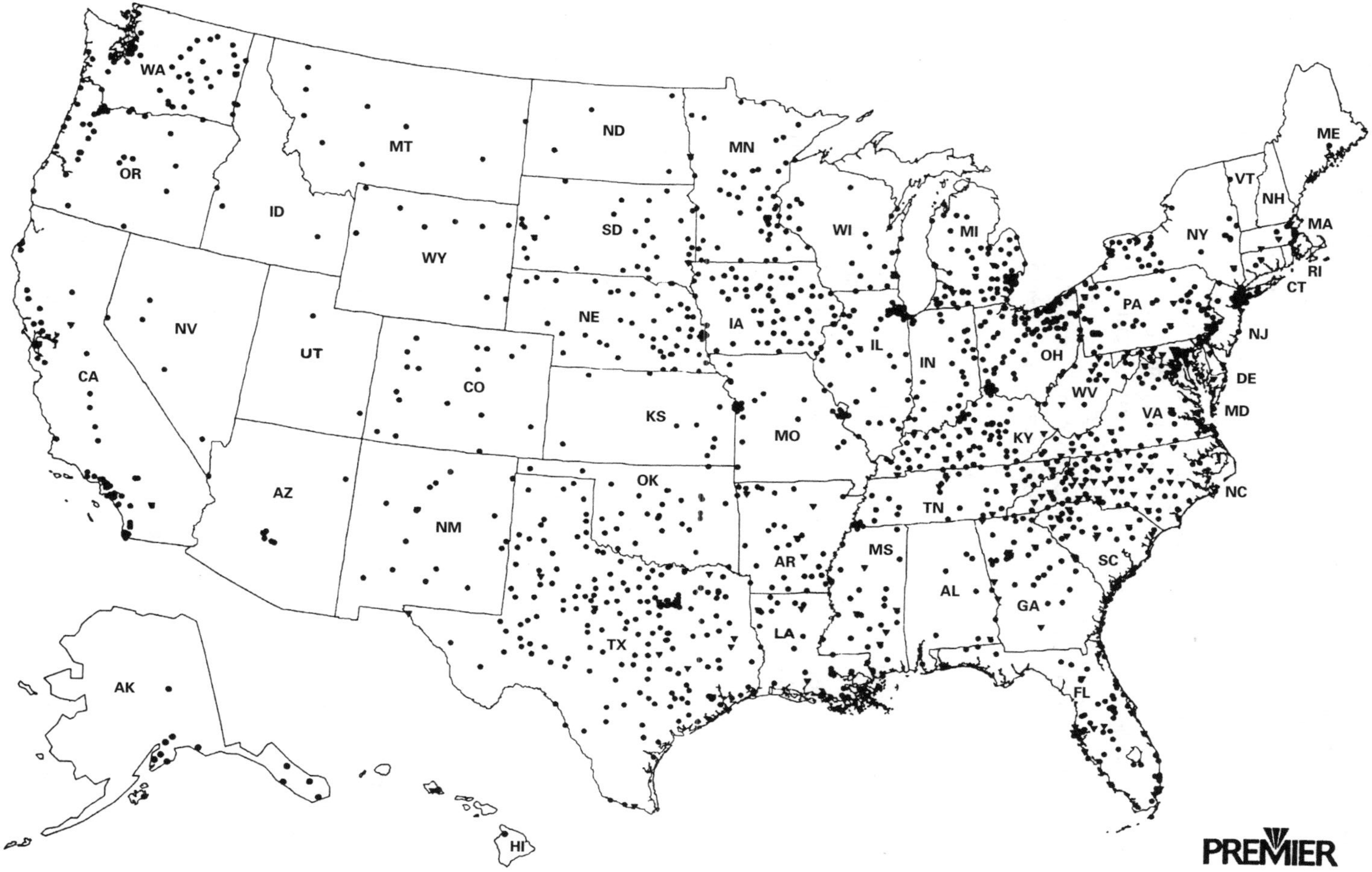

PREMIER

"There was a time in the mid-1980s that we actually became a shareholder in AmHS." Latimer explained, "VHA and Aetna were having conversations about joining together to create a national HMO brand name. AmHS wanted to counter-balance that strong association with one of its own. AmHS offered SunHealth Alliance, Yankee Alliance, Adventists System, and several others an opportunity to develop a national brand name approach to the market through Provident Insurance Company. They only required that SunHealth buy one share of AmHS stock to be a part of the enterprise. We purchased a share as it seemed to be a low-risk opportunity. However, we decided fairly quickly it was not for us. Subsequently, AmHS decided that members of its alliance should be required to do all their purchasing through AmHS and the deal with Provident fell through. We withdrew, as did the Adventists who decided to join with us."

Characteristics of the Three New Partners

Each of the new partners had similarities and differences. Exhibit 18/7 sum-marizes the general characteristics of the organizations before the mergers.

The new leadership team became Robert O'Leary as chairman of the board and chief executive officer, Ben Latimer as vice chairman of the board, and Alan

Exhibit 18/7: Comparison of AmHS, Premier, and SunHealth

	AmHS	PHA	SunHealth
Founded	*1984*	*1983*	*1969*
Leadership	1984–1986, Charles Ewell 1986–1995, M. Trout, MD 1995– , Robert O'Leary	1983– , Alan Weinstein	1969– , Ben Latimer
Stakeholder Terminology	Shareholder	Owner	Partner
Geographic Strength	Northeast, Midwest, Northwest	Major metropolitan markets	Southeast
Number of Stakeholders	40 Shareholders	55 Owners	152 Partners
Number of Owner and Affiliate Hospital Units	925	280	355
Orientation Toward Fee-for-Service	Low	Medium	High
Number of Employees	100	130	650
Purchasing Compliance	100% required, but dual source	Moving toward 80% required	Sole source with incentives
Corporate Structure	Parent corporation and LLP	Cooperative corporation C(6)	Cooperative corporation C(6)
Revenues of Stakeholders	$36 billion	n/a	$24.8 billion
Collected Revenues of Division	$78.6 million	$28 million	$61.5 million

Weinstein as president and chief operating officer. The first board of directors meeting was held in February 1996. Each of the organizations provided five members to the board that also included O'Leary, Latimer, and Weinstein for a total of eighteen members. The organization used AmHS/Premier/SunHealth until March 1996 when the name Premier and the corporate logo were adopted.

Competition

Alliances were created to offer independent members the same buying clout and economies of scale enjoyed by national investor-owned systems plus the opportunity to contract with employers as part of a national health care delivery network.[8] For a variety of reasons many independent hospitals belonged to more than one alliance or purchasing group. Nationally hospitals belonged to an average of 2.8 purchasing groups, although in New York and Pennsylvania, they averaged belonging to four buying organizations.[9]

Industry Competitors

Within the industry there were over 200 purchasing groups. The undercutting of prices led some industry analysts to comment that group purchasing was turning into a commodity industry.[10] However, a purchasing group differed from an alliance in that there was usually no financial or leadership commitment to the purchasing group. An alliance expected member organizations to participate in its governance, sharing of information, and assisting other members as well as paying membership fees.

Many hospital systems and networks were large enough to obtain their own volume buying discounts. Some questioned whether there was still a need for alliances.

There were five major alliances in the United States: AmHS, Premier, SunHealth, University Hospital Consortium (UHC), and VHA. After the merger, Premier became the largest, followed by VHA. UHC was the smallest. Exhibit 18/8 provides a comparison of Premier with its two major competitors.

University HealthSystem Consortium

University HealthSystem Consortium, located in Oakbrook, Illinois, was started as University Hospital Consortium in 1980 by several CEOs of university hospitals. UHC targeted a specific group of hospitals, those owned by universities and whose staffs were controlled by medical schools. It began a group purchasing program in 1984 to provide university institutions with increased clout in purchasing pharmaceuticals, insurance, supplies, and services. In 1993 UHC surpassed $1 billion in group purchases on behalf of its members. Sixty-five university hospitals in the United States were members of UHC.[11] According to Samuel Schultz II, PhD,

Exhibit 18/8: Competitive Organizational Comparison

	Premier	Columbia/HCA	VHA
Total number of acute care hospitals	1,757	307	1,136
Total membership	1,757	363	1,332
Shareholders	131	n/a	97
States	50	36	47
Beds	276,000	61,400	253,000
Admissions	9.3 million	1.9 million	7.8 million
Surgical operations	6.8 million	0.6 million	5.7 million
Emergency visits	26.8 million	0.5 million	21.8 million
Percentage of community hospital beds	30.5%	6.8%	28.0%
Estimated purchasing volume 1996	$6–10 billion	$2.5 billion	$7 billion

Source: "The New Premier: One Year After the Merger," *IN VIVO The Business and Medicine Report* (July/August 1996), p. 25.

vice president for information services at UHC, the organization had grown so much because its member hospitals were "in dire straits."[12] General university funding was severely restricted across the United States during this period of a weakened economy. University hospitals, as part of the university, were affected as well.

University hospitals tended to see their mission in terms of being on the cutting edge of health care as they saw patients, gathered data, and performed research. Thus, they had specific needs for the very newest technology and in fact were often involved with developing that technology. Many academic health centers faced the dilemma of being the site not only where new drugs and technologies were first used but also where the cost ramifications first emerged. Therefore UHC was very involved in cost and reimbursement assessments. UHC did not offer consulting services for investments in technology or services designed to acquire patients. Services included group purchasing, materials management, a national traveling nurse placement service, a nurse recruiting service, risk-management insurance services, advice on winning contracts for clinical research with pharmaceutical companies, managed care planning, and information-sharing services.[13]

Strategic goals recently formulated for UHC included an aggressive quality agenda, with a dozen programs in management reengineering and quality of care plus development of tools for members to perform market assessments.[14] A major growth area was development of information services for clinical and technology assessment. UHC served as a clearinghouse for information on new technology and was setting up information-sharing systems that would assist member hospitals in clinical research by sharing outcomes information. UHC was developing a clinical information network – a vehicle for collecting members' clinical, financial, and administrative data to investigate quality of care and resource management issues.[15] The ability to share data among academic centers, whose information system architecture varied from archaic paper systems to PC LANs to minis to mainframes to client-server setups, was a challenging task but one that was being tackled at UHC.

Voluntary Hospitals of America

Voluntary Hospitals of America, located in Irving, Texas, was the nation's largest hospital alliance in number of beds prior to the Premier merger. It was founded by 30 hospitals in 1977 and grew to include 97 shareholders and more than 1,300 members at the end of 1995.[16] In 1989, VHA Enterprises divested a variety of business activities that were considered strategically less valuable: VHA Physician Services that offered physician bonding products; VHA Capital; VHA Consulting Services, sold to Arthur Andersen and Co., Chicago; VHA Long-Term Care and VHA Physician Placement Services to their respective managements; and VHA Diagnostic Services to a group of outside investors.[17]

At that time, VHA renewed its emphasis on managed care. "We're probably the only alliance that is appropriately in the managed-care business on a national level, because we have the broadest national presence," according to Bruce Brennen, VHA's vice president for communication.[18] VHA retained a 50 percent stake in Partners National Health Plans, a joint venture with Aetna Life Insurance Company of Hartford, Connecticut. With substantially over 2 million members enrolled in 33 states, Partners was the third-largest managed-care program in the United States (Kaiser Permanente was the largest). Brennen said that VHA was keeping its managed-care operations because it helped hospitals in local markets and would be strategically important in the future. About 90 percent of VHA members were involved with Partners, which operated a number of PPOs and HMOs.[19] However, by the end of 1993, VHA sold its 50 percent share to Aetna.[20]

New initiatives for VHA included an in-house educational program on implementing best practices, a separate satellite network program for educating top executives, a program to help its members choose and implement information technologies, and a joint program with the Catholic Health Association to market a software program that measured the benefits that hospitals provided for their communities.

VHA was not pleased with SunHealth's decision to merge with Premier. It released a statement that read, "Over the past year, VHA initiated a relationship with SunHealth by participating in task forces and jointly developing a community-ownership advocacy initiative. These joint activities led to further discussions of how a merger might bring value to our members. VHA did not view a potential merger as crucial to its long-term success and acknowledged that several local market conflicts presented potential roadblocks. Despite these challenges, our conversations with SunHealth focused on the potential benefits of bringing our organizations together. During our discussions, SunHealth, without prior notification, began exclusive negotiations with AmHS/Premier that resulted in their recent decision to merge."

The Future of Alliances

Not all hospital CEOs are satisfied with alliances. The primary disadvantage reported is that programs did not meet the needs of individual hospitals.[21] The larger the alliance, which was good for purchasing volume, the more challenging it became to tailor services that met the needs of individual partners.

For alliances to survive, they had to think strategically for their members, be financially sound, and provide the desired services. Specific factors that appeared to be important for alliances to survive included:

- the ability to drive compliance;
- the ability to provide successful, comprehensive services beyond purchasing;
- the willingness to take risks and be creative in finding solutions for their members;
- homogeneity in alliance members;
- the ability to provide value added services to both members and vendors;
- the ability to focus on the "top-down sell" (meaning hospital CEO involvement); and
- ability to implement at the local level.[22]

Because of the complexity of current agreements, it was becoming increasingly difficult for hospitals to determine the real value of individual contracts. Hospitals more often were finding that their best strategy was to make a commitment to the group that they believed could best meet their needs on an overall basis – price was not the only criterion. Hospitals might not be able to assess the actual value of group purchasing contracts because they had to weigh the value of available services such as inventory management, electronic data interchange, in-service programs, and remote order entry.

Manufacturers' attitudes toward groups were changing, as well.[23] Vendors were becoming more selective in their dealings. They were targeting groups that could best deliver compliance and market share. This selectivity prompted some manufacturers to refuse to sign contracts with certain groups if they could not deliver the business in return for price concessions. As a result, some groups might have closed. This made it even more important for hospitals to develop an understanding of which groups could best serve their needs. The consequence of not understanding a group's direction was that a hospital paid higher prices for the products and services it purchased, which could mean clinical and competitive obsolescence.[24]

Sandwiched between trade associations and multihospital systems, facing aggressive competition from the proliferation of shared service and group purchasing, not-for-profit alliances were searching for unique identities and strategies that provided a sustainable competitive advantage for their members. The diversity of needs and interests among members of an alliance made consensus building, setting priorities, and strategic planning efforts very difficult. The alliances that survived would be those that achieved value for member organizations.

Gerald McManis believed that successful alliances would:

- develop and communicate a concise vision for the future and clearly state long-term strategy and objectives;

- establish a member network that shared the vision and had a good structural fit with the alliance's strategy;
- implement programs and services that capitalized on the unique competence of the organization and its membership;
- operate a lean, professionally managed organization, concentrating on adding real value for members, not simply its own growth and self-perpetuation; and
- build long-term relationships with members based on trust, commitment, and value.[25]

Network growth might eliminate the need for purchasing alliances. Some networks grew large enough to buy on their own or at least became a different type customer. Alliances might need to add alternative-site members to grow – clinics, long-term care facilities, and so on. Among purchasing groups, alternative-site members increased 27.5 percent, but hospital membership only grew 1.2 percent.[26]

Looking Toward the Future of the Premier Alliance

At the first major meeting of the newly merged organization, Rob O'Leary "vowed the giant group would produce the best prices and the most innovative programs. Our role and our responsibility now is to help reshape the American delivery system."[27] He predicted that Premier would launch a physician equity company – Premier Practice Management – that would go public, a similar company that would be an alternative to selling to a for-profit chain, and use the organization's tremendous leverage to reduce prices to member organizations. In addition, Premier offered a full complement of services for its shareholders and affiliates (see Exhibit 18/9).

The first renegotiated contracts were signed in June 1996. DuPont offered a 30 percent lower price to be the sole supplier of film. Glaxo Wellcome agreed to use the same pricing for acute care drugs and outpatient care drugs, something the pharmaceutical industry had been resisting. This was an important breakthrough for those organizations that managed care.

In October 1996, Premier announced agreements with Alliant Foodservice, Inc., and Cerner Corporation. Alliant won the sole-source contract valued at approximately $1 billion. Premier agreed to exclusively endorse Cerner as the preferred supplier of clinical data repository systems. Cerner provided Premier members a package named "Premier Foundations," an open clinical data foundation that supported a desktop management information system for clinicians as well as support applications. The use of this architecture by over 30 percent of US hospitals had far-reaching implications.

Things were happening rapidly within Premier, but the melding of the organizations would take some time. As a first step in integrating the three different organizations, each one appointed committee members to tackle important issues in merging the organizations. One of the first outcomes was a statement

Cost Reduction Tools
Purchasing program
- Supplies group purchasing for medical/surgical, laboratory, operating room, food service, cardiology, and support services
- Materials management consulting
- Support services including contract management consulting and operations improvement consulting
- Pharmacy group purchasing
- Pharmacy benefit management services
- Pharmaceutical biotechnology information program
- Drug Intelligence Center
- Regional clinical pharmacy coordinators

Clinical and operational design
- Benchmarking (clinical and operational)
- Process design and reengineering consulting
- Clinical operations consulting
- Premier CareLinks (clinical resource management)
- On-site management engineering and consulting (community-based performance services)
- Emergency room design using simulation software
- Care management/clinical pathways programs
- Collaborative groups consulting

Insurance management services
Risk bearing
- Excess liability
- Directors and officers liability
- Excess workers' compensation
Group sponsored
- Property
- Managed care liability
- Employee medical benefit stop loss
- Long-term disability
- Group life and accidental death and dismemberment insurance
- Payroll deduction universal life insurance
- Group self-insured workers' compensation
- Universal life insurance program

Financial resources
- Business office management services
- Consulting and analysis for ambulatory patient groupings classification
- GE medical tax-exempt financing

System Development and Integration Strategies
Strategic planning, managed-care, and operations services
- Strategy and business planning
- Managed care consulting
- Integrated delivery system development
- Government contracting
- Managed care organization development
- Implementation management
- Medical management
- Physician practice management
- *Integrated HealthCare Report*

Technology Management Resources
Clinical equipment management
- Biomedical equipment repair
- Imaging equipment repair
- Technology assessment
- Technology life cycle management
- Buying, selling, upgrading, de-installation, and disposal of preowned equipment
- Network Technologies biomedical and imaging equipment accessories and parts dealership
- Clinical engineering department support and management
- Capital Asset Protection Program for lower capital equipment maintenance costs
- Capital equipment purchase negotiations and group buys

Clinical research

Facilities management
- Facilities consulting
- Cable Healthcare
- Energy monitoring and conservation

Information technology resources and management
- Support materials – A health information network white paper, readiness assessment tool kit, planning and deployment methodology, and a managed-care information technology white paper
- An alliance information technology directory and vendor catalog
- Information system strategic planning
- Information technology network consulting
- Vendor selection and contract negotiation assistance
- Information technology system integration and implementation
- Operations redesign following systems implementation
- Telecommunications consulting

Exhibit 18/9: (cont'd)

Networking and Knowledge Transfer Opportunities

Advocacy
- Grassroots program initiation
- Policy development
- Advocacy publications

Education and experience sharing
- Continuing medical education
- Customized workshops, seminars, and retreats
- Managed care and IDS education
- Nurse leadership courses
- Physician education
- Physician practice manager training
- Technology Futures Panel conference
- Research and library services
- Peer group networking meetings

Human resources management
- Custom local and regional wage and salary surveys
- Human resources reference desk
- Annual wage and salary surveys
- Physician incentive program design

Legal, regulatory, and JCAHO compliance
- JCAHO/NCQA accreditation preparation services are available and JCAHO decision grid score reports are prepared and compared with those of other organizations, mock surveys and staff training also can be arranged
- Employment, labor law, and other specialized services can be accessed through discounted arrangements negotiated by Premier staff

Market and customer research
- A comprehensive, modular health assessment involving quantitative and qualitative evaluation of health needs, risks, behaviors, and existing community resources
- Research services focusing on customer perceptions including community psychographics, focus group facilitation, moderator training, and patient, physician, and employer survey tools

Measuring and comparing performance
- Comparing clinical and financial data with that of other health care facilities
- Critical care decision support (APACHE)
- Decision support and cost accounting system assistance
- A functional assessment tool to measure a patient's physical and mental well-being
- A quality indicator comparative database
- A service quality satisfaction survey

Organizational effectiveness
- Organizational effectiveness training
- Change management consultation
- Self-managed team development
- Organizational diagnosis
- Mission, vision, and values development
- Executive team building
- Health care organizational performance self-assessment
- Strategic visioning conferences

of values developed by the employees of the new Premier and adopted by the board in April 1996 (see Exhibit 18/10).

Each of the former CEOs knew that merging the three separate organizations to accomplish the synergy they wanted was going to be a real challenge. Using Jim Collins and Jerry Porras's "core ideology" and "envisioned future" framework, Premier was developing a draft of its foundation statements.[28] The organizational leadership had a draft of core values, core purpose, and core roles (see Exhibit 18/11). Using these as a point of departure, they were working on refining and gaining consensus on the core ideology and the development of Premier's "envisioned future."

"For us to focus on survival of the acute-care hospital is wrong," Ben Latimer emphatically stated. "Success will be increasing the health status of our partners' communities without acute care. It is our task to help our partners achieve this paradigm shift and deliver care – wellness promotion as well as illness care – in new ways that lead to improved health status."

Exhibit 18/10: Premier Values Statement

Premier consists of leading systems and networks of healthcare organizations that have created this enterprise to further their responsibility for improving the health of communities. *Premier exists to bring value to its owners and affiliates.* We provide value through quantifiable economic advantage and meaningful strategic solutions to the management and clinical issues facing our constituency. Premier's strength comes from its ability to provide leveraged solutions while recognizing the need for market flexibility.

Values

We believe our success is dependent on creating partnerships that bring value. We think of every encounter as an opportunity for a partner relationship. This includes encounters with our owners, affiliates, business partners, and employees. We are a responsible and accountable organization within the healthcare industry and the larger society. We work together to achieve our mission through the following core values:

We act ethically
- We are honest and fair
- We treat individuals with equality and respect
- We are accountable, both individually and corporately, for our actions
- We use our influence responsibly
- We actively embrace our fiduciary responsibility

We deliver exemplary and customized service
- We ask and listen to our partners
- We provide meaningful and timely products and services to meet our partners' needs
- We work as a team to provide coordinated services
- We openly communicate meaningful and timely information
- We empower employees to make decisions

We enhance value
- We optimize revenue growth and owner return on investment
- We deliver cost-effective performance improvement in our operations and our business solutions
- We are committed to maximizing profitability
- We develop strategic solutions through knowledge transfer

We lead and embrace change
- We are visionary, yet respectful of our heritage
- We deliver innovative solutions
- We reward creative thinking and responsible risk taking
- We actively challenge our assumptions and the way we conduct business
- We work beyond traditional norms and practices
- We commit to personal and organizational development, recognizing individual accountability for our own growth
- We commit to transforming the industry to benefit the broader society

We Commit to be The Best
- We attract and retain the best partners
- We deliver the best products and services
- We create the best work environment and support the balance between work and personal life
- We continually raise our standards as we try for new levels of excellence
- We invest in developing leadership expertise throughout the organization

We celebrate our accomplishments and have fun in what we do while serving our communities and patients.

April 4, 1996

Exhibit 18/11: Premier Core Ideology (Draft)

Foundation Statements

Core Ideology

Core Values
- Integrity that shines in the individual and the enterprise
- Enduring respect for others' worth and for the principles that uphold our communities
- A passion for performance and a bias for action: creating real value, engaging change, leading the pace

Core Purpose
- To improve the health of communities

Core Roles of the Enterprise
- Producing cost savings and quality improvements
- Providing alternative revenue sources
- Providing strategic vehicles
- Facilitating the rapid transfer of knowledge and experience

NOTES

1. Adjusted occupied bed (AOB) is computed by multiplying total annual patient care revenues by the average 12-month census and dividing by total annual inpatient revenues: AOB = total annual patient care revenues × average 12-month census ÷ total annual inpatient revenues.
2. Much of the information for this section was taken from *Building Value for Our Systems,* an American Healthcare Systems brochure.
3. Howard Larkin, "Alliances: Changing Focus for Changing Times," *Hospitals* 63 (December 20, 1989), pp. 34–35.
4. Howard Larkin, "Alliances Argue Merits of Compliance Incentives," *Hospitals* 63 (December 20, 1989), p. 37.
5. Much of the information for this section was taken from a Premier Health Alliance brochure.
6. Larkin, "Alliances: Changing Focus for Changing Times," pp. 34–35.
7. "Collaborative Efforts Enhance Program Development," *Health Care Strategic Management* 11, no. 2 (February 1993), p. 23.
8. Gerald L. McManis, "Not-for-Profit Alliances Need to Focus on Value," *Modern Healthcare* (October 15, 1989), p. 20; and Larkin, "Alliances: Changing Focus for Changing Times," pp. 34–38.
9. Lisa Scott, "Group Purchasing Evolution," *Modern Healthcare* (September 27, 1993), p. 52.
10. Jim Montague, "Can Purchasing Alliances Adapt?" *Hospitals and Health Networks* 69, no. 16 (August 20, 1995), pp. 30–34.
11. Membership information was provided by University Hospital Consortium corporate offices in a telephone interview.
12. Carolyn Dunbar, "A New Era Dawns for the University Hospital Consortium," *Computers in Healthcare* 13, no. 13 (December 1992), p. 32.
13. Ibid., p. 34.
14. Ibid.
15. Ibid.
16. Current membership information was supplied by VHA corporate offices in a telephone interview.
17. Larkin, "Alliances: Changing Focus for Changing Times," p. 35.
18. Ibid.
19. Ibid.
20. Information supplied in a telephone interview.
21. Larkin, "Alliances: Changing Focus for Changing Times," p. 35.
22. John A. Henderson, "Hospitals Should Reassess Group Purchasing," *Modern Healthcare* (March 10, 1989), p. 80.
23. Ibid.
24. Ibid.
25. McManis, "Not-for-Profit Alliances," p. 20.
26. Scott, "Group Purchasing Evolution," p. 58.
27. Lisa Scott, "Giant Alliance Shares New Name, Bold Plans with Hospital Members," *Modern Healthcare* (March 18, 1996), p. 5.
28. For a complete discussion see James C. Collins and Jerry I. Porras, "Building Your Company's Vision," *Harvard Business Review* 88, no. 5 (September/October 1996), pp. 65–77.

19 *CASE*

The Case for Open Heart Surgery at Cabarrus Memorial Hospital

Situation

It was a clear, crisp October morning in Concord, North Carolina. The board of trustees of Cabarrus Memorial Hospital gathered in the windowless, walnut paneled boardroom for its monthly meeting (see Exhibit 19/1 for board members). Board chairman George Batte opened the meeting saying, "Because we do not have an open heart surgery program, patients needing open heart surgery or coronary angioplasty have to be transferred to another hospital, causing inconvenience to the patient's families and risks from delayed treatment. There are several questions we have to answer in addressing this issue. Should we add open heart surgery to the mix of cardiac services we offer? Does the hospital's existing service area provide adequate patient volumes to support the program? What role should the Duke University Medical Center play in the proposed program? Will we be able to obtain the required certificate of need [CON] from the State of North Carolina's Department of Health and Human Services? Will there be opposition to the CON from surrounding hospitals?

This case was written by Fred H. Campbell, The University of North Carolina at Charlotte, and Darise D. Caldwell, Executive Vice President and Chief Operating Officer, Northeast Medical Center. It is intended as a basis for classroom discussion rather than to illustrate either effective or ineffective handling of an administrative situation. Used with permission from Fred Campbell.

What costs are likely to be incurred in the required renovation, construction, medical equipment, and staffing?"

He continued, "As you all know, one of the factors pressing a quick decision is the desire of Dr. R. S. "Chris" Christy to return to the staff of the hospital after completing his fellowship in cardiovascular surgery. He is being heavily recruited by other medical centers."

Mr. Batte then asked Bob Wall, president of Cabarrus Memorial Hospital (CMH), to address the board on the issue. Mr. Wall said, "As we all know, our cardiac catheterization service is run by a Duke Medical Center physician. Our intent has been for the surgical portion of the heart program to be provided by Duke. Dr. Christy is completing a heart surgery residency through the Sanger Clinic and wants to return to Concord to practice. Needless to say, we face a dilemma and there are very different points of view in our medical staff as to the structure and relationship involved in developing a full-fledged heart program at CMH. I bring this to your attention now because Dr. Christy has to make a career choice before January 1st."

Trustee Batte reminded everyone, "Dr. Christy grew up in our community and worked part-time in the hospital while in high school and college. After medical school and a residency in general surgery, he practiced here at CMH prior to leaving to complete his fellowship in cardiovascular surgery. Dr. Christy was very popular among the staff and patients and I, for one, very much want to see him return." (See Exhibit 19/2 for Dr. Christy's biography.)

The board had to make its decision about the future of the cardiac program at CMH before offering Dr. Christy a position; however, it was clear that Dr. Christy could not wait too much longer to be offered a position by CMH. He had received multiple offers but, if he delayed, the offers might be withdrawn.

History of Cabarrus Memorial Hospital

The General Assembly of North Carolina passed legislation in 1935 that enabled Cabarrus County to establish a public hospital. Through the guidance of Mr. Charles A. Cannon, owner of Cannon Mills, the area's largest employer, and other community leaders, Cabarrus Memorial Hospital was established and opened for

Exhibit 19/2: Dr. R. S. "Chris" Christy

Ralph S. "Chris" Christy was born July 26, 1957 at Cabarrus Memorial Hospital. He was one of two children born to Steve and Rachel Christy, hardworking owners of Christy's Nursery in Concord. Chris was educated in the Cabarrus County School system and played football for NorthWest Cabarrus High School. He married Kay Moore, also from Concord, in 1977 and together they embarked on the adventure of Chris becoming a physician. Chris graduated from Davidson College with a BS and the University of North Carolina at Chapel Hill with a medical degree. He then attended a surgical residency program at Memorial Medical Center in Savannah. After his residency, Chris returned to Concord and joined the surgical practice of Flowe, Crooke and Chalfant. Two years later, Chris entered the Cardio-Thoracic and Vascular Fellowship program at Carolinas Medical Center in Charlotte, North Carolina. Under the tutelage of Dr. Frances Robicsek, a well-known and respected pioneer in open-heart surgery, Dr. Christy developed the expert cardiac surgery skills that he wanted to bring to Cabarrus Memorial Hospital.

patients on July 26, 1937. The original facility had 50 inpatient beds and a staff of 19 employees. The first addition of 100 beds was completed in 1940. A second addition opened in 1951 and brought the total bed capacity to 339. A construction and renovation program, started in 1969, expanded the total licensed capacity to 350 acute care beds and 30 bassinets. The adult bed capacity was increased to 457 beds through a 1982 construction project that modernized and consolidated many of the hospital's services.

Duke Medical Center – CMH Affiliation

CMH had several educational affiliation programs and extensive in-service and continuing education programs, including a unique teaching arrangement with Duke University Medical Center. The formal affiliation with Duke included regular sessions on general and specialty medical topics and patient-directed teaching conferences used as an additional education tool (see Exhibit 19/3). This Duke affiliation had begun to seed many specialists at CMH, including a cardiologist, whose practice was rapidly growing.

CMH was a modern, well-equipped facility. Mr. Cannon, as owner of the large Cannon Mills, had wanted the thousands of Cannon Mills' employees to have the very best health care. His generosity and interest in the hospital had made the Duke affiliation possible. It has been said that he carried the hospital on the mill's books as "plant 13." Certainly his philanthropy had in fact made it a much more advanced medical center than those in other communities the size of Cabarrus County.

The Cardiac Program at CMH

For several years, Cabarrus Memorial Hospital had increased the availability of diagnostic and therapeutic cardiovascular services to the community. CMH had as members of the active medical staff one invasive cardiologist and three

Exhibit 19/3: Cabarrus Memorial Hospital – Duke University Medical Center Education
Affiliation

As early as 1966, the United States government launched a series of planning grants for regional medical programs for heart, cancer, and stroke patients. Under this federal proposal Cabarrus Memorial Hospital was to be affiliated with Duke University Medical Center. The Duke–CMH program began in 1968 with Duke faculty members leading training sessions for CMH's doctors and nurses at Salisbury's Rowan Technical Institute.

Dr. George Engstrom recalled, "CMH medical staff wanted a more direct educational affiliation with Duke. Dr. Ladd Hamrick, CMH internist, talked with Dr. Eugene Stead at Duke and a stronger affiliation was proposed. After the discussions with Duke, CMH president Wall, Dr. Bob Hammonds, and Dr. Hamrick took the proposal for the expanded educational affiliation proposals to George Batte, chairman of CMH board's executive committee." Dr. Engstrom continued, "They presented the program in 15 minutes and Mr. Batte's response was, 'Do you think it will work?' The answer was 'yes' and his response was, 'I think we can get the money . . .' The critical funding for the program came from The Cannon Foundation through the leadership of Mr. Batte."

As Dr. Hamrick said, "The affiliation forged in 1972 became 'a powerhouse.'" The successful Duke–Cabarrus liaison was to become a model program for other health centers, for it brought not only Duke medical specialists to CMH, but also spurred seminars, classes, and studies with other nationally recognized physicians and researchers.

The basic agreement was that fellows "from five of Duke's divisions of internal medicine began to travel for two 48-hour periods per month to function as educational consultants to the general internists." Actually, Duke faculty members from other departments began to travel to Cabarrus. The affiliation required that patient contact with Duke physicians be educational for Cabarrus doctors. The Cabarrus activities were to include consultations on educational matters, presenting conferences, reviewing clinical studies, assisting in surgery, and teaching new or different procedures and techniques, among others.

In 1973, Dr. Galen Wagner of Duke's Cardiology faculty, was appointed Department of Medicine coordinator. In 1974, Dr. Tom Long of Duke's gastroenterology faculty was named Cabarrus-based coordinator for the Department of Medicine. He ultimately moved to Cabarrus County where he continued his medical practice and affiliation work.

Under the affiliation, visiting medical professors from such highly regarded universities as Harvard, Stanford, Vanderbilt, University of Pittsburgh, and even medical leaders from foreign countries, came to teach and consult at Cabarrus Memorial Hospital.

According to Dr. Long, "By 1992 there had been 14,703 Duke visits to Cabarrus; 55,826 clinical consultations; 7,636 physicians conferences; and 77,792 continuing medical education hours credited to CMH physicians." He further noted the many benefits to CMH: "Cabarrus doctors received continuing education through Duke conferences; quality physicians were attracted to the community; conferences between Duke and Cabarrus doctors about patients were free; medical expertise and new skills were provided; doctor interest in sophisticated patient care was maintained; and new 'cutting edge' technology was developed."

internists that specialized in treatment of heart diseases. A second invasive cardiologist and another noninvasive cardiologist were expected to join the staff in the next year. Dr. Christy would potentially become the first cardiovascular surgeon on the staff if the board elected to proceed and was successful in receiving the CON.

The scope of the CMH cardiology services included an emergency room staffed and equipped for treatment of cardiac emergencies, an eight-bed coronary care unit, cardiac catheterization, and cardiac rehabilitation. (See Exhibit 19/4 for a glossary of related medical terms.) In addition, the hospital had capabilities for numerous cardiovascular diagnostic and therapeutic services. Electro-diagnostic services included electrocardiograms, cardiac Doppler studies, echo EKGs, exercise EKG studies, and Holter monitoring. The magnetic resonance imaging (MRI) unit had cardiac imaging capabilities. The nuclear medicine department had equipment for nuclear cardiac and thallium scanning. Temporary and permanent pacemaker insertions, thrombolytic therapy through streptokinase and TPA infusions, and Swan Ganz catheter insertions were examples of the hospital's treatment capabilities.

The new program being considered would include one open heart surgical suite for adult procedures, with the capacity for 400 procedures per year. Angioplasty would be offered in the existing cardiac catheterization laboratory. It was projected that by the end of the third year, three dedicated cardiac surgical ICU beds and seven telemetry beds would be required to support the open heart

Exhibit 19/4: Glossary

Angioplasty – The insertion of a catheter into the coronary arteries including inflation of a balloon to squeeze coronary artery plaque formation to decrease blockages

Cardiac Doppler Studies – An imaging study of the heart using ultrasound that involved measurement of pressures in different chambers of the heart, also used to evaluate the valves of the heart

Cardiologist – A physician who attained fellowship training in diseases of the heart and cardiovascular system

Certificate of Need (CON) – Authorization by the State of North Carolina, Department of Health and Human Services, Division of Facility Services to proceed with expenditures for new health facility/equipment

Echocardiography – Diagnostic heart study using ultrasound technology to demonstrate the physical functioning of the heart

Electrocardiogram (EKG) – A trace of the electrical currents that initiated the heartbeat; used to diagnose possible heart disorders

Epidemiology – The study of the health and diseases of populations

Exercise EKG – An electrocardiogram performed when the patient was exercising, usually on a treadmill

Holter Monitor – A diagnostic tool that utilized an extended wearing of an electrocardiogram monitor with which the patient transmitted events telephonically

Intensive Care Unit (ICU) – A specialized patient care unit within a hospital utilized by patients who required constant, high level of care

Invasive Cardiologist – A cardiologist who performed invasive procedures such as angioplasty

Noninvasive Cardiologist – A cardiologist who specialized in medical treatment of heart disease rather than performing invasive procedures

Nuclear Medicine – A field of diagnostic imaging that utilized nucleotide particles injected into the patient, then evaluated with a nuclear camera to produce an image

Swan Ganz Catheter – A pressure catheter that was inserted into the right side of the heart to measure the performance of the heart

Telemetry – The monitoring of the conduction patterns of the heart through radio wave transmission from a remote area to a central location

Thrombolytic Therapy – The use of "clot dissolving" drugs to open blocked arteries

surgery program. Existing space would need to be renovated to accommodate the various service components.

The additional cardiac service being considered would provide patients of CMH with a full-service cardiology program consistent with programs available at other community hospitals and with service areas comparable in size to the CMH service area. The programs and large expenditures would assure continuity of care for patients who received initial cardiac care at CMH. If the board decided not to commit to expanding the cardiac program, CMH patients needing open heart surgery or coronary angioplasty would continue to be transferred to another hospital in the region, such as Duke.

Decision Factors

A major part of the board of trustees' consideration was whether or not there existed a large enough service area to sufficiently support open heart surgery and the expansion of the existing cardiac services. They wanted to know what population threshold would be required. Did they have enough population in the hospital's existing service area? The trustees, in making their expansion decision, looked at a number of factors. They included: (1) the primary and secondary service areas based on historical data; (2) population growth; (3) population epidemiology; (4) availability of existing open heart surgery medical centers; (5) accessibility to cardiac surgery programs; (6) continuity of cardiology care; and (7) rate of demand for open heart surgery. The hospital's planning staff, directed by vice president Glenn Reed, provided data on each of the areas.

1. Primary and Secondary Service Areas

To determine the service area for the proposed heart program expansion, the existing service area for the hospital was identified by examining the hospital's patient database and noting the patients' residential addresses, particularly zip codes. Second, they mapped this service area and evaluated the road and transportation network, travel times, and other hospitals in the region. (See Exhibits 19/5 and 19/6.)

In board discussions, president Wall advised the trustees that hospital planners had looked at patient origins for an existing tertiary program – radiation oncology. This study showed that its major source of patients had been Concord and Kannapolis, with the remainder widely spread over 23 other communities. Mr. Wall asked, "Does this give us reason to believe we can expect referrals to CMH for open heart surgery to come from a wider service area than the hospital average?" (See Exhibits 19/7 and 19/8.)

To further look at the question of patient origins, CMH studied zip code origins for its cardiac catheterization patients. Again, a large number of patients had Concord and Kannapolis zip codes and generally reflected patient origins

Exhibit 19/5 Cabarrus Memorial Hospital Patient Origin

County	% Patient Origin
Cabarrus	80.1
Rowan	9.4
Stanly	7.2
Other	3.3
TOTAL	100.0

Note: "Other" includes Union, Mecklenburg, Davie, Davidson, Iredell, and Lincoln counties.
Source: Hospital Patient Origin Report (North Carolina Medical Database Commission).

Exhibit 19/6: Map of CMH Service Area

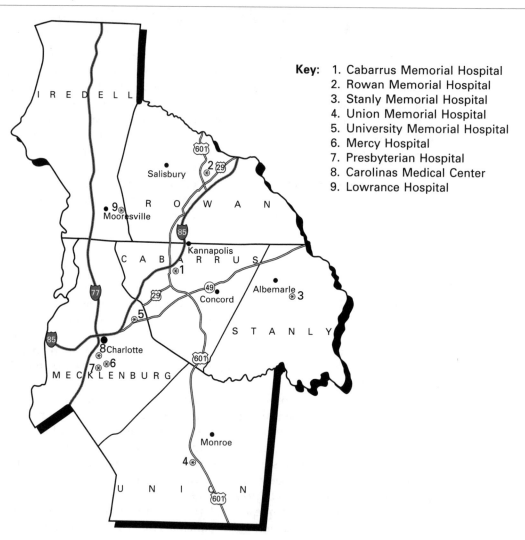

Key: 1. Cabarrus Memorial Hospital
2. Rowan Memorial Hospital
3. Stanly Memorial Hospital
4. Union Memorial Hospital
5. University Memorial Hospital
6. Mercy Hospital
7. Presbyterian Hospital
8. Carolinas Medical Center
9. Lowrance Hospital

Exhibit 19/7: CMH Patient Origin (%) Previous Year

County	Radiation Oncology	Heart Catheterization
Cabarrus	57.4	59.3
Rowan	16.0	30.4
Stanly	19.7	7.3
Other	6.9	3.0
TOTAL	100.0	100.0

Exhibit 19/8: Proposed CMH Open Heart Service Population

County	Population	Market
Cabarrus	69,255	70.0
Rowan	40,813	36.9
Stanly	7,661	14.8
Union	1,516	1.8
Mecklenburg	1,534	0.3
Iredell	651	0.7

similar to those of the radiation oncology program. Again the board wondered if this indicated the open heart program would draw patients from a service area that would include parts or all of six counties: Cabarrus, Rowan, Stanly, Union, Iredell, and Mecklenburg. The outside boundaries of these counties are within 60 miles of Concord, the site of CMH.

Mr. Wall questioned, "What would further analysis of the historical data lead planners to conclude about the program's primary service area? Could it serve as much as 70 percent of Cabarrus and a third of Rowan County? Would the secondary service area include parts of Stanly, Union, Mecklenburg, and Iredell Counties? What percentage of the population in those counties lived within 40 miles of CMH? Would this comprise a secondary service area large enough?"

A major demographic factor driving the perceived demand for open heart surgery at CMH was population growth. According to the Government and Business Services Branch of the State Library of North Carolina, total population for these six counties was expected to increase 18.3 percent over the next ten years. Therefore, even if open heart surgery usage rates remained constant each year, counties in this service area could have expected at least 18 percent more open heart surgery cases over the ten year period. (See Exhibit 19/9.)

2. Growth of At-Risk Population

A second major demographic factor driving the demand for open heart surgery was growth of the at-risk population. According to projections from the recent census, the number of people aged 45 to 64, the population most likely to

Exhibit 19/9: Ten-Year Projection: Service Area Population Growth

County	Year 1	Year 2	Change (%)
Cabarrus	98,935	112,802	14.0
Rowan	110,605	122,268	10.5
Stanly	51,765	55,185	6.6
Union	84,211	99,644	18.3
Mecklenburg	511,433	630,005	23.2
Iredell	92,931	103,820	11.7
TOTAL	949,880	1,123,724	18.3

Exhibit 19/10: Growth of At-Risk Population: Aged 45 to 64

	Previous Year	10 years	Change (%)
Cabarrus	20,419	26,797	31.2
Rowan	22,729	28,348	24.7
Stanly	10,691	12,761	19.4
Union	16,458	23,290	41.5
Mecklenburg	91,747	135,154	47.3
Iredell	19,950	25,504	27.8
TOTAL	181,994	251,854	38.4

suffer occlusive coronary artery disease, was predicted to grow by 38.3 percent in the next ten years, a rate more than twice that of the general population. (See Exhibit 19/10.)

3. Population Epidemiology

Based on the latest available data, all the proposed service area counties, with the exception of Union and Mecklenburg, had evidence of a heart disease mortality rate higher than that of the state as a whole (see Exhibit 19/11). According to the data that had been recently reported by the North Carolina Database Commission, open heart surgery usage rates in Cabarrus County were higher than that of the entire state. The previous year North Carolina had experienced a procedure rate of 1.39 per 1,000 population.

4. Availability of Existing Services for Patients in CMH Service Area

North Carolina had 16 open heart surgery programs located in 11 counties. None of these programs was in the proposed CMH primary service area. Those closest to the CMH service area were located in Charlotte. They were Mercy

Exhibit 19/11: Heart Disease Mortality Rates: Two Years Previous

County	Death Rate/1,000 Population
Rowan	375.8
Cabarrus	320.7
Stanly	326.0
Union	246.5
Mecklenburg	225.0
Iredell	325.2
North Carolina	288.6

Hospital, Presbyterian Hospital, and Carolinas Medical Center, all located about 25 miles from CMH.

Only one of the state's 16 programs had claimed Cabarrus County in its primary service area. That claim had been made eight years earlier by Carolinas Medical Center when it opened its service. Since that time, Carolinas Medical Center had drawn only 5.6 percent of its patients from Cabarrus County, suggesting to the CMH board that Cabarrus patient volumes at Carolinas Medical Center did not warrant being included in Carolinas Medical Center's primary service area.

The three Charlotte programs had reported previous year operating room utilization for cardiac surgery as follows: Mercy Hospital, 36.3 percent; Presbyterian Hospital, 78.5 percent; and Carolinas Medical Center, 84.5 percent. Procedure volume had increased yearly at both Presbyterian and Carolinas Medical Center. Presbyterian, with its two open heart surgery suites operating at 78.5 percent of nominal capacity, apparently needed its operating rooms.

Carolinas Medical Center, with its six rooms classified as combined "open heart surgery/thoracic suites," had submitted a CON application for an additional open heart surgery room. However, earlier in the year, it had subsequently withdrawn its application for a CON. For the Department of Facilities Services to award a CON, the existing utilization rate for the cardiac surgery suite was required to be at 80 percent or higher.

Procedure volume at Mercy Hospital had not followed a year-to-year growth pattern. Room utilization had been well under 50 percent each year for the previous ten years. Moreover, Mercy did not appear to reach the proposed CMH open heart service area. In the previous year only 9 percent of the 174 people from Cabarrus County, and none from Rowan County, had received open heart surgery at Mercy. The pattern indicated a perceived or real barrier to access at Mercy by people in the CMH area counties. Generally, Mercy appeared to serve a population that was more south and east of Charlotte.

5. Accessibility to Cardiac Surgery Programs

The existing open heart surgery programs in Charlotte, Winston-Salem, and Greensboro were 25 to 60 miles from the service population. Although this seemed relatively close for a one-time procedure, it was inconvenient for persons traveling repeatedly for diagnosis, family support, and follow-up care.

"Driving to Charlotte is becoming more and more of a problem," commented a board member. "I am often asked why we can't provide more care in Cabarrus County."

Heart patients from the CMH area had to travel to existing services along combinations of country roads and heavily congested traffic arteries. Travel time was from one to two hours. Congestion and delay were expected to further increase the time as the Charlotte metropolitan area continued to grow 3 percent per year, a rate triple that of the state.

Moreover, to many residents of the CMH service area, Charlotte was a big city and confusing for drivers from out of town. Its perceived distance was farther than its actual distance because of the delays in city travel. This had been noted with the opening of radiation oncology at CMH. Patient volumes were much higher than expected. Surveys of patients and families cited distance, lack of transportation, and fear of the city as reasons for not having obtained radiation treatments at distant sites that had been recommended by their physicians.

As part of the affiliation between Duke University Medical Center and Cabarrus Memorial hospital, two Duke open heart surgeons, Jim Lowe, MD, and Peter Smith, MD, participated in monthly conferences at CMH and consulted on patient candidates for open heart surgery. Those patient consultations became referrals to Duke when surgery was indicated. The medical staff suggested that the patient trip of 120 miles to Duke would be eliminated if open heart surgery of equal quality could be performed at CMH, as was being proposed. However, it was expected that a few cases needing specialized care would still be referred to Duke (or other medical centers) after the CMH program was opened. Approximately 40 percent of CMH cardiac catheterization referrals were going to Duke.

6. Continuity of Cardiology Care

Continuity of care for the cardiology patient was critical. Quality was enhanced when patient transfers were minimized, medical and nursing staff were constant, and staff and technology for diagnostic and therapeutic interventions were maintained. To obtain the desired level of care, CMH patients were being transferred to other facilities when cardiac surgery was indicated. This transfer disrupted continuity.

According to the North Carolina Database Commission, for the previous year, 174 Cabarrus County and 118 Rowan County residents received open heart surgery in one of the following hospitals: Duke University Medical Center, Presbyterian Hospital, Carolinas Medical Center, NC Baptist Hospitals, and a few others. For many of those 292 patients, a CMH-based open heart surgery service would have avoided transfers and ensured continuity of cardiology care. (See Exhibit 19/12.)

The scope and comprehensiveness of cardiology services at CMH had expanded yearly. Two years previously, CMH had initiated its cardiac catheterization

Exhibit 19/12: Where Cabarrus-Rowan Residents Received Open Heart Surgery: Previous
Year

Destination Hospital	Cabarrus Residents	Rowan Residents	Total
Duke University Medical Center	28	16	44
Presbyterian Hospital	68	25	93
Mercy Hospital	9	0	9
Carolinas Medical Center	66	44	110
NC Baptist Hospitals	0	28	28
Unknown	3	5	8
TOTAL	174	118	292

program. In the past year, the CMH program referred 117 patients to open
heart surgery and 82 to angioplasty. In addition, Rowan Memorial Hospital, located
in Salisbury (a half-hour's drive to the north), had opened a cardiac catheterization service and could have been considered another referral source for the
proposed CMH program. The next logical step in the continuity of cardiac
care was argued to be the open heart surgery program. Availability of open heart
surgery and angioplasty would have provided invasive options for treatment
of coronary artery disease and reduced outside referrals to a small percentage
of patients. A physician board member commented, "It is time this becomes
a full-service hospital. Cabarrus County deserves it and cardiac surgery will be
just the beginning."

7. Growth in Demand

Over the previous ten years, North Carolina open heart surgery volume had
increased an average of 26 percent a year. Moreover, statistical forecasts had predicted continued increases in use rate per 1,000 population for the next five years.
The rate of 0.43 open heart surgeries per 1,000 population ten years ago had
increased to 1.39 per 1,000. Cardiac catheterization was the major diagnostic procedure that resulted in a recommendation for open heart surgery. Changes in
cardiac catheterization volumes were, therefore, important to predict open heart
demand at a particular location. North Carolina cardiac catheterization volume
had grown at an average annual rate of 16.2 percent over the prior nine years.
Although the rate of growth was slowing, anecdotal projections and trended
forecasts predicted continued growth for the next five years.

The state's cardiac catheterization to open heart procedure ratio had also
increased annually. Over the past year, the ratio had increased to 4.54 adult catheterizations for each open heart procedure. Similar to the annual growth rate for open
heart surgery procedures, this ratio was also growing.

Exhibit 19/13: CMH Open Heart Staffing Plan

	Year 1 53 Procedures	Year 2 106 Procedures	Year 3 211 Procedures
Operating Room			
Nurse Manager	1.00	1.00	1.00
RN	2.50	3.50	6.00
OR Tech	2.00	2.00	3.00
OR Aide/Transport	0.50	0.50	1.00
CRNA	1.00	1.50	3.00
Anesthesia Tech	0.50	0.50	1.00
Respiratory Therapist	1.00	1.50	3.00
Subtotal	8.50	10.50	18.00
Surgery/Recovery			
Nurse Manager	0.50	0.50	0.50
RN	4.00	4.00	7.00
Ward Secretary	0.50	0.50	0.50
Subtotal	5.00	5.00	8.00
Telemetry Unit			
Nurse Manager	0.50	0.50	0.50
RN	3.00	4.00	7.00
Monitor Tech	3.00	3.00	3.00
Ward Secretary	0.50	0.50	0.50
Subtotal	7.00	8.00	11.00
Nurse Educator	0.50	0.50	0.50
Angioplasty RN	1.00	1.00	1.00
Angioplasty Tech	1.00	1.00	1.00
Subtotal	2.50	2.50	2.50
TOTAL	23.00	26.00	39.50

Financial Considerations

In addition to market demand and trend analysis, the board was faced with the financial aspect of the decision. President Wall asked the CFO to present the financial data. An open heart surgery program would incur a number of expenses. In addition to Dr. Christy and his surgical team, there would be a need for 23 additional employees in year 1, growing to 39 in year 3 (see Exhibit 19/13).

It was projected there would be a need for ten beds licensed as acute care beds, not then being utilized, to become operational as coronary care beds. Additionally there would be a need for three intensive care unit (ICU) beds, and the one new open heart operating suite.

A total of 5,811 sq. ft. of hospital space would require renovation. Projected capital costs, including construction and equipment, were $3,273,180. The hospital had sufficient reserve funds to underwrite the renovation project and the additional equipment without borrowing money.

Exhibit 19/14: Open Heart Program Costs

	Year 1	Year 2	Year 3
Direct Costs			
Clinical Personnel	$711,793	$910,878	$1,695,457
Administrative Personnel	136,565	147,490	159,289
Support Personnel	52,764	56,985	61,544
Personnel Taxes/Benefits	180,224	223,071	383,258
Medical Supplies	315,947	746,439	1,749,771
Other Supplies	15,950	68,980	75,445
Depreciation, Equipment	243,376	243,376	243,376
Plant Operations and Maintenance	48,087	52,415	57,132
Other Associated Expenses (Angioplasty)	449,965	534,033	615,723
Other Associated Expenses	99,543	99,212	99,212
Contracted Services	110,000	134,860	298,185
Total Direct Costs	2,364,214	3,217,739	5,438,392
Indirect Costs			
General and Administrative	255,966	302,376	416,862
Other Overhead	73,200	88,630	175,473
Depreciation, Building	43,525	43,525	43,525
Other Property, Ownership and Use Expense	2,036	2,402	2,835
Consultant Services	122,740	153,399	154,699
Rowan Community Outreach	6,183	6,739	7,346
Total Indirect Costs	503,650	597,071	800,740
Total Costs	$2,867,864	$3,814,810	$6,239,132

Direct costs for the open heart program were projected to be $2,364,214 in year 1, $3,217,739 in year 2, and $5,438,392 in year 3 (see Exhibit 19/14). Average length of stay per open heart patient was projected to be nine days.

Projected average open heart surgery fees per case were $13,000 without catheterization and $15,000 with catheterization. These estimates represented full, nonprofessional fees and the surgeon's fee, as well as other professional components such as anesthesia, pathology, and radiology.

Average room and board charges were estimated at $826 per day. All ancillaries were projected at $3,725 per day. Total average projected charge for each open heart surgery procedure was $40,957.

The Meeting Draws to a Close

President Wall and various members of the hospital staff had presented the findings to the trustees. The data and information had been collected, tabulated, and analyzed. It was time to make a decision. Should CMH go ahead with an application for a certificate of need for an open heart surgery program? As they sat there waiting for someone to speak, Mrs. West asked, "Mr. Batte, what do you think we should do? Do we go for the CON?"

20 CASE

Sunshine County Health Department: Strategy Implementation

Introduction

Liz Rogers, the new administrator of Sunshine County Health Department (SCHD), had just completed her first staff meeting. Many of the staff had voiced concerns about patient waiting times, length of times to make appointments, and overall patient flow through the facility. On the table was a proposal from senior staff to consider using open access scheduling. Open access scheduling, also known as advanced access scheduling, accommodated patients as they arrived. As Liz looked around the room she knew that there were many issues to be explored in addition to patient scheduling. SCHD's strategic plan (created before she arrived by the people in the room) indicated that in the coming year they would have to serve a larger patient population with fewer resources.

This case was prepared by Dr. Donna Malvey and Dr. Eileen Hamby of the University of Central Florida. It is intended to be used as a basis for class discussion rather than to illustrate either effective or ineffective handling of an administrative situation. The names of organizations, individuals, and locations have been disguised to preserve the anonymity of the organization. This work is based on research funded by the IBM Center for Healthcare Management. The opinions and conclusions expressed herein are entirely those of the authors. Used with permission from Eileen Hamby and Donna Malvey.

Liz thought to herself, "The staff has put so much energy into the strategic plan. It seems like they're tired and just want to get back to their normal jobs. I think they are experiencing 'strategic fatigue.' But I don't want a strategic plan that just sits on a shelf . . ."

The state health department provided all of its local health departments, including SCHD, a preset format on what was to be included in each strategic plan. After having read the plan, Liz realized that despite all of the work put into it, the SCHD strategic plan did not actually address all of the key issues that the department faced. There was considerably more work to be done.

Liz thought, "I have too much to do and I need to make the right start with the staff – understand the culture, the key informal leaders, and more. If I use some consultants to help with the strategic plan, they might be able to provide further direction as to what to do with what has been done and what still needs to be done. Based on the information in the strategic plan, I'd like to know what they think about performing a patient flow analysis at SCHD. It would provide information on the flow of patients through the health department. . . ."

Several weeks later, after meeting with the consultants and the staff, Liz determined that SCHD needed more than the application of a technique such as patient flow analysis. The consultants had proposed applying a strategic model of flow management that would assist in achieving a fit between SCHD's formulated strategies and strategy implementation. Liz wondered, "How are we going to achieve our strategic goals?"

Overview of SCHD

SCHD was located in a rapidly growing county – the population had increased 10 percent per year since 2000. The 2004 population of Sunshine County was approximately 85,000. The mean age of the residents was 55 years. One-fifth of the population were Medicaid recipients. Of these low-income residents, 10 percent, or 8,500, had family incomes below the poverty level established by the federal government. Over 20 percent of the children in the county were identified as falling below the poverty level. SCHD's service area consisted of 60 sq. miles and was largely composed of residences and small retail businesses.

Sunshine County ranked below the standard for minimal physician requirements established by the US Department of Health and Human Services. Access to health care was compromised because, in general, there were few medical providers available in Sunshine County to treat low-income patients. In addition, there were no migrant health facilities although migrant workers frequently resided in the county, albeit temporarily, during periods of seasonal employment. Consequently, SCHD was the primary access point for care for low-income patients.

SCHD was a component of the larger state health department. As such, its budget was determined at the state level. Requests for additional money could be made to the local county commission, who used local taxpayer funds to financially support projects that would benefit the community.

The SCHD facility was relatively small in size, being approximately 6,500 sq. feet. It was normally open five days per week, plus an occasional Saturday before the start of the school year, when proof of immunizations was required. Its hours were 7:30 A.M. to 4:30 P.M. on Monday, Tuesday, and Friday, and from 8:30 A.M. to 5:30 P.M. on Wednesday and Thursday. It employed 48 full-time equivalent positions: one full-time physician, four advanced registered nurse practitioners that handled family practice and women's health, one dentist, ten registered nurses, five licensed practical nurses, and support staff.

The search committee responsible for appointing the new administrator for SCHD prepared a bio on Liz Rogers when she was introduced to the staff during the interview process (see Exhibit 20/1). A letter of recommendation from the director of the state health department stated that Liz "was well respected at all levels of the state health department and regularly attended meetings with other health providers in the community."

As the organizational chart in Exhibit 20/2 demonstrated, SCHD was organized into five divisions: medical; dental; environmental; women, infants and children (WIC); and fiscal/business. The administrator of SCHD reported to the director of the state health department.

The function of the medical division was public health, primary care, and epidemiology, including monitoring and treatment of sexually transmitted diseases (STDs), tuberculosis (TB) control, chronic disease management, breast and cervical cancer screenings, an epilepsy program, adult comprehensive care, family planning, and immunizations. Dental's function was also public health, whereas the environmental division focused on environmental safety: sewage treatment and disposal, rabies, and food, as well as pools and coastal water bacteria. WIC provided nutrition services to woman, infants, and children, including counseling and distribution of food vouchers. WIC provided nutrition counseling services to patients from the medical division as well. WIC reported directly to a neighboring health department and indirectly to the SCHD administrator. The WIC supervisor from the neighboring county made two visits a month to SCHD. In addition, the department was involved in emergency and disaster planning and operations. Personnel of SCHD staffed the local special needs shelters during events such as hurricanes.

Exhibit 20/1: Welcome Liz Rogers

Liz Rogers has a Bachelor of Science degree in nursing and a Master of Science degree in health services administration from Fuller University. She has ten years of experience as a public health nurse, and was formerly the assistant administrator of Shaw County Health Department. She has experience in strategic planning and strategy change and served on the state health department's quality improvement committee. Ms. Rogers won the Gilbert Productivity Award from the state health department twice, once for her work on preemptive strategies for bioterror events and second for her work with decreasing the number of cancellations at the Shaw County Health Department.

Exhibit 20/2: SCHD Organizational Chart

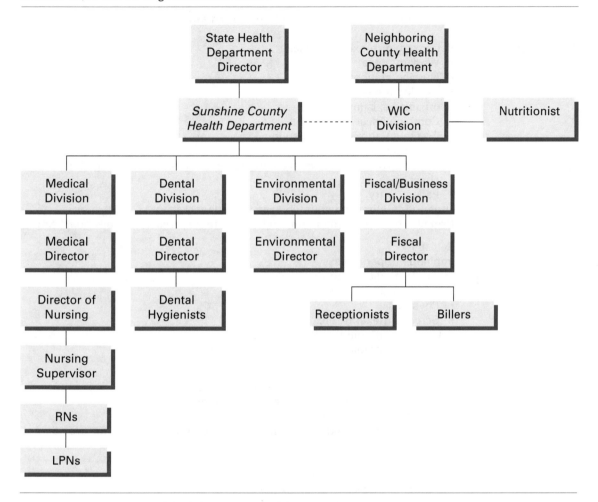

Internal Analysis

The challenges and opportunities for the SCHD were recently revealed in an internal analysis that was validated using focus groups of all staff at SCHD. Exhibit 20/3 presents key findings of the focus group meetings.

A primary challenge involved meeting the demands of the rapidly growing community and providing access to care for a large number of low-income families. Additionally, staffing to meet the demands of emergency response and preparedness posed a test for current staff workloads. Immunization programs represented growing demands in light of the increase in number of school-age children, especially those below the poverty level. An increase in the

Exhibit 20/3: Summary of Key Findings of Focus Group Meetings

Item	Comment as to how to improve current situation
Physical Layout	Better organize existing space • Workup areas • Nursing stations • Waiting areas Reorganize existing space • Combine fiscal offices • Create an administrative suite • Group by functionality • Perform routine facilities planning to accommodate emerging situational changes • Patient entry Organize to eliminate staff workspace bottlenecks Organize to reduce, minimize, and eliminate unnecessary "walkabout" time
Scheduling System	Revise it Implement open access Integrate medical records Create specialty clinics • Physicals • Screening exams, etc. Establish nontraditional Saturday hours Establish nontraditional "late" hours for clinics
Staff Bottlenecks	Working supervisors (two-hats) • Clinicians who also function as administrators • Nurses who also perform case management duties Fiscal/financial advisors Create backup for medically complex patients to compensate for providers who are • Unavailable • No shows or not on time Try triaging medically complex patients Try only scheduling medically complex patients at the end of the day
Patient Bottlenecks	• Waiting for provider • Translation services (cultural) • Phone-loops
Time	Retrain staff to use time management (set priorities) Match provider time with appointment time (support staff) Have the maintenance person "open" the building and turn equipment on prior to official start time
Convenience	Staff • Do not schedule clients for the first 10–15 minutes, instead use this time for morning meetings • Reverse the "flow" – move the staff around vs. moving the patients around

non-English speaking population, especially Romanians, Russians, Portuguese, and Vietnamese, taxed the existing interpretive service capabilities and created a pressing demand for translation services.

Opportunities for SCHD seemed less obvious, but nevertheless were present. For example, although SCHD was currently providing medical care to approximately 3,000 Medicaid patients, there were almost 14,000 additional Medicaid patients in the county that had yet to access care through SCHD. This number represented significant increases in patient workloads, funding possibilities for SCHD, and potential for staffing increases. Of course, the downside – or possible threat – emerged if all 17,000 decided to access care through SCHD; current resources could not meet the increase in demand.

An emergent threat to SCHD was similar to threats facing other health departments throughout the United States – bioterrorism that might involve biologic and chemical incidents in the community. However, although SCHD prepared for such unknown events, its day-to-day challenges included lack of a centralized county funding source for indigent care. Another challenge was the absence of local community health centers and clinics to meet the needs of the underinsured and uninsured.

Strengths and weaknesses were identified by SCHD through the focus group process. Weaknesses included insufficient physician coverage, insufficient space, and less than optimal facility layout that resulted in service bottlenecks. For example, it could take a patient as long as two hours to move from the waiting room through the appropriate treatment areas. Patients moved through an average of four different service points during each visit. Walk-in patients had waiting times of up to several hours.

Another weakness that emerged in the focus groups was the duplication of tasks resulting from the number of providers with whom the patient actually came into contact. Of particular concern to the staff was the weakness involving length of waiting time for a patient to receive an appointment. For example, in the dental division, the waiting time averaged three months for an appointment. In addition, a problem with "no-shows" – patients who failed to keep their appointments and did not call and cancel – existed. At SCHD, 48 percent of appointments were "no-shows." The proposal from senior staff had identified productivity problems because of "no-shows" and suggested that productivity was negatively affected by SCHD's failure to adopt e-technologies such as electronic medical records and scheduling software. For example, scheduling software could be used by both patients and staff to keep apprised of the status of appointments and to facilitate notice of cancellations.

The strengths that were reported through the focus groups included a dedicated, highly qualified, and extremely hard working staff with many years of experience and tenure at SCHD. In addition, the administrator's talents, education, experience, and leadership abilities held promise for making the tough decisions and changes necessary for SCHD to become a center of excellence among county health departments in the state. Because previous satisfaction surveys involving both patients and staff were positive, everyone at SCHD was viewed as having a "can do" attitude.

Strategic Planning Process

The strategic planning process was mandated by the state and had been ongoing prior to the arrival of Liz Rogers. The process had involved all staff as well as patient and community members through focus groups and surveys as a means of assuring effective environmental scanning. The previous administrator had left the "strategic plan" on his desk as a guide for his successor. Exhibit 20/4 summarizes the SCHD strategies developed in the plan.

Strategic goals included serving a larger patient population with fewer resources. SCHD used these goals in linking the formulation strategies with subsequent strategies in the process. The stated mission of SCHD was to provide quality care and ensure the health and well-being of the residents of Sunshine County. The directional strategies were guided by this purposeful statement as well as by the strong public health values exhibited by the staff.

The selection of adaptive strategies was a combination of expansion of scope/market penetration and maintenance of scope/enhancement. This combination was believed to be the best way to perform SCHD's mission and fulfill its vision of becoming a center of excellence among county health departments in the state. In so doing, SCHD aimed to improve its market share by better satisfying existing customers with current products and revising organizational processes to achieve operational efficiencies.

The market entry strategies involved developing an alliance with other providers to achieve a referral network. Because other county health departments formed alliances with hospital emergency departments as a means of creating referrals, SCHD was confident in its ability to fulfill this strategy. In terms of competitive strategies, SCHD determined that the appropriate strategic alternative would be a positioning strategy that relied on differentiation.

Strategic Flow Management Analysis

Flow management models have been much used in industrial settings, primarily to alleviate operational inefficiencies and enhance productivity but also to

Exhibit 20/4: Results of Strategic Thinking for SCHD

Formulation Strategies	Strategic Alternatives	Strategy Types Selected
Directional Strategies	Mission, Vision, Values, and Goals	N/A
Adaptive Strategies	• Expansion of Scope • Maintenance of Scope	• Market Penetration • Enhancement
Market Entry Strategies	Cooperation	Alliance
Competitive Strategies	Positioning	Differentiation

address issues of safety and quality. In health care, flow management gained attention because of overcrowding in emergency departments (EDs). Problems of overcrowding placed the focus increasingly on aspects of capacity or demand management relative to patient flows. As a result, patient flow analysis was emphasized. However, analyzing patient flows represented an operational focus. Although an operational focus was critical in implementing strategy, it could not be considered in isolation from the strategy. To do so imperiled the organization. Therefore, a more comprehensive analysis was required for SCHD.

Rationale for Using Strategic Flow Management Perspective

During the course of ongoing research, the consultants developed a strategic flow management model that presented a broader strategic approach, reflected a systems perspective, and simultaneously responded to the complex and dynamic demands of health care organizations. As illustrated in Exhibit 20/5, the model was an input–throughput–output conceptual model of strategic flow management.

The model illustrated the need for a systems approach with integrated – rather than piecemeal – solutions. The input component consisted of factors that contributed to strategically managing flow. These factors were classified according to resources, competencies, and capabilities. The throughput component of the model identified both the internal and external systems that interacted with the input factors. For example, the collaborative systems that included community partners, such as local hospitals, might serve as a referral network for patients and ultimately contribute to increased workloads. The output component of the model represented important outcomes, not only for the patients and SCHD, but also for the community as a whole.

Thus, in using the strategic flow management model, the consultants studied and analyzed organizational problems within a strategic framework and identified any deficiencies in terms of strategic linkages among activities, especially with respect to implementation. Because many of the issues that surfaced during the focus groups seemed to relate to service delivery strategies, the strategic flow management model offered an opportunity to address operational inefficiencies within the context of these strategies.

Using the strategic flow management model in Exhibit 20/5, the consultants performed a strategic flow management analysis. The analysis was performed by observation, review of records, and interviews with key informants. The flow inputs as specified in the model were assessed for the medical and dental divisions. A decision was made to exclude the environmental division because of its offsite location. Additionally, the WIC division was not evaluated because another local health department was responsible for its administration. Integrated into the strategic flow management analysis was a patient flow study. This study was performed using PFA for Windows (WinPFA) 1.0 – a computer application software package produced in 2004 by the Centers for Disease Control and Prevention (CDC)

Exhibit 20/5: Strategic Flow Management Model

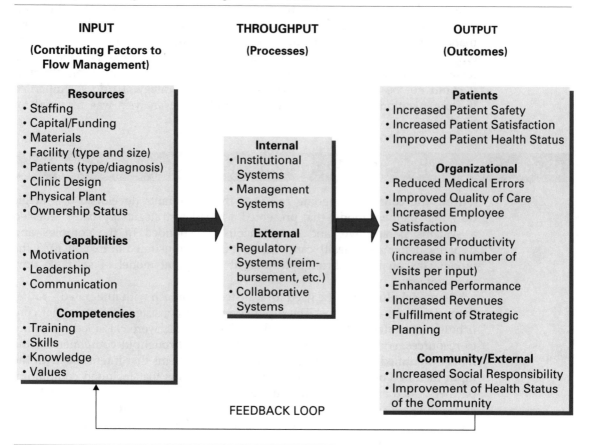

INPUT	THROUGHPUT	OUTPUT
(Contributing Factors to Flow Management)	(Processes)	(Outcomes)

Resources
- Staffing
- Capital/Funding
- Materials
- Facility (type and size)
- Patients (type/diagnosis)
- Clinic Design
- Physical Plant
- Ownership Status

Capabilities
- Motivation
- Leadership
- Communication

Competencies
- Training
- Skills
- Knowledge
- Values

Internal
- Institutional Systems
- Management Systems

External
- Regulatory Systems (reimbursement, etc.)
- Collaborative Systems

Patients
- Increased Patient Safety
- Increased Patient Satisfaction
- Improved Patient Health Status

Organizational
- Reduced Medical Errors
- Improved Quality of Care
- Increased Employee Satisfaction
- Increased Productivity (increase in number of visits per input)
- Enhanced Performance
- Increased Revenues
- Fulfillment of Strategic Planning

Community/External
- Increased Social Responsibility
- Improvement of Health Status of the Community

FEEDBACK LOOP

to analyze patient flows. The specifics of the patient flow study included providing staff with data collection forms that documented the following:

- Patient arrival time vs. appointment time;
- Actual patient service time vs. time spent in clinic by visit type;
- Personnel use in clinic by task;
- Patient load per individual staff member; and
- Sequential order of patient flow.

Results of Strategic Flow Management Analysis

Exhibit 20/6 summarizes the findings of the analysis of the dental division. Patient scheduling issues were identified. For example, appointments were currently scheduled three months out. Emergencies were accommodated daily,

Exhibit 20/6: Summary of the Findings of the Strategic Flow Management Analysis:
Dental

Item	Finding
Patient Privacy	• No patient privacy because the waiting area, which includes patient sign-in and appointments, is open and available to all who walk by
Patient Scheduling	• Appointments for both dental and dental assistant visits were being scheduled about three months out. The delays were attributed to missed "scheduled" appointments
Productivity	• Levels of productivity for all three years are extremely low based on comparative data with other health departments
Staffing	• No staffing performance standards exist for dental
Equipment	• Adequate for workload, but will not be adequate for increased workload. Purchase additional equipment as workload increases
Facility Layout	Patients are moving through restricted clinical areas, which poses possible "contamination" and patient safety as well as infection control problems. Interference with clinical care delivery
Information Technology	• No electronic medical record. Medical records for each day are pulled the day before the patient visit • Current electronic database is not integrated with other e-systems. No electronic applications of mail functions; all appointment reminders and mailings are done manually • Everything is recorded by hand multiple times

usually as the first appointment of the day. Walk-in patients were not accepted. Although the dental receptionist was required to phone patients the day before their scheduled visit as a reminder of their appointments, the analysis showed that the phone reminders were performed only about 22 percent of the time.

Productivity levels were extremely low. The "no-show" rate for dental was 48 percent – that negatively affected productivity and created high standby costs. The productivity rate based on all patients scheduled was 4.2 visits per day for the dental hygienist, and 3.3 visits per day for the dentist. Other health departments in the state averaged a rate of 7.2 visits per day for the dental assistant and 7.4 visits per day for the dentist.

The overall productivity of all employees in the dental division was 31 percent (nearly one-third of their working hours were billable hours). There were no set productivity requirements for the dental division. The dental equipment was evaluated as sufficient for the patient activity level, but as more Medicaid patients accessed the health department's dental services, the equipment needs would have to be reevaluated.

E-technology was severely underutilized. For example, there were no electronic medical records and everything was recorded by hand – multiple times. Patient records were pulled each day from a centralized medical records area. The records were returned at the end of each day. There was no integration of software functions, and much time was spent maneuvering among different software programs to access necessary information.

Exhibit 20/7 reveals the results of the strategic flow management analysis for the medical division. Patient privacy emerged as a critical issue. Patient records

Exhibit 20/7: Summary of the Findings of the Strategic Flow Management Analysis: Medical

Item	Finding
Patient Privacy	• Patients are called by name in the public waiting room. Clinical charts are held in the hallway that is accessible to both patients and all staff
Patient Scheduling	• Length of time between patient contact and appointment date can be several months depending on specific service area within the medical division • High rate of no-shows and cancellations disrupt daily schedules • Although there is the high rate of no-shows and cancellations, nursing supervisors routinely discourage walk-in patients by not fitting walk-ins into cancellation and no-show scheduling slots • Fifty percent of patients arrive early despite staff reports that late arriving patients created scheduling problems. Even those patients who arrive late are within a five-minute range
Productivity	• Productivity levels are low primarily because of the time it takes patients to move through the care process at SCHD • Time spent in recording patient history for each visit negatively affects productivity. Staff typically spends on average about 15–30 minutes performing this function
Staffing	• Physician coverage is inadequate: 25 hours per week are scheduled, but in reality only 20 hours are provided. • The mean salary for physician coverage is below average for the service area
Equipment	• Equipment (clinical and business) is adequate. However, the location of some of the equipment is not conducive to efficient operations. For example, weight scales are found in hallways instead of in exam rooms
Facility Layout	• Layout is less than optimal. Patients typically move through four service areas during the course of a visit with the result of a two-hour visit instead of a one-hour visit • Some rooms, such as the physician exam rooms, are not used when the physician is not present • Bottleneck areas have been created. For example, nurses congregate at the front desk waiting for their patients to arrive
Information Technology	• Need to upgrade to electronic medical records and use electronic databases to support their work

were kept in a file holder on the wall in the middle of the hallway that was accessible to all patients and staff. Patient privacy was impacted when patients were called by name from the waiting room.

Patient scheduling similarly emerged as a critical area for the medical division and underscored a lack of customer service orientation towards patients. The average time to schedule an appointment for the medical areas was 6.5 weeks. The no-show rate was 36 percent of all visits. Only urgent-need walk-in patients, such as those with sexually transmitted diseases, were seen the same day but, because they were worked into the schedule, they waited an average of 3.2 hours to be seen. Of those who did show up for their appointments, approximately 50 percent of patients arrived early, another 25 percent arrived just on time, 20 percent arrived within five minutes after their appointment time, and 5 percent arrived more than five minutes late.

The productivity rate for the advanced registered nurse practitioners (ARNPs) was 41 percent, with each ARNP averaging 3.9 visits per day. The overall productivity rate of the medical division was 33 percent (one-third of their working hours were billable hours). Productivity rates were low in part because of the time it took patients to move through the entire care process at SCHD. Patients were moved from station to station and sometimes to a waiting area as an intermediate step in the process. They often moved through four or five service areas; the average length of a visit was 2.1 hours. Patient information was updated after the patient was called into the treatment area. The patient history was taken after the patient was taken to the first station – the interview room. The patient's vital signs were normally taken at the first station as well. Next, the patient typically was brought to the lab, where the blood work was drawn. Then the patient was brought to an exam room to wait for an examination by the physician or ARNP. After patients were examined, they were moved to the exit station where counseling about their prescriptions or other types of patient education was provided.

The facility layout was not ideal and each care provider worked out of only two assigned examination rooms, instead of any available room. Bottlenecks existed. Nurses congregated at the front desk awaiting their next patients and internal waiting areas were sometimes jammed with patients awaiting a vacant exam room. Exhibit 20/8 depicts the facility layout.

Although the physician was full-time, only 25 hours of patient contact time were scheduled and actual billed time was about 20 hours. The salary of the physician was below average for the service area compared with other local physicians and other county health departments within the state.

There were no electronic medical records used in the medical division. As with dental, patient charts had to be pulled daily from the medical records department. There was no integration of software functions. Reminders of patient visits were mandatory for certain patient diagnostic categories, but the receptionist responsible for calling or sending the reminders was not completing the task. Letters sent to new Medicaid patients to inform them of health department services were running at least two months behind.

Exhibit 20/8: Facility Layout, Sunshine County Health Department

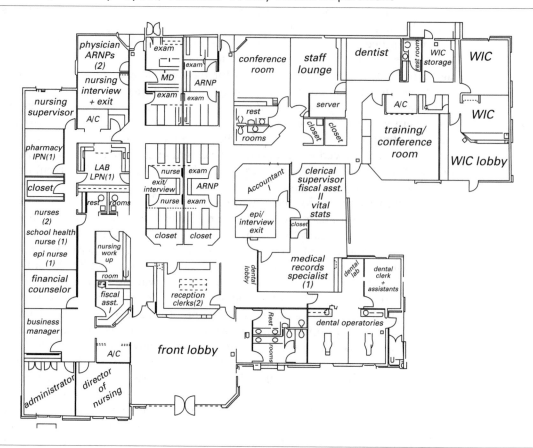

The Future of SCHD

Liz Rogers looked out her window at a number of patients entering the facility. She thought, "SCHD really does perform a needed service in this community, but there are many fixes required if we are going to serve an even larger number of patients with reduced resources. Some of the changes are not going to sit well with the staff, but they are really committed to the patients. I need to engage them in making the changes that need to be made." She began to compose an e-mail message to the staff announcing a strategy implementation meeting.

Index